INTRODUCTION

Everybody has seen the effects of diabetes, either directly or indirectly. I have many family members who suffer from various types of diabetes. I see the suffering and constant battle to keep the diabetes under control. Therefore, I felt that it would be appropriate to create a resource containing pertinent information and diet plans, which are easy to follow. I do not claim to be an expert on this topic. However, I have put in many hours of research, in order to compile information that I hope you find useful and relevant. I understand that many of you have been planning meals for years and I respect that. Even if you learn a few new things, it would be a triumph in my eyes. This book provides a useful compilation of diabetic meal plans, which are effective and simple enough for anybody to follow. It contains 28 day and 7 day meal plans at various caloric levels. All recipes are included with the meal plans and nutritional information is provided with certain recipes. Valuable information on diabetes and control methods are also explained, in an understandable yet detailed style. Images of certain recipes are incorporated to break up an otherwise text heavy compilation. Unfortunately, it was not feasible to obtain images of all the recipes that are mentioned. I am also aware that certain recipes are repeated for the 28 day meal plans. This is the case because the 28 day meal plans are designed similarly but the different caloric levels results in a few new recipes to be introduced. I could have omitted the repeated recipes, but I wanted to stay true to the style in which I wanted the information presented. I do not take credit for or hold responsibility for any of the meal plans presented. The hyperlinked table of contents provides an easy way to navigate this wealth of information. It is hoped that this book takes you on a journey to better health and an improved understanding of diabetes.

CONTENTS

INTRODUCTION i
LEGAL NOTES 1
WHAT IS DIABETES? 2
TYPES OF DIABETES 3
    Type 1 diabetes 3
    Type 2 diabetes 3
SIGNS AND SYMPTOMS OF DIABETES 5
SIGNS OF LOW BLOOD SUGAR LEVELS 6
SIGNS OF HIGH BLOOD SUGAR LEVELS 6
MEDICATION 7
    Insulin injections 7
    Other Medication 8
NOTES ON MONITORING YOUR DIABETES 9
    Checking of Blood Glucose Levels 9
    Blood Glucose Level target range 9
    A1C Testing 10
    Ketone tests 10
TAKING CARE OF YOUR DIABETES 12
    In the event of sickness 12
    At a school or work environment 13
    When not at home 13
    When on a plane 14
    In the event of an Emergency or Natural Disaster 14
TIPS TO KEEP BLOOD GLUCOSE AT A HEALTHY LEVEL 16
BALANCING CARBOHYDRATES 17
    Balancing Carbohydrates 17
GLYCEMIC INDEX 18

1200 CALORIE MEAL PLAN 21

DAY 1 22
DAY 1 RECIPES 22
- Morning Smoothie 22
- Plum spread 23
- Grape and Feta Mixed Green Special 24
- Shrimp French Brisque 25
- Sautéed Fish Fillets 27
- Hot and Spicy Halibut 27
- Coffee Peppercorn Steak 28
- Barley & Wild Rice Pilaf 29
- Mango Sorbet 31

DAY 2 32
DAY 2 RECIPES 33
- Tofu Scrambled Egg 33
- Spicy Red Lentil Soup 33
- Amazon Bean Soup with Winter Squash & Greens 34
- The Diet House Salad 35
- Turkey Cutlets with Sage & Lemon 36
- Glazed Mini Carrots 37
- Warm Red Cabbage Salad 38
- Spring Green Salad with Rouille Dressing 39
- Buttermilk-Herb Mashed Potatoes 40

DAY 3 41
DAY 3 RECIPES 41
- Cranberry Muesli 41
- Pasta & Bean Soup 42
- Egg Thread Soup with Asparagus 44
- Spinach, Avocado & Mango Salad 45
- Berry Frozen Yogurt 46

- Curry-Roasted Shrimp with Oranges 47
- Sesame Green Beans 48
- Chile-Spiced Asparagus 49

DAY 4 50
DAY 4 RECIPES 50
- Tropical Fruit Smoothie 50
- Plum spread 51
- Lettuce Wraps with Spiced Pork 52
- Five-Spice Duck Stir-Fry 54
- Green Papaya Salad 56
- Chicken Breasts with Roasted Lemons 57
- Oven-Poached Salmon Fillets 58
- Arugula-Mushroom Salad 59

DAY 5 60
DAY 5 RECIPES 61
- Baked Asparagus & Cheese Frittata 61
- Curried Corn Bisque 62
- Chilled Tomato Soup with Cilantro-Yogurt Swirl 63
- Spicy Chicken Tacos 65
- Grilled Pork Tenderloin with Mustard, Rosemary & Apple Marinade 66
- Herb-Roasted Turkey 68
- Salad of Boston Lettuce with Creamy Orange-Shallot Dressing 69

DAY 6 70
DAY 6 RECIPES 71
- Berry Rich Muffins 71
- Cranberry Pancakes 72
- The Taco 73
- Calabacitas 75
- Tofu with Peanut-Ginger Sauce 76
- Tuscan Pork Loin 77

Spinach Salad with Black Olive Vinaigrette 79

DAY 7 79

DAY 7 RECIPES 80

Crustless Crab Quiche 80

Curried Corn Bisque 81

Herbed Zucchini Soup 83

Asian Slaw with Tofu & Shiitake Mushrooms 84

Wasabi Salmon Burgers 85

Scallion & Ginger Spiced Chicken 87

Mint-Pesto Rubbed Leg of Lamb 88

DAY 8 89

DAY 8 RECIPES 90

Overnight Oatmeal 90

Chicken, Escarole & Rice Soup 91

The Diet House Salad 92

Baby Spinach Salad with Raspberry Vinaigrette 93

Southwestern Steak & Peppers 94

Oven Sweet Potato Fries 95

Pineapple with Mango Coulis 96

Peach-Lime Sorbet 97

DAY 9 98

DAY 9 RECIPES 98

Pear Butter 98

Greek Lemon Rice Soup 99

Asparagus Soup 100

Tuna & White Bean Salad 102

Korean-Style Steak & Lettuce Wraps 103

Garlic-Roasted Pork (Pernil) 104

Cucumber Salad 105

DAY 10 106

DAY 10 RECIPES 106

- Eggs Baked Over a Spicy Vegetable Ragout 106
- Breakfast Pigs in a Blanket 108
- Pasta, Tuna & Roasted Pepper Salad 109
- Turkey & Tomato Panini 110
- Pork Tenderloin with Roasted Plums & Rosemary 111
- Steamed Vegetable Ribbons 113

DAY 11 114

DAY 11 RECIPES 114

- Blueberry Corn Muffins 114
- Honey-Mustard Turkey Burgers 115
- Broccoli Slaw 116
- Orange-Scented Green Beans with Toasted Almonds 117
- Frosted Grapes 118
- Herbed Scallop Kebabs 118
- Ginger-Coconut Chicken 119
- Strawberry Frozen Yogurt 120

DAY 12 121

DAY 12 RECIPES 121

- Banana-Bran Muffins 122
- Pasta, Tuna & Roasted Pepper Salad 124
- Shrimp Cobb Salad 125
- Grilled Chicken Breasts with Salsa Verde 126
- North African Spiced Carrots 127

DAY 13 128

DAY 13 RECIPES 129

- Baked Asparagus & Cheese Frittata 129
- Pasta with Eggplant Ragu 130
- Gnocchi with Zucchini Ribbons & Parsley Brown Butter 131
- Broiled Pineapple 132

- Oven-Fried Fish Fillets 133
- Grilled Salmon with North African Flavors 134
- Tarragon Tartar Sauce 135
- Salad of Boston Lettuce with Creamy Orange-Shallot Dressing 136

DAY 14 137

DAY 14 RECIPES 138

- Eggs Baked Over a Spicy Vegetable Ragout 138
- Roasted Red Pepper Subs 138
- Cranberry & Herb Turkey Burgers 139
- The Diet House Salad 140
- Roasted Vegetable Pasta 141
- Spinach Salad with Black Olive Vinaigrette 142
- Bold Winter Greens Salad 143

DAY 15 144

DAY 15 RECIPES 145

- Pear Butter 145
- Romaine Salad with Chicken, Apricots & Mint 146
- Fresh Tuna Salad with Tropical Fruits 148
- Pacific Sole with Oranges & Pecans 150
- Steamed Vegetable Ribbons 151
- Roasted Broccoli with Lemon 152

DAY 16 153

DAY 16 RECIPES 153

- Cocoa-Date Oatmeal 153
- Five-Spice Chicken & Orange Salad 154
- Buffalo Chicken Wrap 156
- Pork Medallions with a Port-&-Cranberry Pan Sauce 158
- Roasted Florets 159
- Miso-Glazed Peas & Carrots 160
- The Diet House Salad 161

DAY 17	162
DAY 17 RECIPES	162
Greek Potato & Feta Omelet	162
Quesadillas con Frijoles Refritos	163
Irish Lamb Stew	164
Chicken Tabbouleh	165
Sliced Tomato Salad	166
Rainbow Pepper Saute	166
Hawaiian Smoothie	167
DAY 18	168
DAY 18 RECIPES	168
Overnight Oatmeal	168
Five-Spice Chicken & Orange Salad	169
Tomato, Tuna & Tarragon Salad	170
Slow-Cooker Turkish Lamb & Vegetable Stew	171
Roasted Chicken Tenders with Peppers & Onions	172
Mexican Coleslaw	173
DAY 19	174
DAY 19 RECIPES	174
Tofu Scrambled Egg	174
Turkey & Balsamic Onion Quesadillas	175
Roasted Corn, Black Bean & Mango Salad	176
Roasted Savoy Cabbage with Black Bean-Garlic Sauce	177
Salmon on a Bed of Lentils	177
Grandma Ginger's Fish Casserole	178
Shredded Brussels Sprouts with Bacon & Onions	179
Vegetable Stir-Fry	180
DAY 20	181
DAY 20 RECIPES	181
Cranberry Muesli	181

    Fettuccine with Shiitake Mushrooms & Basil 182

    Southwestern Cheese Panini 183

    Pampered Chicken 183

    Cajun Crab Croquettes 184

    Sliced Fennel Salad 185

DAY 21 186

DAY 21 RECIPES 186

    Crunchy Cereal Trail Mix 186

    Curried Tofu Salad 187

    BLT Salad 188

    Roast Salmon with Salsa 188

    Wild Rice with Shiitakes & Toasted Almonds 189

    North African Spiced Carrots 190

    Bok Choy-Apple Slaw 190

DAY 22 191

DAY 22 RECIPES 192

    Pocket Eggs with Soy-Sesame Sauce 192

    Ravioli with Bell Pepper Sauce 193

    Pork, White Bean & Kale Soup 193

    Chicken, Broccoli Rabe & Feta on Toast 194

    Picadillo 195

    Spiced Corn & Rice Pilaf 197

DAY 23 198

DAY 23 RECIPES 198

    Bacony Barley Salad with Marinated Shrimp 198

    Warm Salad with Chicken Paillards & Chèvre 199

    Rosemary & Garlic Crusted Pork Loin with Butternut Squash & Potatoes 200

    Chicken Tacos with Charred Tomatoes 202

DAY 24 203

DAY 24 RECIPES 203

    Shrimp & Plum Kebabs 203

    Roasted Tomato Soup 204

    Amazing Pea Soup 205

    Ginger-Orange Biscotti 206

    Plum & Apple Compote with Vanilla Custard 207

    Sausage, Mushroom & Spinach Lasagna 208

    Sliced Tomato Salad 210

DAY 25 211

DAY 25 RECIPES 211

    Lemon-Raspberry Muffins 211

    Spicy Tofu Hotpot 212

    Creamy Herb Dip 213

    Baba Ganouj 214

    Turkey Cutlets with Peas & Spring Onions 215

    Black Bean-Salmon Stir-Fry 215

DAY 26 217

DAY 26 RECIPES 217

    Overnight Oatmeal 217

    Stir-Fry of Pork with Vietnamese Flavors 218

    Quick Kimchi 219

    Crunchy Bok Choy Slaw 220

    Korean Chicken Soup 220

    Sausage Soup 221

    Arugula-Mushroom Salad 222

    Sliced Tomato Salad 223

    Salsa Cornbread 223

Day 27 225

DAY 27 RECIPES 225

    Morning Smoothie 225

    Plum spread 226

Fillet of Sole with Spinach & Tomatoes 227

Tofu with Tomato-Mushroom Sauce 228

Penne with Tomato & Sweet Pepper Sauce (Penne Saporite "Il Frantoio") 228

Really Low-Fat Garlic Bread 229

Herbed Potato Bread 230

The Diet House Salad 231

Strawberry Fool 232

DAY 28 233

DAY 28 RECIPES 233

Zucchini-Walnut Loaf 233

Chicken Potpie 234

Gnocchi with Tomatoes, Pancetta & Wilted Watercress 236

Pizza-Style Meatloaf 236

Halibut with Herbs & Capers 237

The Wedge 238

1500 CALORIE MEAL PLAN 240

DAY 1 241

DAY 1 RECIPES 241

Morning Smoothie 241

Plum spread 242

Grape and Feta Mixed Green Special 243

Shrimp French Brisque 244

Roasted Cod, Tomatoes, Orange & Onions 245

Hot and Spicy Halibut 246

Barley & Wild Rice Pilaf 246

Green Beans with Toasted Nuts 248

Lemon Lovers' Asparagus 248

Chocolate Malted Ricotta 249

DAY 2 249

DAY 2 RECIPES 250

Tofu Scrambled Egg 250

Salsa Cornbread 250

Spicy Red Lentil Soup 251

Mixed Greens with Berries & Honey-Glazed Hazelnuts 252

Raspberry, Avocado & Mango Salad 254

Turkey Cutlets with Sage & Lemon 255

Grilled Salmon with Mustard & Herbs 255

Glazed Mini Carrots 256

Spring Green Salad with Rouille Dressing 257

Buttermilk-Herb Mashed Potatoes 258

Dark Fudgy Brownies 258

DAY 3 260

DAY 3 RECIPES 260

Cranberry Muesli 260

Pasta & Bean Soup 261

Spinach, Avocado & Mango Salad 262

Berry Frozen Yogurt 263

Curry-Roasted Shrimp with Oranges 265

Slow-Cooker Braised Pork with Salsa 266

Sesame Green Beans 267

DAY 4 268

DAY 4 RECIPES 269

Apricot Smoothie 269

Roasted Apple Butter 269

Lettuce Wraps with Spiced Pork 270

Mediterranean Tuna Panini 271

Sweet & Tangy Watermelon Salad 272

Feta & Herb Dip 273

Creamy Dill Sauce 273

Chicken Breasts with Roasted Lemons 274

- Arugula-Mushroom Salad ... 275
- Almond Cream with Strawberries ... 276

DAY 5 ... 276
DAY 5 RECIPES ... 277
- Baked Asparagus & Cheese Frittata ... 277
- Broccoli-Cheese Chowder ... 278
- Chicken Tabbouleh ... 279
- Cuban-Style Pork & Rice ... 280
- Grilled Pork Tenderloin with Mustard, Rosemary & Apple Marinade ... 281
- Roasted Cod with Warm Tomato-Olive-Caper Tapenade ... 282
- Salad of Boston Lettuce with Creamy Orange-Shallot Dressing ... 283
- Smashed Spiced Sweet Potatoes ... 284

DAY 6 ... 285
DAY 6 RECIPES ... 285
- Jam-Filled Almond Muffins ... 285
- Blueberry-Ricotta Pancakes ... 286
- The Taco ... 287
- Calabacitas ... 289
- Sloppy Joes ... 289
- Vinegary Coleslaw ... 290
- Plum Fool ... 291
- Farmer's Cheese & Strawberries ... 292

DAY 7 ... 292
DAY 7 RECIPES ... 292
- Crustless Crab Quiche ... 292
- Curried Corn Bisque ... 294
- Lebanese Potato Salad ... 295
- Asian Slaw with Tofu & Shiitake Mushrooms ... 295
- Apricot-Almond Bars with Chocolate ... 296
- Tofu with Peanut-Ginger Sauce ... 297

    Tandoori Chicken 299

    Spinach Salad with Black Olive Vinaigrette.. 300

DAY 8 300

DAY 8 RECIPES 301

    Overnight Oatmeal.. 301

    Spiced Creamy Wheat with Cashews.. 302

    Chicken, Escarole & Rice Soup 302

    Strawberry, Melon & Avocado Salad 303

    Southwestern Steak & Peppers 304

    Oven "Fries" 305

    Roasted Corn with Basil-Shallot Vinaigrette 306

    Mocha-Almond Biscotti 306

DAY 9 307

DAY 9 RECIPES 308

    Pear Butter 308

    Creamy Tomato Bisque with Mozzarella Crostini................................. 309

    Tuna & White Bean Salad 309

    Chewy Chocolate Brownies 310

    Outrageous Macaroons 312

    Korean-Style Steak & Lettuce Wraps.. 313

    Wok-Seared Chicken Tenders with Asparagus & Pistachios 314

    Cucumber Salad 315

    Strawberry-Rhubarb Tart... 315

DAY 10... 317

DAY 10 RECIPES 318

    Eggs Baked Over a Spicy Vegetable Ragout.. 318

    Asian Chicken Salad 319

    Roasted Tomato Soup... 320

    Watermelon Gazpacho 322

    Grilled Lamb with Fresh Mint Chutney 323

    Pork Roast with Walnut-Pomegranate Filling 323

    Green Beans with Poppy Seed Dressing 325

    Orange Slices with Warm Raspberries 326

DAY 11 326

DAY 11 RECIPES 327

    Spiced Apple Butter Bran Muffins 327

    Honey-Mustard Turkey Burgers 328

    Chicken & Blueberry Pasta Salad 329

    Broccoli Slaw 330

    Oatmeal Chocolate Chip Cookies 331

    Frosted Grapes 332

    Herbed Scallop Kebabs 332

    Whole-Wheat Couscous with Parmesan & Peas 333

    Butternut & Barley Pilaf 334

    Stuffed Nectarines 335

DAY 12 335

DAY 12 RECIPES 336

    Date-Oat Muffins 336

    Vegetable Cream Cheese 337

    Pasta, Tuna & Roasted Pepper Salad 337

    Pampered Chicken 338

    Southwestern Stuffed Acorn Squash 339

    Carrot Saute with Ginger & Orange 340

    Cranberry & Ruby Grapefruit Compote 341

DAY 13 342

DAY 13 RECIPES 342

    Healthy Pancakes 342

    Chicken & White Bean Soup 344

    Oven-Fried Fish Fillets 345

    Honey-Soy Broiled Salmon 345

- Tarragon Tartar Sauce 346
- Roasted Asparagus with Pine Nuts 347
- Kale with Apples & Mustard 348
- Salad of Boston Lettuce with Creamy Orange-Shallot Dressing 349

DAY 14 349
DAY 14 RECIPES 350
- Sunday Sausage Strata 350
- Barbecued Chicken Burritos 351
- Tomato & Smoked Mozzarella Sandwiches 352
- The Diet House Salad 353
- Roasted Vegetable Pasta 353
- Chicken & Sweet Potato Stew 354
- Spinach Salad with Black Olive Vinaigrette 355

DAY 15 355
DAY 15 RECIPES 356
- Morning Smoothie 356
- Pear Butter 356
- Romaine Salad with Chicken, Apricots & Mint 357
- Pacific Sole with Oranges & Pecans 358
- Turkey Mushroom Loaves 359
- Steamed Vegetable Ribbons 361
- Rice Pilaf with Lime & Cashews 361
- Mashed Roots with Buttermilk & Chives 362

DAY 16 364
DAY 16 RECIPES 364
- Cocoa-Date Oatmeal 364
- Five-Spice Chicken & Orange Salad 365
- Pork Medallions with a Port-&-Cranberry Pan Sauce 366
- Grilled Sea Scallops with Cilantro & Black Bean Sauce 367
- Roasted Florets 369

- The Diet House Salad 369
- Blueberry Torte 370
- Frozen Raspberry Pie 371

DAY 17 372
DAY 17 RECIPES 373
- Greek Potato & Feta Omelet 373
- Steak Salad-Stuffed Pockets 373
- Burgers with Caramelized Onions 375
- Cucumbers & Cottage Cheese 376
- Chicken Tabbouleh 377
- Portobello "Philly Cheese Steak" Sandwich 378
- Sliced Tomato Salad 380
- Chocolate Velvet Pudding 380

DAY 18 381
DAY 18 RECIPES 382
- Overnight Oatmeal 382
- Grilled Chicken Caesar Salad 383
- Chicken-Sausage & Kale Stew 383
- Puerto Rican Fish Stew (Bacalao) 384
- Mexican Coleslaw 385
- Strawberry Frozen Yogurt 386
- Chocolate Bark with Pistachios & Dried Cherries 387

DAY 19 388
DAY 19 RECIPES 388
- Tofu Scrambled Egg 388
- Salsa Cornbread 389
- Turkey & Balsamic Onion Quesadillas 390
- Arugula & Chicken Sausage Bread Pudding 390
- The Diet House Salad 391
- Salmon on a Bed of Lentils 392

- Scallop Piccata on Angel Hair ... 393
- Sesame Green Beans ... 394
- Plum Fool ... 395

DAY 20 ... 396
DAY 20 RECIPES ... 396
- Cranberry Muesli ... 396
- Penne with Braised Squash & Greens ... 397
- Southwestern Beef & Bean Burger Wraps ... 398
- Pampered Chicken ... 399
- Seared Scallops with Grapefruit Sauce ... 400
- Sliced Fennel Salad ... 401
- One-Bowl Chocolate Cake ... 401

DAY 21 ... 402
DAY 21 RECIPES ... 403
- Zucchini-Walnut Loaf ... 403
- Curried Tofu Salad ... 404
- Roast Salmon with Salsa ... 405
- Pan-Roasted Chicken & Gravy ... 405
- North African Spiced Carrots ... 406
- Rainbow Chopped Salad ... 407
- Frozen Raspberry Mousse ... 408
- Raspberry-Chocolate Chip Frozen Yogurt ... 410

DAY 22 ... 410
DAY 22 RECIPES ... 411
- Banana-Nut-Chocolate Chip Quick Bread ... 411
- Vegetable Cream Cheese ... 412
- Bistro Beef Salad ... 413
- Toasted Pita Crisps ... 414
- Chicken, Broccoli Rabe & Feta on Toast ... 414
- Gorgonzola & Prune Stuffed Chicken ... 415

    Spiced Corn & Rice Pilaf 417

DAY 23 418
DAY 23 RECIPES 418
    Bacony Barley Salad with Marinated Shrimp 418

    Warm Salad with Chicken Paillards & Chèvre 419

    Rosemary & Garlic Crusted Pork Loin with Butternut Squash & Potatoes 420

    Chicken Tacos with Charred Tomatoes 421

DAY 24 423
DAY 24 RECIPES 423
    Healthy Pancakes 423

    Shrimp & Plum Kebabs 424

    Beef Tataki 425

    Roasted Tomato Soup 426

    Ginger-Orange Biscotti 427

    Sausage, Mushroom & Spinach Lasagna 428

    Penne with Vodka Sauce & Capicola 430

    Sliced Tomato Salad 430

DAY 25 431
DAY 25 RECIPES 431
    Spiced Apple Cider Muffins 431

    Nouveau Niçoise 433

    Blackened Salmon Sandwich 434

    Turkey Cutlets with Peas & Spring Onions 435

    Miso Chicken Stir-Fry 436

DAY 26 437
DAY 26 RECIPES 437
    Overnight Oatmeal 437

    Stir-Fry of Pork with Vietnamese Flavors 438

    Shrimp Banh Mi 439

    Quick Kimchi 440

  Corn & Broccoli Calzones 441

  Peanut Noodles with Shredded Chicken & Vegetables 442

  Arugula-Mushroom Salad 443

  Sliced Tomato Salad 444

  Mango Sorbet 444

 DAY 27 445

 DAY 27 RECIPES 446

  Morning Smoothie 446

  Plum spread 446

  Tuna & Bean Salad in Pita Pockets.. 447

  Chicken Parmesan Sub 448

  Turkey Cutlets with Peas & Spring Onions 449

  Edamame Succotash with Shrimp 450

  The Diet House Salad 451

  Berry Frozen Yogurt 452

 DAY 28 453

 DAY 28 RECIPES 453

  Sunday Sausage Strata 453

  Chicken Salad Wraps 454

  Lamb Kafta Pockets 455

  Pizza-Style Meatloaf 456

  Yukon Gold & Sweet Potato Mash 457

  The Wedge 458

1800 CALORIE DIET PLAN 459

 DAY 1 460

 DAY 1 RECIPES 460

  Apricot Smoothie 460

  Plum spread 461

  Grape and Feta Mixed Green Special 462

  Shrimp French Brisque... 462

Hot and Spicy Halibut	464
Simple Roast Chicken	464
Barley & Wild Rice Pilaf	465
Farro with Pistachios & Herbs	466
Green Beans with Toasted Nuts	467
Bread & Tomato Salad	468
Quick "Cheesecake"	469

DAY 2 469
DAY 2 RECIPES 470

Tofu Scrambled Egg	470
Salsa Cornbread	470
Spicy Red Lentil Soup	471
Curried Waldorf Salad	472
Turkey Cutlets with Sage & Lemon	473
Brazilian Grilled Flank Steak	474
Glazed Mini Carrots	475
Cool Fresh Corn Relish	476
Light Ranch Dressing	476
Buttermilk-Herb Mashed Potatoes	477
Fresh Fruit with Lemon-Mint Cream	477

DAY 3 478
DAY 3 RECIPES 479

Cranberry Muesli	479
Pasta & Bean Soup	479
Spinach, Avocado & Mango Salad	480
Sesame Carrots	481
Curry-Roasted Shrimp with Oranges	481
Orange-Rosemary Glazed Chicken	482
Pesto Latkes	483
Sesame Green Beans	484

    Snap Pea Salad with Radish & Lime 484

    Strawberries with Sour Cream & Brown Sugar 485

DAY 4 485

DAY 4 RECIPES 486

    Tropical Fruit Smoothie 486

    Roasted Apple Butter 486

    Lettuce Wraps with Spiced Pork 487

    Turkey & Fontina Melts 488

    Sweet & Tangy Watermelon Salad 489

    Chicken Breasts with Roasted Lemons 490

    Arugula-Mushroom Salad 491

    Brussels Sprouts & Chestnuts 492

    Grilled Pineapple with Coconut Black Sticky Rice 493

    Strawberry Cream 494

DAY 5 495

DAY 5 RECIPES 495

    Baked Asparagus & Cheese Frittata 495

    Broccoli-Cheese Chowder 496

    Chicken Tabbouleh 497

    Spaghetti Squash & Pork Stir-Fry 499

    Ginger-Orange Biscotti 500

    Roasted Eggplant Dip 501

    Grilled Pork Tenderloin with Mustard, Rosemary & Apple Marinade 501

    Salad of Boston Lettuce with Creamy Orange-Shallot Dressing 503

    Sweet Pea Mash 503

    Roasted Pear Trifle 504

    Pear & Dried Cranberry Strudel 505

DAY 6 507

DAY 6 RECIPES 507

    Jam-Filled Almond Muffins 507

 Berry-Almond Quick Bread 508

 The Taco 510

 Calabacitas 511

 Real Cornbread 512

 Sloppy Joes 512

 Turkey Scallopini with Apricot Sauce 513

 Barbecue Bean Salad 514

 Vinegary Coleslaw 515

 Plum Fool 516

DAY 7 516

DAY 7 RECIPES 517

 Crustless Crab Quiche 517

 Curried Corn Bisque 518

 Grilled Chicken Caesar Salad 519

 Chopped Salad al Tonno 520

 Tofu with Peanut-Ginger Sauce 520

 Mock Ceviche 521

 Spinach Salad with Black Olive Vinaigrette 522

 Tropical Fruit Ice 523

DAY 8 524

DAY 8 RECIPES 524

 Overnight Oatmeal 524

 Chicken, Escarole & Rice Soup 525

 Strawberry, Melon & Avocado Salad 526

 Southwestern Steak & Peppers 527

 Roasted Pork Tenderloin with Cherry & Tomato Chutney 528

 Oven "Fries" 529

 Broccoli with Caramelized Onions & Pine Nuts 530

 Rustic Berry Tart 530

 Dried Fruit Compote 532

- DAY 9 533
- DAY 9 RECIPES 534
  - Pear Butter 534
  - Creamy Tomato Bisque with Mozzarella Crostini 534
  - Tuna & White Bean Salad 535
  - Pumpkin Popovers 536
  - Avocado Tea Sandwiches 537
  - Korean-Style Steak & Lettuce Wraps 537
  - Broccoli with Black Bean-Garlic Sauce 538
  - Strawberry Bruschetta 539
  - Cookie Cups with Lemon Thyme-Scented Berry Compote 540
- DAY 10 542
- DAY 10 RECIPES 542
  - Eggs Baked Over a Spicy Vegetable Ragout 542
  - Honey Oat Quick Bread 543
  - Asian Chicken Salad 545
  - Smoked Salmon Salad Niçoise 546
  - Roasted Tomato Soup 547
  - White Bean Spread 548
  - Grilled Lamb with Fresh Mint Chutney 549
  - Raspberry-Balsamic Chicken with Shallots 549
  - Green Beans with Poppy Seed Dressing 550
  - Orange Slices with Warm Raspberries 551
- DAY 11 552
- DAY 11 RECIPES 552
  - Spiced Apple Butter Bran Muffins 552
  - Honey-Mustard Turkey Burgers 553
  - Grilled Lobster Rolls 554
  - Broccoli Slaw 555
  - Oatmeal Chocolate Chip Cookies 556

- Frosted Grapes 557
- Herbed Scallop Kebabs 558
- Five-Spice Roasted Duck Breasts 559
- Whole-Wheat Couscous with Parmesan & Peas 560
- Sliced Fennel Salad 560
- Almond Cream with Strawberries 561

DAY 12 562

DAY 12 RECIPES 562
- Vegetable Cream Cheese 562
- Pasta, Tuna & Roasted Pepper Salad 563
- Lima Bean Spread with Cumin & Herbs 564
- Toasted Pita Crisps 564
- Pampered Chicken 565
- Ham & Swiss Rosti 566
- Carrot Saute with Ginger & Orange 567
- Parsley Tabbouleh 567
- Feta-Herb Spread 568
- Squash Pie 569

DAY 13 571

DAY 13 RECIPES 571
- Healthy Pancakes 571
- Chicken & White Bean Soup 573
- Oven-Fried Fish Fillets 573
- Golden Baked Pork Cutlets 574
- Tarragon Tartar Sauce 575
- Blueberry Ketchup 576
- Roasted Asparagus with Pine Nuts 576
- Endive & Watercress Salad with Pomegranate Dressing 577
- Watermelon-Yogurt Ice 578

DAY 14 579

DAY 14 RECIPES 579

- Sunday Sausage Strata 579
- Barbecued Chicken Burritos 580
- Turkey Sausage & Arugula Pasta 581
- Roasted Corn, Black Bean & Mango Salad 582
- Roasted Vegetable Pasta 583
- Five-Spice Turkey & Lettuce Wraps 584
- Spinach Salad with Black Olive Vinaigrette 585
- Blueberries with Lemon Cream 585

DAY 15 586

DAY 15 RECIPES 587

- Morning Smoothie 587
- Whole-Wheat Irish Soda Bread 587
- Pear Butter 588
- Romaine Salad with Chicken, Apricots & Mint 589
- Pacific Sole with Oranges & Pecans 590
- Saute of Chicken with Apples & Leeks 591
- Roasted Snap Peas with Shallots 592
- Chard with Shallots, Pancetta & Walnuts 592
- Rice Pilaf with Lime & Cashews 593
- Polenta Biscotti 595

DAY 16 596

DAY 16 RECIPES 596

- Cocoa-Date Oatmeal 596
- Five-Spice Chicken & Orange Salad 597
- Light Salade aux Lardons 598
- White Bean Spread 599
- Pork Medallions with a Port-&-Cranberry Pan Sauce 600
- Bistro Beef Tenderloin 601
- Roasted Florets 602

- Grape and Feta Mixed Green Special 602
- Honeyed Couscous Pudding 603

DAY 17 604
DAY 17 RECIPES 604
- Savory Breakfast Muffins 604
- Greek Potato & Feta Omelet 605
- Tomato & Ham Breakfast Melt 606
- Steak Salad-Stuffed Pockets 607
- Winter Squash & Chicken Tzimmes 608
- Chicken Tabbouleh 609
- Sliced Tomato Salad 610
- Baked Apples 610

DAY 18 611
DAY 18 RECIPES 611
- Overnight Oatmeal 611
- Grilled Chicken Caesar Salad 612
- Endive & Pomegranate Salad 613
- Chicken-Sausage & Kale Stew 614
- Turkey with Blueberry Pan Sauce 615
- Mexican Coleslaw 616
- Strawberry Frozen Yogurt 617

DAY 19 618
DAY 19 RECIPES 618
- Tofu Scrambled Egg 618
- Salsa Cornbread 619
- Turkey & Balsamic Onion Quesadillas 620
- Salad of Boston Lettuce with Creamy Orange-Shallot Dressing 620
- Salmon on a Bed of Lentils 621
- Pork Fajitas 622
- Sesame Green Beans 624

 Easy Black Beans 624

 Japanese Cucumber Salad 625

DAY 20 627

DAY 20 RECIPES 627

 Cranberry Muesli 627

 Penne with Braised Squash & Greens 628

 Tangy Cauliflower Salad 629

 Peas & Lettuce 630

 Oatmeal Chocolate Chip Cookies 630

 Pampered Chicken 631

 Cider-Brined Pork Chops 632

 Sliced Fennel Salad 634

 Pina Colada Yogurt Parfait 634

DAY 21 635

DAY 21 RECIPES 635

 Cranberry Muesli 635

 Curried Tofu Salad 636

 Grilled Smoky Eggplant Salad 637

 Roasted Corn, Black Bean & Mango Salad 638

 Roast Salmon with Salsa 639

 North African Spiced Carrots 640

 Rainbow Chopped Salad 640

 Grilled Apples with Cheese & Honey 641

 Summer Berry Pudding 642

DAY 22 643

DAY 22 RECIPES 644

 Vegetable Cream Cheese 644

 Bistro Beef Salad 644

 King Crab & Potato Salad 645

 Black Bean Dip 646

    Chicken, Broccoli Rabe & Feta on Toast 646

    The Cobb Salad 648

    Green Tea Rice 649

    Mixed Berry Sundaes 650

DAY 23 650

DAY 23 RECIPES 651

    Cocoa-Date Oatmeal 651

    Bacony Barley Salad with Marinated Shrimp 651

    Barbecued Raspberry-Hoisin Chicken 652

    Broccoli-Cheese Chowder 654

    Rosemary & Garlic Crusted Pork Loin with Butternut Squash & Potatoes 655

    Fennel-Crusted Salmon on White Beans 656

    Blueberries with Lemon Cream 657

DAY 24 658

DAY 24 RECIPES 658

    Healthy Pancakes 658

    Shrimp Salad-Stuffed Tomatoes 660

    Roasted Pear-Butternut Soup with Crumbled Stilton 660

    Wild Rice with Dried Apricots & Pistachios 661

    Ginger-Orange Biscotti 662

    Sausage, Mushroom & Spinach Lasagna 663

    Chicken Divan 665

    Sliced Tomato Salad 666

    Winter Fruit Salad 666

DAY 25 667

DAY 25 RECIPES 667

    Spiced Apple Cider Muffins 667

    Nouveau Niçoise 669

    Seafood Salad with Citrus Vinaigrette 670

    Cottage Cheese Veggie Dip 671

    Turkey Cutlets with Peas & Spring Onions 671

    Mixed Greens with Berries & Honey-Glazed Hazelnuts 672

    Crunchy Pear & Celery Salad 673

DAY 26 674

DAY 26 RECIPES 675

    Southwestern Omelet Wrap 675

    Stir-Fry of Pork with Vietnamese Flavors 676

    Provolone & Olive Stuffed Chicken Breasts 677

    Quick Kimchi 678

    Rolled Sugar Cookies 678

    Corn & Broccoli Calzones 679

    Lentil & Chicken Stew 681

    Arugula-Mushroom Salad 682

    Sliced Tomato Salad 682

    Mango Sorbet 683

DAY 27 684

DAY 27 RECIPES 684

    Morning Smoothie 684

    Plum spread 685

    Tuna & Bean Salad in Pita Pockets 686

    Chicken Parmesan Sub 687

    Ranch Dip & Crunchy Vegetables 688

    Turkey Cutlets with Peas & Spring Onions 688

    Asian "Salisbury" Steak 689

    Arugula & Strawberry Salad 690

    Mango Bread Pudding with Chai Spices 691

DAY 28 692

DAY 28 RECIPES 693

    Sunday Sausage Strata 693

    Ham & Cheese Breakfast Casserole 694

Chicken Salad Wraps 695
  Toasted Pita Crisps 696
  Pizza-Style Meatloaf 696
  Barbecue Pulled Chicken 697
  Creamy Herb Dip 698
  Red & White Salad 699
  Buttermilk Biscuits 700
  Chewy Chocolate Brownies 701

7 DAY 1500 CALORIE MEAL PLAN 1 (WITH RECIPES) 703
  DAY 1 704
  DAY 2 705
  DAY 4 707
  DAY 5 708
  DAY 6 709
  DAY 7 710

RECIPES FOR 7 DAY 1500 CALORIE MEAL PLAN 711
  30-Day Muffins 711
  Bircher Muesli 712
  Crumble Bars 713
  Fruit Smoothie 714
  Spicy Chicken Fillets 715
  Tuna and Tomato Pasta 716
  Salmon Cakes 717

7 DAY 1400 CALORIE MEAL PLAN 718
  DAY 1 719
  DAY 2 719
  DAY 3 720
  DAY 4 720
  DAY 5 721
  DAY 6 721

  DAY 7 722
ANOTHER 7 DAY MEAL PLAN 723
  DAY 1 724
  DAY 2 724
  DAY 3 725
  DAY 4 725
  DAY 5 726
  DAY 6 726
  DAY 7 727
ABOUT THE AUTHOR 728

LEGAL NOTES

All rights reserved, including the right to reproduce this book or portions thereof in any form whatsoever. This book is not intended as a substitute for the medical advice of physicians. The reader should regularly consult a physician, in matters relating to his/her health and particularly with respect to any symptoms, which may require diagnosis or medical attention. Neither the author nor the publisher claim responsibility for adverse effects resulting from the use of the recipes and/or information found within this book. This book is a compilation of diabetic diet plans and recipes. It also contains pertinent information about diabetes. If there are any queries about copyright, please contact the author to have any portion of the book removed. Information will be removed if it infringes on anyone's copyright. The intention was to compile copyright free material and other useful information, into one book.

WHAT IS DIABETES?

You can say that you have diabetes when blood glucose levels are too high. Our blood contains a glucose which is an important type of sugar. Glucose can be seen as a primary energy source. Glucose is known to be manufactured in your muscles and liver. Various foods that we consume provide us with glucose as well. Your blood pumps throughout your body and carries glucose to all the body cells. The glucose carried into the cells acts as a source of energy that we use in our daily activities.

The pancreas is approximately 6 inches long and it sits across the rear of the abdomen, behind the stomach. The pancreas produces and secretes enzymes, or digestive juices, into the small intestine to break down food, after it exits the stomach. The gland is also responsible for producing a hormone known as insulin, which it secretes into the bloodstream. Insulin is meant to regulate blood glucose levels.

In certain people, the body does not produce enough insulin or the insulin does not function as it should. Therefore, glucose remains in the blood and sometimes does not reach the cells. The result of this is elevated blood glucose levels that cause diabetes or prediabetes. Over a period of time, having too much glucose in your blood can cause health serious problems.

Prediabetes is when your blood glucose levels are elevated, but not at a high enough level to be officially called diabetes. With regards to prediabetes, the risk of getting heart disease, stroke and type two diabetes are significantly higher. It is advisable to take up a form of exercise or sport to prevent or delay getting type two diabetes. It is even possible to reduce glucose levels to normal, by embracing a healthier and more active lifestyle.

TYPES OF DIABETES

Type 1 diabetes

Type 1 diabetes is commonly known to develop in younger individuals. However, it is possible for type 1 diabetes to occur in adults. The pancreas is generally responsible for insulin production. Insulin is needed to help send glucose to the body's cells. When the body produces little or no glucose, type 1 diabetes occurs because not enough glucose can enter the body cells and blood glucose levels are high. The lack of insulin production is due to the immune system destroying cells that are needed to produce insulin. We generally know that the immune system helps us fight off illness and bacteria. However, in this case it acts in a negative way which results in type 1 diabetes.

Treatment for type 1 diabetes includes:

-Taking injections of insulin.

-Oral ingestion of medication.

-Healthy eating.

-Adopting an active lifestyle.

-Keeping blood pressure levels under control.

-Managing cholesterol levels.

Type 2 diabetes

This type of diabetes is known to mainly affect people who are older or middle ages. However, type two diabetes can occur in younger people. . If you are overweight and you do not exercise regularly, you are at a greater risk of developing type 2 diabetes. Type 2 diabetes usually begins with a form of insulin resistance by the body. Insulin resistance is a condition that occurs when the various body cells in vital organs no longer utilize insulin to carry glucose into the body's cells to use as a source of energy. Therefore, the body requires a much greater production of insulin to help glucose enter cells and to compensate for the lack of use of insulin. Initially the pancreas is able to keep up with insulin production demand but eventually it becomes overwhelmed. The blood sugar levels generally spike after meals. Furthermore, over time the pancreas is unable to produce enough insulin to compensate for the post meal glucose level spikes. Once your pancreas becomes overwhelmed and is no longer able to keep up with insulin demand, the patient is now diagnosed with type 2 diabetes.

Treatment for type 2 diabetes includes:

-Taking medication for diabetes.

- Healthy eating.

- Physical activity.

- Managing blood pressure levels.

- Keeping cholesterol levels under control.

Gestational diabetes is a temporary type of diabetes and is one of the most common health problems for pregnant women. Glucose intolerance is an early stage of the condition. Gestational diabetes is not your fault it's caused by the way the hormones in pregnancy affect you. It occurs in about five to seven percent of all pregnancies. During pregnancy an organ called the placenta develops in the uterus. The placenta connects the mother and baby and makes sure the baby has enough food and water. The placenta also makes several hormones. Some of these hormones make it hard for insulin to do its job by controlling blood glucose levels. Insulin opens your cell so that glucose can get in. During your pregnancy your body have to make about three times its normal amount of insulin. Gestational diabetes develops when the organ that makes insulin, the pancreas, can't make enough insulin for pregnancy. Without enough insulin, your blood sugar can't leave the blood and be converted to energy. This causes extra sugar to build up in the blood. Most women which is gestational diabetes will have a healthy baby. If you keep your blood sugars in the safe range the chances of you or your baby having problems are the same as if you didn't have gestational diabetes but if left untreated

gestational diabetes can cause health problems. Keep blood sugar levels in a safe range by following a healthy eating plan.

SIGNS AND SYMPTOMS OF DIABETES

The signs and symptoms of diabetes are:

-Thirst

-Urinating too often

-Hunger

-Tiredness

-Unexplained or rapid weight loss

-Slow healing of sores

-Dry and irritable skin

-A sensation of pins and needles in your feet

-Loss of feeling in feet

-Blurry vision

Some people with diabetes do not display any of these signs or symptoms. The only way to know if you have diabetes is to have your doctor do a blood test. Rather be safe and have yourself checked by a professional as diabetes needs to be treated as soon as possible.

SIGNS OF LOW BLOOD SUGAR LEVELS

Sometimes, medicines taken for other health problems can cause blood glucose levels to drop.

Signs showing that blood glucose levels may be too low are the following:

-Hunger

-Dizziness or shakiness

-Confusion

-Being pale

-Sweating more

-Weakness

-Anxiety or moodiness

-Headaches

-A fast heartbeat

SIGNS OF HIGH BLOOD SUGAR LEVELS

Signs showing that blood glucose levels may be too high are the following:

-Thirst

-Tiredness of weakness

-Headaches

-Regular desire to Urinate

-Attention and focusing problems

-Blurred vision

-Yeast infections

MEDICATION

Type 2 diabetes is usually treated with medication that is in pill form. Type 1 diabetes patients have to generally take insulin. People with type 2 diabetes use medication prescribed by doctors to help control blood glucose levels. Certain people take multiple medications to control blood glucose levels if their pancreas produces insulin but the inulin produced does not help reduce glucose levels.

Diabetes medication comes in two forms which is generally in an injection or pill. The frequency that a patient takes medication will depend on the doctor, with some people taking it twice in a day whilst others take their medication once daily. Sometimes, people who take diabetes medication may also require insulin shots for a period of time to help improve results.

If you have an adverse reaction to any form of medication, it would be wise to contact and inform your doctor. Like any other medication, diabetes medication has certain side effects that you have to tolerate in order to manage your blood glucose levels.

Insulin injections
Only a doctor can prescribe insulin. Your doctor can tell you how much insulin you should take and which of the following ways to take insulin is best for you, as described below.

Insulin shot- Generally a hollow needle which is attached to a syringe is used. The insulin is contained within the syringe and passes into your bloodstream through the hollow needle once you penetrate the skin. In certain cases an insulin pen is used. This is a device that looks like a pen but contains a needle and an insulin cartridge. Avoid sharing needles as there are many diseases that can be transmitted in this way.

Insulin pump- This device is filled with a dose of insulin and can be placed on your belt or even in your pocket due to its compact size. The pump is connected to a small plastic tube and a tiny needle. Any qualified personal can insert the needle under your skin. The needle can stay in for a period of one week.

Insulin jet injector- This injector is known to send a fine mist or spray of insulin through your skin. This is done using very high-pressure air as an alternative to a traditional needle.

Insulin injection port- In this case a small tube is placed just beneath the skin. It remains there for a period of one week. You can inject insulin into the end of the tube instead which will allow it to enter the bloodstream.

Other Medication

Your doctor may prescribe other medication to help with problems related to diabetes, such as:

-Aspirin

-Cholesterol lowering medication

-High blood pressure medication

It is important to remember to take your medication at the right times. This can be a challenge therefore it is wise to keep a 7 day pill box with separate compartments for each day of the week. Certain boxes even offer the ability to separate pills for the morning and evening. Also, ask a medical professional to update your list of medication at each visit. This will ensure that you always have an accurate list of what medication to take.

NOTES ON MONITORING YOUR DIABETES

Checking of Blood Glucose Levels

Checking your blood sugar involves sticking your finger with the lancet and testing your blood with a glucose meter. Your health care provider will tell you when and how often to check your blood sugar. They will also give you a blood sugar target range. Try to keep your blood sugar within your target range as much as possible. You will need soap and water, a lancet which is a small needle that fits into the lancet device, test strips, a blood glucose meter and a log book.

Step 1: Wash your hands with soap and water and then dry them. You could also use an alcohol wipe to clean the finger you will use for the testing site.

Step 2: Remove a test strip from a container and put the cap back on to protect the strips. Be sure to use a new test strip each time you check your blood sugar.

Step 3: Insert the test strip into your glucose meter.

Step 4: Place a new lancet into your lancet device. Always use a new lancet every time you check your blood sugar.

Step 5: Stick the side of your finger with the Lancet to get a drop of blood. Sticking the side of your finger rather than the tip hurts less. Use a different finger for each test to help prevent sore spots. You may need to gently massage or squeeze the blood out of your finger. Squeezing your finger too hard may give an inaccurate reading. Most lancet devices have a dial that lets you select how deep the lancet goes into the skin. If you get more blood than you need, dial the number down so the lancet does not go as deep. If you do not get enough blood, dial the number up so the lancet goes in deeper.

Step 6: Touch the correct part of the test strip to the drop of blood but not your skin. The meter will display your blood sugar level on a screen.

Step 7: Write the number into your logbook. Be sure to record your blood sugar level every time you check it. Make sure you use your blog to record things that may affect your blood sugar such as illness, exercise stress, and eating food at a party. Follow up with your doctor regularly and bring your logbook to all of your doctor appointments. You and your doctor may need to discuss changes to your meal plan, physical activity or diabetes medications.

Blood Glucose Level target range

This normal target range is about 70 to 130 and your aim should be for your blood glucose levels to be close to that of a normal person who does not suffer from diabetes. You are at a lower risk of developing health problems if your blood glucose levels are closer to the normal range. Reaching your target range all of the time can be very difficult for most people but you have to keep trying so that you feel better.

A1C Testing

This is a very simple blood test that addresses an epidemic that's been growing larger with every passing year, diabetes. You might be surprised to learn the twenty six million children and adults in the United States have diabetes. That's over eight percent of our population, but did you know that close to eighty million people have pre diabetes and most don't even know it. Those are frightening statistics. So how do you know if you're at risk? It's actually a lot easier than most people think. There's a very simple blood test that helps one to assess the relative risk for blood sugar issues and it's called the hemoglobin A1C test. Hemoglobin is a type of protein found in your red blood cells and glucose is a type of sugar which helps to provide energy for your body. When too much glucose is in your bloodstream it cross links to the hemoglobin in your red blood cells. This crosslinking of a protein and sugar molecule is called glycation, which is not a desirable reaction. The glycated hemoglobin is now called A1C. We need to have a general understanding as to how hemoglobin A1C works. So let's just suppose that last week your blood sugar was running a little high and more glucose linked to your hemoglobin. The next week you've been good and your glucose is under better control, but your red blood

cells still carry the memory of last week's high glucose in the form of A1C. However, these memories are constantly changing as old red blood cells are being replaced with new ones. In simple terms, the amount of A1C in your blood reflects blood sugar control over the past three to four months, which is the life of the red blood cells. This is different from the standard fasting glucose which is just a single snapshot in time. The A1C test is unique and great because it looks at how your glucose has been doing over this three to four month time period. This is powerful and helpful information.

Ketone tests

Check blood or urine for ketones if you happen to feel sick, or if your blood glucose levels are at a level greater than 240. The body produces ketones during fat burn instead of glucose for that is required for energy. If ketone levels are too high, you may have a very serious condition known as ketoacidosis. ketoacidosis can result in death if it goes untreated.

Signs of ketoacidosis are:

-Vomiting

-Weakness

-Fast breathing

-Sweet-smelling breath

Ketoacidosis is more prevalent people who have type 1 diabetes. A healthcare professional will teach you how to test for ketones.

TAKING CARE OF YOUR DIABETES

Once you are diagnosed with diabetes, it becomes a part of your everyday life. You need to learn how to take care of your diabetes in various life circumstances. This will ensure that you are never caught unprepared.

In the event of sickness

Being ill or having an infection can elevate blood glucose levels. Illness and infection puts abnormal stress on the body. The body is tasked with releasing hormones to handle the extra stress and fight any form of illness. The now higher hormone levels can result in high blood glucose levels. Therefore, it is important to know how to deal with your diabetes when you are unwell.

Speak to a healthcare professional and write down:

-How regularly should blood glucose levels be checked.

-If required to test for ketones in blood or urine.

-If your medication dosage should be changed.
-Which foods and drinks to consume.

-The point when you need to contact a doctor.

When we are sick we sometimes have a loss of appetite or feel an urge to vomit. This lower intake of food can result in low blood glucose levels. It is wise to have snacks or high carb drinks to combat low blood glucose levels.

If you are sick the following is recommended:

1) Check and keep a record of blood glucose levels four times a day. Keep your results safe, so you can produce it for a health care professional.
2) Do not stop taking your diabetes medication.
3) Drink at least 1 cup of water or other liquid that does not contain calories or caffeine for every hour that you stay awake.

Your doctor may ask that you call immediately in the following cases:

-Blood glucose levels are above 240 even after taking medication
-Ketone or urine levels are above normal
-Vomiting than one time

-More than 6 hours of diarrhea

-Breathing problems

-High fever
-Drowsiness and a lack of focus

Contact your doctor if you have questions about taking care of yourself.

At a school or work environment

Diabetes care when at school or at work:

1) Continue to follow a healthy eating plan.

2) Ensure that you take medication and monitor blood glucose levels.

3) Inform all people that interact with you regularly about your diabetes diagnosis. Educate them about the signs of low glucose levels. You might require their help if your glucose levels suddenly drop too low.

4) In the event of low blood glucose levels, keep snacks with you.

5) Certain workplaces have people trained to deal with people who have diabetes. Make sure that you inform them of your diagnosis.

6) Have an identification card that says you have diabetes.

When not at home
The following tips are for managing glucose levels when you are away from home:

1) It is wise to get all vaccines, immunizations and shots before travelling. Make sure you get the correct shots that are relevant to the area that you are visiting.

2) Try to stick to your healthy eating plan as often as possible. Always carry a snack with you, in case you have to wait a long period of time to be served.

3) Try to reduce alcohol intake as much as possible. Find out the recommended amount that you can consume. It is a good idea to eat while drinking, this can help avoid low blood glucose.

4) It is a good idea to check your blood glucose if you are the driver in a long journey. Try to stop every 2 hours and check blood glucose levels.

5) It is highly recommended that you carry your diabetes medication and supplies in the car in case your blood glucose levels drop too low.

6) Keep your medical insurance card, emergency phone numbers and a first aid kit on hand.

When on a plane

These tips can help you when on a plane:

1) Get advised on how to adjust your medication, especially your insulin, if you're possibly going to travel across time zones.

2) Always carry a letter from your doctor stating that you have diabetes. The letter should contain a list of all the medical supplies and medicines
you would require on a plane. The letter should include a list of any possible devices that they must not put through an x-ray machine at an airport.

3) Be sure to carry your diabetes medication and your personal blood testing supplies with you onto the plane. In no circumstances should you put these items in your checked baggage. You may need them in event of an emergency.

4) Carry diabetic friendly food and snacks onto the plane.

5) Ask airport security to check your insulin pump by hand. X-ray machines can cause damage insulin pumps.

In the event of an Emergency or Natural Disaster

Everyone with diabetes should be prepared for emergencies and natural disasters, such as power outages or hurricanes. Always have a kit ready that you can use in event of a disaster. These kits need to contain all things that you need to treat and manage your diabetes, such as:

1) A blood glucose meter, lancets and testing strips your diabetes medicines.

2) Insulin, syringes and an insulated bag to keep insulin cool, if you take insulin.

3) A glucagon kit if you take insulin or if recommended by your doctor.

4) Glucose tablets, food and drinks used to remedy low blood glucose.

5) Antibiotic cream or ointments.

6) A copy of your medical information, including your conditions, medication and latest lab test results.

7) A page containing names of your prescription with information on dosages and phone numbers for disaster relief groups.

TIPS TO KEEP BLOOD GLUCOSE AT A HEALTHY LEVEL

1) Consume a combined total of at least 7 servings of fruit and veggies daily.

2) Try to add whole-grain starchy foods at each meal in small portions.

3) Consume foods that are known to have a lower glycemic index.

4) Decide to eat lower fat food. Try not to fry your foods and control amounts of add on fats, such as oils, margarine and butter. Add ones are often disguises in things such as dressings and sauces.

5) Increase activity and decide to move the body for a minimum of 30 minutes daily. Walking or light jogging is excellent for you.

6) If you are overweight, try to lose 5 to 10% of your present weight. Extra weight increases your chances of getting type 2 diabetes.

7) Eat three balanced meals per day, no more than six hours apart. Limit added sugars and sweets. Stay consistent with the times that you consume your meals each day.

8) Drink water instead of fizzy and fruit drinks. Tea, coffee and low calorie juices and beverages are great too. Fizzy drinks and fruit juices usually contain high amounts of sugar.

9) Include lean protein choices at each of your meals. Lean cuts contain less fat and lowers risk of elevated cholesterol and gaining weight.

BALANCING CARBOHYDRATES

Balancing Carbohydrates

It is important to understand and control the amount of carbohydrates you eat and drink, to better manage your blood glucose. Managing your carbohydrate intake is essential when it comes to controlling your blood glucose levels. It is wise to be very strict about what you eat and when.

Here are some tips:

Carbohydrate is the nutritional term that is commonly utilized for starch, sugar and fibre. Managing or spacing your carbohydrate intake during the day will help your body to keep a stable glucose level. It is not desirable to have glucose levels fluctuating a lot during the day. Starchy food choices that are higher in fibre do not raise your blood glucose levels, as much as lower fibre options. Attempt to make a choice of cereal, bread, crackers, rice and other grain or starch choices that are known to contain at least 2 grams of fibre per serving. Breakfast should be 1/3 starch or grain, 1/3 fruit and 1/3 protein. Lunch and supper should be 1/2 vegetables, 1/4 starch and 1/4 protein. Choose snacks wisely as this can help prevent a drop blood glucose, which can occur if your meals are more than than 4 hours apart or if you are a person who leads a very active lifestyle. Choose snacks that contain about 20 grams of carbohydrate. Fruit, vegetables, high fibre granola bars and whole grain crackers with cheese or peanut butter are just some of the better options.

GLYCEMIC INDEX

Glycemic index is measured on a scale of (0-100). This scale ranking indicates how quickly or slowly a carbohydrate containing food will digest and convert into glucose in our blood. High GI foods break down very rapidly, whereas low GI foods break down at a slower pace. With low GI foods, you feel full for longer periods of time and your body's insulin has more time to do its job and remove glucose from the blood.

Vegetables - Basically, all vegetables are considered to have a medium to high GI besides the following:

-Beets

-Corn

-Leeks

-Sweet Potatoes

-Potatoes

Fruits -The majority of fruits, besides the following, are considered to have a medium GI:

-Apricots

-Cantaloupe

-Figs

-Papaya

-Pineapple

-Raisins

-Watermelon

Nuts and Seeds -The following are rated as low GI foods:

-Flaxseeds

-Sesame Seeds

-Almonds

-Cashews

-Peanuts

-Pumpkin and Sunflower Seeds

-Walnuts

Beans and Legumes -The following are rated as low GI foods:

-Soybeans

-Tofu

-Dried Peas

-Kidney Beans

-Garbanzo Beans

-Lentils

-Navy Beans

Meat and Seafood- The following are rated as low GI foods:

-Cod

-Salmon

-Sardines

-Shrimp

-Tuna

-Grass fed beef

-Pasture raised chicken and turkey

-Grass fed lamb

Dairy Products- Some of low GI dairy products include the following:

-Cheese from grass fed cows

-Pasture raised eggs

-Grass fed cow's milk and yogurt

Grains- Some of low GI grains include the following:

-Barley

-Brown Rice

-Buckwheat

-Oats

-Quinoa

-Rye

-Whole Wheat

1200 CALORIE MEAL PLAN

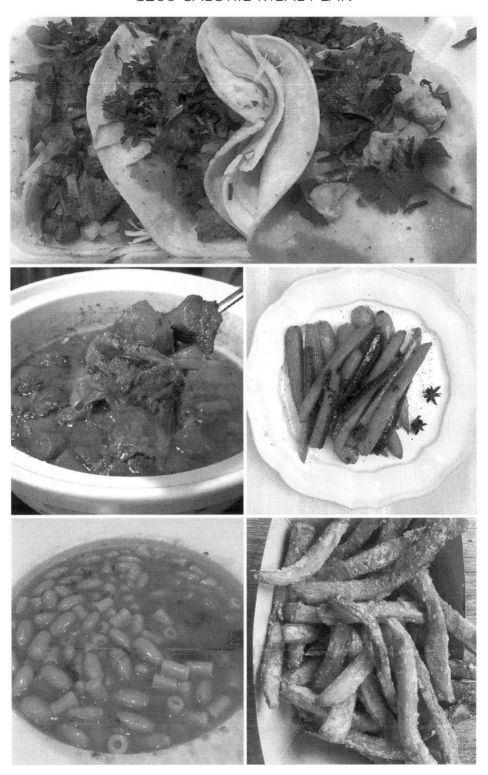

DAY 1
BREAKFAST
Morning Smoothie
Whole-wheat toast
Plum spread

LUNCH
Grape and Feta Mixed Green Special
Shrimp French Brisque or Sautéed Fish Fillets
Wasa crispbread (2 crackers)

SNACK
Apple (1 cup, quartered)
Fat-Free Cheese Slice

DINNER
Hot and Spicy Halibut or Coffee Peppercorn Steak
Barley & Wild Rice Pilaf
Steamed broccoli (1/2 cup)
Mango Sorbet

DAY 1 RECIPES

Morning Smoothie
INGREDIENTS
- 1 1/4 cups orange juice, preferably calcium-fortified
- 1 banana
- 1 1/4 cups frozen berries, such as raspberries, blackberries, blueberries and/or strawberries
- 1/2 cup low-fat silken tofu, or low-fat plain yogurt
- 1 tablespoon sugar, or Splenda Granular (optional)

PREPARATION
1. Mix together the orange juice, banana, berries, tofu (or yogurt) and sugar (or Splenda). If you are using a blender, cover and serve immediately.

NUTRITION

Per serving: 139 calories; 2 g fat (0 g sat, 0 g mono); 0 mg cholesterol; 33 g carbohydrates; 0 g added sugars; 4 g protein; 4 g fiber; 19 mg sodium; 421 mg potassium.
Nutrition Bonus: Vitamin C (110% daily value), Fiber (16% dv).
Carbohydrate Servings: 2

Exchanges: 2 fruit, 1/2 low-fat milk

Plum spread

INGREDIENTS
- 5 pounds plums, pitted and sliced (14-15 cups)
- 3 Granny Smith apples, washed and quartered (not cored)
- 1/4 cup white grape juice, or other fruit juice
- 2 tablespoons lemon juice
- 3/4 cup sugar, or Splenda Granular
- 1/4 teaspoon ground cinnamon, or ginger (optional)

PREPARATION

1. Place a plate in the freezer for testing consistency later.
2. Combine plums, apples, grape juice (or fruit juice) and lemon juice in a large, heavy-bottomed, nonreactive Dutch oven. Bring to a boil over medium-high heat, stirring. Cover and boil gently, stirring occasionally, until the fruit is softened and juicy, 15 to 20 minutes. Uncover and boil gently, stirring occasionally, until the fruit is completely soft, about 20 minutes. (Adjust heat as necessary to maintain a gentle boil.)
3. Pass the fruit through a food mill to remove the skins and apple seeds.
4. Return the strained fruit to the pot. Add sugar (or Splenda) and cinnamon (or ginger), if using. Cook over medium heat, stirring frequently, until a spoonful of jam dropped onto the chilled plate holds its shape, about 15 minutes longer. (See Tip.) Remove from heat and skim off any foam.

TIPS & NOTES

- **Make Ahead Tip**: Store in an airtight container in the refrigerator for up to 2 months.
- **To test the consistency of the spread:** Drop a dollop of cooked spread onto a chilled plate. Carefully run your finger through the dollop. If the track remains unfilled, the jam is done.

NUTRITION

Per tablespoon with sugar: 14 calories; 0 g fat (0 g sat, 0 g mono); 0 mg cholesterol; 4 g carbohydrates; 0 g protein; 0 g fiber; 0 mg sodium; 30 mg potassium.

Exchanges: free food

Grape and Feta Mixed Green Special

INGREDIENTS

DRESSING

- 1/4 cup extra-virgin olive oil
- 2 tablespoons red-wine vinegar
- 1/4 teaspoon salt, or to taste and Freshly ground pepper, to taste

SALAD

- 8 cups mesclun salad greens, (5 ounces)
- 1 head radicchio, thinly sliced
- 2 cups halved seedless grapes, (about 1 pound), preferably red and green
- 3/4 cup crumbled feta, or blue cheese

PREPARATION

1. To prepare dressing: Whisk (or shake) oil, vinegar, salt and pepper in a small bowl (or jar) until blended.
2. To prepare salad: Just before serving, toss greens and radicchio in a large bowl. Drizzle the dressing on top and toss to coat. Divide the salad among 8 plates. Scatter grapes and cheese over each salad; serve immediately.

TIPS & NOTES

- **Make Ahead Tip**: The dressing will keep, covered, in the refrigerator for up to 2 days.

NUTRITION

Per serving: 133 calories; 10 g fat (3 g sat, 6 g mono); 13 mg cholesterol; 9 g carbohydrates; 3 g protein; 1 g fiber; 239 mg sodium; 183 mg potassium.

Nutrition Bonus: Vitamin C (15% daily value), Folate (9% dv).

Carbohydrate Servings: 1/2

Exchanges: 1/2 fruit, 1 vegetable, 2 fat

Shrimp French Brisque

INGREDIENTS

- 12 ounces shrimp (30-40 per pound), shell-on
- 1 onion, chopped, divided
- 1 carrot, peeled and sliced
- 1 stalk celery (with leaves), sliced
- 1/2 cup dry white wine
- 1/2 teaspoon black peppercorns
- 1 bay leaf
- 3 cups water
- 1 tablespoon extra-virgin olive oil
- 4 ounces mushrooms, wiped clean and sliced (about 1 1/2 cups)
- 1/2 green bell pepper, chopped
- 1/4 cup chopped scallions
- 2 tablespoons chopped fresh parsley
- 1/4 cup all-purpose flour
- 1 1/2 cups low-fat milk
- 1/4 cup reduced-fat sour cream
- 1/4 cup dry sherry
- 1 tablespoon lemon juice

- 1/4 teaspoon salt
- Freshly ground pepper to taste
- Dash of hot sauce

PREPARATION

1. Peel and devein shrimp, reserving the shells. Cut the shrimp into 3/4-inch pieces; cover and refrigerate.
2. Combine the shrimp shells with about half the onion, all the carrot, celery, wine, peppercorns and bay leaf in a large heavy saucepan. Add water and simmer over low heat for about 30 minutes. Strain through a sieve, pressing on the solids to extract all the juices; discard the solids. Measure the shrimp stock and add water, if necessary, to make 1 1/2 cups.
3. Heat oil in the same pan over medium heat. Add mushrooms, bell pepper, scallions, parsley and the remaining onion. Cook, stirring, until the mushrooms are soft, about 5 minutes. Sprinkle with flour and cook, stirring constantly, until it starts to turn golden, 2 to 3 minutes. Slowly stir in milk and the shrimp stock. Cook, stirring to loosen any flour sticking to the bottom of the pot, until the soup returns to a simmer and thickens, about 5 minutes. Add the reserved shrimp and cook until they turn opaque in the center, about 2 minutes more. Add sour cream, sherry and lemon juice; stir over low heat until heated through, do not let it come to a boil. Taste and adjust seasonings with salt, pepper and hot sauce.

TIPS & NOTES

- **Make Ahead Tip**: Cover and refrigerate for up to 1 day.

NUTRITION

Per serving: 163 calories; 5 g fat (2 g sat, 2 g mono); 92 mg cholesterol; 12 g carbohydrates; 13 g protein; 1 g fiber; 241 mg sodium; 255 mg potassium.

Nutrition Bonus: Selenium (30% daily value), Vitamin A (26% dv), Vitamin C (24% dv).

Carbohydrate Servings: 1

Exchanges: 1 starch; 2 very lean meat; 1 fat

Sautéed Fish Fillets

INGREDIENTS

- 1/3 cup all-purpose flour
- 1/2 teaspoon salt
- 1/4 teaspoon freshly ground pepper
- 1 pound catfish, tilapia, haddock or other white-fish fillets (see "Choose Sustainable Fish," opposite), cut into 4 portions
- 1 tablespoon extra-virgin olive oil

PREPARATION

Combine flour, salt and pepper in a shallow dish. Thoroughly dredge fillets; discard any leftover flour.

Heat oil in a large nonstick skillet over medium-high heat. Add the fish, working in batches if necessary, and cook until lightly browned and just opaque in the center, 3 to 4 minutes per side. Serve immediately.

NUTRITION

Per serving: 163 calories; 8 g fat (2 g sat, 5 g mono); 43 mg cholesterol; 8 g carbohydrates; 0 g added sugars; 13 g protein; 0 g fiber; 368 mg sodium; 249 mg potassium.

Carbohydrate Servings: 1/2

Exchanges: 1/2 starch, 3 very lean meat, 1/2 fat

Hot and Spicy Halibut

INGREDIENTS

- 1 1/4 pounds halibut, striped bass or tilapia fillet, cut into 4 portions
- 1 teaspoon ground cumin, divided
- 1/4 teaspoon salt
- Freshly ground pepper, to taste

- 1 10-ounce can diced tomatoes with green chiles
- 1/4 cup sliced green olives with pimientos
- 2 tablespoons chopped fresh cilantro
- 1 teaspoon extra-virgin olive oil

PREPARATION

1. Preheat oven to 450°F. Coat a baking sheet with cooking spray. Arrange fish on baking sheet. Season with 1/2 teaspoon cumin, salt and pepper.
2. Combine tomatoes, olives, cilantro, oil and the remaining 1/2 teaspoon cumin in a small bowl. Spoon over the fish.
3. Bake the fish until flaky and opaque in the center, 12 to 15 minutes. Serve immediately.

NUTRITION

Per serving: 188 calories; 7 g fat (1 g sat, 4 g mono); 45 mg cholesterol; 4 g carbohydrates; 30 g protein; 1 g fiber; 758 mg sodium; 638 mg potassium.

Nutrition Bonus: Potassium (18% daily value).

Exchanges: 4 very lean meat, 1 fat (mono)

Coffee Peppercorn Steak

INGREDIENTS

- 1 small clove garlic
- 1/4 teaspoon kosher salt, divided
- 1 tablespoon strong freshly brewed coffee
- 1 tablespoon balsamic vinegar
- Freshly ground pepper, to taste
- 1 tablespoon whole coffee beans, (not flavored beans)
- 1 teaspoon whole black peppercorns

- 1/2 teaspoon extra-virgin olive oil
- 8 ounces sirloin steak, about 1-inch thick, trimmed of fat

PREPARATION

1. Preheat grill to high.
2. Smash and peel garlic clove, sprinkle with 1/8 teaspoon salt and mash into a paste with a spoon or the side of a chef's knife. Transfer to a small bowl and whisk in coffee and vinegar. Season with pepper.
3. Place coffee beans and peppercorns on a cutting board; coarsely crush with the bottom of a heavy pan. Mix the crushed coffee beans and peppercorns together. Rub steaks with oil, sprinkle with the remaining 1/8 teaspoon salt and coat with the coffee-peppercorn mixture, pressing it into the meat. Grill 4 to 5 minutes per side for medium rare.
4. Transfer the steak to a cutting board and let rest 5 minutes. Thinly slice across the grain. Serve with the vinaigrette.

NUTRITION

Per serving: 190 calories; 8 g fat (3 g sat, 4 g mono); 55 mg cholesterol; 2 g carbohydrates; 0 g added sugars; 25 g protein; 0 g fiber; 195 mg sodium; 347 mg potassium.

Nutrition Bonus: Selenium (39% daily value), Zinc (33% dv).

Exchanges: 3 1/2 lean meat

Barley & Wild Rice Pilaf

INGREDIENTS

- 2 teaspoons extra-virgin olive oil
- 1 medium onion, finely chopped
- 1/2 cup wild rice, rinsed
- 1/2 cup pearl barley
- 3 cups reduced-sodium chicken broth, or vegetable broth

- 1/3 cup pine nuts
- 1 cup pomegranate seeds, (1 large fruit; see Tip)
- 2 teaspoons freshly grated lemon zest
- 2 tablespoons chopped flat-leaf parsley

PREPARATION

1. Heat oil in a large saucepan over medium heat. Add onion and cook, stirring often, until softened. Add wild rice and barley; stir for a few seconds. Add broth and bring to a simmer. Reduce heat to low, cover and simmer until the wild rice and barley are tender and most of the liquid has been absorbed, 45 to 50 minutes.
2. Meanwhile, toast pine nuts in a small, dry skillet over medium-low heat, stirring constantly, until light golden and fragrant, 2 to 3 minutes. Transfer to a small bowl to cool.
3. Add pomegranate seeds, lemon zest, parsley and the toasted pine nuts to the pilaf; fluff with a fork. Serve hot.

TIPS & NOTES

- **Make Ahead Tip**: Prepare through Step 2. Cover and refrigerate for up to 2 days. To reheat, place in a baking dish, add 1/4 cup water and cover. Microwave on High for 10 to 15 minutes or bake at 350°F or 25 to 30 minutes.
- **Tip:** To seed a pomegranate and avoid the enduring stains of pomegranate juice, work under water. Fill a large bowl with water. Hold the pomegranate in the water and slice off the crown. Lightly score the fruit into quarters, from crown to stem end. Keeping the fruit under water, break it apart, gently separating the plump seeds from the outer skin and white pith. The seeds will drop to the bottom of the bowl and the pith will float to the surface. Discard the pith. Pour the seeds into a colander. Rinse and pat dry. The seeds can be frozen in an airtight container or sealable bag for up to 3 months.

NUTRITION

Per serving: 209 calories; 7 g fat (1 g sat, 3 g mono); 3 mg cholesterol; 31 g carbohydrates; 0 g added sugars; 7 g protein; 4 g fiber; 75 mg sodium; 250 mg potassium.

Nutrition Bonus: Magnesium (15% dv)

Carbohydrate Servings: 2

Exchanges: 2 starch, 1 fat

Mango Sorbet

INGREDIENTS

- 3 ripe mangoes
- 1/2 cup sugar
- 1/2 cup water
- 1/3 cup coarsely mashed banana, (1 small)
- 2 tablespoons lime juice

PREPARATION

1. Preheat oven to 350°F. Place whole mangoes in a shallow baking pan and roast until very soft, 70 to 90 minutes. Refrigerate until cool, about 1 hour.

2. Meanwhile, combine sugar and water in a small saucepan. Bring to a boil, stirring to dissolve sugar. Remove from heat and refrigerate until cold, about 1 hour.

3. When the mangoes are cool enough to handle, remove skin and coarsely chop pulp, discarding pit. Place the mango pulp and accumulated juices in a food processor. Add banana and lime juice; process until very smooth. Transfer to a large bowl and stir in the sugar syrup. Cover and refrigerate until cold, 40 minutes or overnight.

4. Freeze the mixture in an ice cream maker according to manufacturer's directions. (Alternatively, freeze the mixture in a shallow metal pan until solid, about 6 hours. Break into chunks and process in a food processor until smooth.) Serve immediately or transfer to a storage container and let harden in the freezer for 1 to 1 1/2 hours. Serve in chilled dishes.

TIPS & NOTES

- **Make Ahead Tip**: Store in an airtight container in the freezer for up to 1 week. Let soften in the refrigerator for 1/2 hour before serving. Equipment: Ice cream maker or food processor

NUTRITION

Per serving: 108 calories; 0 g fat (0 g sat, 0 g mono); 0 mg cholesterol; 28 g carbohydrates; 1 g protein; 2 gfiber; 2 mg sodium; 159 mg potassium.

Nutrition Bonus: Vitamin C (40% daily value).

Carbohydrate Servings: 2

Exchanges: 2 fruit

DAY 2
BREAKFAST
Tofu Scrambled Egg
Whole-wheat toast (1 slice)
Strawberries (1 cup)
LUNCH
Spicy Red Lentil Soup or Amazon Bean Soup with Winter Squash & Greens
The Diet House Salad
Wasa crispbread (2 crackers)
SNACK
Nectarine (1 small)
DINNER
Turkey Cutlets with Sage & Lemon
Glazed Mini Carrots or Warm Red Cabbage Salad
Spring Green Salad with Rouille Dressing
Steamed broccoli (1/2 cup)
Buttermilk-Herb Mashed Potatoes
Skim Milk 8 oz

DAY 2 RECIPES

Tofu Scrambled Egg

INGREDIENTS
- 1 large egg
- 1/2 teaspoon dried tarragon
- Dash of hot sauce, such as
- Pinch of salt
- Freshly ground pepper, to taste
- 1 teaspoon extra-virgin olive oil, or canola oil
- 2 tablespoons crumbled tofu, (silken or regular)

PREPARATION
1. Blend egg, tarragon, hot sauce, salt and pepper in a small bowl with a fork. Heat oil in a small nonstick skillet over medium-low heat. Add tofu and cook, stirring, until warmed through, 20 to 30 seconds. Add egg mixture and stir until the egg is set, but still creamy, 20 to 30 seconds. Serve immediately.

NUTRITION
Per serving: 140 calories; 11 g fat (2 g sat, 6 g mono); 212 mg cholesterol; 2 g carbohydrates; 0 g added sugars; 9 g protein; 1 g fiber; 230 mg sodium; 93 mg potassium.
Nutrition Bonus: Selenium (23% daily value).
Exchanges: 1 medium-fat meat. 1 fat (mono)

Spicy Red Lentil Soup

INGREDIENTS
- 6 teaspoons extra-virgin olive oil, divided
- 2 onions, chopped (1 1/2 cups)
- 3 cloves garlic, minced
- 2 teaspoons ground cumin
- 8 cups reduced-sodium chicken broth, or vegetable broth
- 1 1/2 cups red lentils, rinsed (see Tip)
- 1/3 cup bulgur
- 2 tablespoons tomato paste
- 1 bay leaf
- 3 tablespoons lemon juice
- Freshly ground pepper to taste
- 1 teaspoon paprika
- 1 teaspoon cayenne pepper

PREPARATION

1. Heat 2 teaspoons oil in a soup pot or Dutch oven over medium heat. Add onions and cook, stirring, until softened, 3 to 5 minutes. Add garlic and cumin; cook for 1 minute. Add broth, lentils, bulgur, tomato paste and bay leaf; bring to a simmer, stirring occasionally. Cover and cook over low heat until the lentils and bulgur are very tender, 25 to 30 minutes. Discard the bay leaf.
2. Ladle about 4 cups of the soup into a food processor and puree. Return the pureed soup to the soup pot and heat through. Stir in lemon juice and season with pepper.
3. Just before serving, ladle the soup into bowls. Heat remaining 4 teaspoons oil in a skillet and stir in paprika and cayenne. Drizzle about 1/2 teaspoon of the sizzling spice mixture over each bowl.

TIPS & NOTES

- **Make Ahead Tip**: Prepare through Step 2. Cover and refrigerate for up to 2 days or freeze for up to 2 months.
- **Tip:** You can replace red lentils with brown lentils; add 1/2 cup water and simmer 40 to 45 minutes.

NUTRITION

Per serving: 218 calories; 5 g fat (1 g sat, 3 g mono); 5 mg cholesterol; 31 g carbohydrates; 0 g added sugars; 15 g protein; 7 g fiber; 151 mg sodium; 406 mg potassium.
Nutrition Bonus: Fiber (29% daily value), Iron (15% dv).
Carbohydrate Servings: 2
Exchanges: 1 1/2 starch, 1 vegetable, 1 lean meat

Amazon Bean Soup with Winter Squash & Greens

INGREDIENTS

- 1 tablespoon butter
- 4 cloves garlic, minced
- 2 carrots, chopped
- 1 medium onion, chopped
- 6 cups reduced-sodium chicken broth
- 3 pounds buttercup squash, peeled and diced (about 6 cups)
- 1 plum tomato, chopped
- 1/4 teaspoon crushed red pepper
- 1/4 teaspoon salt
- 1/8 teaspoon freshly ground pepper
- 2 15-ounce cans pinto or other brown beans, rinsed
- 10 ounces spinach, stemmed and coarsely chopped
- 1 lime, cut into wedges

PREPARATION

1. Melt butter in a Dutch oven over medium-high heat. Add garlic, carrots and onion and cook, stirring occasionally, until the vegetables are tender and lightly browned, 5 to 7 minutes. Add broth and scrape up any browned bits with a wooden spoon. Add squash, tomato, crushed red pepper, salt and pepper and bring to a boil. Reduce heat to a simmer and cook until the squash is very soft and almost breaking apart, about 20 minutes.
2. Transfer 3 cups of the soup to a blender and puree until smooth. (Use caution when pureeing hot liquids.) Return the pureed soup to the pot. Stir in beans and spinach and cook over medium heat until the beans are heated through and the spinach is wilted, about 5 minutes. Serve with lime wedges.

TIPS & NOTES
- **To make squash bowls:**
- Preheat oven to 425°F. Slice about an inch off the top of each buttercup squash. Scoop out seeds and loose flesh. Pour 1/2 inch water into a glass baking dish (or two) large enough to hold the squash. Place squash cut-side down in the water. Bake until the flesh is tender when gently poked with a knife and the squash still holds its shape, about 30 minutes.

NUTRITION
Per serving: 223 calories; 3 g fat (2 g sat, 0 g mono); 8 mg cholesterol; 43 g carbohydrates; 0 g added sugars; 11 g protein; 10 g fiber; 310 mg sodium; 927 mg potassium.
Nutrition Bonus: Vitamin A (510% daily value), Vitamin C (90% dv), Folate (46% dv), Potassium (34% dv).
Carbohydrate Servings: 2
Exchanges: 2 1/2 starch, 1 1/2 vegetable, 1 lean meat

The Diet House Salad

INGREDIENTS
- 4 cups torn green leaf lettuce
- 1 cup sprouts
- 1 cup tomato wedges
- 1 cup peeled, sliced cucumber
- 1 cup shredded carrots
- 1/2 cup chopped radishes
- 1/2 cup Sesame Tamari Vinaigrette (recipe follows), or other dressing

PREPARATION

Toss lettuce, sprouts, tomato, cucumber, carrots and radishes in a large bowl with the dressing until the vegetables are coated.

NUTRITION

Per serving: 71 calories; 3 g fat (0 g sat, 1 g mono); 0 mg cholesterol; 11 g carbohydrates; 2 g protein; 3 g fiber; 334 mg sodium; 428 mg potassium.
Nutrition Bonus: Vitamin A (140% daily value), Vitamin C (30% dv), Folate (16% dv).
Carbohydrate Servings: 1
Exchanges: 2 vegetable, 1/2 fat

Turkey Cutlets with Sage & Lemon

INGREDIENTS

- 3 tablespoons all-purpose
- 1 pound turkey breast cutlets
- 1/4 teaspoon salt
- Freshly ground pepper, to taste
- 3 teaspoons extra-virgin olive oil, divided
- 2 cloves garlic, minced
- 2 teaspoons chopped fresh sage
- 1/4 cup dry white wine
- 3/4 cup reduced-sodium chicken broth
- 1 teaspoon lemon juice
- 1 teaspoon butter

PREPARATION

1. Spread flour on a large plate. Cut several small slits in outer edges of the turkey to prevent curling. Pat dry with paper towels and season with salt and pepper. Dredge lightly in flour. Discard any remaining flour.

2. Heat 1 teaspoon oil in a large nonstick skillet over medium-high heat. Add half the turkey and cook until golden outside and no longer pink inside, 1 to 2 minutes per side. Transfer to a platter and tent with foil to keep warm. Saute the remaining turkey in another 1 teaspoon oil until golden; transfer to platter.

3. Add the remaining 1 teaspoon oil to the pan. Add garlic and sage; cook, stirring, until fragrant, about 1 minute. Add wine and cook, scraping up any browned bits, until reduced by half, about 1 minute. Add broth and cook until the liquid is reduced by half, 4 to 5 minutes. Stir in lemon juice and any juices accumulated from the turkey and simmer for 1 minute more. Remove from heat and swirl in butter. Serve, spooning the sauce over the turkey.

NUTRITION

Per serving: 205 calories; 5 g fat (1 g sat, 3 g mono); 48 mg cholesterol; 6 g carbohydrates; 0 g added sugars; 29 g protein; 0 g fiber; 273 mg sodium; 358 mg potassium.

Nutrition Bonus: Selenium (47% daily value).

Exchanges: 4 very lean meat, 1 fat

Glazed Mini Carrots

INGREDIENTS

- 3 cups mini carrots, (1 pound)
- 1/3 cup water
- 1 tablespoon honey
- 2 teaspoons butter
- 1/4 teaspoon salt, or to taste
- 1 tablespoon lemon juice
- Freshly ground pepper, to taste
- 2 tablespoons chopped fresh parsley

PREPARATION

Combine carrots, water, honey, butter and salt in a large skillet. Bring to a simmer over medium-high heat. Cover and cook until tender, 5 to 7 minutes. Uncover and cook, stirring often, until the liquid is a syrupy glaze, 1 to 2 minutes. Stir in lemon juice and pepper. Sprinkle with parsley and serve.

NUTRITION

Per serving: 74 calories; 2 g fat (1 g sat, 1 g mono); 5 mg cholesterol; 14 g carbohydrates; 1 g protein; 2 g fiber; 236 mg sodium; 287 mg potassium.

Nutrition Bonus: Vitamin A (320% daily value), Vitamin C (23% dv).

Carbohydrate Servings: 1

Exchanges: 1 vegetable, 1/2 fat

Warm Red Cabbage Salad

INGREDIENTS

- 1 tablespoon extra-virgin olive oil
- 4 cups red cabbage, thinly sliced (about 1/4 large head)
- 3/4 teaspoon caraway seeds
- 1/2 teaspoon salt
- 1 crisp, sweet apple, such as Braeburn or Gala, cut into matchsticks
- 1 shallot, minced
- 1 tablespoon red-wine vinegar
- 1/2 teaspoon Dijon mustard
- 1/2 teaspoon freshly, ground pepper
- 2 tablespoons chopped walnuts, toasted (see Tip)

PREPARATION

1. Heat oil in a large saucepan over medium heat. Add cabbage, caraway seeds and salt. Cook, covered, stirring occasionally, until tender, 8 to 10 minutes. Remove from the heat. Add apple, shallot, vinegar, mustard and pepper and stir until combined. Serve sprinkled with toasted walnuts.

TIPS & NOTES

- **Tip:** To toast chopped walnuts, heat a small dry skillet over medium-low heat. Add nuts and cook, stirring, until lightly browned and fragrant, 2 to 3 minutes.

NUTRITION

Per serving: 76 calories; 4 g fat (1 g sat, 2 g mono); 0 mg cholesterol; 10 g carbohydrates; 0 g added sugars; 2 g protein; 2 g fiber; 216 mg sodium; 183 mg potassium.

Nutrition Bonus: Vitamin C (60% daily value), Vitamin A (15% dv), source of omega-3s.

Carbohydrate Servings: 1/2

Exchanges: 1 1/2 vegetable, 1 fat

Spring Green Salad with Rouille Dressing

INGREDIENTS

- 1/3 cup chopped hazelnuts
- 1/2 cup jarred pimiento peppers, rinsed
- 1/2 teaspoon chopped garlic
- 2 tablespoons water
- 1 1/2 tablespoons white balsamic vinegar, (see Note)
- 1/2 teaspoon salt
- 1/2 teaspoon freshly ground pepper
- 1 large cucumber, peeled, halved, seeded and cut into thin half-moons
- 2 stalks celery, thinly sliced
- 4 cups romaine lettuce, cut or torn into bite-size pieces (about 6 ounces)
- 1 cup baby spinach leaves and 24 leaves fresh basil, chopped

PREPARATION

1. Toast hazelnuts in a small dry skillet over medium heat, stirring often, until lightly browned, about 4 minutes. Transfer to a foodprocessor and let cool for 5 minutes. Add pimientos, garlic, water, vinegar, salt and pepper. Process until smooth.

2. Combine cucumber, celery, romaine, spinach and basil in a salad bowl. Add the dressing, toss gently, and serve.

TIPS & NOTES

- **Note:** White balsamic vinegar is unaged balsamic made from Italian white wine grapes and grape musts (unfermented crushed grapes). Its mild flavor and clear color make it ideal for salad dressing.

NUTRITION

Per serving: 64 calories; 4 g fat (0 g sat, 3 g mono); 0 mg cholesterol; 7 g carbohydrates; 0 g added sugars;3 g protein; 2 g fiber; 362 mg sodium; 243 mg potassium.

Nutrition Bonus: Vitamin A (60% daily value), Vitamin C (20% dv), Folate (18% dv).

Carbohydrate Servings: 1/2

Exchanges: 1 vegetable, 1/2 f

Buttermilk-Herb Mashed Potatoes

INGREDIENTS

- 1 large Yukon Gold potato, peeled and cut into chunks
- 1 clove garlic, peeled and 1 teaspoon butter
- 2 tablespoons nonfat buttermilk
- 1 1/2 teaspoons chopped fresh herbs
- Salt & freshly ground pepper, to taste

PREPARATION

Place potato in a small saucepan and cover with water. Add garlic. Bring to a boil; cook until the potato is tender. Drain; add butter and buttermilk, and mash with a potato masher to the desired consistency. Stir in herbs. Season with salt and freshly ground pepper.

NUTRITION

Per serving: 85 calories; 2 g fat (1 g sat, 0 g mono); 5 mg cholesterol; 14 g carbohydrates; 0 g added sugars; 2 g protein; 1 g fiber; 87 mg sodium; 416 mg potassium.

Carbohydrate Servings: 1

Exchanges: 1 starch

DAY 3
BREAKFAST
Cranberry Muesli
Skim Milk (1 cup)
LUNCH
Pasta & Bean Soup or Egg Thread Soup with Asparagus
Spinach, Avocado & Mango Salad
SNACK
Berry Frozen Yogurt
DINNER
Curry-Roasted Shrimp with Oranges
Brown rice (1/2 cup)
Sesame Green Beansor Chile-Spiced Asparagus
Raspberries (1/2 cup)

DAY 3 RECIPES

Cranberry Muesli

INGREDIENTS

- 1/2 cup low-fat plain yogurt
- 1/2 cup unsweetened or fruit-juice-sweetened cranberry juice
- 6 tablespoons old-fashioned rolled oats, (not quick-cooking or steel-cut)
- 2 tablespoons dried cranberries
- 1 tablespoon unsalted sunflower seeds
- 1 tablespoon wheat germ
- 2 teaspoons honey

- 1/4 teaspoon vanilla extract
- 1/8 teaspoon salt

PREPARATION

1. Combine yogurt, juice, oats, cranberries, sunflower seeds, wheat germ, honey, vanilla and salt in a medium bowl; cover and refrigerate for at least 8 hours and up to 1 day.

TIPS & NOTES

- **Make Ahead Tip**: Cover and refrigerate for up to 1 day.

NUTRITION

Per serving: 209 calories; 4 g fat (1 g sat, 1 g mono); 4 mg cholesterol; 37 g carbohydrates; 8 g protein; 3 gfiber; 190 mg sodium; 266 mg potassium.

Nutrition Bonus: Calcium (15% daily value)

Carbohydrate Servings: 2 1/2

Exchanges: 1 starch, 1 fruit, 1/2 other carbohydrate, 1/2 fat

Pasta & Bean Soup

INGREDIENTS

- 4 14-ounce cans reduced-sodium chicken broth
- 6 cloves garlic, crushed and peeled
- 4 4-inch sprigs fresh rosemary, or 1 tablespoon dried
- 1/8-1/4 teaspoon crushed red pepper
- 1 15-1/2-ounce or 19-ounce can cannellini, (white kidney) beans, rinsed, divided
- 1 14-1/2-ounce can diced tomatoes
- 1 cup medium pasta shells, or orecchiette
- 2 cups individually quick-frozen spinach, (6 ounces) (see Ingredient note)

- 6 teaspoons extra-virgin olive oil, (optional)
- 6 tablespoons freshly grated Parmesan cheese

PREPARATION

1. Combine broth, garlic, rosemary and crushed red pepper in a 4- to 6-quart Dutch oven or soup pot; bring to a simmer. Partially cover and simmer over medium-low heat for 20 minutes to intensify flavor. Meanwhile, mash 1 cup beans in a small bowl.

2. Scoop garlic cloves and rosemary from the broth with a slotted spoon (or pass the soup through a strainer and return to the pot). Add mashed and whole beans to the broth, along with tomatoes; return to a simmer. Stir in pasta, cover and cook over medium heat, stirring occasionally, until the pasta is just tender, 10 to 12 minutes.

3. Stir in spinach, cover and cook just until the spinach has thawed, 2 to 3 minutes. Ladle the soup into bowls and garnish each serving with a drizzle of oil, if desired, and a sprinkling of Parmesan. Variation: Substitute chickpeas (garbanzo beans) for the cannellini beans; use a food processor to puree them.

TIPS & NOTES

- **Ingredient Note:** Individually quick-frozen (IQF) spinach is sold in convenient plastic bags. If you have a 10-ounce box of spinach on hand, use just over half of it and cook according to package directions before adding to the soup in Step 3.

NUTRITION

Per serving: 133 calories; 2 g fat (1 g sat, 0 g mono); 6 mg cholesterol; 21 g carbohydrates; 9 g protein; 4 gfiber; 356 mg sodium; 29 mg potassium.

Nutrition Bonus: Vitamin A (35% daily value), Fiber (16% dv).

Carbohydrate Servings: 1

Exchanges: 1 1/ 2 starch, 1 vegetable, 1 lean meat

Egg Thread Soup with Asparagus

INGREDIENTS

- 8 cups homemade chicken broth, fat skimmed, or reduced-sodium chicken broth
- 1/2 cup pastina, or other tiny pasta, such as alphabet or stars
- 12 ounces asparagus, trimmed and cut into 1 1/2-inch diagonal pieces (2 cups)
- 4 large eggs
- 1/2 teaspoon lemon juice
- 1/4 teaspoon salt, optional

PREPARATION

1. Bring broth to a boil in a Dutch oven or soup pot. Stir in pasta. Cook, uncovered, over medium-high heat, stirring occasionally, until pasta is just tender, about 5 minutes. Stir in asparagus; cook for 2 minutes. Reduce heat to medium.

2. Break eggs into a large measuring cup and whisk until well blended. Add to the gently boiling soup in a thin, steady stream, stirring constantly with a fork. (Slow stirring will produce large threads; rapid stirring will break the threads up into small pieces.) Take off heat and add lemon juice.

NUTRITION

Per serving: 116 calories; 4 g fat (2 g sat, 1 g mono); 110 mg cholesterol; 11 g carbohydrates; 9 g protein; 1 g fiber; 217 mg sodium; 138 mg potassium.

Nutrition Bonus: Calcium (25% daily value), Folate (23% dv).

Carbohydrate Servings: 1

Exchanges: 1/2 starch, 1/2 vegetable, 1 lean protein, 1/2 fat

Spinach, Avocado & Mango Salad

INGREDIENTS

DRESSING

- 1/3 cup orange juice
- 1 tablespoon red-wine vinegar
- 2 tablespoons hazelnut oil, almond oil or canola oil
- 1 teaspoon Dijon mustard
- 1/4 teaspoon salt, or to taste
- Freshly ground pepper, to taste

SALAD

- 10 cups baby spinach leaves, (about 8 ounces)
- 1 1/2 cups radicchio, torn into bite-size pieces
- 8-12 small red radishes, (1 bunch), sliced
- 1 small ripe mango, sliced
- 1 medium avocado, sliced

PREPARATION

To prepare dressing: Whisk juice, vinegar, oil, mustard, salt and pepper in a bowl.

To prepare salad: Just before serving, combine spinach, radicchio, radishes and mango in a large bowl. Add the dressing; toss to coat. Garnish each serving with avocado slices.

NUTRITION

Per serving: 210 calories; 14 g fat (2 g sat, 2 g mono); 0 mg cholesterol; 10 g carbohydrates; 3 g protein; 6 g fiber; 258 mg sodium; 479 mg potassium.

Nutrition Bonus: Vitamin C (70% daily value), Vitamin A (40% dv), Fiber (26% dv).

Carbohydrate Servings: 1

Exchanges: 3 vegetable, 3 fat (mono)

Berry Frozen Yogurt

INGREDIENTS

- 3 cups fresh or frozen and partially thawed blackberries, or raspberries or a mixture of blackberries, raspberries and blueberries (see Tip)
- 6 tablespoons sugar
- 1 tablespoon lemon juice
- 3/4 cup low-fat plain yogurt

PREPARATION

1. Combine berries, sugar and lemon juice in a food processor; process until smooth. Add yogurt and pulse until mixed in. If using fresh berries, transfer the mixture to a medium bowl, cover and refrigerate until chilled, about 1 hour.

2. Transfer the berry mixture to an ice cream maker and freeze according to manufacturer's directions. (Alternatively, freeze the mixture in a shallow metal pan until solid, about 6 hours. Break into chunks and process in a food processor until smooth and creamy.) Serve immediately or transfer to a storage container and let harden in the freezer for 1 to 1 1/2 hours.

TIPS & NOTES

- **Make Ahead Tip**: Store in an airtight container in the freezer for up to 1 week. Let soften in the refrigerator for 1/2 hour before serving. | Equipment: Ice cream maker or food processor
- **Tip:** To freeze fresh berries: Wash berries and pat dry. Spread in a single layer on a tray, cover with plastic wrap and freeze until solid. Pack frozen fruit into ziplock bags, taking care to remove air from the bags. Freeze for up to 1 year.

NUTRITION

Per serving: 106 calories; 1 g fat (0 g sat, 0 g mono); 2 mg cholesterol; 22 g carbohydrates; 3 g protein; 4 gfiber; 22 mg sodium; 192 mg potassium.

Nutrition Bonus: Vitamin C (28% daily value), Fiber (16% dv).

Carbohydrate Servings: 1 1/2

Exchanges: 1 1/2 fruit

Curry-Roasted Shrimp with Oranges

INGREDIENTS

- 2 large seedless oranges
- 1/2 teaspoon kosher salt, divided
- 1 1/2 pounds shrimp, (30-40 per pound), peeled and deveined
- 1 tablespoon extra-virgin olive oil
- 1 tablespoon curry powder, preferably Madras (see Note)
- 1/2 teaspoon freshly ground pepper

PREPARATION

1. Preheat oven to 400°F. Line a baking sheet (with sides) with parchment paper. Finely grate the zest of 1 orange; set aside. Using a sharp knife, peel both oranges, removing all the bitter white pith. Thinly slice the oranges crosswise, then cut the slices into quarters. Spread the orange slices on the prepared baking sheet and sprinkle with 1/4 teaspoon salt. Roast until the oranges are slightly dry, about 12 minutes.

2. Meanwhile, toss shrimp with oil, curry powder, pepper, the orange zest and the remaining 1/4 teaspoon salt in a large bowl. Transfer the shrimp to the baking sheet with the oranges and roast until pink and curled, about 6 minutes. Divide the oranges and the shrimp among 4 plates and serve.

TIPS & NOTES

- **Make Ahead Tip:** Refrigerate for up to 4 days. Reheat before serving.

- **Note:** Madras curry powder is made with a hotter blend of spices than standard curry powder.

NUTRITION

Per serving: 253 calories; 7 g fat (1 g sat, 3 g mono); 259 mg cholesterol; 13 g carbohydrates; 0 g added sugars; 35 g protein; 4 g fiber; 548 mg sodium; 338 mg potassium.

Nutrition Bonus: Selenium (93% daily value), Vitamin C (70% dv).

Carbohydrate Servings: 1

Exchanges: 1 fruit, 5 very lean meat, 1 fat (mono)

Sesame Green Beans

INGREDIENTS

- 1 pound green beans, trimmed
- 2 teaspoons extra-virgin olive oil
- 2 teaspoons toasted sesame seeds, (see Tip)
- 1 teaspoon sesame oil
- Salt & freshly ground pepper, to taste

PREPARATION

1. Preheat oven to 500°F.
2. Toss green beans with olive oil. Spread in an even layer on a rimmed baking sheet. Roast, turning once halfway through cooking, until tender and beginning to brown, about 10 minutes. Toss with sesame seeds, sesame oil, salt and pepper.

TIPS & NOTES

- **Tip:** To toast sesame seeds: Place in a small dry skillet and cook over medium-low heat, stirring constantly, until fragrant and lightly browned, 2 to 4 minutes.

NUTRITION

Per serving: 67 calories; 4 g fat (1 g sat, 3 g mono); 0 mg cholesterol; 7 g carbohydrates; 0 g added sugars; 2 g protein; 4 g fiber; 73 mg sodium; 280 mg potassium.

Nutrition Bonus: Vitamin C (15% daily value).

Carbohydrate Servings: 1/2

Exchanges: 1 vegetable

Chile-Spiced Asparagus

INGREDIENTS

- 1 tablespoon extra-virgin olive oil
- 2 bunches asparagus, tough ends trimmed, cut into 1-inch pieces
- 1 tablespoon water
- 1 1/2 teaspoons chili powder or 1 teaspoon smoked paprika
- 3/4 teaspoon garlic powder
- 1/2 teaspoon salt
- 2 tablespoons sherry vinegar or red-wine vinegar

PREPARATION

1. Heat oil in a large nonstick skillet over medium-high heat. Add asparagus and water; cook, stirring often, 4 to 5 minutes. Add chili powder (or paprika), garlic powder and salt; cook until the asparagus is tender-crisp, about 1 minute. Remove from heat, add vinegar and stir to coat.

TIPS & NOTES

- **Shopping Tip:** Smoked paprika can be purchased in gourmet markets.

NUTRITION

Per serving: 62 calories; 4 g fat (1 g sat, 3 g mono); 0 mg cholesterol; 6 g carbohydrates; 0 g added sugars;3 g protein; 3 g fiber; 321 mg sodium; 275 mg potassium.

Nutrition Bonus: Folate (42% daily value), Vitamin A (30% dv), Vitamin C (15% dv).

Carbohydrate Servings: 1/2

Exchanges: 1 vegetable, 1 fat

DAY 4
BREAKFAST
Tropical Fruit Smoothie
Whole-wheat toast (1 slice)
Plum spread
LUNCH
Lettuce Wraps with Spiced Pork or Five-Spice Duck Stir-Fry
Green Papaya Salad
Whole-wheat toast (1 slice)
Fat-free cheese Slice
SNACK
Skim milk (1 cup)
DINNER
Chicken Breasts with Roasted Lemons or Oven-Poached Salmon Fillets
Arugula-Mushroom Salad
Baked potato (1/2 medium)
Strawberries (1 cup)

DAY 4 RECIPES

Tropical Fruit Smoothie

INGREDIENTS
- 1 cup cubed fresh or canned pineapple
- 1 banana, sliced
- 1/2 cup silken tofu, or low-fat plain yogurt
- 1/3 cup frozen passion fruit concentrate
- 1/2 cup water
- 2 ice cubes
- 1 tablespoon wheat bran, or oat bran (optional)

PREPARATION

1. Combine pineapple, banana, tofu (or yogurt), passion fruit concentrate, water, ice cubes and wheat bran (or oat bran), if using, in a blender; cover and blend until creamy. Serve immediately.

NUTRITION

Per serving: 109 calories; 2 g fat (0 g sat, 0 g mono); 0 mg cholesterol; 21 g carbohydrates; 4 g protein; 2 gfiber; 26 mg sodium; 281 mg potassium.

Nutrition Bonus: Vitamin C (40% daily value).

Carbohydrate Servings: 1 1/2

Exchanges: 1 fruit, 1/2 low-fat milk

Plum spread

INGREDIENTS

- 5 pounds plums, pitted and sliced (14-15 cups)
- 3 Granny Smith apples, washed and quartered (not cored)
- 1/4 cup white grape juice, or other fruit juice
- 2 tablespoons lemon juice
- 3/4 cup sugar, or Splenda Granular
- 1/4 teaspoon ground cinnamon, or ginger (optional)

PREPARATION

1. Place a plate in the freezer for testing consistency later.
2. Combine plums, apples, grape juice (or fruit juice) and lemon juice in a large, heavy-bottomed, nonreactive Dutch oven. Bring to a boil over medium-high heat, stirring. Cover and boil gently, stirring occasionally, until the fruit is softened and juicy, 15 to 20 minutes. Uncover and boil gently, stirring occasionally, until the fruit is completely soft, about 20 minutes. (Adjust heat as necessary to maintain a gentle boil.)

3. Pass the fruit through a food mill to remove the skins and apple seeds.

4. Return the strained fruit to the pot. Add sugar (or Splenda) and cinnamon (or ginger), if using. Cook over medium heat, stirring frequently, until a spoonful of jam dropped onto the chilled plate holds its shape, about 15 minutes longer. (See Tip.) Remove from heat and skim off any foam.

TIPS & NOTES

- **Make Ahead Tip**: Store in an airtight container in the refrigerator for up to 2 months.
- **To test the consistency of the spread:** Drop a dollop of cooked spread onto a chilled plate. Carefully run your finger through the dollop. If the track remains unfilled, the jam is done.

NUTRITION

Per tablespoon with sugar: 14 calories; 0 g fat (0 g sat, 0 g mono); 0 mg cholesterol; 4 g carbohydrates; 0 g protein; 0 g fiber; 0 mg sodium; 30 mg potassium.

Exchanges: free food

Nutrition Note: Per tablespoon with Splenda: 0 Carbohydrate Servings; 12 calories; 3 g carbohydrate.

Lettuce Wraps with Spiced Pork

INGREDIENTS

SAUCE

- 2 tablespoons oyster sauce
- 2 tablespoons water
- 1 tablespoon hoisin sauce
- 1 tablespoon rice vinegar
- 1 tablespoon dry sherry, or rice wine
- 2 teaspoons cornstarch

- 1 teaspoon brown sugar
- 1 teaspoon reduced-sodium soy sauce
- 1 teaspoon sesame oil

STIR-FRY

- 3 teaspoons canola oil, divided
- 1 pound thin center-cut boneless pork chops, trimmed of fat and cut into thin julienne strips
- 2 cloves garlic, minced
- 1 tablespoon minced fresh ginger
- 1 8-ounce can sliced water chestnuts, rinsed and coarsely chopped
- 1 8-ounce can sliced bamboo shoots, rinsed and coarsely chopped
- 8 ounces shiitake mushrooms, stemmed, cut into julienne strips
- 4 scallions, greens only, sliced
- 1 head iceberg lettuce, leaves separated

PREPARATION

1. To prepare sauce: Combine oyster sauce, water, hoisin sauce, vinegar, sherry (or rice wine), cornstarch, brown sugar, soy sauce and sesame oil in a small bowl.

2. To prepare stir-fry: Heat 2 teaspoons canola oil over medium-high heat in a large nonstick skillet or wok. Add pork; cook, stirring constantly, until no longer pink, about 4 minutes. Transfer to a plate. Wipe out the pan.

3. Add remaining 1 teaspoon oil, garlic and ginger; cook, stirring constantly, until fragrant, 30 seconds. Add water chestnuts, bamboo shoots and mushrooms; cook, stirring often, until the mushrooms have softened, about 4 minutes. Return the pork to the pan and add the sauce. Cook, stirring constantly, until a thick glossy sauce has formed, about 1 minute. Serve sprinkled with scallions and wrapped in lettuce leaves.

TIPS & NOTES

- **Make Ahead Tip**: The sauce will keep, covered, in the refrigerator for up to 2 days.

NUTRITION

Per serving: 350 calories; 16 g fat (5 g sat, 8 g mono); 59 mg cholesterol; 29 g carbohydrates; 25 g protein; 7 g fiber; 810 mg sodium; 675 mg potassium.

Nutrition Bonus: Vitamin C (20% daily value), Iron (15% dv).

Carbohydrate Servings: 1

Exchanges: 1/2 other carbohydrate, 2 vegetable, 3 medium-fat meat

Five-Spice Duck Stir-Fry

INGREDIENTS

- 1/4 cup dry sherry, (see Note)
- 2 tablespoons plum sauce
- 1/4 teaspoon salt and Pinch of cayenne pepper
- 1 tablespoon canola oil
- 8 ounces boneless duck breast, (see Note), skin removed, sliced in half lengthwise, then cut into 1/4-inch thick slices
- 2 tablespoons minced garlic
- 2 teaspoons minced fresh ginger
- 1 1/2 cups trimmed, halved green beans
- 2 cups purchased julienne-cut carrots, (8 ounces)
- 1/4 teaspoon five-spice powder, or to taste (see Note)

PREPARATION

1. Combine sherry, plum sauce, salt and cayenne in a small bowl.

2. Heat oil in a large nonstick skillet over medium-high heat. Add duck; cook, stirring often, until browned, 1 to 3 minutes. Transfer to a plate with a slotted spatula.

3. Add garlic and ginger to the pan and cook, stirring constantly, until fragrant, about 30 seconds. Add green beans, carrots and five-spice powder, and cook, stirring, until the carrots are slightly softened, about 1 minute. Add the plum sauce mixture; stir to coat, cover, reduce heat to medium and cook until the green beans are tender, 3 to 4 minutes. Add the cooked duck, toss to combine and serve immediately.

TIPS & NOTES

- **Notes:** Sherry is a type of fortified wine originally from southern Spain. Don't use the "cooking sherry" sold in many supermarkets as it can be surprisingly high in sodium. Instead, purchase dry sherry that's sold with other fortified wines in your wine or liquor store.

- Boneless duck breast halves range widely in weight, from about 1/2 to 1 pound, depending on the breed. They can be found in most supermarkets in the poultry or specialty-meat sections.

- Often a blend of cinnamon, cloves, fennel seed, star anise and Szechuan peppercorns, five-spice powder was originally considered a cure-all miracle blend encompassing the five elements (sour, bitter, sweet, pungent, salty). Look for it in the supermarket spice section.

NUTRITION

Per serving: 336 calories; 12 g fat (2 g sat, 6 g mono); 87 mg cholesterol; 26 g carbohydrates; 26 g protein;6 g fiber; 537 mg sodium; 885 mg potassium.

Nutrition Bonus: Vitamin A (390% daily value), Vitamin C (45% dv), Iron (35% dv), Potassium (25% dv), Folate (19% dv).

Carbohydrate Servings: 1

Exchanges: 1/2 other carbohydrate, 3 vegetable, 3 lean meat, 1 1/2 fat

Green Papaya Salad

INGREDIENTS

- 1/4 teaspoon freshly grated lime zest
- 1/4 cup lime juice
- 2 tablespoons finely chopped palm sugar, or packed brown sugar (see Tip)
- 2 tablespoons fish sauce
- Hawaiian chiles, or any fresh hot chiles, minced, to taste
- 3 cups matchstick-cut or julienned green papaya, (see Tip)
- 1/2 cup very thinly sliced Maui or other sweet onion
- 1/2 cup pea shoots, cut into 3-inch pieces, or bean sprouts
- Freshly ground pepper, to taste

PREPARATION

1. Whisk lime zest, lime juice, sugar, fish sauce and chiles in a large bowl.
2. Add papaya, onion and pea shoots (or sprouts) to the vinaigrette; toss to combine. Sprinkle with pepper just before serving.

TIPS & NOTES

- **Make Ahead Tip**: The vinaigrette (Step 1) will keep, covered, in the refrigerator for up to 1 week.
- **Tips:** Palm sugar is an unrefined sweetener similar in flavor to brown sugar. It's sold in "pods" or as a paste in Asian markets or at importfood.com.
- Green papaya is papaya that is not ripe and firm. Look for it in Asian markets. If you can't find one, a ripe papaya will still taste delicious in this salad.

NUTRITION

Per serving: 59 calories; 0 g fat (0 g sat, 0 g mono); 0 mg cholesterol; 15 g carbohydrates; 1 g protein; 1 gfiber; 403 mg sodium; 58 mg potassium.

Nutrition Bonus: Vitamin C (60% daily value).

Carbohydrate Servings: 1

Exchanges: 1 fruit

Chicken Breasts with Roasted Lemons

INGREDIENTS

ROASTED LEMONS

- 3 medium lemons, thinly sliced and seeded
- 1 teaspoon extra-virgin olive oil
- 1/8 teaspoon salt

CHICKEN

- 4 boneless, skinless chicken breast halves, (about 1 pound total), trimmed
- 1/8 teaspoon salt
- Freshly ground pepper, to taste
- 1/4 cup all-purpose flour
- 2 teaspoons extra-virgin olive oil
- 1 1/4 cups reduced-sodium chicken broth
- 2 tablespoons drained capers, rinsed
- 2 teaspoons butter
- 3 tablespoons chopped fresh parsley, divided

PREPARATION

1. To prepare roasted lemons: Preheat oven to 325°F. Line a baking sheet with parchment paper. Arrange lemon slices in a single layer on it. Brush the lemon slices with 1 tablespoon oil and sprinkle with 1/8 teaspoon salt. Roast the

lemons until slightly dry and beginning to brown around the edges, 25 to 30 minutes.

2. Meanwhile, prepare chicken: Cover chicken with plastic wrap and pound with a rolling pin or heavy skillet until flattened to about 1/2 inch thick. Sprinkle the chicken with 1/8 teaspoon salt and pepper. Place flour in a shallow dish and dredge the chicken to coat both sides; shake off excess (discard remaining flour).

3. Heat 2 teaspoons oil in a large nonstick skillet over medium-high heat. Add the chicken and cook until golden brown, 2 to 3 minutes per side. Add broth and bring to a boil, scraping up any browned bits. Stir in capers. Boil until the liquid is reduced to syrup consistency, 5 to 8 minutes, turning the chicken halfway. Add the roasted lemons, butter, 2 tablespoons parsley and more pepper, if desired; simmer until the butter melts and the chicken is cooked through, about 2 minutes. Transfer to a platter. Sprinkle with the remaining 1 tablespoon parsley and serve.

TIPS & NOTES

- **Make Ahead Tip**: Cover and refrigerate the roasted lemons (Step 1) for up to 2 days.

NUTRITION

Per serving: 219 calories; 7 g fat (2 g sat, 3 g mono); 72 mg cholesterol; 6 g carbohydrates; 0 g added sugars; 28 g protein; 1 g fiber; 396 mg sodium; 376 mg potassium.

Nutrition Bonus: Vitamin C (40% daily value).

Carbohydrate Servings: 1/2

Exchanges: 1/2 fruit, 4 very lean meat, 1 fat.

Oven-Poached Salmon Fillets

INGREDIENTS

- 1 pound salmon fillet, cut into 4 portions, skin removed, if desired
- 2 tablespoons dry white wine

- 1/4 teaspoon salt
- Freshly ground pepper, to taste
- 2 tablespoons finely chopped shallot, (1 medium)
- Lemon wedges, for garnish

PREPARATION

Preheat oven to 425°F. Coat a 9-inch glass pie pan or an 8-inch glass baking dish with cooking spray.

Place salmon, skin-side (or skinned-side) down, in the prepared pan. Sprinkle with wine. Season with salt and pepper, then sprinkle with shallots. Cover with foil and bake until opaque in the center and starting to flake, 15 to 25 minutes, depending on thickness.When the salmon is ready, transfer to dinner plates. Spoon any liquid remaining in the pan over the salmon and serve with lemon wedges.

NUTRITION

Per serving: 216 calories; 12 g fat (2 g sat, 4 g mono); 67 mg cholesterol; 1 g carbohydrates; 0 g added sugars; 23 g protein; 0 g fiber; 213 mg sodium; 432 mg potassium.

Nutrition Bonus: 433 mg potassium (22% dv).

Exchanges: 3 1/2 lean protein

Arugula-Mushroom Salad

INGREDIENTS

- 1 clove garlic, peeled
- 1/4 teaspoon salt
- 1 tablespoon lemon juice
- 1 tablespoon reduced-fat mayonnaise
- 1 tablespoon extra-virgin olive oil
- 1 tablespoon chopped fresh parsley

- Freshly ground pepper, to taste
- 6 cups arugula leaves
- 2 cups sliced mushrooms

PREPARATION

Place garlic on a cutting board and crush. Sprinkle with salt and use the flat of a chef's knife blade to mash the garlic to a paste; transfer to a serving bowl. Whisk in lemon juice, mayonnaise, oil and parsley. Season with pepper. Add arugula and mushrooms; toss to coat with the dressing.

NUTRITION

Per serving: 62 calories; 4 g fat (1 g sat, 3 g mono); 1 mg cholesterol; 3 g carbohydrates; 0 g added sugars; 2 g protein; 1 g fiber; 188 mg sodium; 235 mg potassium. Nutrition Bonus: Vitamin C (15% daily value).

Exchanges: 1 vegetable, 1 fat (mono)

DAY 5
BREAKFAST

Baked Asparagus & Cheese Frittata
Skim milk (1 cup)
Apple (1 cup, quartered)
LUNCH

Curried Corn Bisqu or Chilled Tomato Soup with Cilantro-Yogurt Swirl
Spicy Chicken Tacos
Melon (1 cup, cubes)
SNACK

Fat-free Cheese slice
DINNER

Grilled Pork Tenderloin with Mustard, Rosemary & Apple Marinade or Herb-Roasted Turkey
Salad of Boston Lettuce with Creamy Orange-Shallot Dressing
Brown rice (1/2 cup)

DAY 5 RECIPES

Baked Asparagus & Cheese Frittata

INGREDIENTS

- 2 tablespoons fine dry breadcrumbs
- 1 pound thin asparagus
- 1 1/2 teaspoons extra-virgin olive oil
- 2 onions, chopped
- 1 red bell pepper, chopped
- 2 cloves garlic, minced
- 1/2 teaspoon salt, divided
- 1/2 cup water
- Freshly ground pepper, to taste
- 4 large eggs
- 2 large egg whites
- 1 cup part-skim ricotta cheese
- 1 tablespoon chopped fresh parsley
- 1/2 cup shredded Gruyère cheese

PREPARATION

1. Preheat oven to 325°F. Coat a 10-inch pie pan or ceramic quiche dish with cooking spray. Sprinkle with breadcrumbs, tapping out the excess.

2. Snap tough ends off asparagus. Slice off the top 2 inches of the tips and reserve. Cut the stalks into 1/2-inch-long slices.

3. Heat oil in a large nonstick skillet over medium-high heat. Add onions, bell pepper, garlic and 1/4 teaspoon salt; cook, stirring, until softened, 5 to 7 minutes.

4. Add water and the asparagus stalks to the skillet. Cook, stirring, until the asparagus is tender and the liquid has evaporated, about 7 minutes (the mixture should be very

dry). Season with salt and pepper. Arrange the vegetables in an even layer in the prepared pan.

5. Whisk eggs and egg whites in a large bowl. Add ricotta, parsley, the remaining 1/4 teaspoon salt and pepper; whisk to blend. Pour the egg mixture over the vegetables, gently shaking the pan to distribute. Scatter the reserved asparagus tips over the top and sprinkle with Gruyère.

6. Bake the frittata until a knife inserted in the center comes out clean, about 35 minutes. Let stand for 5 minutes before serving.

NUTRITION

Per serving: 195 calories; 11 g fat (5 g sat, 4 g mono); 164 mg cholesterol; 10 g carbohydrates; 15 g protein; 2 g fiber; 357 mg sodium; 310 mg potassium.

Nutrition Bonus: Vitamin C (70% daily value), Vitamin A (30% dv).

Carbohydrate Servings: 1/2

Exchanges: 2 vegetable, 1 medium-fat meat, 1/2 high-fat meat

Curried Corn Bisque

INGREDIENTS

- 2 teaspoons canola oil
- 1 cup fresh or frozen chopped onions
- 1 tablespoon curry powder
- 1/2 teaspoon hot sauce, or to taste
- 1/4 teaspoon salt, or to taste
- 1/4 teaspoon freshly ground pepper
- 2 16-ounce packages frozen corn, or 3 10-ounce boxes
- 2 cups reduced-sodium chicken broth
- 2 cups water
- 1 cup "lite" coconut milk, (see Ingredient note)

PREPARATION

1. Heat oil in a large saucepan over medium-high heat. Add onions and cook, stirring occasionally, until soft, about 3 minutes. Add curry powder, hot sauce, salt and pepper and stir to coat the onions. Stir in corn, broth and water; increase the heat to high and bring the mixture to a boil. Remove from the heat and puree in a blender or food processor (in batches, if necessary) into a homogeneous mixture that still has some texture. Pour the soup into a clean pot, add coconut milk and heat through. Serve hot or cold. Make Curried Sweet Pea Bisque by substituting frozen peas for the corn.

TIPS & NOTES

- **Make Ahead Tip**: Cover and refrigerate for up to 2 days or freeze for up to 2 months.
- **Ingredient Note**: Look for reduced-fat coconut milk (labeled "lite") in the Asian section of your market.

NUTRITION

Per serving: 138 calories; 4 g fat (2 g sat, 1 g mono); 1 mg cholesterol; 24 g carbohydrates; 0 g added sugars; 5 g protein; 3 g fiber; 121 mg sodium; 291 mg potassium.

Nutrition Bonus: Fiber (13% daily value).

Carbohydrate Servings: 1 1/2

Exchanges: 1 1/2 starch, 1 fat

Chilled Tomato Soup with Cilantro-Yogurt Swirl

INGREDIENTS

- 2 teaspoons ground cumin
- 2 pounds ripe tomatoes, coarsely chopped (about 5 cups)
- 1/2 cup chopped red onion
- 2 tablespoons plus 1/4 cup chopped fresh cilantro, divided

- 2 teaspoons chopped chipotle pepper in adobo sauce, (see Note)
- 1 cup fresh corn kernels, (from about 2 ears; see Note)
- 1 cup ice water
- 2 tablespoons lime juice, or to taste
- 1 teaspoon kosher salt and 1 cup low-fat plain yogurt

PREPARATION

1. To prepare soup: Toast cumin in a small skillet over low heat, stirring, until just fragrant, 1 to 2 minutes.
2. Combine tomatoes, onion, 2 tablespoons cilantro and chipotle in a blender or food processor. Puree until smooth. Transfer to a large bowl. Add the toasted cumin, corn, ice water, lime juice and salt; stir to combine. Refrigerate until chilled, about 1 hour or until ready to serve.
3. To prepare cilantro yogurt: Puree yogurt and the remaining 1/4 cup cilantro in a blender or food processor until smooth. Refrigerate until ready to serve (it will thicken slightly as it stands).
4. To serve, divide the soup among 4 bowls and garnish each with a generous swirl of cilantro yogurt.

TIPS & NOTES

- **Make Ahead Tip**: Refrigerate the soup and cilantro yogurt in separate containers for up to 1 day.
- **Notes:** Chipotle chiles in adobo sauce are smoked jalapeños packed in a flavorful sauce. Look for the small cans with the Mexican foods in large supermarkets. Once opened, they'll keep up to 2 weeks in the refrigerator or 6 months in the freezer.
- **To remove corn from the cob:** Stand an uncooked ear of corn on its stem end in a shallow bowl and slice the kernels off with a sharp, thin-bladed knife. This technique produces whole kernels that are good for adding to salads and salsas. If you want to use the corn kernels for soups, fritters or puddings, you can add another step to the process. After cutting the kernels off, reverse the knife and,

using the dull side, press it down the length of the ear to push out the rest of the corn and its milk.

NUTRITION

Per serving: 128 calories; 2 g fat (1 g sat, 0 g mono); 4 mg cholesterol; 24 g carbohydrates; 7 g protein; 5 gfiber; 667 mg sodium; 827 mg potassium.

Nutrition Bonus: Vitamin C (110% daily value), Vitamin A (30% dv), Potassium (22% dv), Calcium (15% dv)

Carbohydrate Servings: 1

Exchanges: 1/2 starch, 2 vegetable, 1/2 reduced fat milk

Spicy Chicken Tacos

INGREDIENTS

- 8 corn tortillas
- 1 pound boneless, skinless chicken breasts, trimmed of fat and cut into thin strips
- 1/4 teaspoon salt, or to taste
- 2 teaspoons canola oil, divided
- 1 large onion, sliced
- 1 large green bell pepper, seeded and sliced
- 3 large cloves garlic, minced
- 1 jalapeño pepper, seeded and minced
- 1 tablespoon ground cumin
- 1/2 cup prepared hot salsa, plus more for garnish
- 1/4 cup chopped fresh cilantro
- Sliced scallions, chopped fresh tomatoes and reduced-fat sour cream, for garnish

PREPARATION

1. Preheat oven to 300°F. Wrap tortillas in foil and bake until heated through, 10 to 15 minutes. Meanwhile, season chicken with salt. Heat 1 teaspoon oil in a large heavy skillet over high heat until very hot. Add chicken and cook, stirring until browned on all sides, about 6 minutes. Transfer to a bowl.

2. Reduce heat to medium and add the remaining 1 teaspoon oil to skillet. Add onion and cook, stirring, until they start to brown around the edges, 3 to 5 minutes. Add bell pepper, garlic, jalapeño and cumin. Cook, stirring, until peppers are bright green but still crisp, 2 to 3 minutes more.

3. Stir in salsa and reserved chicken. Cook, stirring, until chicken is heated through, about 2 minutes. Remove from heat and stir in cilantro. Spoon into warmed tortillas and garnish with scallions, tomatoes and sour cream.

NUTRITION

Per serving (without garnishes): 303 calories; 6 g fat (1 g sat, 2 g mono); 66 mg cholesterol; 32 g carbohydrates; 1 g added sugars; 31 g protein; 5 g fiber; 421 mg sodium; 533 mg potassium.

Nutrition Bonus: Vitamin C (68% daily value); Folate (25% dv); Fiber (20% dv).

Carbohydrate Servings: 2

Exchanges: 2 starch, 1 vegetable, 31/2 very lean meat

Grilled Pork Tenderloin with Mustard, Rosemary & Apple Marinade

INGREDIENTS

- 1/4 cup frozen apple juice concentrate
- 2 tablespoons plus 1 1/2 teaspoons Dijon mustard
- 2 tablespoons extra-virgin olive oil, divided
- 2 tablespoons chopped fresh rosemary, or thyme
- 4 cloves garlic, minced
- 1 teaspoon crushed peppercorns
- 2 12-ounce pork tenderloins, trimmed of fat

- 1 tablespoon minced shallot
- 3 tablespoons port, or brewed black tea
- 2 tablespoons balsamic vinegar
- 1/4 teaspoon salt, or to taste
- Freshly ground pepper, to taste

PREPARATION

1. Whisk apple juice concentrate, 2 tablespoons mustard, 1 tablespoon oil, rosemary (or thyme), garlic and peppercorns in a small bowl. Reserve 3 tablespoons marinade for basting. Place tenderloins in a shallow glass dish and pour the remaining marinade over them, turning to coat. Cover and marinate in the refrigerator for at least 20 minutes or for up to 2 hours, turning several times.
2. Heat a grill or broiler.
3. Combine shallot, port (or tea), vinegar, salt, pepper and the remaining 1 1/2 teaspoons mustard and 1 tablespoon oil in a small bowl or a jar with a tight-fitting lid; whisk or shake until blended. Set aside.
4. Grill or broil the tenderloins, turning several times and basting the browned sides with the reserved marinade, until just cooked through, 15 to 20 minutes. (An instant-read thermometer inserted in the center should register 155°F. The temperature will increase to 160° during resting.)
5. Transfer the tenderloins to a clean cutting board, tent with foil and let them rest for about 5 minutes before carving them into 1/2-inch-thick slices. Arrange the pork slices on plates and drizzle with the shallot dressing. Serve immediately.

TIPS & NOTES

- **Make Ahead Tip**: The pork can be marinated (Step 1) for up to 2 hours.

NUTRITION

Per serving: 165 calories; 5 g fat (1 g sat, 2 g mono); 63 mg cholesterol; 5 g carbohydrates; 0 g added sugars; 23 g protein; 0 g fiber; 186 mg sodium; 397 mg potassium.

Nutrition Bonus: Vitamin C (20% daily value).

Carbohydrate Servings: 1/2

Exchanges: 1/2 other carbohydrate, 3 lean meat

Herb-Roasted Turkey

INGREDIENTS

- 1 10-12-pound turkey
- 1/4 cup fresh herbs, plus 20 whole sprigs, such as thyme, rosemary, sage, oregano and/or marjoram, divided
- 2 tablespoons canola, oil
- 1 teaspoon salt
- 1 teaspoon freshly ground pepper
- Aromatics, onion, apple, lemon and/or orange, cut into 2-inch pieces (1 1/2 cups)
- 3 cups water, plus more as needed

PREPARATION

1. Position a rack in the lower third of the oven; preheat to 475°F.
2. Remove giblets and neck from turkey cavities and reserve for making gravy. Place the turkey, breast-side up, on a rack in a large roasting pan; pat dry with paper towels. Mix minced herbs, oil, salt and pepper in a small bowl. Rub the herb mixture all over the turkey, under the skin and onto the breast meat. Place aromatics and 10 of the herb sprigs in the cavity. Tuck the wing tips under the turkey. Tie the legs together with kitchen string. Add 3 cups water and the remaining 10 herb sprigs to the pan.

3. Roast the turkey until the skin is golden brown, 45 minutes. Remove the turkey from the oven. If using a remote digital thermometer, insert it into the deepest part of the thigh, close to the joint. Cover the breast with a double layer of foil, cutting as necessary to conform to the breast. Reduce oven temperature to 350° and continue roasting for 11/4 to 13/4 hours more. If the pan dries out, tilt the turkey to let juices run out of the cavity into the pan and add 1 cup water. The turkey is done when the thermometer (or an instant-read thermometer inserted into the thickest part of the thigh without touching bone) registers 165°F.

4. Transfer the turkey to a serving platter and cover with foil. Let the turkey rest for 20 minutes. Remove string and carve.

TIPS & NOTES

- **Make Ahead Tip**: Equipment: Large roasting pan, roasting rack, kitchen string, thermometer

NUTRITION

Per serving (without skin): 155 calories; 5 g fat (1 g sat, 2 g mono); 63 mg cholesterol; 0 g carbohydrates;0 g added sugars; 25 g protein; 0 g fiber; 175 mg sodium; 258 mg potassium.

Carbohydrate Servings: 0

Exchanges: 3 1/2 lean meat

Salad of Boston Lettuce with Creamy Orange-Shallot Dressing

INGREDIENTS

DRESSING

- 1/4 cup reduced-fat mayonnaise
- 1/2 teaspoon Dijon mustard and 1/4 cup orange juice
- 2 teaspoons finely chopped shallot
- Freshly ground pepper, to taste

SALAD

- 1 large head Boston lettuce, torn into bite-size pieces (5 cups)
- 1 cup julienned or grated carrot, (1 carrot)
- 1 cup cherry or grape tomatoes, rinsed and cut in half
- 2 tablespoons snipped fresh tarragon, or chives (optional)

PREPARATION

To prepare dressing: Whisk mayonnaise and mustard in a small bowl. Slowly whisk in orange juice until smooth. Stir in shallot. Season with pepper.

To prepare salad: Divide lettuce among 4 plates and scatter carrot and tomatoes on top. Drizzle the dressing over the salads and sprinkle with tarragon (or chives), if desired. Serve immediately.

NUTRITION

Per serving: 64 calories; 1 g fat (0 g sat, 0 g mono); 0 mg cholesterol; 12 g carbohydrates; 1 g added sugars; 2 g protein; 2 g fiber; 182 mg sodium; 386 mg potassium.

Nutrition Bonus: Vitamin A (120% daily value), Vitamin C (30% dv), Folate (16% dv).

Carbohydrate Servings: 1

Exchanges: 2 vegetable

DAY 6
BREAKFAST
Berry Rich Muffins or Cranberry Pancakes
Skim milk (1 cup)
Melon (1 cup, cubes)
LUNCH
The Taco
Calabacitas
SNACK
Apple (1 cup, quartered)
Fat-free cheese (1 slice)
DINNER

Tofu with Peanut-Ginger Sauce or Tuscan Pork Loin
Brown rice (1/2 cup, cooked)
Spinach Salad with Black Olive Vinaigrette

DAY 6 RECIPES

Berry Rich Muffins

INGREDIENTS
- 1 cup whole-wheat flour
- 1 cup all-purpose flour
- 1 teaspoon baking powder
- 1/2 teaspoon baking soda and 1/4 teaspoon salt
- 1 large egg
- 1 large egg white
- 2/3 cup packed light brown sugar, or 1/3 cup Splenda Sugar Blend for Baking
- 1 cup buttermilk, or equivalent buttermilk powder and water
- 1/4 cup canola oil
- 1 1/2 teaspoons grated lemon or orange zest
- 1 teaspoon vanilla extract
- 1 1/2 cups mixed fresh berries, such as blueberries, raspberries and/or blackberries
- 1/4 cup dried blueberries, or dry cherries and 1 tablespoon sugar

PREPARATION

1. Preheat oven to 400°F. Coat 12 standard 2 1/2-inch muffin cups with cooking spray.
2. Whisk whole-wheat flour, all-purpose flour, baking powder, baking soda and salt in a large bowl.
3. Whisk egg, egg white and brown sugar (or Splenda) in a medium bowl until smooth. Add buttermilk, oil, lemon (or orange) zest and vanilla; whisk until blended.
4. Make a well in the center of the dry ingredients. Add the wet ingredients; stir with a rubber spatula until just combined. Gently stir in mixed berries and dried fruit. Scoop the batter into the prepared pan and sprinkle sugar over the tops.
5. Bake the muffins until the tops spring back when touched lightly, 20 to 25 minutes. Let cool in the pan for 5 minutes. Loosen the edges and turn the muffins out onto a wire rack to cool slightly before serving.

TIPS & NOTES
- **Ingredient note:** You can use buttermilk powder in place of fresh buttermilk. Or make "sour milk": mix 1 tablespoon lemon juice or vinegar to 1 cup milk.

- **Substituting with Splenda:** In the test Kitchen, sucralose is the only alternative sweetener we test with when we feel the option is appropriate. For nonbaking recipes, we use Splenda Granular (boxed, not in a packet). For baking, we use Splenda Sugar Blend for Baking, a mix of sugar and sucralose. It can be substituted in recipes (1/2 cup of the blend for each 1 cup of sugar) to reduce sugar calories by half while maintaining some of the baking properties of sugar. If you make a similar blend with half sugar and half Splenda Granular, substitute this homemade mixture cup for cup.
- When choosing any low- or no-calorie sweetener, be sure to check the label to make sure it is suitable for your intended use.

NUTRITION
Per muffin: 196 calories; 6 g fat (1 g sat, 3 g mono); 18 mg cholesterol; 35 g carbohydrates; 5 g protein; 3 gfiber; 174 mg sodium; 119 mg potassium.
Carbohydrate Servings: 2
Exchanges: 2 starch, 1 fat
Nutrition Note: Per muffin with Splenda: 2 Carbohydrate Servings, 183 calories, 27 g carbohydrate.

Cranberry Pancakes

INGREDIENTS

- 1/2 cup fresh cranberries
- 1/4 cup all-purpose flour
- 2 tablespoons plus 2 teaspoons whole-wheat flour
- 1 tablespoon yellow cornmeal
- 1 tablespoon sugar
- 1/2 teaspoon baking powder
- 1/8 teaspoon salt
- 1/8 teaspoon ground nutmeg, or 1/4 teaspoon vanilla extract
- 6 tablespoons nonfat milk
- 2 tablespoons pasteurized egg substitute, such as Egg Beaters
- 1 1/2 teaspoons walnut or canola oil

PREPARATION

1. Bring 2 inches of water to a boil in a small saucepan. Add cranberries; boil for 2 minutes. Drain and cool for 5 minutes.

2. Meanwhile, whisk all-purpose flour, whole-wheat flour, cornmeal, sugar, baking powder, salt and nutmeg (if using) in a large bowl.

3. Whisk milk, egg substitute, oil and vanilla (if using) in a small bowl until combined.

4. Coarsely chop the cranberries; stir into the milk mixture. Stir the milk mixture into the dry ingredients just until combined.

5. Coat a griddle or large nonstick skillet with cooking spray; heat over medium heat. Using 1/4 cup of batter for each pancake, cook 2 pancakes at a time until bubbles dot the surface, 2 to 3 minutes. Flip and continue cooking until browned, 1 to 2 minutes more. Repeat with the remaining batter.

NUTRITION

Per serving: 189 calories; 4 g fat (0 g sat, 1 g mono); 1 mg cholesterol; 34 g carbohydrates; 6 g protein; 3 g fiber; 336 mg sodium; 185 mg potassium.

Carbohydrate Servings: 2

Exchanges: 2 starch, 1 fat

The Taco

INGREDIENTS

HOMEMADE TACO SHELLS

- 12 6-inch corn tortillas
- Canola oil cooking spray
- 3/4 teaspoon chili powder, divided
- 1/4 teaspoon salt, divided

TACO MEAT

- 8 ounces 93%-lean ground beef
- 8 ounces 99%-lean ground turkey breast

- 1/2 cup chopped onion
- 1 10-ounce can diced tomatoes with green chiles, preferably Rotel brand (see Tip), or 1 1/4 cups petite-diced tomatoes
- 1/2 teaspoon ground cumin
- 1/2 teaspoon ground chipotle chile or 1 teaspoon chili powder
- 1/2 teaspoon dried oregano

TOPPINGS

- 3 cups shredded romaine lettuce
- 3/4 cup shredded reduced-fat Cheddar cheese
- 3/4 cup diced tomatoes
- 3/4 cup prepared salsa
- 1/4 cup diced red onion

PREPARATION

1. To prepare taco shells: Preheat oven to 375°F.
2. Working with 6 tortillas at a time, wrap in a barely damp cloth or paper towel and microwave on High until steamed, about 30 seconds. Lay the tortillas on a clean work surface and coat both sides with cooking spray; sprinkle a little chili powder and salt on one side. Carefully drape each tortilla over two bars of the oven rack. Bake until crispy, 7 to 10 minutes. Repeat with the remaining 6 tortillas.
3. To prepare taco meat: Place beef, turkey and onion in a large nonstick skillet over medium heat. Cook, breaking up the meat with a wooden spoon, until cooked through, about 10 minutes. Transfer to a colander to drain off fat. Wipe out the pan. Return the meat to the pan and add tomatoes, cumin, ground chipotle (or chili powder) and oregano. Cook over medium heat, stirring occasionally, until most of the liquid has evaporated, 3 to 6 minutes.
4. To assemble tacos: Fill each shell with a generous 3 tablespoons taco meat, 1/4 cup lettuce, 1 tablespoon each cheese, tomato and salsa and 1 teaspoon onion.

TIPS & NOTES

- **Make Ahead Tip**: Store taco shells in an airtight container for up to 2 days. Reheat at 375°F for 1 to 2 minutes before serving. Cover and refrigerate taco meat for up to 1 day. Reheat just before serving.

- **Tip:** Look for Rotel brand diced tomatoes with green chiles—original or mild, depending on your spice preference—and set the heat level with either ground chipotle chile (adds smoky heat) or chili powder (adds rich chili taste without extra spice).

NUTRITION

Per serving: 252 calories; 5 g fat (1 g sat, 1 g mono); 38 mg cholesterol; 30 g carbohydrates; 0 g added sugars; 24 g protein; 5 g fiber; 576 mg sodium; 254 mg potassium.

Nutrition Bonus: Vitamin A (49% daily value), Vitamin C & Zinc (17% dv)

Carbohydrate Servings: 2

Exchanges: 1 1/2 starch, 1 vegetable, 3 lean meat

Calabacitas

INGREDIENTS

- 1 tablespoon extra-virgin olive oil
- 1 medium onion, chopped
- 1 poblano or Anaheim chile pepper, seeded and diced
- 2 cups diced zucchini
- 2 cups diced summer squash
- 1/2 teaspoon salt
- 2 tablespoons chopped fresh cilantro, (optional)

PREPARATION

Heat oil in a large nonstick skillet over medium heat. Add onion and chile; cook, stirring, until soft, about 4 minutes. Add zucchini, summer squash and salt; cover and cook, stirring once or twice, until tender, about 3 minutes. Remove from the heat and stir in cilantro (if using).

NUTRITION

Per serving: 40 calories; 2 g fat (0 g sat, 2 g mono); 0 mg cholesterol; 4 g carbohydrates; 0 g added sugars; 1 g protein; 1 g fiber; 199 mg sodium; 201 mg potassium.

Nutrition Bonus: Vitamin C (30% dv).

Exchanges: 1 vegetable, 1/2 fat

Tofu with Peanut-Ginger Sauce

INGREDIENTS

SAUCE

- 5 tablespoons water
- 4 tablespoons smooth natural peanut butter
- 1 tablespoon rice vinegar, (see Ingredient note) or white vinegar
- 2 teaspoons reduced-sodium soy sauce
- 2 teaspoons honey
- 2 teaspoons minced ginger
- 2 cloves garlic, minced

TOFU & VEGETABLES

- 14 ounces extra-firm tofu, preferably water-packed
- 2 teaspoons extra-virgin olive oil
- 4 cups baby spinach, (6 ounces) and 4 scallions, sliced (1 cup)
- 1 1/2 cups sliced mushrooms, (4 ounces)

PREPARATION

1. To prepare sauce: Whisk water, peanut butter, rice vinegar (or white vinegar), soy sauce, honey, ginger and garlic in a small bowl.

2. To prepare tofu: Drain and rinse tofu; pat dry. Slice the block crosswise into eight 1/2-inch-thick slabs. Coarsely crumble each slice into smaller, uneven pieces.

3. Heat oil in a large nonstick skillet over high heat. Add tofu and cook in a single layer, without stirring, until the pieces begin to turn golden brown on the bottom, about 5 minutes. Then gently stir and continue cooking, stirring occasionally, until all sides are golden brown, 5 to 7 minutes more.

4. Add spinach, mushrooms, scallions and the peanut sauce and cook, stirring, until the vegetables are just cooked, 1 to 2 minutes more.

TIPS & NOTES

- **Ingredient Note:** Rice vinegar (or rice-wine vinegar) is mild, slightly sweet vinegar made from fermented rice. Find it in the Asian section of supermarkets and specialty stores.

NUTRITION

Per serving: 221 calories; 14 g fat (2 g sat, 3 g mono); 0 mg cholesterol; 15 g carbohydrates; 3 g added sugars; 12 g protein; 4 g fiber; 231 mg sodium; 262 mg potassium.

Nutrition Bonus: Calcium (16% daily value), Iron (16% dv).

Carbohydrate Servings: 1

Exchanges: 2 vegetable, 2 medium-fat meat

Tuscan Pork Loin

INGREDIENTS

- 1 3-pound pork loin, trimmed
- 1 teaspoon kosher salt
- 3 cloves garlic, crushed and peeled

- 2 tablespoons extra-virgin olive oil
- 2 tablespoons chopped fresh rosemary
- 1 tablespoon freshly grated lemon zest
- 3/4 cup dry vermouth, or white wine
- 2 tablespoons white-wine vinegar

PREPARATION

1. Tie kitchen string around pork in three places so it doesn't flatten while roasting. Place salt and garlic in a small bowl and mash with the back of a spoon to form a paste. Stir in oil, rosemary and lemon zest; rub the mixture into the pork. Refrigerate, uncovered, for 1 hour.
2. Preheat oven to 375°F.
3. Place the pork in a roasting pan. Roast, turning once or twice, until a thermometer inserted into the thickest part registers 145°F, 40 to 50 minutes. Transfer to a cutting board; let rest for 10 minutes.
4. Meanwhile, add vermouth (or wine) and vinegar to the roasting pan and place over medium-high heat. Bring to a simmer and cook, scraping up any browned bits, until the sauce is reduced by half, 2 to 4 minutes. Remove the string and slice the roast. Add any accumulated juices to the sauce and serve with the pork.

TIPS & NOTES

- **Make Ahead Tip**: Equipment: Kitchen string

NUTRITION

Per 3-ounce serving: 221 calories; 11 g fat (3 g sat, 6 g mono); 69 mg cholesterol; 1 g carbohydrates; 0 gadded sugars; 24 g protein; 0 g fiber; 156 mg sodium; 368 mg potassium.

Nutrition Bonus: Thiamin (58% daily value), Selenium (50% dv).

Exchanges: 3.5 lean meat

Spinach Salad with Black Olive Vinaigrette

INGREDIENTS

- 3 tablespoons extra-virgin olive oil
- 1 1/2 tablespoons red-wine vinegar, or lemon juice
- 6 pitted Kalamata olives, finely chopped
- 1/4 teaspoon salt
- Freshly ground pepper, to taste
- 6 cups torn spinach leaves
- 1/2 cucumber, seeded and sliced
- 1/2 red onion, thinly sliced

PREPARATION

Whisk oil, vinegar (or lemon juice) and olives in a salad bowl. Season with salt and pepper. Add spinach, cucumbers and onions; toss well. Serve immediately.

NUTRITION

Per serving: 128 calories; 12 g fat (2 g sat, 9 g mono); 0 mg cholesterol; 3 g carbohydrates; 2 g protein; 1 g fiber; 271 mg sodium; 284 mg potassium.

Nutrition Bonus: Vitamin A (80% daily value), Folate (22% dv), Vitamin C (20% dv).

Exchanges: 1 vegetable, 2 fat

DAY 7
BREAKFAST
Crustless Crab Quiche
Strawberries (1 cup)
Whole-wheat toast (1 slice)
LUNCH
Curried Corn Bisqueor Herbed Zucchini Soup
Asian Slaw with Tofu & Shiitake Mushrooms or Wasabi Salmon Burgers
Skim milk (1 cup)

SNACK

Celery sticks (1 cup)
Fat-free cheese (1 slice)

DINNER

Scallion & Ginger Spiced Chicken or Mint-Pesto Rubbed Leg of Lamb
Whole-wheat couscous (1/2 cup, cooked)
Steamed cauliflower (1/2 cup)
Skim Milk (1 cup)
Apricot (1/2 cup)

DAY 7 RECIPES

Crustless Crab Quiche

INGREDIENTS

- 2 teaspoons extra-virgin olive oil, divided
- 1 onion, chopped
- 1 red bell pepper, chopped
- 12 ounces mushrooms, wiped clean and sliced (about 4 1/2 cups)
- 2 large eggs and 2 large egg whites
- 1 1/2 cups low-fat cottage cheese
- 1/2 cup low-fat plain yogurt
- 1/4 cup all-purpose flour
- 1/4 cup freshly grated Parmesan cheese
- 1/4 teaspoon cayenne pepper
- 1/4 teaspoon salt
- 1/4 teaspoon freshly ground pepper
- 8 ounces cooked lump crabmeat, (fresh or frozen and thawed), drained and picked over (about 1 cup)
- 1/2 cup grated sharp Cheddar cheese, (2 ounces)
- 1/4 cup chopped scallions

PREPARATION

1. Preheat oven to 350°F. Coat a 10-inch pie pan or ceramic quiche dish with cooking spray. Heat 1 teaspoon oil in large nonstick skillet over medium-high heat. Add onion and bell pepper; cook, stirring, until softened, about 5 minutes; transfer to a large bowl. Add the remaining 1 teaspoon oil to the skillet and heat over high heat. Add mushrooms and cook, stirring, until they have softened and most of their liquid has evaporated, 5 to 7 minutes. Add to the bowl with the onion mixture.

2. Place eggs, egg whites, cottage cheese, yogurt, flour, Parmesan, cayenne, salt and pepper in a food processor or blender; blend until smooth. Add to the vegetable mixture, along with crab, Cheddar and scallions; mix with a rubber spatula. Pour into the prepared baking dish.

3. Bake the quiche until a knife inserted in the center comes out clean, 40 to 50 minutes. Let stand for 5 minutes before serving.

NUTRITION

Per serving: 225 calories; 10 g fat (4 g sat, 3 g mono); 122 mg cholesterol; 14 g carbohydrates; 27 g protein; 2 g fiber; 661 mg sodium; 355 mg potassium.

Nutrition Bonus: Vitamin C (70% daily value), Calcium (25% dv), Vitamin A (20% dv).

Carbohydrate Servings: 1

Exchanges: 2 1/2 vegetable, 1 1/2 very lean meat, 1 high-fat meat

Curried Corn Bisque

INGREDIENTS

- 2 teaspoons canola oil
- 1 cup fresh or frozen chopped onions
- 1 tablespoon curry powder
- 1/2 teaspoon hot sauce, or to taste
- 1/4 teaspoon salt, or to taste
- 1/4 teaspoon freshly ground pepper
- 2 16-ounce packages frozen corn, or 3 10-ounce boxes

- 2 cups reduced-sodium chicken broth
- 2 cups water
- 1 cup "lite" coconut milk, (see Ingredient note)

PREPARATION

1. Heat oil in a large saucepan over medium-high heat. Add onions and cook, stirring occasionally, until soft, about 3 minutes. Add curry powder, hot sauce, salt and pepper and stir to coat the onions. Stir in corn, broth and water; increase the heat to high and bring the mixture to a boil. Remove from the heat and puree in a blender or food processor (in batches, if necessary) into a homogeneous mixture that still has some texture. Pour the soup into a clean pot, add coconut milk and heat through. Serve hot or cold. Make Curried Sweet Pea Bisque by substituting frozen peas for the corn.

TIPS & NOTES

- **Make Ahead Tip**: Cover and refrigerate for up to 2 days or freeze for up to 2 months.
- **Ingredient Note:** Look for reduced-fat coconut milk (labeled "lite") in the Asian section of your market.

NUTRITION

Per serving: 138 calories; 4 g fat (2 g sat, 1 g mono); 1 mg cholesterol; 24 g carbohydrates; 0 g added sugars; 5 g protein; 3 g fiber; 121 mg sodium; 291 mg potassium.

Nutrition Bonus: Fiber (13% daily value).

Carbohydrate Servings: 1 1/2

Exchanges: 1 1/2 starch, 1 fat

Herbed Zucchini Soup

INGREDIENTS

- 3 cups reduced-sodium chicken broth
- 1 1/2 pounds zucchini, (about 3 medium), cut into 1-inch pieces
- 1 tablespoon chopped fresh tarragon, or dill or 1 teaspoon dried
- 3/4 cup shredded reduced-fat Cheddar cheese, (3 ounces)
- 1/4 teaspoon salt
- 1/4 teaspoon freshly ground pepper

PREPARATION

1. Place broth, zucchini and tarragon (or dill) in a medium saucepan; bring to a boil over high heat. Reduce to a simmer and cook, uncovered, until the zucchini is tender, 7 to 10 minutes. Puree in a blender (see Tip), in batches if necessary, until smooth. Return the soup to the pan and heat over medium-high, slowly stirring in cheese until it is incorporated. Remove from heat and season with salt and pepper. Serve hot or chilled.

TIPS & NOTES

- **Make Ahead Tip**: Cover and refrigerate for up to 3 days. Serve chilled or reheat.
- Hot liquids can splatter out of a blender when it's turned on. To avoid this, remove the center piece of the lid. Loosely cover the hole with a folded kitchen towel and turn the blender on. Better airflow will keep the contents from spewing all over the kitchen.

NUTRITION

Per serving: 115 calories; 5 g fat (3 g sat, 0 g mono); 19 mg cholesterol; 7 g carbohydrates; 0 g added sugars; 10 g protein; 2 g fiber; 448 mg sodium; 452 mg potassium.

Carbohydrate Servings: 1/2

Exchanges: 1 1/2 vegetable, 1 medium-fat meat

Asian Slaw with Tofu & Shiitake Mushrooms

INGREDIENTS

- 1/4 cup reduced-sodium soy sauce
- 2 1/2 tablespoons lemon juice
- 1 teaspoon wasabi powder, (see Note)
- 1 clove garlic, minced
- 12 ounces firm silken tofu, drained and cut into 1/2-inch cubes
- 4 cups lightly packed shredded napa cabbage, (see Ingredient note)
- 2 cups lightly packed shredded bok choy, (see Ingredient note)
- 2 tablespoons canola oil
- 2 cups sliced shiitake mushroom caps
- 2 teaspoons sesame oil

PREPARATION

1. Whisk soy sauce, lemon juice, wasabi powder and garlic in a medium bowl. Gently stir in tofu. Cover and marinate in the refrigerator for 15 minutes, stirring occasionally.
2. Place cabbage and bok choy in a large serving bowl.
3. Drain the tofu, reserving the marinade. Heat canola oil in a large skillet or wok over medium-high heat. Add mushrooms and sesame oil; cook, stirring often, for 2 minutes. Add the tofu; cook, stirring often, until the tofu is lightly browned, about 4 minutes.
4. Spoon the tofu mixture over cabbage. Add the reserved marinade to the pan and bring to a boil, stirring. Pour the hot marinade over the salad and toss gently to coat. Serve immediately.

TIPS & NOTES

- **Note:** Wasabi, a fiery condiment similar to horseradish, is made from the root of an Asian plant. It is available, as both a paste and a powder, in specialty stores and Asian markets.

- **Ingredient Notes:** Look for heads of napa that are tight, without any browned leaves.

- The best bok choy has large dark green leaves and small white stem. More leaf and less stem makes for a less bitter taste.

NUTRITION

Per serving: 178 calories; 12 g fat (1 g sat, 6 g mono); 0 mg cholesterol; 11 g carbohydrates; 0 g added sugars; 9 g protein; 2 g fiber; 598 mg sodium; 330 mg potassium.

Nutrition Bonus: Vitamin C (63% daily value), Selenium (27% dv).

Carbohydrate Servings: 1/2

Exchanges: 2 vegetable, 1 medium-fat meat, 2 fat (mono)

Wasabi Salmon Burgers

INGREDIENTS

- 2 tablespoons reduced-sodium soy sauce
- 1 1/2 teaspoons wasabi powder, (see Note)
- 1/2 teaspoon honey
- 1 pound salmon fillet, skinned (see Tip)
- 2 scallions, finely chopped
- 1 egg, lightly beaten
- 2 tablespoons minced peeled fresh ginger
- 1 teaspoon toasted sesame oil

PREPARATION

1. Whisk soy sauce, wasabi powder and honey in a small bowl until smooth. Set aside.

2. With a large chef's knife, chop salmon using quick, even, straight-up-and-down motions (do not rock the knife through the fish or it will turn mushy). Continue chopping, rotating the knife, until you have a mass of roughly 1/4-inch pieces. Transfer to a large bowl. Add scallions, egg, ginger and oil; stir to combine. Form the mixture into 4 patties. The mixture will be moist and loose, but holds together nicely once the first side is cooked.

3. Coat a large nonstick skillet with cooking spray and heat over medium heat for 1 minute. Add the patties and cook for 4 minutes. Turn and continue to cook until firm and fragrant, about 3 minutes. Spoon the reserved wasabi glaze evenly over the burgers and cook for 15 seconds more. Serve immediately.

TIPS & NOTES

- **Ingredient Note:** Wasabi powder, when mixed with water, becomes the green paste most of us know from sushi restaurants. The powder is available in jars in the Asian aisle of most supermarkets or in almost all Asian markets. Store at room temperature for up to 1 year.

- **Tip:** To skin a salmon fillet: Place it on a clean cutting board, skin side down. Starting at the tail end, slip the blade of a long, sharp knife between the fish flesh and the skin, holding the skin down firmly with your other hand. Gently push the blade along at a 30 degree angle, separating the fillet from the skin without cutting through either. Or have your fishmonger do it for you.

NUTRITION

Per serving: 174 calories; 7 g fat (2 g sat, 2 g mono); 100 mg cholesterol; 3 g carbohydrates; 1 g added sugars; 25 g protein; 0 g fiber; 342 mg sodium; 484 mg potassium.

Nutrition Bonus: Selenium (84% daily value), omega-3s.

Exchanges: 4 lean meat

Scallion & Ginger Spiced Chicken

INGREDIENTS

- 4 boneless, skinless chicken breasts, (1-1 1/4 pounds total), trimmed
- Salt & freshly ground pepper
- 1 tablespoon extra-virgin olive oil, divided
- 1/4 cup minced scallion whites plus 1/2 cup sliced scallion greens, divided
- 3 cloves garlic, minced
- 1 tablespoon minced fresh ginger
- 3/4 cup reduced-sodium chicken broth
- 1/3 cup red-wine vinegar
- 2 tablespoons hoisin sauce
- 2 teaspoons sugar
- Reduced-sodium soy sauce, to taste

PREPARATION

1. Season chicken on both sides with salt and pepper. Heat 1 1/2 teaspoons oil in a large heavy skillet over medium-high heat. Add the chicken and sear until well browned, about 3 minutes per side. Transfer the chicken to a plate and tent with foil.

2. Reduce heat to medium and add the remaining 1 1/2 teaspoons oil to the pan. Add scallion whites, garlic and ginger. Cook, stirring, for 1 minute. Add broth, vinegar, hoisin sauce and sugar. Bring to a simmer. Cook until slightly thickened, about 3 minutes.

3. Return the chicken and any accumulated juices to the pan; reduce heat to low. Simmer until the chicken is cooked through, about 4 minutes. Transfer the chicken to a warmed platter. Season sauce with soy sauce to taste and spoon over the chicken. Garnish with scallion greens.

NUTRITION

Per serving: 192 calories; 5 g fat (1 g sat, 2 g mono); 64 mg cholesterol; 12 g carbohydrates; 4 g added sugars; 24 g protein; 1 g fiber; 526 mg sodium; 277 mg potassium.

Nutrition Bonus: Selenium (31% daily value).

Carbohydrate Servings: 1

Exchanges: 3 lean meat

Mint-Pesto Rubbed Leg of Lamb

INGREDIENTS

- 1/2 cup packed fresh basil leaves
- 1/4 cup packed fresh mint leaves
- 1/4 cup packed fresh parsley leaves
- 2 tablespoons toasted pine nuts, (see Tip)
- 2 tablespoons grated Parmigiano-Reggiano cheese
- 2 tablespoons extra-virgin olive oil
- 1 clove garlic, peeled and 1 teaspoon salt, divided
- 1/2 teaspoon freshly ground pepper
- 1 3 1/2-pound boneless leg of lamb, butterflied (see Tip) and trimmed

PREPARATION

1. Preheat oven to 350°F.
2. Place basil, mint, parsley, pine nuts, cheese, oil, garlic, 1/2 teaspoon salt and pepper in a food processor and process until fairly smooth. Sprinkle lamb all over with the remaining 1/2 teaspoon salt. Reserve 2 tablespoons of the pesto; spread the rest over the top side of the lamb and roll it closed. (It will not be a perfect cylinder.) Tie kitchen string around the roast in five places; do not tie too tightly or the pesto will squeeze out. Rub the reserved pesto over the outside of the lamb and place in a roasting pan.
3. Roast the lamb until a thermometer inserted into the thickest part registers 140°F for medium-rare, about 1 hour 20 minutes. Transfer to a cutting board; let rest for 10 minutes. Carve the lamb, leaving the string in place to help hold the roast together.

TIPS & NOTES

- **Make Ahead Tip**: Equipment: Kitchen string
- **Tips:** To toast pine nuts, cook in a small dry skillet over medium-low heat, stirring constantly, until fragrant and lightly browned, 2 to 5 minutes.
- Have your butcher "butterfly" a boneless leg of lamb (that is, open it up to a large, flat cut of meat); ask that any visible fat be trimmed off.

NUTRITION

Per 3-ounce serving: 192 calories; 10 g fat (3 g sat, 5 g mono); 76 mg cholesterol; 1 g carbohydrates; 0 gadded sugars; 25 g protein; 0 g fiber; 228 mg sodium; 313 mg potassium.

Nutrition Bonus: Selenium (37% daily value), Zinc (29% dv).

Exchanges: 3 lean meat

DAY 8

BREAKFAST

Overnight Oatmeal
Apricot (1 cup, halves)
Skim milk (1 cup)

LUNCH

Chicken, Escarole & Rice Soup
The Diet House Salad or Baby Spinach Salad with Raspberry Vinaigrette
Wasa crispbread (1 cracker)
Melon (1 cup, cubes)

SNACK

Skim milk (1 cup)

DINNER

Southwestern Steak & Peppers
Oven Sweet Potato Fries
Steamed aparagus (1/2 cup)
Pineapple with Mango Coulis or Peach-Lime Sorbet

DAY 8 RECIPES

Overnight Oatmeal

INGREDIENTS

- 8 cups water
- 2 cups steel-cut oats, (see Ingredient note)
- 1/3 cup dried cranberries
- 1/3 cup dried apricots, chopped
- 1/4 teaspoon salt, or to taste

PREPARATION

1. Combine water, oats, dried cranberries, dried apricots and salt in a 5- or 6-quart slow cooker. Turn heat to low. Put the lid on and cook until the oats are tender and the porridge is creamy, 7 to 8 hours. Stovetop Variation Halve the above recipe to accommodate the size of most double boilers: Combine 4 cups water, 1 cup steel-cut oats, 3 tablespoons dried cranberries, 3 tablespoons dried apricots and 1/8 teaspoon salt in the top of a double boiler. Cover and cook over boiling water for about 1 1/2 hours, checking the water level in the bottom of the double boiler from time to time.

TIPS & NOTES

- **Ingredient Note:** Steel-cut oats, sometimes labeled "Irish oatmeal," look like small pebbles. They are toasted oat groats for which the oat kernel that has been removed from the husk that have been cut in 2 or 3 pieces. Do not substitute regular rolled oats, which have a shorter cooking time, in the slow-cooker oatmeal recipe.
- For easy cleanup, try a slow-cooker liner. These heat-resistant, disposable liners fit neatly inside the insert and help prevent food from sticking to the bottom and sides of your slow cooker.

NUTRITION

Per serving: 193 calories; 3 g fat (0 g sat, 1 g mono); 0 mg cholesterol; 34 g carbohydrates; 0 g added sugars; 6 g protein; 9 g fiber; 77 mg sodium; 195 mg potassium.

Nutrition Bonus: Fiber (36% daily value).

Carbohydrate Servings: 2

Exchanges: 2 starch, 1/2 fruit

Chicken, Escarole & Rice Soup

INGREDIENTS

- 1 tablespoon extra-virgin olive oil
- 1 large onion, chopped
- 2 cloves garlic, minced
- 1 head escarole, trimmed and thinly sliced
- 3 14-ounce cans reduced-sodium chicken broth
- 1 14-ounce can diced tomatoes
- 1/2 cup long-grain white rice
- 1 pound boneless, skinless chicken breasts, trimmed and cut into 1/2-inch pieces
- Freshly ground pepper, to taste
- 6 tablespoons freshly grated Romano or Parmesan cheese

PREPARATION

1. Heat oil in a large pot over medium high heat. Add onion and garlic; cook, stirring frequently, until they soften and begin to brown, 5 to 7 minutes. Add escarole and cook, stirring occasionally, until wilted, 2 to 3 minutes. Add broth, tomatoes and rice; bring to a boil. Reduce heat to low, cover and simmer until the rice is almost tender, 12 to 15 minutes.

2. Add chicken and simmer until it is no longer pink in the center and the rice is tender, about 5 minutes. Season with pepper. Serve hot, sprinkled with Romano (or Parmesan).

TIPS & NOTES

- **Make Ahead Tip**: Cover and refrigerate for up to 2 days or freeze for up to 2 months.

NUTRITION

Per serving: 157 calories; 4 g fat (1 g sat, 2 g mono); 30 mg cholesterol; 15 g carbohydrates; 16 g protein; 2 g fiber; 166 mg sodium; 337 mg potassium.

Nutrition Bonus: Folate (21% daily value), Vitamin A (20% dv).

Carbohydrate Servings: 1

Exchanges: 1 starch, 1 1/2 lean meat

The Diet House Salad

INGREDIENTS

- 4 cups torn green leaf lettuce
- 1 cup sprouts
- 1 cup tomato wedges
- 1 cup peeled, sliced cucumber
- 1 cup shredded carrots
- 1/2 cup chopped radishes
- 1/2 cup Sesame Tamari Vinaigrette, or other dressing

PREPARATION

Toss lettuce, sprouts, tomato, cucumber, carrots and radishes in a large bowl with the dressing until the vegetables are coated.

NUTRITION

Per serving: 71 calories; 3 g fat (0 g sat, 1 g mono); 0 mg cholesterol; 11 g carbohydrates; 2 g protein; 3 g fiber; 334 mg sodium; 428 mg potassium.

Nutrition Bonus: Vitamin A (140% daily value), Vitamin C (30% dv), Folate (16% dv).

Carbohydrate Servings: 1

Exchanges: 2 vegetable, 1/2 fat

Baby Spinach Salad with Raspberry Vinaigrette

INGREDIENTS

VINAIGRETTE

- 1/3 cup canola oil
- 1/4 cup raspberry vinegar or red-wine vinegar
- 3 tablespoons orange juice
- 1/4 teaspoon salt
- Freshly ground pepper to taste

SALAD

- 6 cups prewashed baby spinach
- 1 small red bell pepper, thinly sliced
- 1 ripe, but firm, nectarine, cut into 1-inch chunks
- 3 tablespoons Raspberry Vinaigrette

PREPARATION

1. To prepare vinaigrette: Add oil, vinegar, orange juice, salt and pepper to a jar with a tight-fitting lid; shake well to combine.
2. To prepare salad: Combine spinach, bell pepper and nectarine in a large bowl; toss with 3 tablespoons of the vinaigrette.

TIPS & NOTES

- **Make Ahead Tip**: Cover and refrigerate the leftover dressing for up to 1 week.

NUTRITION

Per serving: 72 calories; 5 g fat (0 g sat, 3 g mono); 0 mg cholesterol; 6 g carbohydrates; 0 g added sugars;2 g protein; 2 g fiber; 74 mg sodium; 350 mg potassium.

Nutrition Bonus: Vitamin A (98% daily value), Vitamin C (65% dv), Folate (25% dv).

Carbohydrate Servings: 1/2

Exchanges: 1 vegetable, 1 fat

Southwestern Steak & Peppers

INGREDIENTS

- 1/2 teaspoon ground cumin
- 1/2 teaspoon ground coriander
- 1/2 teaspoon chili powder
- 1/4 teaspoon salt, or to taste
- 3/4 teaspoon coarsely ground pepper, plus more to taste
- 1 pound boneless top sirloin steak, trimmed of fat
- 3 cloves garlic, peeled, 1 halved and 2 minced
- 3 teaspoons canola oil, or extra-virgin olive oil, divided
- 2 red bell peppers, thinly sliced
- 1 medium white onion, halved lengthwise and thinly sliced
- 1 teaspoon brown sugar
- 1/2 cup brewed coffee, or prepared instant coffee
- 1/4 cup balsamic vinegar
- 4 cups watercress sprigs

PREPARATION

1. Mix cumin, coriander, chili powder, salt and 3/4 teaspoon pepper in a small bowl. Rub steak with the cut garlic. Rub the spice mix all over the steak.

2. Heat 2 teaspoons oil in a large heavy skillet, preferably cast iron, over medium-high heat. Add the steak and cook to desired doneness, 4 to 6 minutes per side for medium-rare. Transfer to a cutting board and let rest.

3. Add remaining 1 teaspoon oil to the skillet. Add bell peppers and onion; cook, stirring often, until softened, about 4 minutes. Add minced garlic and brown sugar; cook, stirring often, for 1 minute. Add coffee, vinegar and any accumulated meat juices; cook for 3 minutes to intensify flavor. Season with pepper.

4. To serve, mound 1 cup watercress on each plate. Top with the sauteed peppers and onion. Slice the steak thinly across the grain and arrange on the vegetables. Pour the sauce from the pan over the steak. Serve immediately.

NUTRITION

Per serving: 226 calories; 12 g fat (3 g sat, 5 g mono); 60 mg cholesterol; 12 g carbohydrates; 1 g added sugars; 26 g protein; 3 g fiber; 216 mg sodium; 606 mg potassium.

Nutrition Bonus: Vitamin C (210% daily value), Vitamin A (60% dv), Iron (25% dv).

Carbohydrate Servings: 1

Exchanges: 2 vegetable, 3 lean meat

Oven Sweet Potato Fries

INGREDIENTS

1 large sweet potato, peeled and cut into wedges

2 teaspoons canola oil

1/4 teaspoon salt

Pinch of cayenne pepper

PREPARATION

1. Preheat oven to 450°F. Toss sweet potato wedges with oil, salt and pepper. Spread the wedges out on a rimmed baking sheet. Bake until browned and tender, turning once, about 20 minutes total.

NUTRITION

Per serving: 122 calories; 5 g fat (0 g sat, 3 g mono); 0 mg cholesterol; 19 g carbohydrates; 0 g added sugars; 2 g protein; 3 g fiber; 323 mg sodium; 429 mg potassium.

Carbohydrate Servings: 1

Exchanges: 1 starch, 1 fat

Pineapple with Mango Coulis

INGREDIENTS

- 1 small mango, diced
- 1.5 tablespoons dark rum
- 1 1/2 tablespoons lime juice
- 1 teaspoon lime zest
- Sugar, to taste
- Fresh pineapple spears, or chunks

PREPARATION

Puree the mango with the rum, lime juice and lime zest in a food processor or blender. Add sugar to taste. Serve over pineapple

NUTRITION

Per serving: 103 calories; 0 g fat (0 g sat, 0 g mono); 0 mg cholesterol; 24 g carbohydrates; 1 g protein; 3 g fiber; 2 mg sodium; 221 mg potassium.

Nutrition Bonus: Vitamin C (97% daily value).

Carbohydrate Servings: 1 1/2

Exchanges: 1 fruit

Peach-Lime Sorbet

INGREDIENTS

- 1 1/2 cups water
- 2/3 cup sugar
- 2 tablespoons light corn syrup
- 1 pound fresh peaches or nectarines, halved and pitted
- 1 teaspoon freshly grated lime zest
- 6 tablespoons lime juice
- 1/4 teaspoon salt

PREPARATION

1. Stir water, sugar and corn syrup in a large saucepan over medium heat until the sugar dissolves. Add peaches (or nectarines); bring to a simmer. Reduce heat, cover and simmer for 10 minutes.

2. Pour the fruit-syrup mixture into a blender. Add lime zest, juice and salt; blend until smooth. Pour into a large bowl and refrigerate until cold, 4 hours or overnight.

3. Freeze the sorbet mixture in an ice cream maker, according to the manufacturer's directions. (Alternatively, pour the mixture into ice cube trays and freeze until solid, about 4 hours. Unmold cubes, place half in a food processor fitted with the chopping blade, and process, scraping the sides as necessary, until fairly smooth but still icy. Repeat with the remaining cubes.)

TIPS & NOTES

- **Make Ahead Tip**: Freeze in a resealable plastic container for up to 1 week.

NUTRITION

Per serving: 109 calories; 0 g fat (0 g sat, 0 g mono); 0 mg cholesterol; 29 g carbohydrates; 0 g protein; 1 gfiber; 77 mg sodium; 115 mg potassium.

Carbohydrate Servings: 2

Exchanges: 2 other carbohydrates

DAY 9
BREAKFAST
Nonfat plain yogurt (8 oz.)
Whole-wheat toast (1 slice)
Pear Butter
LUNCH
Greek Lemon Rice Soupor Asparagus Soup
Tuna & White Bean Salad
Skim milk (1 cup)
Whole-wheat pita bread (1/2 medium pita)
SNACK
Blueberries (1 cup)
DINNER
Korean-Style Steak & Lettuce Wraps or Garlic-Roasted Pork (Pernil)
Shredded carrots (1 cup)
Cucumber Salad
Raspberries (1 cup)

DAY 9 RECIPES

Pear Butter

INGREDIENTS

- 4 ripe but firm Bartlett pears, (1-1 1/4 pounds), peeled, cored and cut into 1-inch chunks

- 3/4 cup pear nectar

PREPARATION

1. Place pears and pear nectar in a heavy medium saucepan; bring to a simmer. Cover and simmer over medium-low heat, stirring occasionally, until the pears are very tender, 30 to 35 minutes. Cooking time will vary depending on the ripeness of the pears.

2. Mash the pears with a potato masher. Cook, uncovered, over medium-low heat, stirring often, until the puree has cooked down to a thick mass (somewhat thicker than applesauce), 20 to 30 minutes. Stir almost constantly toward the end of cooking. Scrape the pear butter into a bowl or storage container and let cool.

TIPS & NOTES

- **Make Ahead Tip**: Store in an airtight container in the refrigerator for up to 2 weeks or freeze for up to 6 months.

NUTRITION

Per tablespoon: 22 calories; 0 g fat (0 g sat, 0 g mono); 0 mg cholesterol; 6 g carbohydrates; 0 g protein; 1 g fiber; 1 mg sodium; 33 mg potassium.

Carbohydrate Servings: 1/2

Exchanges: 1/2 fruit

Greek Lemon Rice Soup

INGREDIENTS

- 4 cups reduced-sodium chicken broth
- 1/3 cup white rice
- 1 12-ounce package silken tofu, (about 1 1/2 cups)
- 1 tablespoon extra-virgin olive oil
- 1/4 teaspoon turmeric and 1/4 cup lemon juice
- 2 tablespoons chopped fresh dill
- 1/4 teaspoon freshly ground pepper

PREPARATION

1. Bring broth and rice to a boil in a large saucepan. Reduce heat to a simmer and cook until the rice is very tender, about 15 minutes.

2. Carefully transfer 2 cups of the rice mixture to a blender. Add tofu, oil and turmeric; process until smooth. (Use caution when pureeing hot liquids.) Whisk the tofu mixture, lemon juice, dill and pepper into the soup remaining in the pan. Heat through.

TIPS & NOTES

- **Make Ahead Tip**: Cover and refrigerate for up to 2 days.

NUTRITION

Per serving: 163 calories; 6 g fat (1 g sat, 3 g mono); 0 mg cholesterol; 19 g carbohydrates; 9 g protein; 0 gfiber; 559 mg sodium; 395 mg potassium.

Carbohydrate Servings: 1

Exchanges: 1 starch, 1 medium-fat meat, 1/2 fat (mono)

Asparagus Soup

INGREDIENTS

- 1 14-ounce can reduced-sodium chicken broth
- 1/4 cup water
- 1 yellow-fleshed potato, such as Yukon Gold (6 ounces), peeled and cut into 1/2-inch cubes
- 1 medium shallot, thinly sliced
- 1 clove garlic, thinly sliced
- 1/2 teaspoon dried thyme
- 1/2 teaspoon dried savory, or marjoram leaves
- 1/8 teaspoon salt
- 12 ounces asparagus, woody ends removed, sliced into 1-inch pieces

- 1 1/2 ounces thinly sliced prosciutto, chopped
- Freshly ground pepper, to taste

PREPARATION

1. Place broth, water, potato, shallot, garlic, thyme, savory (or marjoram) and salt in a large saucepan. Bring to a boil over high heat. Reduce heat to medium-low, cover, and simmer until the potato is tender, about 8 minutes. Add asparagus, return to a simmer, and cook, covered, until the asparagus is tender, about 5 minutes more.
2. Meanwhile, cook prosciutto in a small skillet over medium heat, stirring, until crisp, about 5 minutes.
3. Pour the soup into a large blender or food processor (see Tip); puree until smooth, scraping down the sides if necessary. Season with pepper. Serve topped with the crisped prosciutto.

TIPS & NOTES

- **Make Ahead Tip**: Prepare the soup (Steps 1 & 3), cover and refrigerate for up to 2 days. Top with prosciutto just before serving.
- Hot liquids can splatter out of a blender when it's turned on. To avoid this, remove the center piece of the lid. Loosely cover the hole with a folded kitchen towel and turn the blender on. Better airflow will keep the contents from spewing all over the kitchen.

NUTRITION

Per serving: 174 calories; 3 g fat (1 g sat, 0 g mono); 20 mg cholesterol; 25 g carbohydrates; 15 g protein; 5 g fiber; 818 mg sodium; 378 mg potassium.

Nutrition Bonus: Vitamin C (50% daily value), Iron (30% dv), Vitamin A (25% dv), Folate (22% dv).

Carbohydrate Servings: 1

Exchanges: 1 starch, 1 vegetable, 1 lean meat

Tuna & White Bean Salad

INGREDIENTS

- 3 tablespoons lemon juice
- 2 tablespoons extra-virgin olive oil
- 1 clove garlic, minced
- 1/8 teaspoon salt
- Freshly ground pepper, to taste
- 1 19-ounce can cannellini (white kidney) beans, rinsed
- 1 6-ounce can chunk light tuna in water, drained and flaked (see Note)
- 1/4 cup chopped red onion
- 3 tablespoons chopped fresh parsley
- 3 tablespoons chopped fresh basil

PREPARATION

1. Whisk lemon juice, oil, garlic, salt and pepper in a medium bowl. Add beans, tuna, onion, parsley and basil; toss to coat well.

TIPS & NOTES

- **Make Ahead Tip**: Cover and refrigerate for up to 2 days.
- **Note:** Chunk light tuna, which comes from the smaller skipjack or yellowfin, has less mercury than canned white albacore tuna. The FDA/EPA advises that women who are or might become pregnant, nursing mothers and young children consume no more than 6 ounces of albacore a week; up to 12 ounces of canned light tuna is considered safe.

NUTRITION

Per serving: 226 calories; 8 g fat (1 g sat, 5 g mono); 13 mg cholesterol; 21 g carbohydrates; 0 g added sugars; 16 g protein; 6 g fiber; 498 mg sodium; 157 mg potassium.

Nutrition Bonus: Fiber (24% daily value), Iron (16% dv), Vitamin C (15% dv).

Carbohydrate Servings: 1

Exchanges: 1 starch, 2 very lean meat, 1 fat (mono)

Korean-Style Steak & Lettuce Wraps

INGREDIENTS

- 1 pound flank steak
- 1/4 teaspoon salt
- 1/4 teaspoon freshly ground pepper
- 1 cup diced peeled cucumber
- 6 cherry tomatoes, halved
- 1/4 cup thinly sliced shallot
- 1 tablespoon finely chopped fresh mint
- 1 tablespoon finely chopped fresh basil
- 1 tablespoon finely chopped fresh cilantro
- 1 tablespoon brown sugar
- 2 tablespoons reduced-sodium soy sauce
- 2 tablespoons lime juice
- 1/2 teaspoon crushed red pepper
- 1 head Bibb lettuce, leaves separated

PREPARATION

1. Preheat grill to medium-high.
2. Sprinkle steak with salt and pepper. Oil the grill rack (see Tip). Grill the steak for 6 to 8 minutes per side for medium. Transfer to a cutting board and let rest for 5 minutes. Cut across the grain into thin slices.
3. Combine the sliced steak, cucumber, tomatoes, shallot, mint, basil and cilantro in a large bowl. Mix sugar, soy sauce, lime juice and

4. crushed red pepper in a small bowl. Drizzle over the steak mixture; toss well to coat. To serve, spoon a portion of the steak mixture into a lettuce leaf and roll into a "wrap."

TIPS & NOTES

- **Make Ahead Tip**: The steak mixture will keep, covered, in the refrigerator for up to 1 day.
- **To oil a grill rack:** Oil a folded paper towel, hold it with tongs and rub it over the rack. Do not use cooking spray on a hot grill.

NUTRITION

Per serving: 199 calories; 7 g fat (3 g sat, 3 g mono); 45 mg cholesterol; 9 g carbohydrates; 3 g added sugars; 24 g protein; 1 g fiber; 465 mg sodium; 542 mg potassium.

Nutrition Bonus: Vitamin A (35% daily value), Vitamin C (20% dv), Iron (15% dv).

Carbohydrate Servings: 1/2

Exchanges: 1 1/2 vegetable, 3 lean meat

Garlic-Roasted Pork (Pernil)

INGREDIENTS

- 6 cloves garlic, crushed and peeled
- 2 tablespoons extra-virgin olive oil
- 1 tablespoon dried oregano
- 1 teaspoon paprika
- 1 teaspoon salt
- 1/2 teaspoon freshly ground pepper
- 1 2-pound boneless pork loin, trimmed

PREPARATION

1. Combine garlic, oil, oregano, paprika, salt and pepper in a food processor or blender and puree. Rub pork all over with the seasoning mix and wrap tightly with plastic wrap or place in a large sealable plastic bag. Let marinate in the refrigerator for at least 20 minutes or up to 1 day.

2. Preheat oven to 350°F.

3. Remove the pork from the plastic and place in a shallow roasting pan. Roast, uncovered, until an instant-read thermometer inserted into the center registers 145°F, 50 minutes to 1 hour. Let rest for 10 minutes, then slice and serve.

TIPS & NOTES

- **Make Ahead Tip**: Prepare through Step 1 up to 1 day ahead.

NUTRITION

Per serving: 203 calories; 11 g fat (3 g sat, 6 g mono); 64 mg cholesterol; 1 g carbohydrates; 0 g added sugars; 23 g protein; 0 g fiber; 337 mg sodium; 361 mg potassium.

Nutrition Bonus: Selenium (40% daily value).

Exchanges: 3 lean meat, 1 fat

Cucumber Salad

INGREDIENTS

- 2 cucumbers, peeled, seeded and cut crosswise into 1/4-inch slices
- 1 tablespoon rice-wine vinegar, or distilled white vinegar
- 1/4 teaspoon sugar
- Cayenne pepper, to taste
- Salt & freshly ground pepper, to taste

PREPARATION

Whisk together vinegar, sugar and a pinch of cayenne pepper. Season with salt and pepper. Add cucumbers and toss to coat. Chill until ready to serve.

NUTRITION

Per serving: 24 calories; 0 g fat (0 g sat, 0 g mono); 0 mg cholesterol; 6 g carbohydrates; 0 g added sugars; 1 g protein; 1 g fiber; 145 mg sodium; 222 mg potassium.

Carbohydrate Servings: 1/2

Exchanges: 1 vegetable

DAY 10
BREAKFAST
Eggs Baked Over a Spicy Vegetable Ragout or Breakfast Pigs in a Blanket
Skim milk (1 cup)
Whole-wheat toast (1 slice)
LUNCH
Pasta, Tuna & Roasted Pepper Salad or Turkey & Tomato Panini
Skim milk (1 cup)
SNACK

Apricot (1/2 cup)
Wasa crispbread (1 cracker)

DINNER

Pork Tenderloin with Roasted Plums & Rosemary
Steamed Vegetable Ribbons
Whole-wheat couscous (1/2 cup, cooked)

DAY 10 RECIPES

Eggs Baked Over a Spicy Vegetable Ragout
INGREDIENTS

- 3 teaspoons extra-virgin olive oil, divided
- 1 small eggplant, cut into 1/2-inch cubes

- 1 medium onion, chopped
- 1 large red bell pepper, diced
- 6 cloves garlic, minced
- 2 teaspoons ground cumin
- 1/8-1/4 teaspoon hot sauce, such as Hot pepper
- 1 medium summer squash, halved lengthwise and thinly sliced
- 1 14-ounce can diced tomatoes
- 1/4 cup water
- 3 tablespoons chopped fresh parsley, divided
- 1/8 teaspoon salt
- Freshly ground pepper to taste
- 4 large large eggs

PREPARATION

1. Preheat oven to 400°F. Coat a shallow 2-quart baking dish with cooking spray.
2. Heat 2 teaspoons oil in a large nonstick skillet over medium-high heat. Add eggplant and cook, stirring frequently, until browned and softened, 5 to 7 minutes. Transfer to a plate.
3. Heat the remaining 1 teaspoon oil in a Dutch oven or large deep sauté pan over medium heat. Add onion and cook, stirring occasionally, until softened, 3 to 5 minutes. Add bell pepper and cook, stirring occasionally, until softened, 3 to 5 minutes. Add garlic, cumin and hot sauce and cook until fragrant, 15 to 30 seconds. Stir in squash, tomatoes, water and the eggplant. Cover and simmer for 10 minutes. Stir in 2 tablespoons parsley, salt and pepper.
4. Spread the vegetable ragout in the prepared baking dish. Make 4 shallow wells in the ragout and gently crack 1 egg into each well, being careful not to break yolks.
5. Bake, uncovered, until the eggs are barely set, 10 to 12 minutes. (Caution: Eggs can overcook very quickly. Check them often and remove from the oven when they still look a little underdone; they will continue to cook in the hot ragout. If

the baking dish is ceramic, the cooking time will be closer to 12 minutes. A glass dish will cook eggs much faster.) Sprinkle with the remaining 1 tablespoon parsley. Serve immediately.

TIPS & NOTES

- **Make Ahead Tip**: Prepare through Step 3, cover and refrigerate for up to 2 days. Reheat before continuing.

NUTRITION

Per serving: 201 calories; 9 g fat (2 g sat, 5 g mono); 212 mg cholesterol; 23 g carbohydrates; 0 g added sugars; 10 g protein; 6 g fiber; 282 mg sodium; 471 mg potassium.

Nutrition Bonus: Vitamin C (170% daily value), Vitamin A (45% dv), Fiber (24% dv), Folate (17% dv), Iron (15% dv).

Carbohydrate Servings: 1

Exchanges: 4 vegetable; 1 medium-fat meat; 1/2 fat (mono)

Breakfast Pigs in a Blanket

INGREDIENTS

- 2 frozen pancakes, preferably whole-grain
- 2 teaspoons raspberry jam
- 2 1/2-ounce slices ham

PREPARATION

1) Heat pancakes in the microwave to soften for about 30 seconds. Spread 1 teaspoon raspberry jam down the center of each. Place one slice of ham on each. Microwave to heat through, about 1 minute. Roll up.

NUTRITION

Per serving: 203 calories; 5 g fat (1 g sat, 1 g mono); 29 mg cholesterol; 31 g carbohydrates; 10 g protein; 1 g fiber; 275 mg sodium; 103 mg potassium.

Carbohydrate Servings: 2

Exchanges: 2 starch, 1 lean meat

Pasta, Tuna & Roasted Pepper Salad

INGREDIENTS

- 1 6-ounce can chunk light tuna in water, drained (see Note)
- 1 7-ounce jar roasted red peppers, rinsed and sliced (2/3 cup), divided
- 1/2 cup finely chopped red onion or scallions
- 2 tablespoons capers, rinsed, coarsely chopped if large
- 2 tablespoons nonfat plain yogurt
- 2 tablespoons chopped fresh basil
- 1 tablespoon extra-virgin olive oil
- 1 1/2 teaspoons lemon juice
- 1 small clove garlic, crushed and peeled
- 1/8 teaspoon salt, or to taste and Freshly ground pepper, to taste
- 6 ounces whole-wheat penne or rigatoni, (1 3/4 cups)

PREPARATION

1. Put a large pot of lightly salted water on to boil.
2. Combine tuna, 1/3 cup red peppers, onion (or scallions) and capers in a large bowl.
3. Combine yogurt, basil, oil, lemon juice, garlic, salt, pepper and the remaining 1/3 cup red peppers in a blender or food processor. Puree until smooth.

4. Cook pasta until just tender, 10 to 14 minutes or according to package directions. Drain and rinse under cold water. Add to the tuna mixture along with the red pepper sauce; toss to coat.

TIPS & NOTES

- **Note:** Chunk light tuna, which comes from the smaller skipjack or yellowfin, has less mercury than canned white albacore tuna. The FDA/EPA advises that women who are or might become pregnant, nursing mothers and young children consume no more than 6 ounces of albacore a week; up to 12 ounces of canned light tuna is considered safe.

NUTRITION

Per serving: 270 calories; 5 g fat (1 g sat, 3 g mono); 13 mg cholesterol; 39 g carbohydrates; 0 g added sugars; 18 g protein; 6 g fiber; 539 mg sodium; 234 mg potassium.

Nutrition Bonus: Vitamin C (30% daily value), Fiber (23% dv), Magnesium (19% dv).

Carbohydrate Servings: 2

Exchanges: 2 starch, 2 very lean meat

Turkey & Tomato Panini

INGREDIENTS

- 3 tablespoons reduced-fat mayonnaise
- 2 tablespoons nonfat plain yogurt
- 2 tablespoons shredded Parmesan cheese
- 2 tablespoons chopped fresh basil
- 1 teaspoon lemon juice
- Freshly ground pepper, to taste
- 8 slices whole-wheat bread
- 8 ounces thinly sliced reduced-sodium deli turkey

- 8 tomato slices
- 2 teaspoons canola oil

PREPARATION

1. Have four 15-ounce cans and a medium skillet (not nonstick) ready by the stove.

2. Combine mayonnaise, yogurt, Parmesan, basil, lemon juice and pepper in a small bowl. Spread about 2 teaspoons of the mixture on each slice of bread. Divide turkey and tomato slices among 4 slices of bread; top with the remaining bread.

3. Heat 1 teaspoon oil in a large nonstick skillet over medium heat. Place 2 panini in the pan. Place the medium skillet on top of the panini, then weight it down with the cans. Cook the panini until golden on one side, about 2 minutes. Reduce the heat to medium-low, flip the panini, replace the top skillet and cans, and cook until the second side is golden, 1 to 3 minutes more. Repeat with another 1 teaspoon oil and the remaining panini.

NUTRITION

Per serving: 286 calories; 6 g fat (1 g sat, 3 g mono); 27 mg cholesterol; 36 g carbohydrates; 10 g protein; 5 g fiber; 681 mg sodium; 136 mg potassium.

Nutrition Bonus: Fiber (20% daily value), Calcium & Iron (15% dv)

Carbohydrate Servings: 2

Exchanges: 2 starch, 1 lean meat

Pork Tenderloin with Roasted Plums & Rosemary

INGREDIENTS

ROASTED PLUMS

- 1 pound black or red plums, pitted and cut into eighths (6-7 plums)
- 2 sprigs fresh rosemary, plus more for garnish
- 1/2 cup water
- 1/2 cup balsamic vinegar

- 6 tablespoons sugar, divided
- 10 black peppercorns, crushed
- 1 vanilla bean, split (see Substitution Tip)

PORK

- 2 teaspoons extra-virgin olive oil
- 1 pound pork tenderloin, trimmed of fat
- 1/4 teaspoon freshly ground pepper
- 1/8 teaspoon salt

PREPARATION

1. To roast plums: Preheat oven to 400°F. Place plums and 2 rosemary sprigs in an 8-inch-square baking dish. Whisk water, vinegar, 4 tablespoons sugar and peppercorns in a small bowl until the sugar dissolves. Scrape seeds from vanilla bean; add the seeds and bean to the vinegar mixture. Pour the mixture over the plums. Sprinkle with the remaining 2 tablespoons sugar.

2. Roast the plums, uncovered, until tender and beginning to break down, 20 to 25 minutes. Discard the rosemary and the vanilla bean. Transfer the plums to a serving platter and cover with foil. Strain the roasting liquid into a small saucepan and bring to a boil. Reduce heat to medium-high; cook until reduced to 1/2 cup, 6 to 8 minutes. Pour the sauce over the plums; keep warm.

3. To prepare pork: Meanwhile, heat oil in a large ovenproof skillet over medium-high heat. Sprinkle pork with pepper and salt. Add to the skillet and brown on all sides, 5 to 8 minutes.

4. Transfer the pan to the oven; bake at 400° until an instant-read thermometer registers 155° and the pork has just a hint of pink in the center, 10 to 15 minutes. Transfer the pork to a cutting board and let rest for 10 minutes. (The internal temperature will increase to 160° during resting.) Cut the pork into thin slices and serve with the roasted plums.

TIPS & NOTES

- **Make Ahead Tip**: Cover and refrigerate the roasted plums for up to 2 days.

- **Substitution Tip:** You can use 1/4 teaspoon vanilla extract instead of the vanilla bean.

NUTRITION

Per serving: 298 calories; 7 g fat (2 g sat, 4 g mono); 63 mg cholesterol; 37 g carbohydrates; 24 g protein; 2 g fiber; 127 mg sodium; 564 mg potassium.

Nutrition Bonus: Selenium (56% daily value), Vitamin C (20% dv).

Carbohydrate Servings: 2 1/2

Exchanges: 2 fruit, 5 lean meat

Steamed Vegetable Ribbons

INGREDIENTS

- 2 large carrots, peeled
- 3 small zucchini
- 2 teaspoons extra-virgin olive oil
- 2 teaspoons lemon juice, or to taste
- 1/4 teaspoon salt, or to taste
- Freshly ground pepper, to taste

PREPARATION

1) With a swivel vegetable peeler, shave carrots lengthwise into wide ribbons. Repeat with zucchini, shaving long, wide strips from all sides until you reach the seedy core. Discard the core.

2) Bring 2 inches of water to a boil in a large saucepan fitted with a steamer basket. Add the carrots; cover and steam for 2 minutes. Place the zucchini over the carrots; cover and steam until the vegetables are just tender, 2 to 3 minutes more. Transfer the vegetables to a large bowl. Toss with oil, lemon juice, salt and pepper.

NUTRITION

Per serving: 51 calories; 3 g fat (0 g sat, 2 g mono); 0 mg cholesterol; 7 g carbohydrates; 0 g added sugars; 1 g protein; 2 g fiber; 179 mg sodium; 350 mg potassium.

Nutrition Bonus: Vitamin A (90% daily value), Vitamin C (30% dv).

Carbohydrate Servings: 1/2

Exchanges: 11/2 vegetable, 1/2 fat (mono)

DAY 11
BREAKFAST

Blueberry Corn Muffins
Skim milk (1 cup)
Strawberries (1 cup)

LUNCH

Honey-Mustard Turkey Burgers
Broccoli Slaw or Orange-Scented Green Beans with Toasted Almonds
Skim milk (1 cup)

SNACK

Frosted Grapes

DINNER

Herbed Scallop Kebabs or Ginger-Coconut Chicken
Quick-cooking barley (1/2 cup)
Steamed cauliflower (1 cup)
Strawberry Frozen Yogurt

DAY 11 RECIPES

Blueberry Corn Muffins

INGREDIENTS
- 2/3 cup whole-wheat flour
- 2/3 cup all-purpose flour
- 2/3 cup cornmeal
- 1 tablespoon baking powder
- 1 teaspoon ground cinnamon
- 1/4 teaspoon salt
- 1 cup blueberries
- 1 large egg

- 2/3 cup low-fat milk
- 1/2 cup honey
- 3 tablespoons canola oil
- 1 teaspoon sugar

PREPARATION
1. Preheat oven to 400°F. Coat 12 standard 21/2-inch muffin cups with cooking spray.
2. Whisk whole-wheat flour, all-purpose flour, cornmeal, baking powder, cinnamon and salt in a large bowl. Add blueberries and toss to coat.
3. Whisk egg in a medium bowl. Add milk, honey and oil, whisking until well combined. Add the wet ingredients to the dry ingredients and stir until just combined. Do not overmix. Scoop the batter into the prepared pan, filling each cup about two-thirds full. Sprinkle the tops with sugar.
4. Bake the muffins until the tops spring back when touched lightly, 18 to 22 minutes Let cool in the pan for 5 minutes. Loosen the edges and turn the muffins out onto a wire rack to cool slightly before serving.

NUTRITION
Per muffin: 172 calories; 5 g fat (0 g sat, 2 g mono); 18 mg cholesterol; 32 g carbohydrates; 4 g protein; 2 gfiber; 162 mg sodium; 72 mg potassium.
Carbohydrate Servings: 2
Exchanges: 2 starch

Honey-Mustard Turkey Burgers

INGREDIENTS
- 1/4 cup coarse-grained mustard
- 2 tablespoons honey
- 1 pound ground turkey breast
- 1/4 teaspoon salt
- 1/4 teaspoon freshly ground pepper
- 2 teaspoons canola oil
- 4 whole-wheat hamburger rolls, split and toasted
- Lettuce, tomato slices and red onion slices, for garnish

PREPARATION
1. Prepare a grill.
2. Whisk mustard and honey in a small bowl until smooth.
3. Combine turkey, 3 tablespoons of the mustard mixture, salt and pepper in a bowl; mix well. Form into four 1-inch-thick burgers.

4. Lightly brush the burgers on both sides with oil. Grill until no pink remains in center, 5 to 7 minutes per side. Brush the burgers with the remaining mustard mixture. Serve on rolls with lettuce, tomato and onion slices.

NUTRITION
Per serving: 317 calories; 11 g fat (3 g sat, 2 g mono); 65 mg cholesterol; 31 g carbohydrates; 26 g protein;3 g fiber; 593 mg sodium; 387 mg potassium.
Nutrition Bonus: Folate (20% daily value), Iron (20% dv), Calcium (15% dv).
Carbohydrate Servings: 2
Exchanges: 2 starch, 4 lean meat

Broccoli Slaw

INGREDIENTS
- 4 slices turkey bacon
- 1 12- to 16-ounce bag shredded broccoli slaw, or 1 large bunch broccoli (about 1 1/2 pounds)
- 1/4 cup low-fat or nonfat plain yogurt
- 1/4 cup reduced-fat mayonnaise
- 3 tablespoons cider vinegar
- 2 teaspoons sugar
- 1/2 teaspoon salt, or to taste
- Freshly ground pepper, to taste
- 1 8-ounce can low-sodium sliced water chestnuts, rinsed and coarsely chopped
- 1/2 cup finely diced red onion, (1/2 medium)

PREPARATION
1. Cook bacon in a large skillet over medium heat, turning frequently, until crisp, 5 to 8 minutes. (Alternatively, microwave on High for 2 1/2 to 3 minutes.) Drain bacon on paper towels. Chop coarsely.
2. If using whole broccoli, trim about 3 inches off the stems. Chop the rest into 1/4-inch pieces.
3. Whisk yogurt, mayonnaise, vinegar, sugar, salt and pepper in a large bowl. Add water chestnuts, onion, bacon and broccoli; toss to coat. Chill until serving time.

TIPS & NOTES
- **Make Ahead Tip**: Cover and chill for up to 2 days.

NUTRITION

Per serving: 80 calories; 3 g fat (1 g sat, 1 g mono); 5 mg cholesterol; 9 g carbohydrates; 1 g added sugars;3 g protein; 3 g fiber; 271 mg sodium; 181 mg potassium.
Nutrition Bonus: Vitamin C (70% daily value).
Carbohydrate Servings: 1/2
Exchanges: 2 vegetable, 1 fat

Orange-Scented Green Beans with Toasted Almonds

INGREDIENTS
- 1 pound green beans, trimmed
- 1 teaspoon extra-virgin olive oil
- 1/2 teaspoon freshly grated orange zest
- 1/4 teaspoon salt
- Freshly ground pepper, to taste
- 1/4 cup sliced almonds, toasted (see Tip)

PREPARATION
1. Place a steamer basket in a large saucepan, add 1 inch of water and bring to a boil. Put green beans in the basket and steam until tender, about 6 minutes. Toss the green beans in a large bowl with oil, orange zest, salt, pepper and almonds.

TIPS & NOTES
- **Tip:** To toast sliced almonds, place in a small dry skillet and cook over medium-low heat, stirring constantly, until fragrant and lightly browned, 2 to 4 minutes.

NUTRITION

Per serving: 84 calories; 4 g fat (0 g sat, 3 g mono); 0 mg cholesterol; 10 g carbohydrates; 0 g added sugars; 3 g protein; 4 g fiber; 147 mg sodium; 206 mg potassium.
Nutrition Bonus: Vitamin C (20% daily value), Vitamin A (15% dv)
Carbohydrate Servings: 1/2
Exchanges: 2 vegetable, 1 fat

Frosted Grapes

INGREDIENTS
- 2 cups seedless grapes

PREPARATION
1. Wash and pat dry grapes. Freeze 45 minutes. Let stand for 2 minutes at room temperature before serving.

NUTRITION

Per serving: 55 calories; 0 g fat (0 g sat, 0 g mono); 0 mg cholesterol; 14 g carbohydrates; 1 g protein; 1 gfiber; 2 mg sodium; 153 mg potassium.
Carbohydrate Servings: 1
Exchanges: 1 fruit

Herbed Scallop Kebabs

INGREDIENTS
- 3 tablespoons lemon juice
- 1 1/2 tablespoons chopped fresh thyme
- 2 teaspoons extra-virgin olive oil
- 2 teaspoons freshly grated lemon zest
- 1 teaspoon freshly ground pepper
- 1/4 teaspoon salt, or to taste
- 1 1/4 pounds sea scallops, trimmed
- 1 lemon, cut into 8 wedges

PREPARATION
1. Preheat grill to medium-high. Place a fine-mesh nonstick grill topper on grill to heat.
2. Whisk lemon juice, thyme, oil, lemon zest, pepper and salt in a small bowl.
3. Toss scallops with 2 tablespoons of the lemon mixture; reserve the remaining mixture for basting the kebabs. Thread the scallops and the lemon wedges onto four 10-inch-long skewers (see Tip), placing 6 to 7 scallops and 2 lemon wedges on each skewer.
4. Lightly oil the grill rack (see Tip). Cook the kebabs, turning from time to time and basting with the reserved lemon mixture, until the scallops are opaque in the center, 8 to 12 minutes. Serve immediately.

TIPS & NOTES
- If using wooden skewers, soak them in water for 20 to 30 minutes first to prevent them from scorching.

- **To oil a grill rack:** Oil a folded paper towel, hold it with tongs and rub it over the rack. Do not use cooking spray on a hot grill.

NUTRITION

Per serving: 152 calories; 3 g fat (0 g sat, 2 g mono); 47 mg cholesterol; 5 g carbohydrates; 0 g added sugars; 24 g protein; 0 g fiber; 374 mg sodium; 478 mg potassium.
Nutrition Bonus: Selenium (44% daily value), Vitamin C (20% dv).
Exchanges: 31/2 very lean meat

Ginger-Coconut Chicken

INGREDIENTS
- 1 tablespoon yellow split peas
- 1 teaspoon coriander seeds
- 1-2 dried red chiles, such as Thai, cayenne or chiles de arbol
- 1/4 cup "lite" coconut milk, (see Ingredient note)
- 2 tablespoons minced fresh ginger
- 4 medium cloves garlic, minced
- 2 tablespoons finely chopped fresh cilantro
- 1/2 teaspoon salt, or to taste
- 4 boneless, skinless chicken breast halves, (1-1 1/4 pounds total), trimmed

PREPARATION
1. Toast split peas, coriander seeds and chiles in a small skillet over medium heat, shaking the pan occasionally, until the split peas turn reddish-brown, the coriander becomes fragrant and the chiles blacken slightly, 2 to 3 minutes. Transfer to a plate to cool for 3 to 5 minutes. Grind in a spice grinder or mortar and pestle until the mixture is the texture of finely ground pepper.
2. Combine coconut milk, ginger, garlic, cilantro, salt and the spice blend in a shallow glass dish. Add chicken and turn to coat. Cover and refrigerate for at least 30 minutes or overnight.
3. Preheat broiler. Coat a broiler-pan rack with cooking spray. Place the chicken (including marinade) on the rack over the broiler pan. Broil chicken 3 to 5 inches from the heat source until it is no longer pink in the center and the juices run clear, 4 to 6 minutes per side.

TIPS & NOTES
- **Make Ahead Tip**: The chicken can be marinated (Steps 1-2) overnight.
- **Ingredient Note:** Look for reduced-fat coconut milk (labeled "lite") in the Asian section of your market.

NUTRITION

Per serving: 152 calories; 3 g fat (1 g sat, 0 g mono); 66 mg cholesterol; 4 g carbohydrates; 0 g added sugars; 27 g protein; 1 g fiber; 371 mg sodium; 327 mg potassium.
Nutrition Bonus: Potassium (16% daily value

Strawberry Frozen Yogurt

INGREDIENTS
- 4 cups strawberries, hulled
- 1/3 cup sugar
- 2 tablespoons orange juice
- 1/2 cup nonfat or low-fat plain yogurt

PREPARATION
1. Place berries in a food processor and process until smooth, scraping down the sides as necessary. Add sugar and orange juice; process for a few seconds. Add yogurt and pulse several times until blended. Transfer to a bowl. Cover and refrigerate until chilled, about 1 hour or overnight.
2. Pour the strawberry mixture into an ice cream maker and freeze according to manufacturer's directions. Serve immediately or transfer to a storage container and let harden in the freezer for 1 to 1 1/2 hours. Serve in chilled dishes.

TIPS & NOTES
- **Make Ahead Tip:** Freeze for up to 1 week. Let soften in the refrigerator for 1/2 hour before serving. | Equipment: Ice cream maker

NUTRITION

Per serving: 82 calories; 0 g fat (0 g sat, 0 g mono); 0 mg cholesterol; 20 g carbohydrates; 1 g protein; 2 gfiber; 12 mg sodium; 170 mg potassium.
Nutrition Bonus: Vitamin C (100% daily value).
Carbohydrate Servings: 1
Exchanges: 1 fruit

DAY 12

BREAKFAST

Blueberry Corn Muffins or Banana-Bran Muffins
Skim milk (1 cup)
Grapefruit (1/2)

LUNCH

Pasta, Tuna & Roasted Pepper Salad or Shrimp Cobb Salad
Whole-wheat pita bread (1/2 medium pita)
Skim milk (1 cup)

SNACK

Melon (1 cup, cubes)

DINNER

Grilled Chicken Breasts with Salsa Verde
Brown rice (1/2 cup, cooked)
North African Spiced Carrots
Blueberries (1 cup)

DAY 12 RECIPES

INGREDIENTS
- 2/3 cup whole-wheat flour
- 2/3 cup all-purpose flour
- 2/3 cup cornmeal
- 1 tablespoon baking powder
- 1 teaspoon ground cinnamon
- 1/4 teaspoon salt
- 1 cup blueberries
- 1 large egg
- 2/3 cup low-fat milk
- 1/2 cup honey
- 3 tablespoons canola oil
- 1 teaspoon sugar

PREPARATION
1. Preheat oven to 400°F. Coat 12 standard 2 1/2-inch muffin cups with cooking spray.
2. Whisk whole-wheat flour, all-purpose flour, cornmeal, baking powder, cinnamon and salt in a large bowl. Add blueberries and toss to coat.
3. Whisk egg in a medium bowl. Add milk, honey and oil, whisking until well combined. Add the wet ingredients to the dry ingredients and stir until just

combined. Do not overmix. Scoop the batter into the prepared pan, filling each cup about two-thirds full. Sprinkle the tops with sugar.
4. Bake the muffins until the tops spring back when touched lightly, 18 to 22 minutes Let cool in the pan for 5 minutes. Loosen the edges and turn the muffins out onto a wire rack to cool slightly before serving.

NUTRITION
Per muffin: 172 calories; 5 g fat (0 g sat, 2 g mono); 18 mg cholesterol; 32 g carbohydrates; 4 g protein; 2 gfiber; 162 mg sodium; 72 mg potassium.
Carbohydrate Servings: 2
Exchanges: 2 starch

Banana-Bran Muffins

INGREDIENTS

- 2 large eggs
- 2/3 cup packed light brown sugar
- 1 cup mashed ripe bananas, (2 medium)
- 1 cup buttermilk, (see Ingredient notes)
- 1 cup unprocessed wheat bran, (see Ingredient notes)
- 1/4 cup canola oil
- 1 teaspoon vanilla extract
- 1 cup whole-wheat flour
- 3/4 cup all-purpose flour
- 1 1/2 teaspoons baking powder
- 1/2 teaspoon baking soda
- 1/2 teaspoon ground cinnamon
- 1/4 teaspoon salt
- 1/2 cup chocolate chips, (optional)
- 1/3 cup chopped walnuts, (optional)

PREPARATION

1. Preheat oven to 400°F. Coat 12 muffin cups with cooking spray.
2. Whisk eggs and brown sugar in a medium bowl until smooth. Whisk in bananas, buttermilk, wheat bran, oil and vanilla.
3. Whisk whole-wheat flour, all-purpose flour, baking powder, baking soda, cinnamon and salt in a large bowl. Make a well in the dry ingredients; add the wet ingredients and stir with a rubber spatula until just combined. Stir in chocolate chips, if using. Scoop the batter into the prepared muffin cups (they'll be quite full). Sprinkle with walnuts, if using.
4. Bake the muffins until the tops are golden brown and spring back when touched lightly, 15 to 25 minutes. Let cool in the pan for 5 minutes. Loosen edges and turn muffins out onto a wire rack to cool slightly before serving.

TIPS & NOTES

- **Ingredient Notes:** You can use buttermilk powder in place of fresh buttermilk. Or make "sour milk": mix 1 tablespoon lemon juice or vinegar to 1 cup milk.
- Unprocessed wheat bran is the outer layer of the wheat kernel, removed during milling. Also known as miller's bran, it can be found in the baking section. Do not substitute bran cereal in this recipe.

.NUTRITION

Per serving: 200 calories; 6 g fat (1 g sat, 3 g mono); 36 mg cholesterol; 32 g carbohydrates; 5 g protein; 4 g fiber; 182 mg sodium; 167 mg potassium.

Nutrition Bonus: Fiber (17% daily value).

Carbohydrate Servings: 2

Exchanges: 2 starch, 1 fat

Pasta, Tuna & Roasted Pepper Salad

INGREDIENTS

- 1 6-ounce can chunk light tuna in water, drained (see Note)
- 1 7-ounce jar roasted red peppers, rinsed and sliced (2/3 cup), divided
- 1/2 cup finely chopped red onion or scallions
- 2 tablespoons capers, rinsed, coarsely chopped if large
- 2 tablespoons nonfat plain yogurt
- 2 tablespoons chopped fresh basil
- 1 tablespoon extra-virgin olive oil
- 1 1/2 teaspoons lemon juice
- 1 small clove garlic, crushed and peeled
- 1/8 teaspoon salt, or to taste
- Freshly ground pepper, to taste
- 6 ounces whole-wheat penne or rigatoni, (1 3/4 cups)

PREPARATION

1. Put a large pot of lightly salted water on to boil.
2. Combine tuna, 1/3 cup red peppers, onion (or scallions) and capers in a large bowl.
3. Combine yogurt, basil, oil, lemon juice, garlic, salt, pepper and the remaining 1/3 cup red peppers in a blender or food processor. Puree until smooth.
4. Cook pasta until just tender, 10 to 14 minutes or according to package directions. Drain and rinse under cold water. Add to the tuna mixture along with the red pepper sauce; toss to coat.

TIPS & NOTES

- **Note:** Chunk light tuna, which comes from the smaller skipjack or yellowfin, has less mercury than canned white albacore tuna. The FDA/EPA advises that women who are or might become pregnant, nursing mothers and young children consume no more than 6 ounces of albacore a week; up to 12 ounces of canned light tuna is considered safe.

NUTRITION

Per serving: 270 calories; 5 g fat (1 g sat, 3 g mono); 13 mg cholesterol; 39 g carbohydrates; 0 g added sugars; 18 g protein; 6 g fiber; 539 mg sodium; 234 mg potassium.

Nutrition Bonus: Vitamin C (30% daily value), Fiber (23% dv), Magnesium (19% dv).

Carbohydrate Servings: 2

Exchanges: 2 starch, 2 very lean meat

Shrimp Cobb Salad

INGREDIENTS

- 3 cups chopped hearts of romaine
- 5 grape or cherry tomatoes
- 1/4 cup sliced cucumber
- 1 hard-boiled egg, sliced (see Tip)
- 5 cooked peeled shrimp, (31-40 per pound)
- Freshly ground pepper, to taste
- 2 tablespoons light blue cheese dressing

PREPARATION

1. Combine lettuce, tomatoes, cucumber, egg and shrimp in a bowl. Season with pepper. Toss with dressing and serve.

TIPS & NOTES

- **Tip:** To hard-boil eggs: Place eggs in a single layer in a saucepan; cover with water. Bring to a simmer over medium-high heat. Reduce heat to low and cook at the barest simmer for 10 minutes. Remove from heat, pour out hot water and run a constant stream of cold water over the eggs until completely cooled.

NUTRITION

Per serving: 273 calories; 13 g fat (3 g sat, 2 g mono); 348 mg cholesterol; 13 g carbohydrates; 1 g added sugars; 27 g protein; 5 g fiber; 556 mg sodium; 894 mg potassium.

Nutrition Bonus: Vitamin A (220% daily value), Vitamin C (90% dv), Folate (67% dv), Iron (20% dv).

Carbohydrate Servings: 1

Exchanges: 2 vegetables, 3 lean meat, 1 fat

Grilled Chicken Breasts with Salsa Verde

INGREDIENTS

SALSA VERDE

- 1/2 cup chopped fresh parsley
- 1 1/2 tablespoons capers, rinsed
- 1 clove garlic, peeled and smashed
- 1 tablespoon extra-virgin olive oil
- 1 tablespoon lemon juice and 1 tablespoon water
- 1 teaspoon anchovy paste
- Freshly ground pepper, to taste

CHICKEN

- 4 boneless, skinless chicken breast halves, (about 1 pound total), trimmed
- 1 teaspoon extra-virgin olive oil
- 1/8 teaspoon salt
- Freshly ground pepper, to taste

PREPARATION

1. To prepare salsa verde: Combine parsley, capers and garlic in a blender or food processor; process until finely chopped. Add oil, lemon juice, water and anchovy paste and process until blended. Season with pepper.

2. To prepare chicken: Prepare a grill or preheat broiler. Rub chicken with oil and season with salt and pepper. Grill or broil until no longer pink inside, 3 to 4 minutes per side. Serve with salsa verde.

TIPS & NOTES

- **Make Ahead Tip**: Cover and refrigerate the salsa verde (Step 1) up to 2 days. Bring to room temperature before serving.

NUTRITION

Per serving: 183 calories; 7 g fat (1 g sat, 4 g mono); 70 mg cholesterol; 1 g carbohydrates; 0 g added sugars; 27 g protein; 0 g fiber; 471 mg sodium; 340 mg potassium.

Nutrition Bonus: Selenium (28% daily value), Vitamin C (20% dv).

Exchanges: 4 very lean meat, 1 fat (mono)

North African Spiced Carrots

INGREDIENTS

- 1 tablespoon extra-virgin olive oil
- 4 cloves garlic, minced
- 2 teaspoons paprika
- 1 teaspoon ground cumin
- 1 teaspoon ground coriander
- 3 cups sliced carrots, (4 medium-large)
- 1 cup water
- 3 tablespoons lemon juice

- 1/8 teaspoon salt, or to taste
- 1/4 cup chopped fresh parsley

PREPARATION

1) Heat oil in a large nonstick skillet over medium heat. Add garlic, paprika, cumin and coriander; cook, stirring, until fragrant but not browned, about 20 seconds. Add carrots, water, lemon juice and salt; bring to a simmer. Reduce heat to low, cover and cook until almost tender, 5 to 7 minutes. Uncover and simmer, stirring often, until the carrots are just tender and the liquid is syrupy, 2 to 4 minutes. Stir in parsley. Serve hot or at room temperature.

NUTRITION

Per serving: 51 calories; 3 g fat (0 g sat, 2 g mono); 0 mg cholesterol; 7 g carbohydrates; 0 g added sugars; 1 g protein; 2 g fiber; 86 mg sodium; 186 mg potassium.

Nutrition Bonus: Vitamin A (210% daily value), Vitamin C (15% dv).

Carbohydrate Servings: 1/2

Exchanges: 1 vegetable, 1/2 fat (mono)

DAY 13
BREAKFAST
Skim milk (1 cup)
Baked Asparagus & Cheese Frittata
LUNCH
Pasta with Eggplant Ragu or Gnocchi with Zucchini Ribbons & Parsley Brown Butter
Orange
SNACK
Broiled Pineapple
DINNER
Oven-Fried Fish Fillets or Grilled Salmon with North African Flavors
Tarragon Tartar Sauce
Steamed broccoli (1/2 cup)
Brown rice (1/2 cup, cooked)
Salad of Boston Lettuce with Creamy Orange-Shallot Dressing

DAY 13 RECIPES

Baked Asparagus & Cheese Frittata

INGREDIENTS
- 2 tablespoons fine dry breadcrumbs
- 1 pound thin asparagus
- 1 1/2 teaspoons extra-virgin olive oil
- 2 onions, chopped
- 1 red bell pepper, chopped
- 2 cloves garlic, minced
- 1/2 teaspoon salt, divided
- 1/2 cup water
- Freshly ground pepper, to taste
- 4 large eggs
- 2 large egg whites
- 1 cup part-skim ricotta cheese
- 1 tablespoon chopped fresh parsley
- 1/2 cup shredded Gruyère cheese

PREPARATION

1. Preheat oven to 325°F. Coat a 10-inch pie pan or ceramic quiche dish with cooking spray. Sprinkle with breadcrumbs, tapping out the excess.
2. Snap tough ends off asparagus. Slice off the top 2 inches of the tips and reserve. Cut the stalks into 1/2-inch-long slices.
3. Heat oil in a large nonstick skillet over medium-high heat. Add onions, bell pepper, garlic and 1/4 teaspoon salt; cook, stirring, until softened, 5 to 7 minutes.
4. Add water and the asparagus stalks to the skillet. Cook, stirring, until the asparagus is tender and the liquid has evaporated, about 7 minutes (the mixture should be very dry). Season with salt and pepper. Arrange the vegetables in an even layer in the prepared pan.
5. Whisk eggs and egg whites in a large bowl. Add ricotta, parsley, the remaining 1/4 teaspoon salt and pepper; whisk to blend. Pour the egg mixture over the vegetables, gently shaking the pan to distribute. Scatter the reserved asparagus tips over the top and sprinkle with Gruyère.
6. Bake the frittata until a knife inserted in the center comes out clean, about 35 minutes. Let stand for 5 minutes before serving.

NUTRITION

Per serving: 195 calories; 11 g fat (5 g sat, 4 g mono); 164 mg cholesterol; 10 g carbohydrates; 15 gprotein; 2 g fiber; 357 mg sodium; 310 mg potassium.
Nutrition Bonus: Vitamin C (70% daily value), Vitamin A (30% dv).
Carbohydrate Servings: 1/2
Exchanges: 2 vegetable, 1 medium-fat meat, 1/2 high-fat meat

Pasta with Eggplant Ragu

INGREDIENTS

- 2 teaspoons extra-virgin olive oil
- 1 onion, coarsely chopped
- 2 cloves garlic, minced
- 1 eggplant, (1-1 1/4 pounds), diced
- Salt & freshly ground pepper, to taste
- 2 cups prepared marinara sauce
- 1 yellow or red bell pepper, diced
- 3 tablespoons chopped fresh basil
- 12 ounces pasta, preferably penne
- 1/2 cup crumbled feta cheese, or 1/4 cup freshly grated Parmesan cheese

PREPARATION

1. Put a large pot of salted water on to boil.

2. Heat oil in a large nonstick skillet over medium heat. Add onion and garlic and cook, stirring, until softened, about 4 minutes. Add eggplant and cook, stirring, for 2 minutes more. Season with salt and pepper. Stir in marinara sauce and bring to a simmer. Cover and cook, stirring occasionally, until eggplant is almost tender, about 20 minutes. Add bell pepper and basil; cover and cook for 5 minutes more.

3. Meanwhile, cook pasta in boiling water until al dente, 8 to 10 minutes. Drain and toss with sauce. Sprinkle with feta (or Parmesan) and serve.

NUTRITION

Per serving: 325 calories; 8 g fat (3 g sat, 2 g mono); 11 mg cholesterol; 57 g carbohydrates; 0 g added sugars; 10 g protein; 10 g fiber; 524 mg sodium; 219 mg potassium.

Carbohydrate Servings: 4

Exchanges: 3 starch, 1 vegetable, 1 fat

Gnocchi with Zucchini Ribbons & Parsley Brown Butter

INGREDIENTS

- 1 pound fresh or frozen gnocchi
- 2 tablespoons butter
- 2 medium shallots, chopped
- 1 pound zucchini, (about 3 small), very thinly sliced lengthwise (see Tip)
- 1 pint cherry tomatoes, halved
- 1/2 teaspoon salt
- 1/4 teaspoon grated nutmeg
- Freshly ground pepper, to taste
- 1/2 cup grated Parmesan cheese
- 1/2 cup chopped fresh parsley

PREPARATION

1. Bring a large saucepan of water to a boil. Cook gnocchi until they float, 3 to 5 minutes or according to package directions. Drain.
2. Meanwhile, melt butter in a large skillet over medium-high heat. Cook until the butter is beginning to brown, about 2 minutes. Add shallots and zucchini and cook, stirring often, until softened, 2 to 3 minutes. Add tomatoes, salt, nutmeg and pepper and continue cooking, stirring often, until the tomatoes are just starting to break down, 1 to 2 minutes. Stir in Parmesan and parsley. Add the gnocchi and toss to coat. Serve immediately.

TIPS & NOTES

- **Tip:** To make "ribbon-thin" zucchini, slice lengthwise with a vegetable peeler or a mandoline slicer.

NUTRITION

Per serving: 424 calories; 10 g fat (6 g sat, 0 g mono); 25 mg cholesterol; 66 g carbohydrates; 17 g protein;5 g fiber; 753 mg sodium; 539 mg potassium.

Nutrition Bonus: Vitamin C (75% daily value), Vitamin A (35% dv), Calcium (28% dv)

Carbohydrate Servings: 4 1/2

Exchanges: 2 1/2 starch, 2 vegetable, 1 medium-fat meat, 1 fat

Broiled Pineapple

INGREDIENTS

- 1 large pineapple
- 2 teaspoons canola oil, divided
- 2 tablespoons brown sugar
- Lime wedges

PREPARATION

Peel pineapple. With a sharp knife, cut it crosswise into 1-inch-thick slices. Brush the slices lightly with 1 teaspoon oil and place in a single layer on a baking sheet. Broil until lightly browned, about 7 minutes. Turn slices over, brush with remaining teaspoon oil and broil for 5 to 7 minutes longer. Immediately sprinkle pineapple with brown sugar. Cut into chunks and serve with lime wedges.

NUTRITION

Per serving: 68 calories; 2 g fat (0 g sat, 1 g mono); 0 mg cholesterol; 14 g carbohydrates; 0 g protein; 1 g fiber; 1 mg sodium; 90 mg potassium.

Nutrition Bonus: Vitamin C (50% daily value).

Carbohydrate Servings: 1

Exchanges: 1 fruit, 1/2 fat

Oven-Fried Fish Fillets

INGREDIENTS

- 1/3 cup fine, dry, unseasoned breadcrumbs
- 1/4 teaspoon salt
- Freshly ground pepper, to taste
- 1 pound Pacific sole fillets
- 1 tablespoon extra-virgin olive oil
- 1/2 cup Tarragon Tartar Sauce, (recipe follows)
- Lemon wedges

PREPARATION

1. Preheat oven to 450°F. Coat a baking sheet with cooking spray.

2. Place breadcrumbs, salt and pepper in a small dry skillet over medium heat. Cook, stirring, until toasted, about 5 minutes. Remove from heat. Brush both sides of each fish fillet with oil and dredge in the breadcrumb mixture. Place on the prepared baking sheet.

3. Bake the fish until opaque in the center, 5 to 6 minutes.

4. Meanwhile, make Tarragon Tartar Sauce.

5. To serve, carefully transfer the fish to plates using a spatula. Garnish with a dollop of the sauce and serve with lemon wedges.

NUTRITION

Per serving: 229 calories; 10 g fat (2 g sat, 4 g mono); 59 mg cholesterol; 11 g carbohydrates; 23 g protein; 1 g fiber; 444 mg sodium; 472 mg potassium.

Nutrition Bonus: Selenium (57% daily value).

Carbohydrate Servings: 1

Exchanges: 1/2 starch, 3 lean meat

Grilled Salmon with North African Flavors

INGREDIENTS

- 1/4 cup low-fat or nonfat plain yogurt
- 1/4 cup chopped fresh parsley
- 1/4 cup chopped fresh cilantro
- 2 tablespoons lemon juice
- 1 tablespoon extra-virgin olive oil
- 3 cloves garlic, minced
- 1 1/2 teaspoons paprika
- 1 teaspoon ground cumin
- 1/4 teaspoon salt, or to taste and Freshly ground pepper, to taste
- 1 pound center-cut salmon fillet, cut into 4 portions (see Tip)
- 1 lemon, cut into wedges

PREPARATION

1. Stir together yogurt, parsley, cilantro, lemon juice, oil, garlic, paprika, cumin, salt and pepper in a small bowl. Reserve 1/4 cup for sauce; cover and refrigerate. Place salmon fillets in a large sealable plastic bag. Pour in the remaining herb mixture, seal the bag and turn to coat. Refrigerate for 20 to 30 minutes, turning the bag over once.
2. Meanwhile, preheat grill to medium-high.
3. Oil the grill rack (see Tip). Remove the salmon from the marinade, blotting any excess. Grill the salmon until browned and opaque in the center, 4 to 6 minutes per side. To serve, top each piece with a dollop of the reserved sauce and garnish with lemon wedges.

TIPS & NOTES

- **Tips:** Keeping the skin on when grilling salmon helps hold the fish together and protects the delicate flesh from the searing heat. Once cooked, the skin slips off easily.

- **To oil a grill:** Oil a folded paper towel, hold it with tongs and rub it over the rack. (Do not use cooking spray on a hot grill.) When grilling delicate foods like tofu and fish, it is helpful to spray the food with cooking spray.

NUTRITION

Per serving: 229 calories; 14 g fat (3 g sat, 6 g mono); 67 mg cholesterol; 1 g carbohydrates; 0 g added sugars; 23 g protein; 0 g fiber; 134 mg sodium; 452 mg potassium.

Nutrition Bonus: 452 mg potassium (23% dv), 9 mg vitamin c (15% dv).

Exchanges: 3 lean protein, 1/2 fat

Tarragon Tartar Sauce

INGREDIENTS

- 1/2 cup nonfat or low-fat plain yogurt
- 1/2 cup reduced-fat mayonnaise
- 1 teaspoon sugar
- 1/2 teaspoon Dijon mustard
- 1/2 teaspoon lemon juice
- 1/4 cup finely chopped dill pickle
- 1 tablespoon drained capers, minced
- 2 tablespoons chopped fresh parsley
- 2 teaspoons chopped fresh tarragon, or 1/2 teaspoon dried
- 1 clove garlic, minced

PREPARATION

1. Whisk yogurt, mayonnaise, sugar, mustard and lemon juice in a small bowl. Stir in pickle, capers, parsley, tarragon and garlic.

TIPS & NOTES

- **Make Ahead Tip**: The sauce will keep, covered, in the refrigerator for up to 4 days.

NUTRITION

Per tablespoon: 22 calories; 2 g fat (0 g sat, 0 g mono); 2 mg cholesterol; 2 g carbohydrates; 0 g protein; 0 g fiber; 71 mg sodium; 6 mg potassium.

Exchanges: Per tablespoon: free food

Salad of Boston Lettuce with Creamy Orange-Shallot Dressing

INGREDIENTS

DRESSING

- 1/4 cup reduced-fat mayonnaise
- 1/2 teaspoon Dijon mustard
- 1/4 cup orange juice
- 2 teaspoons finely chopped shallot
- Freshly ground pepper, to taste

SALAD

- 1 large head Boston lettuce, torn into bite-size pieces (5 cups)
- 1 cup julienned or grated carrot, (1 carrot)
- 1 cup cherry or grape tomatoes, rinsed and cut in half
- 2 tablespoons snipped fresh tarragon, or chives (optional)

PREPARATION

1. **To prepare dressing**: Whisk mayonnaise and mustard in a small bowl. Slowly whisk in orange juice until smooth. Stir in shallot. Season with pepper.

2. **To prepare salad:** Divide lettuce among 4 plates and scatter carrot and tomatoes on top. Drizzle the dressing over the salads and sprinkle with tarragon (or chives), if desired. Serve immediately.

NUTRITION

Per serving: 64 calories; 1 g fat (0 g sat, 0 g mono); 0 mg cholesterol; 12 g carbohydrates; 1 g added sugars; 2 g protein; 2 g fiber; 182 mg sodium; 386 mg potassium.

Nutrition Bonus: Vitamin A (120% daily value), Vitamin C (30% dv), Folate (16% dv).

Carbohydrate Servings: 1

Exchanges: 2 vegetable

DAY 14
BREAKFAST

Eggs Baked Over a Spicy Vegetable Ragout
Skim milk (1 cup)
Orange (1 large)
LUNCH

Roasted Red Pepper Subs or Cranberry & Herb Turkey Burgers
Fat-free cheese (1 slice)
The Diet House Salad
SNACK

Melon (1 cup, cubes)
DINNER

Roasted Vegetable Pasta
Spinach Salad with Black Olive Vinaigrette or Bold Winter Greens Salad
Apricot (1/2 cup, halves)

DAY 14 RECIPES

Eggs Baked Over a Spicy Vegetable Ragout

INGREDIENTS
- 3 teaspoons extra-virgin olive oil, divided
- 1 small eggplant, cut into 1/2-inch cubes
- 1 medium onion, chopped
- 1 large red bell pepper, diced
- 6 cloves garlic, minced
- 2 teaspoons ground cumin
- 1/8-1/4 teaspoon hot sauce, such as Hot pepper
- 1 medium summer squash, halved lengthwise and thinly sliced
- 1 14-ounce can diced tomatoes
- 1/4 cup water
- 3 tablespoons chopped fresh parsley, divided
- 1/8 teaspoon salt
- Freshly ground pepper to taste
- 4 large large eggs

TIPS & NOTES

- **Make Ahead Tip**: Prepare through Step 3, cover and refrigerate for up to 2 days. Reheat before continuing.

NUTRITION
Per serving: 201 calories; 9 g fat (2 g sat, 5 g mono); 212 mg cholesterol; 23 g carbohydrates; 0 g added sugars; 10 g protein; 6 g fiber; 282 mg sodium; 471 mg potassium.
Nutrition Bonus: Vitamin C (170% daily value), Vitamin A (45% dv), Fiber (24% dv), Folate (17% dv), Iron (15% dv).
Carbohydrate Servings: 1
Exchanges: 4 vegetable; 1 medium-fat meat; 1/2 fat (mono)

Roasted Red Pepper Subs

INGREDIENTS
- 1 12-ounce jar roasted red peppers, rinsed
- 1 clove garlic, minced
- 1 tablespoon red-wine vinegar
- 1 teaspoon extra-virgin olive oil
- Pinch of salt
- Freshly ground pepper, to taste
- 1 16- to 20-inch baguette, preferably whole-wheat

- 3 tablespoon olive paste, (olivada)
- 4 ounces creamy goat cheese
- 1 1/2 cups arugula leaves

PREPARATION
1. Combine peppers, garlic, vinegar and oil in a small bowl; toss to combine. Season with salt and pepper.
2. Slice baguette in half lengthwise. Spread one half with olive paste and the other half with goat cheese. Layer pepper mixture and arugula over olive paste. Top with remaining baguette. Cut across into 4 pieces.

TIPS & NOTES
- **Make Ahead Tip**: Wrap in plastic wrap and store in the refrigerator or in a cooler with a cold pack for up to 8 hours.

NUTRITION
Per serving: 221 calories; 15 g fat (5 g sat, 3 g mono); 13 mg cholesterol; 7 g carbohydrates; 7 g protein; 1 g fiber; 262 mg sodium; 59 mg potassium.
Nutrition Bonus: Vitamin A (50% daily value).
Carbohydrate Servings: 1
Exchanges: 1 starch, 1 vegetable, 1 high-fat meat, 1/2 fat

Cranberry & Herb Turkey Burgers

INGREDIENTS
- 1/4 cup plus 2 tablespoons whole-wheat couscous
- 1/2 cup boiling water
- 2 tablespoons extra-virgin olive oil
- 1 small onion, finely chopped
- 1 stalk celery, minced
- 1 tablespoon chopped fresh thyme
- 1 1/2 teaspoons chopped fresh sage
- 1/2 teaspoon salt
- 1/2 teaspoon freshly ground pepper
- 1/4 cup dried cranberries, finely chopped
- 1 pound 93%-lean ground turkey

PREPARATION
1. Place couscous in a large bowl. Pour in boiling water, stir and set aside until the water is absorbed, about 5 minutes. If grilling the burgers, preheat grill to medium-high.

2. Meanwhile, heat oil in a large skillet over medium heat. Add onion and cook, stirring, for 1 minute. Add celery; cook, stirring, until softened, about 3 minutes. Add thyme, sage, salt and pepper; cook until fragrant, about 20 seconds more. Transfer the mixture to the bowl with the couscous, add cranberries and stir to combine. Let cool for 5 minutes. Add turkey and stir until combined; do not overmix. Form the mixture into 6 patties.
3. To cook on the stovetop: Coat a large nonstick skillet, preferably cast-iron, with cooking spray and set over medium-high heat for 2 minutes. Add the patties, reduce heat to medium, and cook for 4 minutes. Turn and cook on the other side for 2 minutes. Cover and continue to cook until lightly browned but still juicy (the juices should run clear, not pink), about 4 minutes more. (An instant-read thermometer inserted in the center should read 165° F.) To grill: Oil the grill rack (see Tip) and grill the burgers for 5 to 6 minutes per side, flipping gently to avoid breaking them. Serve immediately.

TIPS & NOTES
- To oil a grill rack, oil a folded paper towel, hold it with tongs and rub it over the rack. (Do not use cooking spray on a hot grill.)

NUTRITION
Per serving: 217 calories; 10 g fat (2 g sat, 4 g mono); 43 mg cholesterol; 17 g carbohydrates; 0 g added sugars; 17 g protein; 2 g fiber; 256 mg sodium; 49 mg potassium.
Carbohydrate Servings: 1
Exchanges: 1 starch, 2 very lean meat, 1 fat (mono)

The Diet House Salad

INGREDIENTS
- 4 cups torn green leaf lettuce
- 1 cup sprouts
- 1 cup tomato wedges
- 1 cup peeled, sliced cucumber
- 1 cup shredded carrots
- 1/2 cup chopped radishes
- 1/2 cup Sesame Tamari Vinaigrette (recipe follows), or other dressing

PREPARATION
1. Toss lettuce, sprouts, tomato, cucumber, carrots and radishes in a large bowl with the dressing until the vegetables are coated.

NUTRITION

Per serving: 71 calories; 3 g fat (0 g sat, 1 g mono); 0 mg cholesterol; 11 g carbohydrates; 2 g protein; 3 gfiber; 334 mg sodium; 428 mg potassium.

Nutrition Bonus: Vitamin A (140% daily value), Vitamin C (30% dv), Folate (16% dv).

Carbohydrate Servings: 1

Exchanges: 2 vegetable, 1/2 fat

Roasted Vegetable Pasta

INGREDIENTS

- 1 medium zucchini, diced
- 1 red or yellow bell pepper, seeded and diced
- 1 large onion, thinly sliced
- 2 tablespoons extra-virgin olive oil, divided
- Salt & freshly ground pepper, to taste
- 2 large tomatoes, chopped
- 1/4 cup chopped fresh basil
- 2 cloves garlic, minced
- 12 ounces whole-wheat pasta
- 1/2 cup crumbled feta cheese

PREPARATION

1. Preheat oven to 450°F. Put a large pot of lightly salted water on to boil.

2. Toss zucchini, bell pepper and onion with 1 tablespoon oil in a large roasting pan or a large baking sheet with sides. Season with salt and pepper. Roast the vegetables, stirring every 5 minutes, until tender and browned, 10 to 20 minutes.

3. Meanwhile, combine tomatoes, basil, garlic and the remaining 1 tablespoon oil in a large bowl. Season with salt and pepper.

4. Cook pasta until just tender, 8 to 10 minutes. Drain and transfer to the bowl with the tomatoes. Add the roasted vegetables and toss well. Adjust seasoning with salt and pepper. Serve, passing feta cheese separately.

NUTRITION

Per serving: 288 calories; 12 g fat (4 g sat, 6 g mono); 17 mg cholesterol; 75 g carbohydrates; 17 g protein; 6 g fiber; 226 mg sodium; 619 mg potassium.

Nutrition Bonus: Vitamin C (90% daily value), Fiber (34% dv), Vitamin A (25% dv).

Carbohydrate Servings: 2 1/2

Exchanges: 3 starch, 1 vegetable, 1 fat

Spinach Salad with Black Olive Vinaigrette

INGREDIENTS

- 3 tablespoons extra-virgin olive oil
- 1 1/2 tablespoons red-wine vinegar, or lemon juice
- 6 pitted Kalamata olives, finely chopped
- 1/4 teaspoon salt
- Freshly ground pepper, to taste
- 6 cups torn spinach leaves
- 1/2 cucumber, seeded and sliced
- 1/2 red onion, thinly sliced

PREPARATION

Whisk oil, vinegar (or lemon juice) and olives in a salad bowl. Season with salt and pepper. Add spinach, cucumbers and onions; toss well. Serve immediately.

NUTRITION

Per serving: 128 calories; 12 g fat (2 g sat, 9 g mono); 0 mg cholesterol; 3 g carbohydrates; 2 g protein; 1 g fiber; 271 mg sodium; 284 mg potassium.

Nutrition Bonus: Vitamin A (80% daily value), Folate (22% dv), Vitamin C (20% dv).

Exchanges: 1 vegetable, 2 fat

Bold Winter Greens Salad

INGREDIENTS

- 2-3 cloves garlic, minced
- 1/4 teaspoon kosher salt
- 1/4 teaspoon freshly ground pepper, or to taste
- 2 tablespoons lemon juice
- 1 tablespoon sherry vinegar
- 3-4 anchovy fillets, rinsed and chopped
- 1/3 cup extra-virgin olive oil
- 12 cups chopped mixed bitter salad greens, such as chicory, radicchio and escarole, such as chicory, radicchio and escarole
- 3 large hard-boiled eggs, (see Tip)

PREPARATION

1. Place garlic to taste in a large salad bowl and sprinkle with salt and pepper. Add lemon juice and vinegar; let stand for 5 minutes. Stir in anchovies to taste. Whisk in oil in a slow steady stream until well combined.

2. Add salad greens and toss. Shred 3 egg whites and 1 egg yolk through the large holes of a box grater (reserve the remaining yolks for another use or discard). Sprinkle the salad with the grated egg.

TIPS & NOTES

- **Make Ahead Tip**: Prepare the dressing (Step 1), cover and refrigerate for up to 1 day.

- **Tip:** To hard-boil eggs, place eggs in a single layer in a saucepan; cover with water. Bring to a simmer over medium-high heat. Reduce heat to low and cook at the barest simmer for 10 minutes. Remove from heat, pour out hot water and cover the eggs with ice-cold water. Let stand until cool enough to handle before peeling.

NUTRITION

Per serving: 92 calories; 8 g fat (1 g sat, 6 g mono); 20 mg cholesterol; 2 g carbohydrates; 0 g added sugars; 2 g protein; 1 g fiber; 102 mg sodium; 168 mg potassium.

Nutrition Bonus: Vitamin A (120% daily value), Vitamin C (50% dv), Folate (34% dv), Potassium (16% dv)

Exchanges: 1 vegetable, 1 1/2 fat

DAY 15
BREAKFAST
Nonfat plain yogurt (8 oz)
Whole-wheat toast (1 slice)
Pear Butter
LUNCH
Romaine Salad with Chicken, Apricots & Mint or Fresh Tuna Salad with Tropical Fruits
Whole-wheat pita bread (1/2 medium pita)
SNACK
Fat-free cheese (1 slice)
DINNER
Pacific Sole with Oranges & Pecans
Steamed Vegetable Ribbons or Roasted Broccoli with Lemon
Whole-wheat couscous (1/2 cup, cooked)
Melon (1 cup, cubes)

DAY 15 RECIPES

Pear Butter

INGREDIENTS

- 4 ripe but firm Bartlett pears, (1-1 1/4 pounds), peeled, cored and cut into 1-inch chunks
- 3/4 cup pear nectar

PREPARATION

1. Place pears and pear nectar in a heavy medium saucepan; bring to a simmer. Cover and simmer over medium-low heat, stirring occasionally, until the pears are very tender, 30 to 35 minutes. Cooking time will vary depending on the ripeness of the pears.

2. Mash the pears with a potato masher. Cook, uncovered, over medium-low heat, stirring often, until the puree has cooked down to a thick mass (somewhat thicker than applesauce), 20 to 30 minutes. Stir almost constantly toward the end of cooking. Scrape the pear butter into a bowl or storage container and let cool.

TIPS & NOTES

- **Make Ahead Tip**: Store in an airtight container in the refrigerator for up to 2 weeks or freeze for up to 6 months.

NUTRITION

Per tablespoon: 22 calories; 0 g fat (0 g sat, 0 g mono); 0 mg cholesterol; 6 g carbohydrates; 0 g protein; 1 g fiber; 1 mg sodium; 33 mg potassium.

Carbohydrate Servings: 1/2

Exchanges: 1/2 fruit

Romaine Salad with Chicken, Apricots & Mint

INGREDIENTS

MARINADE & DRESSING

- 1/2 cup dried apricots
- 1 cup hot water
- 2 cups loosely packed mint leaves, (about 1 bunch)
- 1 teaspoon freshly grated orange zest
- 1/2 cup orange juice
- 2 tablespoons honey
- 4 teaspoons Dijon mustard
- 4 teaspoons red-wine vinegar
- 1/2 teaspoon salt, or to taste
- Freshly ground pepper, to taste
- 1/4 cup extra-virgin olive oil

SALAD

- 1 pound boneless, skinless chicken breast, trimmed of fat
- 1 large head romaine lettuce, torn into bite-size pieces (10 cups)
- 6 fresh apricots, or plums, pitted and cut into wedges
- 1 cup loosely packed mint leaves, (about 1/2 bunch), roughly chopped
- 1/2 cup sliced almonds, toasted (see Tip)

PREPARATION

1. Preheat grill.
2. To prepare marinade & dressing: Soak dried apricots in hot water for 10 minutes. Drain and transfer apricots to a food processor. Add 2 cups mint, orange zest, orange juice, honey, mustard, vinegar, salt and pepper. Process until smooth. With the motor running, gradually drizzle in oil. Reserve 1 cup for the dressing.

3. To prepare salad: Transfer the remaining marinade to a large sealable plastic bag. Add chicken, seal and turn to coat. Marinate in the refrigerator for 20 minutes.

4. Lightly oil the grill rack (hold a piece of oil-soaked paper towel with tongs and rub it over the grate). Grill the chicken over medium-high

   heat until no longer pink in the center, 6 to 8 minutes per side. (Discard the marinade.)

5. Meanwhile, combine lettuce, apricot (or plum) wedges and chopped mint in a large bowl. Add the reserved dressing and toss to coat. Divide the salad among 4 plates. Slice the chicken and arrange over the salads. Sprinkle with almonds and serve.

TIPS & NOTES

- **Make Ahead Tip**: The dressing will keep, covered, in the refrigerator for up to 2 days.
- **Tip:** To toast almonds: Spread on a baking sheet and bake at 350°F until golden brown and fragrant, 5 to 7 minutes. Toasted almonds will keep, tightly covered, at room temperature for up to 1 week.

NUTRITION

Per serving: 456 calories; 20 g fat (3 g sat, 13 g mono); 66 mg cholesterol; 33 g carbohydrates; 34 gprotein; 10 g fiber; 433 mg sodium; 1281 mg potassium.

Nutrition Bonus: Vitamin A (230% daily value), Vitamin C (110% dv), Fiber (41% dv).

Carbohydrate Servings: 2

Exchanges: 1 fruit, 3 vegetable, 4 lean meat, 1fat (mono)

Fresh Tuna Salad with Tropical Fruits

INGREDIENTS

TUNA SALAD

- 3 tablespoons frozen pineapple juice concentrate
- 1/4 cup water
- 2 tablespoons reduced-sodium soy sauce
- 2 teaspoons honey
- 1/4 teaspoon freshly ground pepper
- 1 pound tuna steak (about 1 inch thick) (see Tips)
- 2 teaspoons extra-virgin olive oil
- 4 cups mixed salad greens
- 1 small head radicchio, cored and shredded (about 2 cups)
- 1 ripe mango, peeled and sliced (see Tips)
- 2 kiwis, peeled and cut into 8 pieces each

PINEAPPLE-MINT VINAIGRETTE

- 3 tablespoons frozen pineapple juice concentrate
- 1 1/2 tablespoons water
- 2 tablespoons cider vinegar
- 2 teaspoons chopped fresh mint
- 1/4 teaspoon salt
- 1/4 teaspoon ground pepper
- 1/4 cup extra-virgin olive oil

PREPARATION

1. To marinate tuna: Whisk 3 tablespoons pineapple juice concentrate, 1/4 cup water, soy sauce, honey and 1/4 teaspoon pepper in a small bowl. Place tuna steak in a shallow pan. Pour the

marinade over the tuna; turn to coat. Cover and marinate in the refrigerator for 45 minutes, turning twice.

2. To prepare the vinaigrette: Whisk pineapple juice concentrate, water, vinegar, mint, salt and pepper in a small bowl; slowly whisk in oil.

3. To cook the tuna: Remove tuna from the marinade and pat dry. Heat 2 teaspoons oil in a large skillet over medium heat. Add tuna; cook until browned and just opaque in the center, 4 to 6 minutes per side. Transfer tuna to a cutting board; let stand for 5 minutes.

4. To finish the salad: Combine greens, radicchio, mango and kiwis in a large bowl. Pour on 1/3 cup of the vinaigrette and toss to coat. Divide salad among 4 plates.

5. Cut tuna into 1/4-inch-thick slices. Top each salad with tuna and drizzle with the remaining vinaigrette. Serve immediately.

.TIPS & NOTES

- **Make Ahead Tip**: The greens and fruit can be tossed together (without the dressing) and stored under a barely moistened paper towel in the refrigerator for up to 3 hours.

- If you prefer your tuna medium-rare, as it is often served in restaurants, use sushi-grade (or sashimi) tuna, if you can find it, and cook it for about 3 minutes per side.

- **To peel and slice a mango:** Slice off both ends, revealing the long, slender seed inside. Set the fruit upright on a work surface and remove the skin with a sharp knife. With the seed perpendicular to you, slice the fruit from both sides of the seed, yielding two large pieces. Turn the seed parallel to you and slice the two smaller pieces of fruit from each side. Cut the fruit into slices.

NUTRITION

Per serving: 421 calories; 18 g fat (3 g sat, 14 g mono); 44 mg cholesterol; 36 g carbohydrates; 3 g added sugars; 30 g total sugars; 31 g protein; 4 g fiber; 486 mg sodium; 1141 mg potassium.

Nutrition Bonus: Vitamin C (140% daily value), Vitamin A (51% dv), Vitamin B12 (40% dv), Folate (34% dv), Potassium (33% dv), Magnesium (21% dv).

Carbohydrate Servings: 2 1/2

Exchanges: 2 fruit, 1 vegetable, 4 very lean protein, 3 1/2 fat

Pacific Sole with Oranges & Pecans

INGREDIENTS

- 1 orange
- 10 ounces Pacific sole, (see Note) or tilapia fillets
- 1/4 teaspoon salt
- 1/4 teaspoon freshly ground pepper
- 2 teaspoons unsalted butter
- 1 medium shallot, minced
- 2 tablespoons white-wine vinegar
- 2 tablespoons chopped pecans, toasted (see Cooking Tip)
- 2 tablespoons chopped fresh dill

PREPARATION

1. Using a sharp paring knife, remove the skin and white pith from orange. Hold the fruit over a medium bowl and cut between the membranes to release individual orange sections into the bowl, collecting any juice as well. Discard membranes, pith and skin.

2. Sprinkle both sides of fillets with salt and pepper. Coat a large nonstick skillet with cooking spray and place over medium heat. Add the fillets and cook 1 minute for sole or 3 minutes for tilapia. Gently flip and cook until the fish is opaque in the center and just cooked through, 1 to 2 minutes for sole or 3 to 5 minutes for tilapia. Divide between 2 serving plates; tent with foil to keep warm.

3. Add butter to the pan and melt over medium heat. Add shallot and cook, stirring, until soft, about 30 seconds. Add vinegar and the orange sections and juice; loosen any browned bits on the bottom of the pan and cook for 30 seconds. Spoon the sauce over the fish and sprinkle each portion with pecans and dill. Serve immediately. Makes 2 servings.

TIPS & NOTES

- **Ingredient Note:** The term "sole" is widely used for many types of flatfish from both the Atlantic and Pacific. Flounder and Atlantic halibut are included in the group that is often identified as sole or grey sole. The best choices are Pacific, Dover or English sole. Other sole and flounder are overfished.
- **Cooking Tip:** To toast chopped nuts or seeds: Cook in a small dry skillet over medium-low heat, stirring constantly, until fragrant and lightly browned, 2 to 4 minutes.

NUTRITION

Per serving: 234 calories; 9 g fat (3 g sat, 3 g mono); 70 mg cholesterol; 11 g carbohydrates; 0 g added sugars; 28 g protein; 2 g fiber; 401 mg sodium; 556 mg potassium.

Nutrition Bonus: Vitamin C (70% daily value); Calcium (20% dv).

Carbohydrate Servings: 1

Exchanges: 1 fruit, 4 very lean meat, 1 fat

Steamed Vegetable Ribbons

INGREDIENTS

- 2 large carrots, peeled
- 3 small zucchini
- 2 teaspoons extra-virgin olive oil
- 2 teaspoons lemon juice, or to taste
- 1/4 teaspoon salt, or to taste
- Freshly ground pepper, to taste

PREPARATION

1. With a swivel vegetable peeler, shave carrots lengthwise into wide ribbons. Repeat with zucchini, shaving long, wide strips from all sides until you reach the seedy core. Discard the core.

2. Bring 2 inches of water to a boil in a large saucepan fitted with a steamer basket. Add the carrots; cover and steam for 2 minutes. Place the zucchini over the carrots; cover and steam until the vegetables are just tender, 2 to 3 minutes more. Transfer the vegetables to a large bowl. Toss with oil, lemon juice, salt and pepper. Serve immediately.

NUTRITION

Per serving: 51 calories; 3 g fat (0 g sat, 2 g mono); 0 mg cholesterol; 7 g carbohydrates; 0 g added sugars; 1 g protein; 2 g fiber; 179 mg sodium; 350 mg potassium.

Nutrition Bonus: Vitamin A (90% daily value), Vitamin C (30% dv).

Carbohydrate Servings: 1/2

Exchanges: 11/2 vegetable, 1/2 fat (mono)

Roasted Broccoli with Lemon

INGREDIENTS

- 4 cups broccoli florets
- 1 tablespoon extra-virgin olive oil
- 1/4 teaspoon salt
- Freshly ground pepper
- Lemon wedges

PREPARATION

1. Preheat oven to 450°F.

2. Toss broccoli with oil, salt and pepper. Place on a large baking sheet (not air-insulated) and roast until the broccoli is tender and blackened on the bottom, 10 to 12 minutes. Serve immediately, with lemon wedges.

NUTRITION

Per serving: 54 calories; 4 g fat (1 g sat, 3 g mono); 0 mg cholesterol; 4 g carbohydrates; 0 g added sugars; 2 g protein; 2 g fiber; 165 mg sodium; 240 mg potassium.

Nutrition Bonus: Vitamin C (120% daily value), Vitamin A (45% dv).

Exchanges: 1 vegetable, 1 fat

DAY 16
BREAKFAST
Cocoa-Date Oatmeal
Skim milk (1 cup)
Melon (1 cup, cubes)
LUNCH
Skim milk (1 cup)
Five-Spice Chicken & Orange Salad or Buffalo Chicken Wrap
Apricot (1/2 cup, halves)
SNACK
Fat-free cheese (1 slice)
Whole-wheat breadsticks (1 8" stick)
DINNER
Pork Medallions with a Port-&-Cranberry Pan Sauce
Quick-cooking barley (1/2 cup)
Roasted Florets or Miso-Glazed Peas & Carrots
The Diet House Salad

DAY 16 RECIPES

Cocoa-Date Oatmeal

INGREDIENTS

- 1/4 cup chopped pitted dates, (10-12 dates)
- 1 cup old-fashioned rolled oats
- 2 tablespoons cocoa
- Pinch of salt
- 2 cups water

PREPARATION

1. Combine dates, oats, cocoa and salt in a 1-quart microwavable container. Slowly stir in the water. Partially cover with plastic wrap. Microwave on Medium for 4 or 5 minutes, then stir. Microwave on Medium again for 3 or 4 minutes, then stir. Continue cooking and stirring until the cereal is creamy.

TIPS & NOTES

- **Note:** The cooking times will vary considerably depending on the power of your microwave. New microwaves tend to cook much faster than older models.

NUTRITION

Per serving: 142 calories; 4 g fat (1 g sat, 1 g mono); 0 mg cholesterol; 61 g carbohydrates; 0 g added sugars; 8 g protein; 9 g fiber; 81 mg sodium; 497 mg potassium.

Nutrition Bonus: Fiber (16% daily value).

Carbohydrate Servings: 2

Exchanges: 11/2 starch, 1/2 fruit

Nutrition Note: Chocolate contains compounds called flavonoids, which can function as antioxidants and also seem to keep blood from clotting. Cocoa is unusually rich in two kinds of flavonoids, flavonols and proanthocyanidins, which appear to be especially potent.

Five-Spice Chicken & Orange Salad

INGREDIENTS

- 6 teaspoons extra-virgin olive oil, divided
- 1 teaspoon five-spice powder, (see Note)
- 1 teaspoon kosher salt, divided
- 1/2 teaspoon freshly ground pepper, plus more to taste
- 1 pound boneless, skinless chicken breasts, trimmed
- 3 oranges

- 12 cups mixed Asian or salad greens
- 1 red bell pepper, cut into thin strips
- 1/2 cup slivered red onion
- 3 tablespoons cider vinegar
- 1 tablespoon Dijon mustard

PREPARATION

1. Preheat oven to 450°F. Combine 1 teaspoon oil, five-spice powder, 1/2 teaspoon salt and 1/2 teaspoon pepper in a small bowl. Rub the mixture into both sides of the chicken breasts.

2. Heat 1 teaspoon oil in a large ovenproof nonstick skillet over medium-high heat. Add chicken breasts; cook until browned on one side, 3 to 5 minutes. Turn them over and transfer the pan to the oven. Roast until the chicken is just cooked through (an instant-read thermometer inserted into the center should read 165°F), 6 to 8 minutes. Transfer the chicken to a cutting board; let rest for 5 minutes.

3. Meanwhile, peel and segment two of the oranges (see Tip), collecting segments and any juice in a large bowl. (Discard membranes, pith and skin.) Add the greens, bell pepper and onion to the bowl. Zest and juice the remaining orange. Place the zest and juice in a small bowl; whisk in vinegar, mustard, the remaining 4 teaspoons oil, remaining 1/2 teaspoon salt and freshly ground pepper to taste. Pour the dressing over the salad; toss to combine. Slice the chicken and serve on the salad.

TIPS & NOTES

- **Make Ahead Tip**: Prepare through Step 2. Store the chicken in an airtight container in the refrigerator for up to 2 days. Slice and serve chilled.
- **Note:** Often a blend of cinnamon, cloves, fennel seed, star anise and Szechuan peppercorns, five-spice powder was originally considered a cure-all miracle blend encompassing the five elements (sour, bitter, sweet, pungent, salty). Look for it in the supermarket spice section.

- **Tip:** To segment citrus: With a sharp knife, remove the skin and white pith from the fruit. Working over a bowl, cut the segments from their surrounding membranes. Squeeze juice into the bowl before discarding the membranes.

NUTRITION

Per serving: 278 calories; 10 g fat (2 g sat, 6 g mono); 63 mg cholesterol; 23 g carbohydrates; 0 g added sugars; 26 g protein; 7 g fiber; 491 mg sodium; 450 mg potassium.

Nutrition Bonus: Vitamin C (170% daily value), Vitamin A (140% dv), Selenium (30% dv), Iron (15% dv).

Carbohydrate Servings: 1

Exchanges: 1 fruit, 1 1/2 vegetable, 3 lean meat, 1 1/2 fat

Buffalo Chicken Wrap

INGREDIENTS

- 2 tablespoons hot pepper sauce, such as Frank's RedHot
- 3 tablespoons white vinegar, divided
- 1/4 teaspoon cayenne pepper
- 2 teaspoons extra-virgin olive oil
- 1 pound chicken tenders
- 2 tablespoons reduced-fat mayonnaise
- 2 tablespoons nonfat plain yogurt
- Freshly ground pepper, to taste
- 1/4 cup crumbled blue cheese
- 4 8-inch whole-wheat tortillas
- 1 cup shredded romaine lettuce
- 1 cup sliced celery
- 1 large tomato, diced

PREPARATION

1. Whisk hot pepper sauce, 2 tablespoons vinegar and cayenne pepper in a medium bowl.

2. Heat oil in a large nonstick skillet over medium-high heat. Add chicken tenders; cook until cooked through and no longer pink in

   the middle, 3 to 4 minutes per side. Add to the bowl with the hot sauce; toss to coat well.

3. Whisk mayonnaise, yogurt, pepper and the remaining 1 tablespoon vinegar in a small bowl. Stir in blue cheese.

4. To assemble wraps: Lay a tortilla on a work surface or plate. Spread with 1 tablespoon blue cheese sauce and top with one-fourth of the chicken, lettuce, celery and tomato. Drizzle with some of the hot sauce remaining in the bowl and roll into a wrap sandwich. Repeat with the remaining tortillas.

TIPS & NOTES

- Eat neat: Keeping the filling inside a wrap or burrito can be a challenge, especially if you're on the go. That's why we recommend wrapping your burrito in foil so you can pick it up and eat it without losing the filling, peeling back the foil as you go.

NUTRITION

Per serving: 275 calories; 8 g fat (2 g sat, 2 g mono); 55 mg cholesterol; 29 g carbohydrates; 24 g protein; 3 g fiber; 756 mg sodium; 266 mg potassium.

Nutrition Bonus: Vitamin A (35% daily value), Selenium (28% dv), Vitamin C (20% dv).

Carbohydrate Servings: 2

Exchanges: 1 1/2 starch, 1 vegetable, 3 very lean meat, 1/2 fat

Pork Medallions with a Port-&-Cranberry Pan Sauce

INGREDIENTS

- 1/4 cup dried cranberries
- 1/4 cup port
- 1 pound pork tenderloin, trimmed
- Salt & freshly ground pepper to taste
- 1 teaspoon extra-virgin olive oil
- 2 cloves cloves garlic, peeled and halved
- 1 teaspoon balsamic vinegar
- 2 sage leaves
- 1/2 cup reduced-sodium chicken broth

PREPARATION

1. Combine cranberries and port in a small bowl. Set aside. Slice tenderloin into medallions 1 1/2 inches thick. Place between 2 layers of plastic wrap, and pound the medallions with the bottom of a saucepan until they are 1/2 inch thick. Season both sides with salt and pepper.

2. Heat oil in a nonstick skillet over medium-high heat. Sear medallions on one side until golden brown, 2 to 3 minutes. Turn and sear on the other side for 4 to 5 minutes; turn medallions again and continue cooking until golden brown and no longer pink in the center, 2 to 3 minutes. Remove to a serving platter and cover loosely to keep warm.

3. Add garlic to the pan and return to medium-high heat. Cook, stirring, 1 minute. Add port with cranberries, vinegar and sage leaves; cook for 1 minute, scraping skillet for browned bits. Pour in broth, swirl the pan and bring to a boil again. Continue cooking until sauce thickens and is reduced

4. by half, about 3 minutes. Remove the garlic and sage. Season the sauce to taste with salt and pepper. Spoon over the pork and serve.

NUTRITION

Per serving: 194 calories; 5 g fat (2 g sat, 2 g mono); 64 mg cholesterol; 9 g carbohydrates; 0 g added sugars; 23 g protein; 0 g fiber; 137 mg sodium; 370 mg potassium.

Nutrition Bonus: Selenium (55% daily value).

Carbohydrate Servings: 1/2

Exchanges: 1/2 fruit, 4 1/2 lean meat

Roasted Florets

INGREDIENTS

- 8 cups bite-size cauliflower florets, or broccoli florets (about 1 head), sliced
- 2 tablespoons extra-virgin olive oil
- 1/2 teaspoon salt, or to taste
- Freshly ground pepper, to taste
- Lemon wedges, (optional)

PREPARATION

Preheat oven to 450°F. Place florets in a large bowl with oil, salt and pepper and toss to coat. Spread out on a baking sheet. Roast the vegetables, stirring once, until tender-crisp and browned in spots, 15 to 25 minutes. Serve hot or warm with lemon wedges, if desired.

NUTRITION

Per serving (cauliflower): 113 calories; 7 g fat (1 g sat, 5 g mono); 0 mg cholesterol; 7 g carbohydrates; 4 g protein; 4 g fiber; 327 mg sodium; 433 mg potassium.

Carbohydrate Servings: 1/2

Exchanges: 2 vegetable, 11/2 fat (mono)

Nutrition Note: Per serving (broccoli): 101 calories; 7 g fat (1 g sat, 5 g mono); 0 mg cholesterol; 7 g carbohydrate; 4 g protein; 4 g fiber; 327 mg sodium.

Miso-Glazed Peas & Carrots

INGREDIENTS

- 3 tablespoons miso, preferably white (see Ingredient note)
- 1 tablespoon mirin
- 2 tablespoons rice vinegar
- 1 teaspoon minced fresh ginger
- 1 teaspoon toasted sesame oil
- 2 cups thinly sliced carrots, fresh or frozen
- 1/4 cup water
- 2 cups frozen peas, (8 ounces)

PREPARATION

1. Combine miso, mirin, vinegar, ginger and oil in a small bowl. Place carrots and water in a large nonstick skillet over medium-high heat; cover and cook, stirring occasionally, until tender-crisp, about 5 minutes. Stir in the miso mixture and peas; cook, stirring occasionally, until the peas are heated through and the sauce is slightly thickened, about 3 minutes.

TIPS & NOTES

- **Ingredient Note:** Miso: Fermented bean paste made from barley, rice or soybeans used in Japanese cooking to add flavor to dishes, such as soups, sauces and salad dressings. Miso is available in different colors; in general, the lighter the color, the more mild the flavor. Look for miso alongside the refrigerated tofu in the supermarket. It will keep, in the refrigerator, for more than a year.

NUTRITION

Per serving: 120 calories; 2 g fat (0 g sat, 1 g mono); 0 mg cholesterol; 20 g carbohydrates; 0 g added sugars; 4 g protein; 5 g fiber; 397 mg sodium; 281 mg potassium.

Nutrition Bonus: Vitamin A (180% daily value), Vitamin C (15% dv).

Carbohydrate Servings: 1

Exchanges: 1 starch, 1 vegetable

The Diet House Salad

INGREDIENTS

- 4 cups torn green leaf lettuce
- 1 cup sprouts
- 1 cup tomato wedges
- 1 cup peeled, sliced cucumber
- 1 cup shredded carrots
- 1/2 cup chopped radishes
- 1/2 cup Sesame Tamari Vinaigrette (recipe follows), or other dressing

PREPARATION

Toss lettuce, sprouts, tomato, cucumber, carrots and radishes in a large bowl with the dressing until the vegetables are coated.

NUTRITION

Per serving: 71 calories; 3 g fat (0 g sat, 1 g mono); 0 mg cholesterol; 11 g carbohydrates; 2 g protein; 3 g fiber; 334 mg sodium; 428 mg potassium.

Nutrition Bonus: Vitamin A (140% daily value), Vitamin C (30% dv), Folate (16% dv).

Carbohydrate Servings: 1

Exchanges: 2 vegetable, 1/2 fat

DAY 17

BREAKFAST

Greek Potato & Feta Omelet
Strawberries (1 cup)

LUNCH

Quesadillas con Frijoles Refritosor Irish Lamb Stew
Skim milk (1 cup)

SNACK

Low-fat cottage cheese (1/2 cup)
Nectarine (1 small)

DINNER

Chicken Tabbouleh
Sliced Tomato Salad or Rainbow Pepper Saute
Hawaiian Smoothie

DAY 17 RECIPES

Greek Potato & Feta Omelet

INGREDIENTS
- 2 teaspoons extra-virgin olive oil, divided
- 1 cup frozen hash brown potatoes, or cooked potatoes cut into 1/2-inch cubes
- 1/3 cup chopped scallions
- 4 large eggs
- 1/8 teaspoon salt
- Freshly ground pepper to taste
- 1/4 cup crumbled feta cheese

PREPARATION
1. Heat 1 teaspoon oil in a medium nonstick skillet over medium-high heat. Add potatoes and cook, shaking the pan and tossing the potatoes, until golden brown, 4 to 5 minutes. Add scallions and cook for 1 minute longer. Transfer to a plate. Wipe out the pan.
2. Blend eggs, salt and pepper in a medium bowl. Stir in feta and the potato mixture.
3. Preheat broiler. Brush the pan with the remaining 1 teaspoon oil; heat over medium heat. Add the egg mixture and tilt to distribute evenly. Reduce heat to medium-low and cook until the bottom is light golden, lifting the the edges to allow uncooked egg to flow underneath, 3 to 4 minutes. Place the pan under the broiler and cook until the top is set, 1 1/2 to 2 1/2 minutes. Slide the omelet onto a plate and cut into wedges.

NUTRITION
Per serving: 294 calories; 17 g fat (5 g sat, 7 g mono); 380 mg cholesterol; 18 g carbohydrates; 16 gprotein; 3 g fiber; 433 mg sodium; 442 mg potassium.
Nutrition Bonus: Vitamin A (15% daily value), Vitamin C (15% dv).
Carbohydrate Servings: 1
Exchanges: 1 starch; 2 medium-fat meat; 1 1/2 fat (mono)

Quesadillas con Frijoles Refritos

INGREDIENTS
- 1 cup fat-free refried beans
- 2 tablespoons hot salsa, plus more for dipping
- 12 6-inch corn tortillas
- 1 cup frozen corn, thawed
- 1/3 cup chopped fresh cilantro
- 1/3 cup chopped scallions
- 3/4 cup finely grated Monterey Jack cheese, (3 ounces)

PREPARATION
1. Preheat oven to 400°F. Line a baking sheet with foil.
2. Combine refried beans and 2 tablespoons salsa in a small bowl.
3. Place a tortilla directly on a stovetop burner (gas or electric), set at medium, and toast, turning frequently with tongs, until softened, about 30 seconds. Wrap in a kitchen towel to keep warm while you soften the remaining tortillas in the same manner.
4. Lay 6 of the softened tortillas on the prepared baking sheet. Divide the bean mixture among these tortillas, spreading evenly. Sprinkle each with corn, cilantro and scallions, then cheese. Top with the remaining softened tortillas and press to seal.
5. Bake until lightly crisped and browned, about 10 minutes. Cut each quesadilla into 4 wedges. Serve hot, with additional salsa for dipping.

NUTRITION
Per serving: 224 calories; 6 g fat (3 g sat, 2 g mono); 13 mg cholesterol; 35 g carbohydrates; 0 g added sugars; 10 g protein; 6 g fiber; 285 mg sodium; 169 mg potassium.
Carbohydrate Servings: 2
Exchanges: 2 1/2 starch, 1/2 high-fat meat

Irish Lamb Stew

INGREDIENTS

- 2 pounds boneless leg of lamb, trimmed and cut into 1-inch pieces
- 1 3/4 pounds white potatoes, peeled and cut into 1-inch pieces
- 3 large leeks, white part only, halved, washed (see Tip) and thinly sliced
- 3 large carrots, peeled and cut into 1-inch pieces
- 3 stalks celery, thinly sliced
- 1 14-ounce can reduced-sodium chicken broth
- 2 teaspoons chopped fresh thyme
- 1 teaspoon salt
- 1 teaspoon freshly ground pepper
- 1/4 cup packed fresh parsley leaves, chopped

PREPARATION

1. Combine lamb, potatoes, leeks, carrots, celery, broth, thyme, salt and pepper in a 6-quart slow cooker; stir to combine. Put the lid on and cook on low until the lamb is fork-tender, about 8 hours. Stir in parsley before serving.

TIPS & NOTES

- **Make Ahead Tip**: Cover and refrigerate for up to 2 days or freeze for up to 1 month. | Equipment: 6-quart slow cooker
- To clean leeks, trim and discard green tops and white roots. Split leeks lengthwise and place in plenty of water. Swish the leeks in the water to release any sand or soil. Drain. Repeat until no grit remains.
- For easy cleanup, try a slow-cooker liner. These heat-resistant, disposable liners fit neatly inside the insert and help prevent food from sticking to the bottom and sides of your slow cooker.

NUTRITION

Per serving: 266 calories; 7 g fat (2 g sat, 3 g mono); 65 mg cholesterol; 27 g carbohydrates; 0 g added sugars; 23 g protein; 4 g fiber; 427 mg sodium; 803 mg potassium.
Nutrition Bonus: Vitamin A (139% daily value), Vitamin C (26% dv), Potassium (23% dv), Folate & Iron (15% dv).
Carbohydrate Servings: 1 1/2
Exchanges: 1 starch, 2 vegetable, 2 lean meat

Chicken Tabbouleh

INGREDIENTS
- 3 cups water
- 1 cup bulgur
- 3 cups cubed skinless cooked chicken, (1-inch cubes)
- 1 cup chopped fresh parsley
- 1 cup chopped scallions
- 1/3 cup currants
- 1/4 cup frozen orange juice concentrate
- 2 tablespoons lemon juice
- 1 tablespoon extra-virgin olive oil
- 1 teaspoon ground cumin
- 1/4 teaspoon cayenne pepper, or to taste
- 1/4 teaspoon salt
- Freshly ground pepper, to taste

PREPARATION

1. Bring water to a boil in a large saucepan. Add bulgur and remove from the heat. Let stand until most of the water is absorbed, 20 to 30 minutes.
2. Drain bulgur well, squeezing out excess moisture. Transfer to a large bowl. Add chicken, parsley, scallions and currants.
3. Whisk orange juice concentrate, lemon juice, oil, cumin and cayenne in a small bowl until blended. Toss with the bulgur mixture. Season with salt and pepper and serve.

TIPS & NOTES
- **To poach chicken breasts:** Place boneless, skinless chicken breasts in a medium skillet or saucepan and add lightly salted water to cover; bring to a boil. Cover, reduce heat to low and simmer gently until chicken is cooked through and no longer pink in the middle, 10 to 12 minutes.
- **Ingredient note:** Bulgur is made by parboiling, drying and coarsely grinding or cracking wheat berries. Don't confuse bulgur with cracked wheat, which is simply that—cracked wheat. Since the parboiling step is skipped, cracked wheat must be cooked for up to an hour whereas bulgur simply needs a quick soak in hot water for most uses. Look for it in the natural-foods section of large supermarkets, near other grains, or online at kalustyans.com, lebaneseproducts.com.

NUTRITION
Per serving: 260 calories; 5 g fat (1 g sat, 3 g mono); 60 mg cholesterol; 31 g carbohydrates; 0 g added sugars; 26 g protein; 6 g fiber; 166 mg sodium; 536 mg potassium.

Nutrition Bonus: Vitamin C (60% daily value), Fiber (24% dv), Potassium (15% dv).
Carbohydrate Servings: 1 1/2
Exchanges: 2 starch, 3 very lean meat

Sliced Tomato Salad

INGREDIENTS
- 4 tomatoes, sliced
- 1/4 cup thinly sliced red onion
- 8 anchovies
- 1/2 teaspoon dried oregano
- Salt & freshly ground pepper, to taste
- 2 tablespoons extra-virgin olive oil
- 1 tablespoon white-wine vinegar

PREPARATION
1. Arrange tomato slices on a platter. Top with onion, anchovies, oregano, salt and pepper. Drizzle with oil and vinegar.

NUTRITION

Per serving: 44 calories; 1 g fat (0 g sat, 0 g mono); 3 mg cholesterol; 8 g carbohydrates; 0 g added sugars;3 g protein; 2 g fiber; 300 mg sodium; 403 mg potassium.
Nutrition Bonus: Vitamin C (35% daily value), Vitamin A (25% dv).
Carbohydrate Servings: 1/2
Exchanges: 1 vegetable, 1 1/2 fat

Rainbow Pepper Saute

INGREDIENTS
- 2 tablespoons extra-virgin olive oil
- 2 medium onions, chopped
- 6 red, yellow and/or orange bell peppers, seeded and cut into 2-inch slivers
- 1 teaspoon dried oregano
- 1/4 teaspoon salt, or to taste
- Freshly ground pepper, to taste

PREPARATION
1. Heat oil in a large nonstick skillet over medium heat. Add onions and cook, stirring often, until softened, 3 to 5 minutes. Add peppers; cook, stirring occasionally, until softened, 7 to 10 minutes. Stir in oregano, salt and pepper; cover. Cook, stirring occasionally and adjusting the heat as necessary so the

mixture doesn't burn, until the peppers are very tender, 15 to 20 minutes. Serve warm or at room temperature.

TIPS & NOTES
- **Make Ahead Tip**: Cover and refrigerate for up to 4 days.

NUTRITION

Per serving: 47 calories; 2 g fat (0 g sat, 2 g mono); 0 mg cholesterol; 6 g carbohydrates; 0 g added sugars;1 g protein; 1 g fiber; 51 mg sodium; 168 mg potassium.
Nutrition Bonus: Vitamin C (190% daily value), Vitamin A (20% dv).
Carbohydrate Servings: 1/2
Exchanges: 1 vegetable

Hawaiian Smoothie

INGREDIENTS
- 1 cup chopped fresh pineapple
- 1/2 cup chopped peeled papaya
- 1/4 cup guava nectar, (see Ingredient Note)
- 1 tablespoon lime juice
- 1 teaspoon grenadine, (see Ingredient Note)
- 1/2 cup ice

PREPARATION
1. Place ingredients in the order listed in a blender. Pulse three times to chop the fruit, then blend until smooth. Serve immediately.

TIPS & NOTES
- **Ingredient Notes:** Grenadine is a red syrup (originally flavored with pomegranate juice) used to color and flavor drinks. Look for it in the bar-mix section of your supermarket.
- Guava nectar is available in most markets, with the juices or in the Latin American section.

NUTRITION

Per serving: 81 calories; 0 g fat (0 g sat, 0 g mono); 0 mg cholesterol; 21 g carbohydrates; 1 g protein; 2 gfiber; 5 mg sodium; 201 mg potassium.
Nutrition Bonus: Vitamin C (100% daily value).
Carbohydrate Servings: 1 1/2
Exchanges: 1 1/2 fruit

DAY 18
BREAKFAST
Overnight Oatmeal
Skim milk (1 cup)
Grapefruit (1/2)
LUNCH
Five-Spice Chicken & Orange Salad or Tomato, Tuna & Tarragon Salad
Whole-wheat pita bread (1/2 medium pita)
SNACK
Blueberries (1 cup)
Nonfat plain yogurt (8 oz.)
DINNER
Slow-Cooker Turkish Lamb & Vegetable Stew or Roasted Chicken Tenders with Peppers & Onions
Mexican Coleslaw
Brown rice (1/2 cup, cooked)

DAY 18 RECIPES

Overnight Oatmeal

INGREDIENTS
- 8 cups water
- 2 cups steel-cut oats, (see Ingredient note)
- 1/3 cup dried cranberries
- 1/3 cup dried apricots, chopped
- 1/4 teaspoon salt, or to taste

PREPARATION
1. Combine water, oats, dried cranberries, dried apricots and salt in a 5- or 6-quart slow cooker. Turn heat to low. Put the lid on and cook until the oats are tender and the porridge is creamy, 7 to 8 hours. Stovetop Variation Halve the above recipe to accommodate the size of most double boilers: Combine 4 cups water, 1 cup steel-cut oats, 3 tablespoons dried cranberries, 3 tablespoons dried apricots and 1/8 teaspoon salt in the top of a double boiler. Cover and cook over boiling water for about 1 1/2 hours, checking the water level in the bottom of the double boiler from time to time.

TIPS & NOTES
- **Ingredient Note:** Steel-cut oats, sometimes labeled "Irish oatmeal," look like small pebbles. They are toasted oat groatsfor which the oat kernel that has been

removed from the husk that have been cut in 2 or 3 pieces. Do not substitute regular rolled oats, which have a shorter cooking time, in the slow-cooker oatmeal recipe.
- For easy cleanup, try a slow-cooker liner. These heat-resistant, disposable liners fit neatly inside the insert and help prevent food from sticking to the bottom and sides of your slow cooker.

NUTRITION
Per serving: 193 calories; 3 g fat (0 g sat, 1 g mono); 0 mg cholesterol; 34 g carbohydrates; 0 g added sugars; 6 g protein; 9 g fiber; 77 mg sodium; 195 mg potassium.
Nutrition Bonus: Fiber (36% daily value).
Carbohydrate Servings: 2
Exchanges: 2 starch, 1/2 fruit

Five-Spice Chicken & Orange Salad

INGREDIENTS
- 6 teaspoons extra-virgin olive oil, divided
- 1 teaspoon five-spice powder, (see Note)
- 1 teaspoon kosher salt, divided
- 1/2 teaspoon freshly ground pepper, plus more to taste
- 1 pound boneless, skinless chicken breasts, trimmed
- 3 oranges
- 12 cups mixed Asian or salad greens
- 1 red bell pepper, cut into thin strips
- 1/2 cup slivered red onion
- 3 tablespoons cider vinegar
- 1 tablespoon Dijon mustard
-

PREPARATION
1. Preheat oven to 450°F. Combine 1 teaspoon oil, five-spice powder, 1/2 teaspoon salt and 1/2 teaspoon pepper in a small bowl. Rub the mixture into both sides of the chicken breasts.
2. Heat 1 teaspoon oil in a large ovenproof nonstick skillet over medium-high heat. Add chicken breasts; cook until browned on one side, 3 to 5 minutes. Turn them over and transfer the pan to the oven. Roast until the chicken is just cooked through (an instant-read thermometer inserted into the center should read 165°F), 6 to 8 minutes. Transfer the chicken to a cutting board; let rest for 5 minutes.

3. Meanwhile, peel and segment two of the oranges (see Tip), collecting segments and any juice in a large bowl. (Discard membranes, pith and skin.) Add the greens, bell pepper and onion to the bowl. Zest and juice the remaining orange. Place the zest and juice in a small bowl; whisk in vinegar, mustard, the remaining 4 teaspoons oil, remaining 1/2 teaspoon salt and freshly ground pepper to taste. Pour the dressing over the salad; toss to combine. Slice the chicken and serve on the salad.

TIPS & NOTES
- **Make Ahead Tip**: Prepare through Step 2. Store the chicken in an airtight container in the refrigerator for up to 2 days. Slice and serve chilled.
- **Note:** Often a blend of cinnamon, cloves, fennel seed, star anise and Szechuan peppercorns, five-spice powder was originally considered a cure-all miracle blend encompassing the five elements (sour, bitter, sweet, pungent, salty). Look for it in the supermarket spice section.
- **Tip:** To segment citrus: With a sharp knife, remove the skin and white pith from the fruit. Working over a bowl, cut the segments from their surrounding membranes. Squeeze juice into the bowl before discarding the membranes.

NUTRITION
Per serving: 278 calories; 10 g fat (2 g sat, 6 g mono); 63 mg cholesterol; 23 g carbohydrates; 0 g added sugars; 26 g protein; 7 g fiber; 491 mg sodium; 450 mg potassium.
Nutrition Bonus: Vitamin C (170% daily value), Vitamin A (140% dv), Selenium (30% dv), Iron (15% dv).
Carbohydrate Servings: 1
Exchanges: 1 fruit, 1 1/2 vegetable, 3 lean meat, 1 1/2 fat

Tomato, Tuna & Tarragon Salad

INGREDIENTS
- 1/2 cup diced red onion
- 1/3 cup reduced-fat mayonnaise
- 1/4 teaspoon kosher salt
- Freshly ground pepper to taste
- 2 6-ounce cans chunk light tuna in olive oil, drained (see Note)
- 2 stalks celery, thinly sliced (about 1 cup)
- 1/4 cup packed coarsely chopped fresh tarragon leaves
- 8 cups torn lettuce, or mixed greens
- 1 pound small ripe tomatoes, cut into wedges
- 1 lemon, cut into 8 wedges

PREPARATION
1. Place onion in a small bowl and cover with cold water. Refrigerate for 20 minutes. Drain.
2. Whisk mayonnaise, salt and pepper in a medium bowl. Add tuna, celery, tarragon and onion; stir to combine. Serve on top of the lettuce (or mixed greens) with tomato and lemon wedges.

TIPS & NOTES
- **Make Ahead Tip**: Store in an airtight container in the refrigerator for up to 1 day.
- **Note:** Chunk light tuna, which comes from the smaller skipjack or yellowfin, has less mercury than canned white albacore tuna. The FDA/EPA advises that women who are or might become pregnant, nursing mothers and young children consume no more than 6 ounces of albacore a week; up to 12 ounces of canned light tuna is considered safe.

NUTRITION
Per serving: 259 calories; 10 g fat (2 g sat, 3 g mono); 15 mg cholesterol; 15 g carbohydrates; 28 g protein; 3 g fiber; 667 mg sodium; 731 mg potassium.
Nutrition Bonus: Vitamin C (50% daily value), Vitamin A (30% dv), Potassium (20% dv).
Carbohydrate Servings: 1
Exchanges: 3 vegetable, 3 lean meat

Slow-Cooker Turkish Lamb & Vegetable Stew

INGREDIENTS
- 1 1/2 pounds lean boneless leg of lamb, trimmed and cut into 1 1/4-inch pieces
- 1 1/4 teaspoons salt, divided
- Freshly ground pepper, to taste
- 1 1/2 tablespoons extra-virgin olive oil, divided
- 2 large onions, thinly sliced
- 4 cloves garlic, minced
- 1/2 teaspoon dried oregano
- 1 14-ounce can diced tomatoes
- 1 large all-purpose potato, preferably Yukon Gold, peeled and cut into 3/8-inch-thick slices
- 1/2 pound green beans, trimmed
- 1 small eggplant, cut into 3/8-inch-thick slices
- 1 medium zucchini, cut into 3/8-inch-thick slices
- 6 bay leaves
- 3 tablespoons chopped fresh parsley

PREPARATION
1. Season lamb with 1/4 teaspoon salt and pepper to taste. Heat 1/2 tablespoon oil in a large heavy skillet over medium-high heat. Add half the lamb and sear, turning, until well browned, 2 to 4 minutes. Transfer to a 4-quart slow cooker. Add another 1/2 tablespoon oil to skillet and brown remaining lamb. Add to slow cooker.
2. Add remaining 1/2 tablespoon oil to skillet and reduce heat to medium. Add onions and cook, stirring, until softened, 3 to 5 minutes. Add garlic and oregano; cook, stirring, for 1 minute more. Add tomatoes and bring to a simmer, mashing with a potato masher or fork. Remove from heat and spoon half the mixture over the lamb.
3. Arrange potatoes in a layer in the pot; season with 1/4 teaspoon salt and pepper to taste. Add green beans, followed by eggplant and zucchini, seasoning each layer with 1/4 teaspoon salt and pepper to taste. Spread remaining tomato-onion mixture over vegetables. Top with bay leaves.
4. Cover and cook on high until lamb and vegetables are very tender, about 4 hours. Discard bay leaves. Serve hot, garnished with parsley.

TIPS & NOTES
- **Make Ahead Tip**: Cover and refrigerate for up to 2 days. Reheat on the stovetop, in a microwave or in the oven.
- Lamb cut from the leg is 19 percent leaner than shoulder meat.
- For easy cleanup, try a slow-cooker liner. These heat-resistant, disposable liners fit neatly inside the insert and help prevent food from sticking to the bottom and sides of your slow cooker.

NUTRITION
Per serving: 179 calories; 7 g fat (2 g sat, 4 g mono); 53 mg cholesterol; 15 g carbohydrates; 0 g added sugars; 17 g protein; 5 g fiber; 466 mg sodium; 554 mg potassium.
Nutrition Bonus: Iron (40% daily value), Potassium (37% dv), Iron (15% dv).
Carbohydrate Servings: 1
Exchanges: 2 vegetable, 2 1/2 lean meat

Roasted Chicken Tenders with Peppers & Onions

INGREDIENTS
- 1/2 teaspoon freshly grated lemon zest
- 3 tablespoons lemon juice
- 2 tablespoons finely chopped garlic
- 2 tablespoons finely chopped fresh oregano, or 1 teaspoon dried
- 2 tablespoons finely chopped pickled jalapeno peppers
- 2 tablespoons extra-virgin olive oil

- 1/2 teaspoon salt
- 1 pound chicken tenders
- 1 red, yellow or orange bell pepper, seeded and thinly sliced
- 1/2 medium onion, thinly sliced

PREPARATION
1. Preheat oven to 425°F. Whisk lemon zest, lemon juice, garlic, oregano, jalapenos, oil and salt in a 9-by-13-inch glass baking dish. Add tenders, bell pepper and onion; toss to coat. Spread the mixture out evenly; cover with foil. Bake until the chicken is cooked through and no longer pink in the middle, 25 to 30 minutes.

NUTRITION
Per serving: 172 calories; 7 g fat (1 g sat, 5 g mono); 49 mg cholesterol; 6 g carbohydrates; 0 g added sugars; 19 g protein; 1 g fiber; 518 mg sodium; 122 mg potassium.
Nutrition Bonus: Vitamin C (100% daily value), Selenium (28% dv), Vitamin A (20% dv).
Carbohydrate Servings: 1/2
Exchanges: 1/2 vegetable, 3 very lean meats, 1 1/2 fat

Mexican Coleslaw

INGREDIENTS
- 6 cups very thinly sliced green cabbage, (about 1/2 head) (see Tip)
- 1 1/2 cups peeled and grated carrots, (2-3 medium)
- 1/3 cup chopped cilantro
- 1/4 cup rice vinegar
- 2 tablespoons extra-virgin olive oil
- 1/4 teaspoon salt

PREPARATION
1. Place cabbage and carrots in a colander; rinse thoroughly with cold water to crisp. Let drain for 5 minutes.
2. Meanwhile, whisk cilantro, vinegar, oil and salt in a large bowl. Add cabbage and carrots; toss well to coat.

TIPS & NOTES
- **Make Ahead Tip**: Cover and refrigerate for up to 1 day. Toss again to refresh just before serving.
- **Tip:** To make this coleslaw even faster, use a coleslaw mix containing cabbage and carrots from the produce section of the supermarket.

NUTRITION
Per serving: 53 calories; 4 g fat (1 g sat, 3 g mono); 0 mg cholesterol; 5 g carbohydrates; 0 g added sugars;1 g protein; 2 g fiber; 97 mg sodium; 199 mg potassium.
Nutrition Bonus: Vitamin A (50% daily value), Vitamin C (30% dv), phytochemicals sulforaphane and indoles.
Exchanges: 1 vegetable, 1/2 fat (mono

DAY 19
BREAKFAST

Tofu Scrambled Egg
Skim milk (1 cup)
Strawberries (1 cup)
LUNCH

Turkey & Balsamic Onion Quesadillas
Roasted Corn, Black Bean & Mango Salad or Roasted Savoy Cabbage with Black Bean-Garlic Sauce
SNACK

Fat-free cheese (1 slice)
Melon (1/2 cup, cubes)
DINNER

Salmon on a Bed of Lentils or Grandma Ginger's Fish Casserole
Shredded Brussels Sprouts with Bacon & Onions
Vegetable Stir-Fry
Melon (1/2 cup)

DAY 19 RECIPES

Tofu Scrambled Egg

INGREDIENTS
- 1 large egg
- 1/2 teaspoon dried tarragon
- Dash of hot sauce, such as
- Pinch of salt
- Freshly ground pepper, to taste
- 1 teaspoon extra-virgin olive oil, or canola oil
- 2 tablespoons crumbled tofu, (silken or regular)

PREPARATION
1. Blend egg, tarragon, hot sauce, salt and pepper in a small bowl with a fork. Heat oil in a small nonstick skillet over medium-low heat. Add tofu and cook, stirring, until warmed through, 20 to 30 seconds. Add egg mixture and stir until the egg is set, but still creamy, 20 to 30 seconds. Serve immediately.

NUTRITION

Per serving: 140 calories; 11 g fat (2 g sat, 6 g mono); 212 mg cholesterol; 2 g carbohydrates; 0 g added sugars; 9 g protein; 1 g fiber; 230 mg sodium; 93 mg potassium.
Nutrition Bonus: Selenium (23% daily value).
Exchanges: 1 medium-fat meat. 1 fat (mono)

Turkey & Balsamic Onion Quesadillas

INGREDIENTS
- 1 small red onion, thinly sliced
- 1/4 cup balsamic vinegar
- 4 10-inch whole-wheat tortillas
- 1 cup shredded sharp Cheddar cheese
- 8 slices deli turkey, preferably smoked (8 ounces)

PREPARATION
1. Combine onion and vinegar in a bowl; let marinate for 5 minutes. Drain, reserving the vinegar for another use, such as salad dressing.
2. Warm 2 tortillas in a large nonstick skillet over medium-high heat for about 45 seconds, then flip. Pull the tortillas up the edges of the pan so they are no longer overlapping. Working on one half of each tortilla, sprinkle one-fourth of the cheese, cover with 2 slices of turkey and top with one-fourth of the onion. Fold the tortillas in half, flatten gently with a spatula and cook until the cheese starts to melt, about 2 minutes. Flip and cook until the second side is golden, 1 to 2 minutes more. Transfer to a plate and cover to keep warm. Make 2 more quesadillas with the remaining ingredients.

NUTRITION

Per serving: 328 calories; 12 g fat (6 g sat, 0 g mono); 56 mg cholesterol; 30 g carbohydrates; 24 g protein; 2 g fiber; 871 mg sodium; 33 mg potassium.

Nutrition Bonus: Calcium (30% daily value).
Carbohydrate Servings: 1 ½

Exchanges: 1 1/2 starch, 3 lean meat

Roasted Corn, Black Bean & Mango Salad

INGREDIENTS
- 2 teaspoons canola oil
- 1 clove garlic, minced
- 1 1/2 cups corn kernels, (from 3 ears)
- 1 large ripe mango, (about 1 pound), peeled and diced
- 1 15-ounce or 19-ounce can black beans, rinsed
- 1/2 cup chopped red onion
- 1/2 cup diced red bell pepper
- 3 tablespoons lime juice
- 1 small canned chipotle pepper in adobo sauce, (see Ingredient Note), drained and chopped
- 1 1/2 tablespoons chopped fresh cilantro
- 1/4 teaspoon ground cumin
- 1/4 teaspoon salt

PREPARATION
1. Heat oil in a large nonstick skillet over medium-high heat. Add garlic and cook, stirring, until fragrant, about 30 seconds. Stir in corn and cook, stirring occasionally, until browned, about 8 minutes. Transfer the corn mixture to a large bowl. Stir in mango, beans, onion, bell pepper, lime juice, chipotle, cilantro, cumin and salt.

TIPS & NOTES
- **Make Ahead Tip**: Cover and refrigerate for up to 8 hours. Serve at room temperature.

- **Ingredient Note:** Chipotle peppers are smoked jalapenos with a fiery taste that are canned in adobo sauce. Look for them in the Hispanic section of large supermarkets and in specialty stores.

NUTRITION
Per serving: 125 calories; 2 g fat (0 g sat, 1 g mono); 0 mg cholesterol; 26 g carbohydrates; 0 g added sugars; 4 g protein; 4 g fiber; 245 mg sodium; 223 mg potassium.
Nutrition Bonus: Vitamin C (70% daily value), Fiber (18% dv).
Carbohydrate Servings: 2
Exchanges: 1 starch, 1 fruit

Roasted Savoy Cabbage with Black Bean-Garlic Sauce

INGREDIENTS
- 1 head Savoy cabbage, (about 1 1/2 pounds), cored and cut into 1-inch squares
- 4 teaspoons canola oil
- 2 tablespoons Shao Hsing rice wine, or dry sherry (see Tip)
- 4 teaspoons black bean-garlic sauce, (see Tip)
- 1 bunch scallions, minced
- 2 teaspoons distilled white vinegar
- 2 teaspoons toasted sesame oil
- 5 dashes hot sauce, or to taste

PREPARATION
1. Preheat oven to 500°F. Toss cabbage and canola oil in a large roasting pan and spread out in an even layer. Roast until beginning to wilt and brown, about 15 minutes.
2. Combine rice wine (or sherry) and black bean sauce in a small bowl; drizzle over the cabbage and toss. Continue roasting until tender, about 5 minutes more. Toss with scallions, vinegar, sesame oil and hot sauce until combined.

TIPS & NOTES
- **Tips:** Shao Hsing (or Shaoxing) is a seasoned rice wine. Both are available in Asian specialty markets and some supermarkets in the Asian section.
- Black bean-garlic sauce is made from fermented black beans, garlic and rice wine.

NUTRITION

Per serving: 123 calories; 8 g fat (1 g sat, 4 g mono); 0 mg cholesterol; 12 g carbohydrates; 4 g protein; 5 gfiber; 485 mg sodium; 406 mg potassium.
Nutrition Bonus: Vitamin C (80% daily value), Vitamin A (35% dv), Folate (32% dv), high omega-3s.
Carbohydrate Servings: 1/2
Exchanges: 2 vegetable, 1 1/2 fat

Salmon on a Bed of Lentils

INGREDIENTS
- 2 teaspoons extra-virgin olive oil
- 1 tablespoon finely chopped shallots
- 2 teaspoons minced garlic
- 2 1/2 cups reduced-sodium chicken broth
- 1 cup green or brown lentils, rinsed
- 1 small onion, peeled and studded with a clove

- 1 1/2 teaspoons chopped fresh thyme, or 1/2 teaspoon dried
- 1/4 teaspoon salt
- Freshly ground pepper, to taste
- 2 carrots, peeled and finely chopped
- 2 small white turnips, peeled and finely chopped
- 1 pound salmon fillet, skin removed, cut into 4 portions
- 2 tablespoons chopped fresh parsley
- 1 lemon, quartered

PREPARATION
1. Heat oil in a Dutch oven or deep sauté pan over medium heat. Add shallots and garlic and cook, stirring, until softened, about 30 seconds. Add broth, lentils, onion, thyme, salt and pepper. Bring to a boil, reduce heat to low and simmer, covered, until the lentils are tender, 25 minutes.
2. Add carrots and turnips; simmer until the vegetables are tender, about 10 minutes more. Remove the onion. Add more broth if necessary; the mixture should be slightly soupy. Taste and adjust seasonings. Lay salmon fillets on top, cover the pan and cook until the salmon is opaque in the center, 8 to 10 minutes.
3. Serve in shallow bowls, garnished with parsley and lemon wedges.

NUTRITION

Per serving: 382 calories; 11 g fat (2 g sat, 4 g mono); 65 mg cholesterol; 35 g carbohydrates; 0 g added sugars; 36 g protein; 9 g fiber; 342 mg sodium; 1142 mg potassium.
Nutrition Bonus: Vitamin A (80% daily value), Potassium (56% dv), Fiber (36% dv), Vitamin C(20% dv), Iron (20% dv).
Carbohydrate Servings: 2
Exchanges: 1 1/2 starch, 1 vegetable, 4 lean meat

Grandma Ginger's Fish Casserole

INGREDIENTS
- 4 teaspoons extra-virgin olive oil, divided
- 1 medium onion, very thinly sliced
- 1/2 cup dry white wine
- 8 ounces cod (see Tip) or tilapia, cut into 2 pieces
- 1 teaspoon chopped fresh thyme or 1/4 teaspoon dried
- 1/4 teaspoon kosher salt and 1/4 teaspoon freshly ground pepper
- 3/4 cup finely chopped whole-wheat country bread, (about 1 slice)
- 1/4 teaspoon paprika
- 1/4 teaspoon garlic powder
- 1/2 cup finely shredded Gruyère or Swiss cheese

PREPARATION
1. Preheat oven to 400°F.
2. Heat 2 teaspoons oil in a medium ovenproof skillet over medium-high heat. Add onion and cook, stirring often, until just starting to soften, 4 to 6 minutes. Add wine, increase heat to high and cook, stirring often, until the wine is slightly reduced, 2 to 4 minutes.
3. Place fish on top of the onion and sprinkle with thyme, salt and pepper. Cover the pan tightly with foil; transfer to the oven and bake for 12 minutes.
4. Toss the bread with the remaining 2 teaspoons oil, paprika and garlic powder in a small bowl. Uncover the fish; top with the bread mixture and cheese. Bake, uncovered, until the fish is just cooked through, 8 to 10 minutes.

TIPS & NOTES

- **Tip:** Overfishing and trawling have drastically reduced the number of cod in the U.S. and Canadian Atlantic Ocean and destroyed its sea floor. For sustainably fished cod, choose U.S. Pacific cod or Atlantic cod from Iceland and the northeast Arctic. For more information, visit Monterey Bay Aquarium Seafood Watch at seafoodwatch.org.

NUTRITION
Per serving: 383 calories; 19 g fat (7 g sat, 10 g mono); 73 mg cholesterol; 15 g carbohydrates; 28 gprotein; 4 g fiber; 337 mg sodium; 346 mg potassium.
Nutrition Bonus: Selenium (48% daily value), Calcium (35% dv), Zinc (20% dv), Magnesium (19% dv).
Exchanges: 1 other carbohydrate, 3 lean meat, 2 fat

Shredded Brussels Sprouts with Bacon & Onions

INGREDIENTS
- 2 slices bacon
- 1 small yellow onion, thinly sliced
- 1/4 teaspoon salt
- 3/4 cup water
- 1 teaspoon Dijon mustard
- 1 pound Brussels sprouts, trimmed, halved and very thinly sliced
- 1 tablespoon cider vinegar

PREPARATION
1. Cook bacon in a large skillet over medium heat, turning once, until crisp, 5 to 7 minutes. Drain on a paper towel. Crumble.
2. Add onion and salt to the drippings in the pan. Cook over medium heat, stirring often, until tender and browned, about 3 minutes. Add water and mustard and

scrape up any browned bits. Add Brussels sprouts and cook, stirring often, until tender, 4 to 6 minutes. Stir in vinegar and top with the crumbled bacon.

NUTRITION

Per serving: 47 calories; 1 g fat (0 g sat, 0 g mono); 2 mg cholesterol; 7 g carbohydrates; 0 g added sugars;3 g protein; 2 g fiber; 171 mg sodium; 292 mg potassium.
Nutrition Bonus: Vitamin K (145% daily value), Vitamin C (70% dv).
Carbohydrate Servings: 1/2
Exchanges: 1 vegetable

Vegetable Stir-Fry

INGREDIENTS

- 1 16-ounce package frozen stir-fry vegetables
- 1 teaspoon peanut oil, or canola oil
- 2 tablespoons oyster sauce, or hoisin sauce
- 1 tablespoon rice vinegar

PREPARATION

1. Heat oil in a large skillet over medium-high heat. Add stir-fry vegetables and cook, stirring often, until hot. Stir in oyster sauce (or hoisin sauce) and vinegar.

NUTRITION

Per serving: 53 calories; 1 g fat (0 g sat, 1 g mono); 0 mg cholesterol; 10 g carbohydrates; 0 g added sugars; 3 g protein; 3 g fiber; 405 mg sodium; 213 mg potassium.
Nutrition Bonus: Vitamin A (90% daily value), Vitamin C (40% dv).
Carbohydrate Servings: 1/2
Exchanges: 1 1/2 vegetable

DAY 20
BREAKFAST

Cranberry Muesli
Skim milk (1 cup)
Grapefruit (1/2)

LUNCH

Skim milk (1 cup)
Fettuccine with Shiitake Mushrooms & Basil or Southwestern Cheese Panini

SNACK

Banana (1/2 cup, sliced)

DINNER

Pampered Chicken or Cajun Crab Croquettes
Sliced Fennel Salad
Quick-cooking barley (1/2 cup)
Steamed aparagus (1 cup)

DAY 20 RECIPES

Cranberry Muesli

INGREDIENTS
- 1/2 cup low-fat plain yogurt
- 1/2 cup unsweetened or fruit-juice-sweetened cranberry juice
- 6 tablespoons old-fashioned rolled oats, (not quick-cooking or steel-cut)
- 2 tablespoons dried cranberries
- 1 tablespoon unsalted sunflower seeds
- 1 tablespoon wheat germ
- 2 teaspoons honey
- 1/4 teaspoon vanilla extract
- 1/8 teaspoon salt

PREPARATION
1. Combine yogurt, juice, oats, cranberries, sunflower seeds, wheat germ, honey, vanilla and salt in a medium bowl; cover and refrigerate for at least 8 hours and up to 1 day.

TIPS & NOTES
- **Make Ahead Tip**: Cover and refrigerate for up to 1 day.

NUTRITION

Per serving: 209 calories; 4 g fat (1 g sat, 1 g mono); 4 mg cholesterol; 37 g carbohydrates; 8 g protein; 3 gfiber; 190 mg sodium; 266 mg potassium.
Nutrition Bonus: Calcium (15% daily value)
Carbohydrate Servings: 2 1/2
Exchanges: 1 starch, 1 fruit, 1/2 other carbohydrate, 1/2 fat

Fettuccine with Shiitake Mushrooms & Basil

INGREDIENTS
- 2 tablespoons extra-virgin olive oil
- 3 cloves garlic, minced
- 2 ounces shiitake mushrooms, stemmed and sliced (1 1/2 cups)
- 2 teaspoons freshly grated lemon zest
- 2 tablespoons lemon juice, juice
- 1/4 teaspoon salt, or to taste
- Freshly ground pepper, to taste
- 8 ounces whole-wheat fettuccine, or spaghetti (see Ingredient note)
- 1/2 cup freshly grated Parmesan cheese, (1 ounce)
- 1/2 cup chopped fresh basil, divided

PREPARATION
1. Bring a large pot of lightly salted water to a boil for cooking pasta.
2. Heat oil in large nonstick skillet over low heat. Add garlic and cook, stirring, until fragrant but not browned, about 1 minute. Add mushrooms and increase heat to medium-high; cook, stirring occasionally, until tender and lightly browned, 4 to 5 minutes. Stir in lemon zest, lemon juice, salt and pepper. Remove from the heat.
3. Meanwhile, cook pasta, stirring occasionally, until just tender, 9 to 11 minutes or according to package directions. Drain, reserving 1/2 cup cooking liquid.
4. Add the pasta, the reserved cooking liquid, Parmesan and 1/4 cup basil to the mushrooms in the skillet; toss to coat well. Serve immediately, garnished with remaining basil.

TIPS & NOTES
- **Ingredient Note:** Whole-wheat pastas are higher in fiber than white pastas. They can be found in health-food stores and some large supermarkets.

NUTRITION
Per serving: 311 calories; 11 g fat (3 g sat, 6 g mono); 9 mg cholesterol; 44 g carbohydrates; 0 g added sugars; 13 g protein; 8 g fiber; 307 mg sodium; 125 mg potassium.
Nutrition Bonus: Fiber (28% daily value), Calcium (14% dv).

Carbohydrate Servings: 2 1/2
Exchanges: 21/2 starch, 1 lean meat, 1 fat

Southwestern Cheese Panini

INGREDIENTS
- 4 ounces shredded sharp Cheddar cheese
- 1 cup shredded zucchini
- 1/2 cup shredded carrot
- 1/4 cup finely chopped red onion
- 1/4 cup prepared salsa
- 1 tablespoon chopped pickled jalapeño pepper, (optional)
- 8 slices whole-wheat bread
- 2 teaspoons canola oil

PREPARATION
1. Have four 15-ounce cans and a medium skillet (not nonstick) ready by the stove.
2. Combine Cheddar, zucchini, carrot, onion, salsa and jalapeño (if using) in a medium bowl. Divide among 4 slices of bread and top with the remaining bread.
3. Heat 1 teaspoon canola oil in a large nonstick skillet over medium heat. Place 2 panini in the pan. Place the medium skillet on top of the panini, then weigh it down with the cans. Cook the panini until golden on one side, about 2 minutes. Reduce the heat to medium-low, flip the panini, replace the top skillet and cans, and cook until the second side is golden, 1 to 3 minutes more. Repeat with another 1 teaspoon oil and the remaining panini.

NUTRITION

Per serving: 331 calories; 14 g fat (5 g sat, 2 g mono); 30 mg cholesterol; 37 g carbohydrates; 16 g protein;5 g fiber; 523 mg sodium; 163 mg potassium.
Nutrition Bonus: Vitamin A (50% daily value), Calcium (30% dv), Vitamin C (20% dv), Iron (15% dv).
Carbohydrate Servings: 2
Exchanges: 2 starch, 1 1/2 vegetable, 1 high-fat meat

Pampered Chicken

INGREDIENTS
- 4 boneless, skinless chicken breast halves, (about 1 pound), trimmed of fat
- 4 slices Monterey Jack cheese, (2 ounces)
- 2 egg whites
- 1/3 cup seasoned (Italian-style) breadcrumbs
- 2 tablespoons freshly grated Parmesan cheese
- 2 tablespoons chopped fresh parsley

- 1/4 teaspoon salt, or to taste
- 1/2 teaspoon freshly ground pepper
- 2 teaspoons extra-virgin olive oil
- Lemon wedges, for garnish

PREPARATION
1. Preheat oven to 400°F. Place a chicken breast, skinned-side down, on a cutting board. Keeping the blade of a sharp knife parallel to the board, make a horizontal slit along the thinner, long edge of the breast, cutting nearly through to the opposite side. Open the breast so it forms two flaps, hinged at the center. Place a slice of cheese on one flap, leaving a 1/2-inch border at the edge. Press remaining flap down firmly over the cheese and set aside. Repeat with the remaining breasts.
2. Lightly beat egg whites with a fork in a medium bowl. Mix breadcrumbs, Parmesan, parsley, salt and pepper in a shallow dish. Holding a stuffed breast together firmly, dip it in the egg whites and then roll in the breadcrumbs. Repeat with the remaining breasts.
3. Heat oil in a large ovenproof skillet over medium-high heat. Add the stuffed breasts and cook until browned on one side, about 2 minutes. Turn the breasts over and place the skillet in the oven.
4. Bake the chicken until no longer pink in the center, about 20 minutes. Serve with lemon wedges.

NUTRITION

Per serving: 255 calories; 11 g fat (4 g sat, 4 g mono); 78 mg cholesterol; 7 g carbohydrates; 31 g protein; 1 g fiber; 518 mg sodium; 268 mg potassium.
Nutrition Bonus: Selenium (40% daily value), Calcium (15% dv).
Carbohydrate Servings: 1/2
Exchanges: 1/2 starch, 4 very lean meat, 1 medium-fat meat

Cajun Crab Croquettes

INGREDIENTS
- 3 teaspoons canola oil, divided
- 1 small onion, finely diced
- 1/2 cup finely diced green bell pepper
- 1/2 cup frozen corn kernels, thawed
- 1 1/2 teaspoons Cajun seasoning, divided
- 1 pound pasteurized crabmeat, drained if necessary
- 1 large egg white
- 3/4 cup plain dry breadcrumbs, divided
- 1/4 cup reduced-fat mayonnaise and 1/2 teaspoon freshly grated lemon zest

PREPARATION
1. Preheat oven to 425nF. Coat a baking sheet with cooking spray.
2. Heat 1 teaspoon oil in a large nonstick skillet over medium heat. Add onion, bell pepper, corn and 1 teaspoon Cajun seasoning and cook, stirring, until the vegetables are softened, about 4 minutes. Transfer to a large bowl. Let cool for 5 minutes. Add crab, egg white, 1/2 cup breadcrumbs, mayonnaise and lemon zest. Mix well.
3. Divide the mixture into 8 equal portions (about 1/2 cup each). Form each portion into an oblong patty that's about 4 inches by 2 inches. Place on the prepared baking sheet. Combine the remaining 1/4 cup breadcrumbs, 1/2 teaspoon Cajun seasoning and 2 teaspoons oil in a small bowl. Sprinkle 1 heaping teaspoon of the breadcrumb mixture over the top of each croquette, then gently press it on.
4. Bake the croquettes until heated through and golden brown on top, about 20 minutes.

NUTRITION

Per serving: 260 calories; 7 g fat (1 g sat, 2 g mono); 132 mg cholesterol; 23 g carbohydrates; 27 g protein;2 g fiber; 942 mg sodium; 148 mg potassium.
Nutrition Bonus: Iron (35% daily value), Vitamin C (25% dv), Calcium (15% dv).
Carbohydrate Servings: 1 1/2
Exchanges: 1 1/2 starch, 3 very lean meat, 1/2 fat

Sliced Fennel Salad

INGREDIENTS
- 1 large fennel bulb
- 1 tablespoon extra-virgin olive oil
- 1 tablespoon lemon juice
- 1/8 teaspoon salt
- Freshly ground pepper, to taste

PREPARATION
1. Trim base from fennel bulb. Remove and discard the fennel stalks; reserve some of the feathery leaves for garnish. Pull off and discard any discolored parts from the bulb. Stand the bulb upright and cut vertically into very thin slices. Arrange the slices on 4 salad plates.
2. Whisk oil, lemon juice and salt in a small bowl. Drizzle the mixture over the fennel and garnish with a grinding of pepper and a few fennel leaves.

NUTRITION

Per serving: 51 calories; 4 g fat (0 g sat, 3 g mono); 0 mg cholesterol; 5 g carbohydrates; 0 g added sugars;1 g protein; 2 g fiber; 103 mg sodium; 247 mg potassium.
Nutrition Bonus: Vitamin C (15% daily value).
Exchanges: vegetable, 1 fat (mono)

DAY 21
BREAKFAST

Skim Milk
Crunchy Cereal Trail Mix
Apple (1 cup, quartered)
LUNCH

Curried Tofu Salad
Whole-wheat pita bread (1/2 medium pita) or BLT Salad
Orange (1 large)
SNACK

Low-fat vanilla yogurt (8 oz.)
DINNER

Roast Salmon with Salsa
Brown rice (1 cup, cooked)or Wild Rice with Shiitakes & Toasted Almonds
North African Spiced Carrots
Bok Choy-Apple Slaw

DAY 21 RECIPES

Crunchy Cereal Trail Mix

INGREDIENTS
- 1/4 cup Cheerios
- 1 tablespoon pepitas
- 2 teaspoons raisins
- 2 teaspoons semisweet mini chocolate chips

PREPARATION
1. Combine Cheerios, pepitas, raisins and chocolate chips in a small bowl.

NUTRITION

Per serving: 98 calories; 3 g fat (2 g sat, 1 g mono); 0 mg cholesterol; 17 g carbohydrates; 2 g protein; 2 gfiber; 78 mg sodium; 161 mg potassium.
Carbohydrate Servings: 1 1/2
Exchanges: 1 1/2 starch, 1 fat

Curried Tofu Salad

INGREDIENTS
- 3 tablespoons low-fat plain yogurt
- 2 tablespoons reduced-fat mayonnaise
- 2 tablespoons prepared mango chutney
- 2 teaspoons hot curry powder, preferably Madras
- 1/4 teaspoon salt
- Freshly ground pepper, to taste
- 1 14-ounce package extra-firm water-packed tofu, drained, rinsed and finely crumbled (see Ingredient note)
- 2 stalks celery, diced
- 1 cup red grapes, sliced in half
- 1/2 cup sliced scallions
- 1/4 cup chopped walnuts

PREPARATION
1. Whisk yogurt, mayonnaise, chutney, curry powder, salt and pepper in a large bowl. Stir in tofu, celery, grapes, scallions and walnuts.

TIPS & NOTES
- **Make Ahead Tip:** Cover and refrigerate for up to 2 days.
- **Ingredient Note:** We prefer water-packed tofu from the refrigerated section of the supermarket. Crumbling it into uneven pieces creates more surface area, improving the texture and avoiding the blocky look that turns many people away.

NUTRITION

Per serving: 140 calories; 8 g fat (1 g sat, 2 g mono); 2 mg cholesterol; 13 g carbohydrates; 3 g added sugars; 7 g protein; 2 g fiber; 241 mg sodium; 271 mg potassium.
Nutrition Bonus: Calcium (15% daily value).
Carbohydrate Servings: 1
Exchanges: 1 other carb, 1 medium-fat meat

BLT Salad

INGREDIENTS
- 1 cup cubed whole-wheat country bread
- 2 teaspoons extra-virgin olive oil
- 4 medium tomatoes, divided
- 3 tablespoons reduced-fat mayonnaise
- 2 tablespoons minced chives, or scallion greens
- 2 teaspoons distilled white vinegar
- 1/4 teaspoon garlic powder
- Freshly ground pepper, to taste
- 5 cups chopped hearts of romaine lettuce
- 3 slices center-cut bacon, cooked and crumbled

PREPARATION
1. Preheat oven to 350°F. Toss bread with oil and spread on a baking sheet. Bake, turning once, until golden brown, 15 to 20 minutes.
2. Cut 1 tomato in half. Working over a large bowl, shred both halves using the large holes on a box grater. Discard the skin. Add mayonnaise, chives (or scallion greens), vinegar, garlic powder and pepper; whisk to combine.
3. Chop the remaining 3 tomatoes. Add the tomatoes, romaine and croutons to the bowl with the dressing; toss to coat. Sprinkle with bacon.

NUTRITION

Per serving: 151 calories; 6 g fat (1 g sat, 3 g mono); 5 mg cholesterol; 20 g carbohydrates; 0 g added sugars; 5 g protein; 4 g fiber; 306 mg sodium; 555 mg potassium.
Nutrition Bonus: Vitamin A (110% daily value), Vitamin C (60% dv), Folate (30% dv), Potassium (16% dv).
Carbohydrate Servings: 1
Exchanges: 1 starch, 1 vegetable, 1 fat

Roast Salmon with Salsa

INGREDIENTS
- 2 medium plum tomatoes, chopped
- 1 small onion, roughly chopped
- 1 clove garlic, peeled and quartered
- 1 fresh jalapeno pepper, seeded and chopped
- 2 teaspoons cider vinegar
- 1 teaspoon chili powder
- 1/2 teaspoon ground cumin

- 1/2 teaspoon salt
- 2-4 dashes hot sauce
- 1 1/2 pounds salmon fillet, skinned and cut into 6 portions

PREPARATION
1. Preheat oven to 400°F.
2. Place tomatoes, onion, garlic, jalapeno, vinegar, chili powder, cumin, salt and hot sauce to taste in a food processor; process until finely diced and uniform.
3. Place salmon in a large roasting pan; spoon the salsa on top. Roast until the salmon is flaky on the outside but still pink inside, about 15 minutes.

NUTRITION
Per serving: 227 calories; 13 g fat (3 g sat, 5 g mono); 65 mg cholesterol; 3 g carbohydrates; 0 g added sugars; 23 g protein; 1 g fiber; 269 mg sodium; 474 mg potassium.
Nutrition Bonus: Good source of omega-3s
Exchanges: 1/2 vegetable, 3.5 lean meat

Wild Rice with Shiitakes & Toasted Almonds

INGREDIENTS
- 2 1/4 cups reduced-sodium chicken broth, or vegetable broth
- 2 cups sliced shiitake mushroom caps, or button mushrooms (3 ounces)
- 1 cup wild rice
- 6 tablespoons sliced almonds
- 1 teaspoon butter
- 1 bunch scallions, trimmed and thinly sliced (about 2 cups)
- Freshly ground pepper, to taste

PREPARATION

1. Bring broth to a boil in a medium saucepan over high heat. Stir in mushrooms and wild rice. Return to a boil. Reduce heat to very low, cover, and simmer until the rice has "blossomed" and is just tender, 45 to 55 minutes. Drain any remaining liquid and transfer the rice to a serving bowl.
2. Meanwhile, toast almonds in a small dry skillet over medium-low heat, stirring constantly until golden brown and fragrant, 2 to 3 minutes. Transfer to a plate to cool.
3. About 5 minutes before the rice is done, melt butter in a medium nonstick skillet over medium heat. Add scallions and cook, stirring often, until softened and still bright green, 2 to 3 minutes. Stir the scallions, almonds and pepper into the rice. Serve warm.

NUTRITION
Per serving: 158 calories; 4 g fat (1 g sat, 2 g mono); 2 mg cholesterol; 26 g carbohydrates; 0 g added sugars; 7 g protein; 4 g fiber; 264 mg sodium; 340 mg potassium.
Nutrition Bonus: Magnesium (18% daily value)
Carbohydrate Servings: 1 1/2
Exchanges: 1 starch, 1 vegetable, 1 fat (mono)

North African Spiced Carrots

INGREDIENTS
- 1 tablespoon extra-virgin olive oil
- 4 cloves garlic, minced
- 2 teaspoons paprika
- 1 teaspoon ground cumin
- 1 teaspoon ground coriander
- 3 cups sliced carrots, (4 medium-large)
- 1 cup water
- 3 tablespoons lemon juice
- 1/8 teaspoon salt, or to taste
- 1/4 cup chopped fresh parsley

PREPARATION
1. Heat oil in a large nonstick skillet over medium heat. Add garlic, paprika, cumin and coriander; cook, stirring, until fragrant but not browned, about 20 seconds. Add carrots, water, lemon juice and salt; bring to a simmer. Reduce heat to low, cover and cook until almost tender, 5 to 7 minutes. Uncover and simmer, stirring often, until the carrots are just tender and the liquid is syrupy, 2 to 4 minutes. Stir in parsley. Serve hot or at room temperature.

NUTRITION
Per serving: 51 calories; 3 g fat (0 g sat, 2 g mono); 0 mg cholesterol; 7 g carbohydrates; 0 g added sugars;1 g protein; 2 g fiber; 86 mg sodium; 186 mg potassium.
Nutrition Bonus: Vitamin A (210% daily value), Vitamin C (15% dv).
Carbohydrate Servings: 1/2

Bok Choy-Apple Slaw

INGREDIENTS
- 1/3 cup reduced-fat sour cream
- 1/3 cup reduced-fat mayonnaise
- 2 tablespoons white-wine vinegar

- 2 teaspoons sugar or honey
- 1/2 teaspoon celery salt
- 1/4 teaspoon salt
- 6 cups very thinly sliced bok choy, (1-pound head, trimmed)
- 1 large Granny Smith apple, julienned or shredded
- 1 large carrot, julienned or shredded
- 1/2 cup slivered red onion

PREPARATION
1. Whisk sour cream, mayonnaise, vinegar, sugar (or honey), celery salt and salt in a large bowl until smooth. Add bok choy, apple, carrot and onion; toss to coat.

NUTRITION
Per serving: 56 calories; 2 g fat (1 g sat, 0 g mono); 3 mg cholesterol; 8 g carbohydrates; 1 g added sugars;2 g protein; 1 g fiber; 272 mg sodium; 224 mg potassium.
Nutrition Bonus: Vitamin A (80% daily value), Vitamin C (45% dv).
Carbohydrate Servings: 1/2
Exchanges: 1 vegetable

DAY 22
BREAKFAST
Pocket Eggs with Soy-Sesame Sauce
Skim milk (1 cup)
LUNCH
Skim milk (1 cup)
Ravioli with Bell Pepper Sauce or Pork, White Bean & Kale Soup
Apricot (1 cup, halves)
SNACK
Carrot sticks (1/2 cup)
Fat-free cheese (1 slice)
DINNER
Chicken, Broccoli Rabe & Feta on Toast or Picadillo
Spiced Corn & Rice Pilaf
Apple (1 cup quartered)

DAY 22 RECIPES

Pocket Eggs with Soy-Sesame Sauce

INGREDIENTS
- 2 tablespoons reduced-sodium soy sauce
- 1 teaspoon toasted sesame oil
- 1 1/2 teaspoons rice vinegar
- 1 tablespoon minced scallion greens
- 4 teaspoons canola oil
- 4 large eggs
- 2 teaspoons black sesame seeds, (see Shopping Tip)
- 1 tablespoon dried basil
- 1/4 teaspoon ground white pepper

PREPARATION
1. Combine soy sauce, sesame oil, vinegar and scallion in a small bowl. Set aside.
2. Heat canola oil in a medium nonstick skillet over medium heat and swirl to coat. Crack 2 eggs into a small bowl; crack the remaining 2 eggs into a second small bowl.
3. Working quickly, pour 2 eggs on one side of the pan and the other 2 on the other side. The egg whites will flow together, forming one large piece.
4. Sprinkle sesame seeds, basil and pepper over the eggs. Cook until the egg whites are crispy and brown on the bottom and the yolks are firmly set, about 3 minutes. Keeping them in one piece, flip the eggs using a wide spatula and cook until the whites turn crispy and brown on the other side, 1 to 2 minutes more.
5. Pour the reserved sauce over the eggs. Simmer for 30 seconds, turning the eggs once to coat both sides with sauce. Serve in wedges, drizzled with the pan sauce.

TIPS & NOTES
- **Shopping Tip:** Black sesame seeds are slightly more flavorful and aromatic than white sesame seeds. Find them in the Asian-foods section of the supermarket or substitute the white variety if they aren't available.

NUTRITION

Per serving: 139 calories; 12 g fat (2 g sat, 5 g mono); 212 mg cholesterol; 2 g carbohydrates; 0 g added sugars; 7 g protein; 1 g fiber; 338 mg sodium; 123 mg potassium.
Exchanges: 1 medium fat meat, 1 fat

Ravioli with Bell Pepper Sauce

INGREDIENTS
- 2 teaspoons extra-virgin olive oil
- 2 cloves garlic, minced
- 2 teaspoons finely chopped fresh rosemary, divided
- 1 16-ounce package frozen stir-fry vegetables, (bell peppers and onions)
- 1 14-ounce can diced tomatoes, undrained
- 1 cup individually quick-frozen spinach
- Freshly ground pepper, to taste
- 24 ounces fresh or frozen cheese ravioli
- 1/2 cup freshly grated Parmesan cheese

PREPARATION
1. Put a large pot of lightly salted water on to boil for cooking ravioli.
2. Heat oil in a large nonstick skillet over medium heat. Add garlic and 1 teaspoon rosemary; cook, stirring, until fragrant, about 1 minute. Add stir-fry vegetables and tomatoes. Bring to a simmer. Cook until vegetables are tender, 5 to 10 minutes. Stir in spinach; cook until tender, about 2 minutes more. Add the remaining 1 teaspoon rosemary and season with pepper.
3. Meanwhile, cook ravioli in the boiling water until they float, 5 to 7 minutes. Drain and transfer to a large bowl. Toss with the sauce. Serve with Parmesan. Substitution: In place of the frozen stir-fry mixture, use 1 onion and 2 bell peppers, sliced.

NUTRITION

Per serving: 267 calories; 8 g fat (4 g sat, 1 g mono); 41 mg cholesterol; 30 g carbohydrates; 12 g protein; 3 g fiber; 332 mg sodium; 10 mg potassium.
Nutrition Bonus: Vitamin A (20% daily value), Vitamin C (20% dv), Calcium (20% dv).
Carbohydrate Servings: 2
Exchanges: 11/2 starch, 1 vegetable, 1 high-fat meat, 1/2 very lean meat

Pork, White Bean & Kale Soup

INGREDIENTS
- 1 tablespoon extra-virgin olive oil
- 1 pound pork tenderloin, trimmed and cut into 1-inch pieces
- 3/4 teaspoon salt
- 1 medium onion, finely chopped
- 4 cloves garlic, minced
- 2 teaspoons paprika, preferably smoked
- 1/4 teaspoon crushed red pepper, or to taste (optional)
- 1 cup white wine

- 4 plum tomatoes, chopped
- 4 cups reduced-sodium chicken broth
- 1 bunch kale, ribs removed, chopped (about 8 cups lightly packed)
- 1 15-ounce can white beans, rinsed (see Tip)

PREPARATION
1. Heat oil in a Dutch oven over medium-high heat. Add pork, sprinkle with salt and cook, stirring once or twice, until no longer pink on the outside, about 2 minutes. Transfer to a plate with tongs, leaving juices in the pot.
2. Add onion to the pot and cook, stirring often, until just beginning to brown, 2 to 3 minutes. Add garlic, paprika and crushed red pepper (if using) and cook, stirring constantly, until fragrant, about 30 seconds. Add wine and tomatoes, increase heat to high and stir to scrape up any browned bits. Add broth and bring to a boil.
3. Add kale and stir just until it wilts. Reduce heat to maintain a lively simmer and cook, stirring occasionally, until the kale is just tender, about 4 minutes. Stir in beans, the reserved pork and any accumulated juices; simmer until the beans and pork are heated through, about 2 minutes.

TIPS & NOTES
- **Tip:** While we love the convenience of canned beans, they tend to be high in sodium. Give them a good rinse before adding to a recipe to rid them of some of their sodium (up to 35 percent) or opt for low-sodium or no-salt-added varieties. (Our recipes are analyzed with rinsed, regular canned beans.) Or, if you have the time, cook your own beans from scratch.

NUTRITION
Per serving: 262 calories; 6 g fat (1 g sat, 3 g mono); 45 mg cholesterol; 26 g carbohydrates; 25 g protein; 7 g fiber; 627 mg sodium; 1024 mg potassium.
Nutrition Bonus: Vitamin A (290% daily value), Vitamin C (190% dv), Potassium (29% dv), Iron (20% dv)
Carbohydrate Servings: 1
Exchanges: 1 starch, 2 vegetable, 2 lean meat

Chicken, Broccoli Rabe & Feta on Toast

INGREDIENTS
- 4 thick slices whole-wheat country bread
- 1 clove garlic, peeled (optional), plus 1/4 cup chopped garlic
- 4 teaspoons extra-virgin olive oil, divided
- 1 pound chicken tenders, cut crosswise into 1/2-inch pieces

- 1 bunch broccoli rabe, stems trimmed, cut into 1-inch pieces, or 2 bunches broccolini, chopped (see Ingredient note)
- 2 cups cherry tomatoes, halved
- 1 tablespoon red-wine vinegar
- 1/8 teaspoon salt
- Freshly ground pepper, to taste
- 3/4 cup crumbled feta cheese

PREPARATION
1. Grill or toast bread. Lightly rub with peeled garlic clove, if desired. Discard the garlic.
2. Heat 2 teaspoons oil in a large nonstick skillet over high heat until shimmering but not smoking. Add chicken; cook, stirring occasionally, until just cooked through and no longer pink in the middle, 4 to 5 minutes. Transfer the chicken and any juices to a plate; cover to keep warm.
3. Add the remaining 2 teaspoons oil to the pan. Add chopped garlic and cook, stirring constantly, until fragrant but not brown, about 30 seconds. Add broccoli rabe (or broccolini) and cook, stirring often, until bright green and just wilted, 2 to 4 minutes. Stir in tomatoes, vinegar, salt and pepper; cook, stirring occasionally, until the tomatoes are beginning to break down, 2 to 4 minutes. Return the chicken and juices to the pan, add feta cheese and stir to combine. Cook until heated through, 1 to 2 minutes. Serve warm over garlic toasts.

TIPS & NOTES
- **Ingredient Note:** Pleasantly pungent and mildly bitter, broccoli rabe, or rapini, is a member of the cabbage family and commonly used in Mediterranean cooking. Broccolini (a cross between broccoli and Chinese kale) is sweet and tender - the florets and stalks are edible.

NUTRITION
Per serving: 313 calories; 11 g fat (5 g sat, 5 g mono); 85 mg cholesterol; 26 g carbohydrates; 35 g protein;4 g fiber; 653 mg sodium; 423 mg potassium.
Nutrition Bonus: Vitamin C (160% daily value), Vitamin A (140% dv), Selenium (28% dv), Calcium (20% dv).
Carbohydrate Servings: 2
Exchanges: 1 starch, 2 vegetable, 4 lean meat

Picadillo

INGREDIENTS
- 2 eggs, (optional)
- 1 pound lean ground beef, or ground turkey breast
- 2 teaspoons extra-virgin olive oil

- 1 medium onion, chopped
- 1/2 cup chopped scallions, divided
- 3 cloves garlic, minced
- 4 teaspoons chili powder
- 1 1/2 teaspoons dried oregano
- 1 1/2 teaspoons ground cumin
- 3/4 teaspoon ground cinnamon
- 1/8 teaspoon cayenne pepper
- 1/2 cup golden raisins
- 1/2 cup chopped pitted green olives
- 2 tablespoons tomato paste
- 1 cup water
- 1/2 teaspoon freshly ground pepper

PREPARATION

1. If using eggs, place in a small saucepan and cover with cold water. Bring to a boil; simmer on medium-low for 15 minutes. Drain; let cool; peel and slice.
2. Meanwhile, cook meat in a large nonstick skillet over medium-high heat, crumbling it with a wooden spoon, until no longer pink, about 5 minutes. Transfer to a colander; drain off fat.
3. Add oil to the skillet. Add onion, 1/4 cup scallions and garlic; cook over medium heat, stirring often, until softened, 2 to 3 minutes. Stir in chili powder, oregano, cumin, cinnamon and cayenne; cook, stirring, until fragrant, about 1 minute. Add raisins, olives, tomato paste, water and the browned meat; stir to blend. Reduce heat to low, cover and simmer, stirring occasionally, for 10 minutes. Season with pepper. Garnish with the remaining scallions and the hard-cooked eggs, if desired.

NUTRITION
Per serving (with beef): 313 calories; 9 g fat (3 g sat, 7 g mono); 45 mg cholesterol; 25 g carbohydrates; 0 g added sugars; 30 g protein; 4 g fiber; 548 mg sodium; 362 mg potassium.
Nutrition Bonus: Iron (25% daily value), Vitamin A (20% dv), Vitamin C (15% dv).
Carbohydrate Servings: 1 1/2
Exchanges: 1 other carbohydrate, 1 vegetable, 4 lean meat
Nutrition Note: Per serving (with turkey): 277 calories; 9 g fat (0 g sat, 5 g mono); 45 mg cholesterol; 25 g carbohydrate; 30 g protein; 4 g fiber; 548 mg sodium.

Spiced Corn & Rice Pilaf

INGREDIENTS
- 2 teaspoons extra-virgin olive oil
- 1/4 cup finely chopped onion
- 1 3-inch cinnamon stick
- 3/4 teaspoon cumin seeds
- 1/4 teaspoon ground cardamom
- 1/4 teaspoon salt
- 1 cup brown basmati or long-grain brown rice
- 2 3/4 cups reduced-sodium chicken broth, or vegetable broth
- 2 tablespoons hulled pumpkin seeds
- 1 cup fresh corn kernels, (from 2 ears) or frozen

PREPARATION
1. Heat oil in a large saucepan over medium-high heat. Add onion and cook, stirring often, until lightly browned, about 3 minutes. Add cinnamon stick, cumin seeds, cardamom, salt and rice; cook, stirring often, until spices are fragrant, about 1 minute.
2. Stir in broth and bring to a boil. Reduce heat to low; cover and simmer until the liquid is absorbed and the rice is tender, 35 to 40 minutes.
3. Meanwhile, toast pumpkin seeds in a small dry skillet over medium-low heat, stirring constantly, until fragrant, 1 to 2 minutes. Transfer to a bowl to cool.
4. When the rice is ready, stir in corn, cover and cook until heated through, about 5 minutes. Remove the cinnamon stick. Fluff the pilaf with a fork and fold in the toasted pumpkin seeds.

NUTRITION

Per serving: 129 calories; 3 g fat (1 g sat, 2 g mono); 2 mg cholesterol; 22 g carbohydrates; 0 g added sugars; 4 g protein; 2 g fiber; 126 mg sodium; 80 mg potassium.
Carbohydrate Servings: 1 1/2
Exchanges: 11/2 starch, 1/2 fat (mono)

DAY 23
BREAKFAST

Skim milk (1 cup)
Cereal (dry, 1 cup)
Blueberries (1 cup)

LUNCH

Bacony Barley Salad with Marinated Shrimp or Warm Salad with Chicken Paillards & Chèvre
Whole-wheat pita bread (1/2 medium pita)
Apricot (1/2 cup, halves)

SNACK

Skim milk (1 cup)
Carrot sticks (1/2 cup)

DINNER

Rosemary & Garlic Crusted Pork Loin with Butternut Squash & Potatoes or Chicken Tacos with Charred Tomatoes
Steamed cauliflower (1/2 cup)

DAY 23 RECIPES

Bacony Barley Salad with Marinated Shrimp

INGREDIENTS
- 3 strips bacon, chopped
- 1 1/3 cups water
- 1/2 teaspoon salt
- 2/3 cup quick-cooking barley
- 1 pound peeled cooked shrimp, (21-25 per pound; thawed if frozen), tails removed, coarsely chopped
- 1/3 cup lime juice
- 2 cups cherry tomatoes, halved
- 1/2 cup finely diced red onion
- 1/2 cup chopped fresh cilantro
- 2 tablespoons extra-virgin olive oil
- Freshly ground pepper, to taste
- 1 avocado, peeled and diced

PREPARATION

1. Cook bacon in a small saucepan over medium heat, stirring often, until crispy, about 4 minutes. Drain on paper towel; discard fat.

2. Add water and salt to the pan and bring to a boil. Add barley and return to a simmer. Reduce heat to low, cover and simmer until all the liquid is absorbed, 10 to 12 minutes.
3. Combine shrimp and lime juice in a large bowl. Add the cooked barley; toss to coat. Let stand for 10 minutes, stirring occasionally, to allow the barley to absorb some of the lime juice. Add tomatoes, onion, cilantro and the bacon; toss to coat. Add oil and pepper and toss again. Stir in avocado and serve.

TIPS & NOTES
- **Make Ahead Tip**: Prepare without avocado, cover and refrigerate for up to 2 days. Stir in the avocado just before serving.

NUTRITION
Per serving: 393 calories; 19 g fat (3 g sat, 11 g mono); 235 mg cholesterol; 3 g carbohydrates; 35 gprotein; 7 g fiber; 752 mg sodium; 859 mg potassium.
Nutrition Bonus: Vitamin C (50% daily value), Fiber (29% dv), Iron (25% dv), Folate (15% dv).
Carbohydrate Servings: 1 1/2
Exchanges: 1 starch, 1 vegetable, 4 very lean meat, 3 fat (mono)

Warm Salad with Chicken Paillards & Chèvre

INGREDIENTS
- 12 cups arugula, tough stems removed (about 8 ounces)
- 8 green olives, pitted and quartered
- 8 large dates, pitted and quartered
- 2 oranges, peeled, sectioned and sliced into chunks
- 1 pound boneless, skinless chicken breasts, trimmed of fat
- 1/3 cup seasoned Italian breadcrumbs
- 4 teaspoons extra-virgin olive oil, divided
- 1/4 cup frozen orange juice concentrate, thawed
- 2 tablespoons water
- 2 tablespoons cider vinegar
- 2 tablespoons Dijon mustard
- 1/8 teaspoon salt
- Freshly ground pepper, to taste
- 3 ounces aged or fresh goat cheese, crumbled (see Note)

PREPARATION
1. Place arugula, olives, dates and orange chunks in a large salad bowl.

2. Lay each chicken breast between 2 large pieces of plastic wrap. Gently pound with the smooth side of a meat mallet or a heavy saucepan until 1/4 inch thick. Place breadcrumbs on a large plate and dredge the chicken in them.
3. Heat 2 teaspoons oil in a large nonstick skillet over medium-high heat. Add 2 chicken breasts and cook until golden and just cooked through, about 2 minutes per side. Transfer to a platter, cover and keep warm. Reduce heat to medium, add the remaining 2 teaspoons oil to the pan and repeat with the remaining chicken. Transfer to the platter and cover.
4. Add orange juice concentrate, water and vinegar to the pan. Stir in mustard and let the dressing boil for 30 seconds. Season with salt and pepper. Add half the warm dressing to the salad; gently toss to mix.
5. To serve, cut chicken into thin slices. Top salad with chicken, goat cheese and the remaining dressing.

TIPS & NOTES
- **Note:** Goat cheese, also known as chèvre (French for goat), is earthy-tasting and slightly tart. Fresh goat cheese is creamy and commonly available. Aged goat cheese has a nutty, sharp flavor and is drier and firmer. Look for aged goat cheese in a well-stocked cheese section at larger supermarkets and specialty cheese shops.

NUTRITION

Per serving: 427 calories; 18 g fat (7 g sat, 8 g mono); 85 mg cholesterol; 35 g carbohydrates; 33 g protein;5 g fiber; 657 mg sodium; 792 mg potassium.
Nutrition Bonus: Vitamin C (110% daily value), Vitamin A (40% dv), Calcium (35% dv), Folate (28% dv), Potassium (23% dv).
Carbohydrate Servings: 2
Exchanges: 1.5 fruit, 2 vegetable, 4 very lean meat, 3.5 fat

Rosemary & Garlic Crusted Pork Loin with Butternut Squash & Potatoes
INGREDIENTS
- 3 tablespoons chopped fresh rosemary, or 1 tablespoon dried
- 4 cloves garlic, minced
- 1 teaspoon kosher salt, divided
- 1/2 teaspoon freshly ground pepper, plus more to taste
- 1 2-pound boneless center-cut pork loin roast, trimmed
- 1 1/2 pounds small Yukon Gold potatoes, scrubbed and cut into 1-inch cubes
- 4 teaspoons extra-virgin olive oil, divided
- 1 pound butternut squash, peeled, seeded and cut into 1-inch cubes
- 1/2 cup port, or prune juice
- 1/2 cup reduced-sodium chicken broth

PREPARATION
1. Preheat oven to 400°F.
2. Combine rosemary, garlic, 1/2 teaspoon salt and 1/2 teaspoon pepper in a mortar and crush with the pestle to form a paste. (Alternatively, finely chop the ingredients together on a cutting board.)
3. Coat a large roasting pan with cooking spray. Place pork in the pan and rub the rosemary mixture all over it. Toss potatoes with 2 teaspoons oil and 1/4 teaspoon salt in a medium bowl; scatter along one side of the pork.
4. Roast the pork and potatoes for 30 minutes. Meanwhile, toss squash with the remaining 2 teaspoons oil, 1/4 teaspoon salt and pepper in a medium bowl.
5. Remove the roasting pan from the oven. Carefully turn the pork over. Scatter the squash along the other side of the pork.
6. Roast the pork until an instant-read thermometer inserted in the center registers 155°F, 30 to 40 minutes more. Transfer the pork to a carving board; tent with foil and let stand for 10 to 15 minutes. If the vegetables are tender, transfer them to a bowl, cover and keep them warm. If not, continue roasting until they are browned and tender, 10 to 15 minutes more.
7. After removing the vegetables, place the roasting pan over medium heat and add port (or prune juice); bring to a boil, stirring to scrape up any browned bits. Simmer for 2 minutes. Add broth and bring to a simmer. Simmer for a few minutes to intensify the flavor. Add any juices that have accumulated on the carving board.
8. To serve, cut the strings from the pork and carve. Serve with the roasted vegetables and pan sauce.

TIPS & NOTES
- By placing the potatoes along one side of the roast and the squash along the other, you have the flexibility of removing one of the vegetables if it is done before the other.

NUTRITION
Per serving: 299 calories; 10 g fat (3 g sat, 5 g mono); 63 mg cholesterol; 23 g carbohydrates; 1 g added sugars; 25 g protein; 3 g fiber; 365 mg sodium; 451 mg potassium.
Nutrition Bonus: Vitamin A (110% daily value), Vitamin C (45% dv).
Carbohydrate Servings: 1 1/2
Exchanges: 11/2 starch, 3 lean meat

Chicken Tacos with Charred Tomatoes

INGREDIENTS

- 2 plum tomatoes, cored
- 8 ounces boneless, skinless chicken breast, trimmed of fat
- 1/4 teaspoon salt
- 1/8 teaspoon freshly ground pepper
- 2 teaspoons canola oil, divided
- 1/2 cup finely chopped white onion
- 1 clove garlic, minced
- 1 small jalapeño pepper, seeded and minced
- 2 teaspoons lime juice, plus lime wedges for garnish
- 2 teaspoons chopped fresh cilantro
- 2 scallions, chopped
- 6 small corn tortillas, heated (see Tip)

PREPARATION

1. Heat a medium skillet over high heat until very hot. Add tomatoes and cook, turning occasionally with tongs, until charred on all sides, 8 to 10 minutes. Transfer to a plate to cool slightly. Cut the tomatoes in half crosswise; squeeze to discard seeds. Remove cores and chop the remaining pulp and skin.
2. Cut chicken into 1-inch chunks; sprinkle with salt and pepper. Add 1 teaspoon oil to the pan and heat over high heat until very hot. Add the chicken and cook, stirring occasionally, until it is browned and no longer pink in the middle, 3 to 5 minutes. Transfer to a plate.
3. Reduce the heat to medium and add the remaining 1 teaspoon oil. Add onion and cook, stirring, until softened, about 2 minutes. Add garlic and jalapeño and cook, stirring, until fragrant, about 30 seconds. Add lime juice, the chicken and tomatoes. Cook, stirring, until heated through, 1 to 2 minutes. Stir in cilantro and scallions. Divide the chicken mixture among tortillas. Serve with lime wedges.

TIPS & NOTES

- **Tip:** Wrap tortillas in barely damp paper towels and microwave on High for 30 to 45 seconds.

NUTRITION
Per serving: 297 calories; 9 g fat (1 g sat, 4 g mono); 63 mg cholesterol; 27 g carbohydrates; 0 g added sugars; 27 g protein; 2 g fiber; 415 mg sodium; 463 mg potassium.
Nutrition Bonus: Selenium & Vitamin C (30% daily value), Vitamin A (20% dv).
Carbohydrate Servings: 2
Exchanges: 2 starch, 3 very lean meat, 1 fat

DAY 24
BREAKFAST
Whole-wheat toast (1 slice)
Strawberries (1 cup)
Low-fat vanilla yogurt (8 oz.)
LUNCH
Shrimp & Plum Kebabs
Roasted Tomato Soup or Amazing Pea Soup
Whole-wheat toast (1 slice)
Ginger-Orange Biscotti
SNACK
Banana (3/4 cup, sliced) or Plum & Apple Compote with Vanilla Custard
DINNER
Sausage, Mushroom & Spinach Lasagna
Sliced Tomato Salad
Steamed asparagus (1/2 cup)
Apricot (1/2 cup, halves)

DAY 24 RECIPES

Shrimp & Plum Kebabs

INGREDIENTS
- 3 tablespoons canola oil, or toasted sesame oil
- 2 tablespoons chopped fresh cilantro
- 1 teaspoon freshly grated lime zest
- 3 tablespoons lime juice
- 1/2 teaspoon salt
- 12 raw shrimp, (8-12 per pound), peeled and deveined
- 3 jalapeño peppers, stemmed, seeded and quartered lengthwise
- 2 plums, pitted and cut into sixths

PREPARATION
1. Whisk oil, cilantro, lime zest, lime juice and salt in a large bowl. Set aside 3 tablespoons of the mixture in a small bowl to use as dressing. Add shrimp, jalapeños and plums to the remaining marinade; toss to coat.
2. Preheat grill to medium-high.
3. Make 4 kebabs, alternating shrimp, jalapeños and plums evenly among four 10-inch skewers. (Discard the marinade.) Grill the kebabs, turning once, until the shrimp are cooked through, about 8 minutes total. Drizzle with the reserved dressing.

TIPS & NOTES
- **Make Ahead Tip**: Equipment: Four 10-inch skewers

NUTRITION
Per serving: 194 calories; 8 g fat (1 g sat, 4 g mono); 221 mg cholesterol; 5 g carbohydrates; 0 g added sugars; 24 g protein; 1 g fiber; 446 mg sodium; 292 mg potassium.
Nutrition Bonus: Selenium (64% daily value), Iron & Vitamin C (20% dv).
Exchanges: 1 vegetable, 3 very lean meat, 1 fat

Roasted Tomato Soup

INGREDIENTS
- 1 1/2 pounds large tomatoes, such as beefsteak, cut in half crosswise
- 1 medium sweet onion, such as Vidalia, peeled and cut in half crosswise
- 3 large cloves garlic, unpeeled
- 1 tablespoon plus 1 teaspoon extra-virgin olive oil, divided
- 1/4 teaspoon salt, or to taste
- Freshly ground pepper, to taste
- 2 cups reduced-sodium chicken broth, or vegetable broth, divided
- 1/4 cup tomato juice
- 1 teaspoon tomato paste
- 1/4 teaspoon Worcestershire sauce
- 1 tablespoon fresh basil, chopped
- Brown sugar, to taste (optional)
- 1/2 cup corn kernels, (fresh, from 1 ear, see Tip) or frozen, thawed

PREPARATION
1. Preheat oven to 400°F. Coat a baking sheet with cooking spray.
2. Toss tomatoes, onion and garlic in a mixing bowl with 1 tablespoon oil. Season with salt and pepper. Spread on the prepared baking sheet and roast until the vegetables are soft and caramelized, about 30 minutes. Let cool.

3. Peel and seed the tomatoes. Trim off the onion ends. Peel the garlic. Place the vegetables in a food processor or blender with 1 cup broth and the remaining 1 teaspoon oil. Pulse to desired thickness and texture.
4. Transfer the vegetable puree to a large heavy pot or Dutch oven. Add the remaining 1 cup broth, tomato juice, tomato pate, Worcestershire sauce, basil and brown sugar (if using). Bring to a simmer over medium heat, stirring often. Ladle into 6 soup bowls, garnish with corn and serve.

TIPS & NOTES
- **Make Ahead Tip**: Cover and refrigerate for up to 2 days or freeze for up to 2 months.
- **Tip:** Removing Corn from the Cob: Stand an uncooked ear of corn on its stem end in a shallow bowl and slice the kernels off with a sharp, thin-bladed knife. This technique produces whole kernels that are good for adding to salads and salsas. If you want to use the corn kernels for soups, fritters or puddings, you can add another step to the process. After cutting the kernels off, reverse the knife and, using the dull side, press it down the length of the ear to push out the rest of the corn and its milk.

NUTRITION
Per serving: 95 calories; 4 g fat (1 g sat, 2 g mono); 1 mg cholesterol; 15 g carbohydrates; 0 g added sugars; 3 g protein; 3 g fiber; 340 mg sodium; 406 mg potassium.
Nutrition Bonus: Vitamin C (35% daily value), Vitamin A (20% dv).
Carbohydrate Servings: 1
Exchanges: 2 vegetable, 1 fat

Amazing Pea Soup

INGREDIENTS
- 12 cups water
- 2 pounds English peas with shells
- 1/3 cup finely chopped fresh dill, plus sprigs for garnish
- 1 teaspoon salt
- Freshly ground pepper, to taste
- 3/4 cup low-fat plain yogurt

PREPARATION
1. Bring water to a boil in a large pot. Add peas, return to a boil and then reduce to a simmer. Cook, stirring occasionally, for 45 minutes.
2. Using a slotted spoon, transfer one-third of the pea pods to a food processor. Add 1/2 cup cooking liquid and process until smooth. (Use caution when pureeing hot liquids.) Pour into a large bowl. Repeat with the remaining pea

pods in 2 batches, with 1/2 cup cooking liquid each time. Pour the pureed peas plus the remaining cooking liquid through a fine-meshed sieve, pressing on the solids to extract as much liquid as possible. (Alternatively, put through a food mill fitted with a fine disc.)
3. Return the soup to the pot, bring to a boil and then simmer until reduced by about a third (to about 6 cups), 30 to 35 minutes. Stir in chopped dill, salt and pepper. Ladle into bowls and top each serving with a swirl or dollop of yogurt and a sprig of dill, if desired.

NUTRITION
Per serving: 79 calories; 1 g fat (0 g sat, 0 g mono); 2 mg cholesterol; 13 g carbohydrates; 0 g added sugars; 6 g protein; 4 g fiber; 429 mg sodium; 364 mg potassium.
Nutrition Bonus: Vitamin C (140% daily value), Vitamin A (30% dv), Folate (16% dv), Calcium & Iron (15% dv).
Carbohydrate Servings: 1
Exchanges: 1 starch

Ginger-Orange Biscotti

INGREDIENTS
- 3/4 cup whole-wheat pastry flour
- 3/4 cup all-purpose flour
- 1 cup sugar, or 1/2 cup Splenda Sugar Blend for Baking
- 1/2 cup cornmeal
- 2 teaspoons ground ginger
- 1 teaspoon baking powder
- 1/2 teaspoon baking soda
- 1/4 teaspoon salt
- 2 large eggs
- 2 large egg whites
- 2 teaspoons freshly grated orange zest
- 1 tablespoon orange juice

PREPARATION
1. Preheat oven to 325°F. Line a baking sheet with parchment paper or a silicone baking mat.
2. Whisk whole-wheat flour, all-purpose flour, sugar (or Splenda), cornmeal, ginger, baking powder, baking soda and salt in a medium bowl. Whisk eggs, egg whites, orange zest and orange juice in a large bowl until blended. Stir in the dry ingredients with a wooden spoon until just combined.

3. Divide the dough in half. With dampened hands, form each piece into a 14-by-1 1/2-inch log. Place the logs side by side on the prepared baking sheet
4. Bake until firm, 20 to 25 minutes. Cool on the pan on a wire rack. Reduce oven temperature to 300°.
5. Slice the logs on the diagonal into cookies 1/2 inch thick. Arrange, cut-side down, on 2 ungreased baking sheets. Bake until golden brown and crisp, 15 to 20 minutes. (Rotate the baking sheets if necessary to ensure even browning.) Transfer the biscotti to a wire rack to cool.

TIPS & NOTES
- **Make Ahead Tip**: Store in an airtight container for up to 2 weeks.

NUTRITION

Per biscotti: 34 calories; 0 g fat (0 g sat, 0 g mono); 8 mg cholesterol; 8 g carbohydrates; 1 g protein; 0 gfiber; 34 mg sodium; 9 mg potassium.
Carbohydrate Servings: 1/2
Exchanges: 1/2 other carbohydrate
Nutrition Note: Per biscotti with Splenda: 0 Carbohydrate Servings; 28 calories; 5 g carbohydrate.

Plum & Apple Compote with Vanilla Custard

INGREDIENTS
COMPOTE
- 12 prune plums, or 8 red or black plums, pitted and chopped
- 1/3 cup apple cider
- 1/4 cup sugar, or
- 1/4 teaspoon ground cinnamon
- 4 large apples, such as Mutsu (Crispin), Fuji or Gala

CUSTARD
- 1 1/2 cups 1% milk, divided
- 1/4 cup sugar, or
- 1 tablespoon cornstarch
- Pinch of salt
- 2 large eggs, lightly beaten
- 1 teaspoon vanilla extract

PREPARATION
1. To prepare compote: Combine plums, cider, 1/4 cup sugar (or Splenda) and cinnamon in a medium saucepan; bring to a simmer over medium heat. Cook, stirring occasionally, until the plums are soft and falling apart, about 5 minutes.

Remove from the heat. Peel and grate apples. Stir the grated apples into the plums. Spoon the compote into a large bowl and chill in the refrigerator.
2. To prepare custard: Heat 1 cup milk in a saucepan over medium heat until steaming; do not boil. Mix 1/4 cup sugar (or Splenda), cornstarch and salt in a medium bowl. Add eggs and whisk until smooth. Whisk in the remaining 1/2 cup cold milk. Add the heated milk to the egg mixture, whisking constantly. Return the mixture to the saucepan. Cook over low heat, whisking constantly, until thickened, about 3 minutes. Remove from the heat and whisk in vanilla. Transfer the custard to a clean bowl and let cool slightly or refrigerate until chilled.
3. To serve, spoon custard into dessert dishes and top each with compote.

TIPS & NOTES
- **Make Ahead Tip**: Refrigerate compote and custard in separate containers for up to 2 days.
- **Ingredient Note:** In the test Kitchen, sucralose is the only alternative sweetener we test with when we feel the option is appropriate. For nonbaking recipes, we use Splenda Granular (boxed, not in a packet). For baking, we use Splenda Sugar Blend for Baking, a mix of sugar and sucralose. It can be substituted in recipes (1/2 cup of the blend for each 1 cup of sugar) to reduce sugar calories by half while maintaining some of the baking properties of sugar. If you make a similar blend with half sugar and half Splenda Granular, substitute this homemade mixture cup for cup.
- When choosing any low- or no-calorie sweetener, be sure to check the label to make sure it is suitable for your intended use.

NUTRITION
Per serving: 119 calories; 1 g fat (0 g sat, 0 g mono); 37 mg cholesterol; 18 g carbohydrates; 3 g protein; 2 g fiber; 37 mg sodium; 210 mg potassium.
Carbohydrate Servings: 1 1/2
Exchanges: 11/2 other carbohydrate

Sausage, Mushroom & Spinach Lasagna

INGREDIENTS
- 8 ounces whole-wheat lasagna noodles
- 1 pound lean spicy Italian turkey sausage, casings removed, or vegetarian sausage-style soy product
- 4 cups sliced mushrooms, (10 ounces)
- 1/4 cup water
- 1 pound frozen spinach, thawed
- 1 28-ounce can crushed tomatoes, preferably chunky

- 1/4 cup chopped fresh basil
- 1/4 teaspoon salt
- Freshly ground pepper, to taste
- 1 pound part-skim ricotta cheese, (2 cups)
- 8 ounces part-skim mozzarella cheese, shredded (about 2 cups), divided

PREPARATION
1. Preheat oven to 350°F. Coat a 9-by-13-inch baking dish with cooking spray.
2. Bring a large pot of water to a boil. Add noodles and cook until not quite tender, about 2 minutes less than the package directions. Drain; return the noodles to the pot, cover with cool water and set aside.
3. Coat a large nonstick skillet with cooking spray and heat over medium-high heat. Add sausage; cook, crumbling with a wooden spoon, until browned, about 4 minutes. Add mushrooms and water; cook, stirring occasionally and crumbling the sausage more, until it is cooked through, the water has evaporated and the mushrooms are tender, 8 to 10 minutes. Squeeze spinach to remove excess water, then stir into the pan; remove from heat.
4. Mix tomatoes with basil, salt and pepper in a medium bowl.
5. To assemble lasagna: Spread 1/2 cup of the tomatoes in the prepared baking dish. Arrange a layer of noodles on top, trimming to fit if necessary. Evenly dollop half the ricotta over the noodles. Top with half the sausage mixture, one-third of the remaining tomatoes and one-third of the mozzarella. Continue with another layer of noodles, the remaining ricotta, the remaining sausage, half the remaining tomatoes and half the remaining mozzarella. Top with a third layer of noodles and the remaining tomatoes.
6. Cover the lasagna with foil and bake until bubbling and heated through, 1 hour to 1 hour 10 minutes. Remove the foil; sprinkle the remaining mozzarella on top. Return to the oven and bake until the cheese is just melted but not browned, 8 to 10 minutes. Let rest for 10 minutes before serving. Vegetarian Variation: Use a sausage-style soy product, such as Gimme Lean, or simply omit the sausage altogether.

TIPS & NOTES
- **Make Ahead Tip**: Prepare through Step 5 up to 1 day ahead.
- **Ingredient Note:** Whole-wheat lasagna noodles are higher in fiber than white noodles. They can be found in health-food stores and some large supermarkets.
- **Vegetarian Variation:** Use a sausage-style soy product, such as Gimme Lean, or simply omit the sausage altogether.

NUTRITION

Per serving: 333 calories; 14 g fat (5 g sat, 3 g mono); 41 mg cholesterol; 28 g carbohydrates; 26 g protein; 7 g fiber; 655 mg sodium; 607 mg potassium.
Nutrition Bonus: Vitamin A (128% daily value), Calcium (23% dv), Iron (21% dv), Folate (19% dv), Potassium (17% dv).
Carbohydrate Servings: 1 1/2
Exchanges: 1 starch, 1 1/2 vegetable, 1 lean meat, 2 medium-fat meat

Sliced Tomato Salad

INGREDIENTS

- 4 tomatoes, sliced
- 1/4 cup thinly sliced red onion
- 8 anchovies
- 1/2 teaspoon dried oregano
- Salt & freshly ground pepper, to taste
- 2 tablespoons extra-virgin olive oil
- 1 tablespoon white-wine vinegar

PREPARATION

1. Arrange tomato slices on a platter. Top with onion, anchovies, oregano, salt and pepper. Drizzle with oil and vinegar.

NUTRITION

Per serving: 44 calories; 1 g fat (0 g sat, 0 g mono); 3 mg cholesterol; 8 g carbohydrates; 0 g added sugars; 3 g protein; 2 g fiber; 300 mg sodium; 403 mg potassium.
Nutrition Bonus: Vitamin C (35% daily value), Vitamin A (25% dv).
Carbohydrate Servings: 1/2
Exchanges: 1 vegetable, 1 1/2 fat

DAY 25
BREAKFAST

Lemon-Raspberry Muffins
Skim milk (1 cup)
Grapefruit (1/2)

LUNCH

Skim milk (1 cup)
Spicy Tofu Hotpot
Wasa crispbread (2 crackers)

SNACK

Creamy Herb Dip or Baba Ganouj
Carrot sticks (1/2 cup)

DINNER

Turkey Cutlets with Peas & Spring Onions or Black Bean-Salmon Stir-Fry
Quick-cooking barley (1/2 cup)
Strawberries (1 cup)

DAY 25 RECIPES

Lemon-Raspberry Muffins

INGREDIENTS
- 1 lemon
- 1/2 cup sugar
- 1 cup nonfat buttermilk (see Tip)
- 1/3 cup canola oil
- 1 large egg
- 1 teaspoon vanilla extract
- 1 cup white whole-wheat flour or whole-wheat pastry flour (see Shopping Tip)
- 1 cup all-purpose flour
- 2 teaspoons baking powder
- 1 teaspoon baking soda
- 1/4 teaspoon salt
- 1 1/2 cups fresh or frozen (not thawed) raspberries

PREPARATION

1. Preheat oven to 400°F. Coat 12 large (1/2-cup) muffin cups with cooking spray or line with paper liners.
2. Use a vegetable peeler to remove the zest from the lemon in long strips. Combine the zest and sugar in a food processor; pulse until the zest is very finely

chopped into the sugar. Add buttermilk, oil, egg and vanilla and pulse until blended.
3. Combine whole-wheat flour, all-purpose flour, baking powder, baking soda and salt in a large bowl. Add the buttermilk mixture and fold until almost blended. Gently fold in raspberries. Divide the batter among the muffin cups.
4. Bake the muffins until the edges and tops are golden, 20 to 25 minutes. Let cool in the pan for 5 minutes before turning out onto a wire rack. Serve warm.

TIPS & NOTES
- **Make Ahead Tip**: Wrap each in plastic and freeze in a freezer bag for up to 1 month. To reheat, remove plastic, wrap muffin in a paper towel and microwave on High for 30 to 60 seconds.
- **Tip:** No buttermilk? Mix 1 tablespoon lemon juice into 1 cup milk.
- **Shopping Tip:** White whole-wheat flour, made from a special variety of white wheat, is light in color and flavor but has the same nutritional properties as regular whole wheat. Whole-wheat pastry flour can be used as a substitute here. Both can be found in the natural-foods section of the supermarket or online from King Arthur Flour, bakerscatalogue.com.

NUTRITION
Per muffin: 185 calories; 7 g fat (1 g sat, 4 g mono); 18 mg cholesterol; 27 g carbohydrates; 4 g protein; 2 gfiber; 245 mg sodium; 42 mg potassium.
Carbohydrate Servings: 2
Exchanges: 1 starch, 1 other carbohydrate, 1 1/2 fat

Spicy Tofu Hotpot

INGREDIENTS
- 14 ounces firm tofu, preferably water-packed
- 2 teaspoons canola oil
- 2 tablespoons grated fresh ginger
- 6 cloves garlic, minced
- 4 ounces fresh shiitake mushrooms, stemmed and sliced (about 2 cups)
- 1 tablespoon brown sugar
- 4 cups vegetable broth, or reduced-sodium chicken broth
- 1/4 cup reduced-sodium soy sauce
- 2 teaspoons chile-garlic sauce, or to taste
- 4 cups thinly sliced tender bok choy greens
- 8 ounces fresh Chinese-style (lo mein) noodles
- 1/2 cup chopped fresh cilantro

PREPARATION
1. Drain and rinse tofu; pat dry. Cut the block into 1-inch cubes.
2. Heat oil in a Dutch oven over medium heat. Add ginger and garlic; cook, stirring, until fragrant, about 1 minute. Add mushrooms and cook until slightly soft, 2 to 3 minutes. Stir in sugar, broth, soy sauce and chile-garlic sauce; cover and bring to a boil. Add bok choy and tofu, cover and simmer until greens are wilted, about 2 minutes. Raise heat to high and add the noodles, pushing them down into the broth. Cook, covered, until the noodles are tender, 2 to 3 minutes. Remove from the heat and stir in cilantro.

TIPS & NOTES
- Chile-garlic sauce is a spicy blend of chiles, garlic and other seasonings; it is found in the Asian section of the market.

NUTRITION
Per serving: 251 calories; 7 g fat (1 g sat, 1 g mono); 0 mg cholesterol; 40 g carbohydrates; 13 g protein; 7 g fiber; 636 mg sodium; 191 mg potassium.
Nutrition Bonus: Vitamin A (45% daily value), Vitamin C (40% dv), Fiber (27% dv), Iron (20% dv).
Carbohydrate Servings: 2
Exchanges: 2 starch, 1 vegetable, 1/2 medium-fat meat, 1 fat

Creamy Herb Dip

INGREDIENTS
- 1/4 cup reduced-fat cream cheese, (Neufchâtel), softened (2 ounces)
- 2 tablespoons buttermilk, or low-fat milk
- 2 tablespoons chopped fresh chives, or scallions
- 1 tablespoon chopped fresh dill, or parsley
- 1 teaspoon prepared horseradish, or more to taste
- Pinch of sugar
- 1/8 teaspoon salt
- Freshly ground pepper, to taste

PREPARATION
1. Place cream cheese in a small bowl and stir in buttermilk (or milk) until smooth. Mix in chives (or scallions), dill (or parsley), horseradish, sugar, salt and pepper.

TIPS & NOTES
- **Make Ahead Tip**: Cover and refrigerate for up to 4 days.

NUTRITION

Per tablespoon: 20 calories; 2 g fat (1 g sat, 0 g mono); 5 mg cholesterol; 1 g carbohydrates; 0 g added sugars; 1 g protein; 0 g fiber; 72 mg sodium; 18 mg potassium.
Exchanges: free food

Baba Ganouj

INGREDIENTS

- 2 medium eggplants, (about 1 pound each)
- 4 cloves garlic, unpeeled
- 1/4 cup lemon juice
- 2 tablespoons tahini, (see Note)
- 1 1/4 teaspoons salt
- Extra-virgin olive oil, for garnish
- Ground sumac, for garnish (see Note)

PREPARATION

1. Preheat grill to high.
2. Prick eggplants all over with a fork. Thread garlic cloves onto a skewer. Grill the eggplants, turning occasionally, until charred and tender, 10 to 12 minutes. Grill the garlic, turning once, until charred and tender, 6 to 8 minutes.
3. Transfer the eggplants and garlic to a cutting board. When cool enough to handle, peel both. Transfer to a food processor. Add lemon juice, tahini and salt; process until almost smooth. Drizzle with oil and sprinkle with sumac, if desired.

TIPS & NOTES

- **Make Ahead Tip**: Cover and refrigerate for up to 3 days. | Equipment: Skewer
- **Notes:** Tahini is a thick paste of ground sesame seeds. Look for it in large supermarkets in the Middle Eastern section or near other nut butters.
- The tart berries of a particular variety of sumac bush add a distinctive element to many Middle Eastern dishes. Find them whole or ground in Middle Eastern markets or online at kalustyans.com or lebaneseproducts.com.

NUTRITION

Per serving: 32 calories; 1 g fat (0 g sat, 1 g mono); 0 mg cholesterol; 5 g carbohydrates; 0 g added sugars;1 g protein; 2 g fiber; 245 mg sodium; 163 mg potassium.
Exchanges: 1 vegetable

Turkey Cutlets with Peas & Spring Onions

INGREDIENTS
- 1/2 cup all-purpose flour
- 1/2 teaspoon salt, divided
- 1/4 teaspoon freshly ground pepper
- 1 pound 1/4-inch-thick turkey breast cutlets, or steaks
- 2 tablespoons extra-virgin olive oil, divided
- 4 ounces shiitake mushrooms, stemmed and sliced (about 1 1/2 cups)
- 1 bunch spring onions, or scallions, sliced, whites and greens separated
- 1 cup reduced-sodium chicken broth
- 1/2 cup dry white wine
- 1 cup peas, fresh or frozen, thawed
- 1 teaspoon freshly grated lemon zest

PREPARATION
1. Whisk flour, 1/4 teaspoon salt and pepper in a shallow dish. Dredge each turkey cutlet (or steak) in the flour mixture. Heat 1 tablespoon oil in a large nonstick skillet over medium-high heat. Add the turkey and cook until lightly golden, 2 to 3 minutes per side. Transfer to a plate; cover with foil to keep warm.
2. Add the remaining 1 tablespoon oil to the pan and heat over medium-high heat. Add mushrooms and onion (or scallion) whites and cook, stirring often, until the mushrooms are browned and the whites are slightly softened, 2 to 3 minutes. Add broth, wine and the remaining 1/4 teaspoon salt; cook, stirring occasionally, until the sauce is slightly reduced, 2 to 3 minutes. Stir in peas and onion (or scallion) greens and cook, stirring, until heated through, about 1 minute. Stir in lemon zest. Nestle the turkey into the vegetables along with any accumulated juices from the plate. Cook, turning the cutlets once, until heated through, 1 to 2 minutes.

NUTRITION

Per serving: 313 calories; 8 g fat (1 g sat, 5 g mono); 45 mg cholesterol; 23 g carbohydrates; 34 g protein; 3 g fiber; 571 mg sodium; 223 mg potassium.
Nutrition Bonus: Iron (15% daily value), Vitamin A & C (20% dv).
Carbohydrate Servings: 1
Exchanges: 1 starch, 1 vegetable, 4 lean meat, 1 fat

Black Bean-Salmon Stir-Fry

INGREDIENTS
- 1/4 cup water
- 2 tablespoons rice vinegar
- 2 tablespoons black bean-garlic sauce, (see Note)

- 1 tablespoon Shao Hsing rice wine or dry sherry, (see Note)
- 2 teaspoons cornstarch
- Pinch of crushed red pepper
- 1 tablespoon canola oil
- 1 pound salmon, skinned (see Tip) and cut into 1-inch cubes
- 12 ounces mung bean sprouts, (6 cups)
- 1 bunch scallions, sliced

PREPARATION

1. Whisk water, vinegar, black bean-garlic sauce, rice wine (or sherry), cornstarch and crushed red pepper in a small bowl until combined.
2. Heat oil in a large nonstick skillet over medium-high heat. Add salmon and cook, stirring gently, for 2 minutes. Add bean sprouts, scallions and the sauce mixture (the pan will be full). Cook, stirring, until the sprouts are cooked down and very tender, 2 to 3 minutes.

TIPS & NOTES

- **Notes:** Black bean-garlic sauce, a savory, salty sauce used in Chinese cooking, is made from fermented black soybeans, garlic and rice wine. Find it in the Asian-foods section of some supermarkets or at Asian markets.
- The "cooking sherry" sold in many supermarkets can be surprisingly high in sodium. We prefer dry sherry, sold with other fortified wines in your wine or liquor store.
- **Tip:** How to skin a salmon fillet: Place salmon fillet on a clean cutting board, skin-side down. Starting at the tail end, slip the blade of a long knife between the fish flesh and the skin, holding down firmly with your other hand. Gently push the blade along a 30° angle, separating the fillet from the skin without cutting through either.

NUTRITION

Per serving: 302 calories; 17 g fat (3 g sat, 6 g mono); 67 mg cholesterol; 12 g carbohydrates; 26 g protein;3 g fiber; 802 mg sodium; 608 mg potassium.
Nutrition Bonus: Selenium (60% daily value), Vitamin C (33% dv), Folate (24% dv), Potassium (17% dv), excellent source of omega-3s.
Carbohydrate Servings: 1
Exchanges: 1 vegetable, 1/2 other carbohydrate, 3 lean meat, 1 fat

DAY 26
BREAKFAST

Skim milk (1 cup)
Overnight Oatmeal
Grapefruit (1/2)

LUNCH

Stir-Fry of Pork with Vietnamese Flavors
Quick Kimchi or Crunchy Bok Choy Slaw
Whole-wheat toast (1 slice)

SNACK

Skim milk (1 cup)

DINNER

Korean Chicken Soup or Sausage Soup
Arugula-Mushroom Salad
Sliced Tomato Salad
Salsa Cornbread
Strawberries (1 cup)

DAY 26 RECIPES

Overnight Oatmeal

INGREDIENTS
- 8 cups water
- 2 cups steel-cut oats, (see Ingredient note)
- 1/3 cup dried cranberries
- 1/3 cup dried apricots, chopped
- 1/4 teaspoon salt, or to taste

PREPARATION
1. Combine water, oats, dried cranberries, dried apricots and salt in a 5- or 6-quart slow cooker. Turn heat to low. Put the lid on and cook until the oats are tender and the porridge is creamy, 7 to 8 hours. Stovetop Variation Halve the above recipe to accommodate the size of most double boilers: Combine 4 cups water, 1 cup steel cut oats, 3 tablespoons dried cranberries, 3 tablespoons dried apricots and 1/8 teaspoon salt in the top of a double boiler. Cover and cook over boiling water for about 1 1/2 hours, check the water level in the bottom of the double boiler.

TIPS & NOTES
- **Ingredient Note:** Steel-cut oats, sometimes labeled "Irish oatmeal," look like small pebbles. They are toasted oat groats—the oat kernel that has been

removed from the husk that have been cut in 2 or 3 pieces. Do not substitute regular rolled oats, which have a shorter cooking time, in the slow-cooker oatmeal recipe.
- For easy cleanup, try a slow-cooker liner. These heat-resistant, disposable liners fit neatly inside the insert and help prevent food from sticking to the bottom and sides of your slow cooker.

NUTRITION
Per serving: 193 calories; 3 g fat (0 g sat, 1 g mono); 0 mg cholesterol; 34 g carbohydrates; 0 g added sugars; 6 g protein; 9 g fiber; 77 mg sodium; 195 mg potassium.
Nutrition Bonus: Fiber (36% daily value).
Carbohydrate Servings: 2
Exchanges: 2 starch, 1/2 fruit

Stir-Fry of Pork with Vietnamese Flavors

INGREDIENTS
- 2 tablespoons finely chopped fresh ginger
- 2 serrano or jalapeño peppers, seeded and finely chopped
- 4 cloves garlic, finely chopped
- 3 tablespoons fish sauce, divided
- 2 tablespoons orange juice, divided
- 1 teaspoon cornstarch
- 1/2 teaspoon freshly ground pepper
- 1 pound pork tenderloin, trimmed and cut across the grain into 1/4-inch-thick slices
- 1 tablespoon sugar and 3 teaspoons canola oil, divided
- 2 cups finely sliced onions, (2-4 onions)
- 1/4 cup sliced fresh cilantro leaves

PREPARATION

1. Combine ginger, peppers, garlic, 1 tablespoon of the fish sauce, 1 tablespoon of the orange juice, cornstarch and black pepper in a shallow dish. Add pork and toss to coat it with marinade. Set aside to marinate for 10 to 20 minutes.
2. Mix sugar, the remaining 2 tablespoons fish sauce and 1 tablespoon orange juice in a small bowl.
3. Heat a wok over high heat. Swirl in 1 teaspoon of the oil. Add onions and cook, stirring, until limp and caramelized, about 5 minutes. Transfer the onions to a plate. Wipe out the pan. Add the remaining 2 teaspoons oil to the pan and increase heat to high. Slowly drop in pork and stir-fry until browned and just cooked through, 2 to 3 minutes. Add the reserved fish sauce/orange juice

mixture and the reserved onions; toss until the pork is coated with sauce. Sprinkle with cilantro and serve over rice.

NUTRITION

Per serving: 243 calories; 7 g fat (1 g sat, 4 g mono); 68 mg cholesterol; 19 g carbohydrates; 3 g added sugars; 25 g protein; 3 g fiber; 575 mg sodium; 615 mg potassium.
Nutrition Bonus: Selenium (44% daily value), Vitamin C (28% dv), Potassium (18% dv).
Carbohydrate Servings: 1
Exchanges: 1 1/2 vegetable, 3 lean meat

Quick Kimchi

INGREDIENTS
- 1 small head napa (Chinese) cabbage, cored and cut into 1-inch squares (about 8 cups)
- 2 cloves garlic, minced
- 1/4 cup water
- 2 tablespoons distilled white vinegar
- 1 tablespoon toasted sesame oil
- 2 teaspoons fresh ginger, finely grated
- 3/4 teaspoon salt
- 1/2 teaspoon sugar
- 1/2 teaspoon crushed red pepper, red
- 3 scallions, sliced
- 1 carrot, peeled and grated

PREPARATION
1. Combine cabbage, garlic and water in a large saucepan and bring to a boil over high heat. Reduce heat to medium-low and cook, stirring once or twice, until tender, 4 to 5 minutes.
2. Meanwhile, whisk vinegar, oil, ginger, salt, sugar and crushed red pepper in a large bowl.
3. Add the cabbage, scallions and carrot to the bowl and toss to combine. Refrigerate for about 25 minutes before serving.

NUTRITION
Per serving: 37 calories; 2 g fat (0 g sat, 1 g mono); 0 mg cholesterol; 4 g carbohydrates; 0 g added sugars;1 g protein; 1 g fiber; 235 mg sodium; 47 mg potassium.
Nutrition Bonus: Vitamin A (50% daily value), Vitamin C (40% dv).
Exchanges: 1 vegetable

Crunchy Bok Choy Slaw

INGREDIENTS
- 1/4 cup rice vinegar
- 1 tablespoon toasted sesame oil
- 2 teaspoons sugar
- 2 teaspoons Dijon mustard
- 1/4 teaspoon salt
- 6 cups very thinly sliced bok choy, (about a 1-pound head, trimmed)
- 2 medium carrots, shredded
- 2 scallions, thinly sliced

PREPARATION
1. Whisk vinegar, oil, sugar, mustard and salt in a large bowl until the sugar dissolves. Add bok choy, carrots and scallions; toss to coat with the dressing.

NUTRITION

Per serving: 33 calories; 2 g fat (0 g sat, 1 g mono); 0 mg cholesterol; 4 g carbohydrates; 1 g added sugars; 1 g protein; 1 g fiber; 132 mg sodium; 185 mg potassium.
Nutrition Bonus: Vitamin A (100% daily value), Vitamin C (40% dv).
Exchanges: 1 vegetable

Korean Chicken Soup

INGREDIENTS
- 8 cups reduced-sodium chicken broth
- 2 tablespoons finely chopped garlic
- 2 tablespoons finely grated fresh ginger
- 1/2 cup uncooked white rice
- 1 tablespoon reduced-sodium soy sauce
- 1 teaspoon toasted sesame oil
- 1-2 teaspoons hot chile paste or hot chile sauce
- 1 cup shredded cooked chicken (see How To)
- 2 scallions, finely chopped
- 1 tablespoon sesame seeds, toasted (see Tip)

PREPARATION
1. Combine broth, garlic and ginger in a Dutch oven; bring to a boil over high heat. Add rice, reduce the heat to medium-low and simmer until the rice is tender, 12 to 15 minutes. Stir in soy sauce and sesame oil; add chile paste (or sauce) to taste. Add chicken and heat through. Garnish with scallions and sesame seeds.

TIPS & NOTES

- **How To Poach Chicken Breasts:** If you don't have leftover chicken but you want to make a recipe that calls for cooked chicken, the easiest way to cook it is to poach it. Place boneless, skinless chicken breasts in a medium skillet or saucepan. Add lightly salted water (or chicken broth) to cover and bring to a boil. Cover, reduce heat to low and simmer gently until the chicken is cooked through and
no longer pink in the middle, 10 to 15 minutes. (1 pound raw chicken = about 2 1/2 cups chopped or shredded cooked chicken)
- **Tip:** To toast sesame seeds, place in a small dry skillet and cook over medium-low heat, stirring constantly, until fragrant and lightly browned, 2 to 4 minutes.

NUTRITION

Per serving: 149 calories; 2 g fat (0 g sat, 1 g mono); 20 mg cholesterol; 18 g carbohydrates; 0 g added sugars; 13 g protein; 1 g fiber; 857 mg sodium; 392 mg potassium.
Nutrition Bonus: Folate (16% daily value)
Carbohydrate Servings: 1
Exchanges: 1 starch, 1 1/2 lean meat

Sausage Soup

INGREDIENTS

- 8 ounces hot Italian turkey sausage, casings removed
- 8 ounces sweet Italian turkey sausage, casings removed
- 5 cups water
- 3 large white potatoes, (about 2 1/2 pounds), cut into 1/2-inch cubes
- 3 stalks celery, sliced
- 1 small zucchini, sliced
- 1 medium onion, chopped
- 1 28-ounce can whole tomatoes, chopped, juice reserved
- 1 15-ounce can kidney beans, undrained
- 3/4 cup sliced California Ripe Olives
- 2 cloves garlic, minced
- 1 teaspoon aniseed
- 1/2 teaspoon freshly ground pepper

PREPARATION

1. Cook hot and sweet sausages in a Dutch oven over medium heat, breaking them up into small pieces with a wooden spoon, until browned and cooked through, about 6 minutes. Drain fat.

2. Stir in water, potatoes, celery, zucchini, onion, tomatoes with their juices, beans, olives, garlic, aniseed and pepper. Bring to a boil. Reduce heat to low, cover and simmer until vegetables are tender, about 30 minutes.

TIPS & NOTES
- **Make Ahead Tip**: Cover and refrigerate for up to 1 day.

NUTRITION
Per serving: 145 calories; 6 g fat (1 g sat, 0 g mono); 23 mg cholesterol; 12 g carbohydrates; 0 g added sugars; 10 g protein; 3 g fiber; 392 mg sodium; 240 mg potassium.
Nutrition Bonus: Vitamin C (16% daily value)
Carbohydrate Servings: 1
Exchanges: 1/2 starch, 1/2 vegetable, 1 lean meat, 1/2 fat

Arugula-Mushroom Salad

INGREDIENTS
- 1 clove garlic, peeled
- 1/4 teaspoon salt
- 1 tablespoon lemon juice
- 1 tablespoon reduced-fat mayonnaise
- 1 tablespoon extra-virgin olive oil
- 1 tablespoon chopped fresh parsley
- Freshly ground pepper, to taste
- 6 cups arugula leaves and 2 cups sliced mushrooms

PREPARATION
1. Place garlic on a cutting board and crush. Sprinkle with salt and use the flat of a chef's knife blade to mash the garlic to a paste; transfer to a serving bowl. Whisk in lemon juice, mayonnaise, oil and parsley. Season with pepper. Add arugula and mushrooms; toss to coat with the dressing.

NUTRITION
Per serving: 62 calories; 4 g fat (1 g sat, 3 g mono); 1 mg cholesterol; 3 g carbohydrates; 0 g added sugars; 2 g protein; 1 g fiber; 188 mg sodium; 235 mg potassium.
Nutrition Bonus: Vitamin C (15% daily value).
Exchanges: 1 vegetable, 1 fat (mono)

Sliced Tomato Salad

INGREDIENTS
- 4 tomatoes, sliced
- 1/4 cup thinly sliced red onion
- 8 anchovies
- 1/2 teaspoon dried oregano
- Salt & freshly ground pepper, to taste
- 2 tablespoons extra-virgin olive oil
- 1 tablespoon white-wine vinegar

PREPARATION
1. Arrange tomato slices on a platter. Top with onion, anchovies, oregano, salt and pepper. Drizzle with oil and vinegar.

NUTRITION
Per serving: 44 calories; 1 g fat (0 g sat, 0 g mono); 3 mg cholesterol; 8 g carbohydrates; 0 g added sugars;3 g protein; 2 g fiber; 300 mg sodium; 403 mg potassium.
Nutrition Bonus: Vitamin C (35% daily value), Vitamin A (25% dv).
Carbohydrate Servings: 1/2
Exchanges: 1 vegetable, 1 1/2 fat

Salsa Cornbread

INGREDIENTS
- 1 cup all-purpose flour
- 1/2 cup whole-wheat flour
- 1/2 cup cornmeal
- 2 teaspoons baking powder
- 1/2 teaspoon salt
- Freshly ground pepper, to taste
- 3 large eggs, lightly beaten
- 1/2 cup buttermilk, or equivalent buttermilk powder
- 1 tablespoon butter, melted
- 1 tablespoon honey
- 1/2 cup drained canned corn kernels
- 1 small onion, diced
- 1/2 cup chopped tomato
- 1 clove garlic, minced
- 1 jalapeno pepper, seeded and minced
- 1/2 cup grated Cheddar cheese

PREPARATION
1. Preheat oven to 425° F. Place a 9-inch cast-iron skillet (or similar ovenproof skillet, see Tip) in the oven to heat.
2. Whisk all-purpose flour, whole-wheat flour, cornmeal, baking powder, salt and pepper in a large mixing bowl.
3. Whisk eggs, buttermilk, butter and honey in a medium bowl. Add the egg mixture to the dry ingredients; mix with a rubber spatula. Stir in corn, onion, tomato, garlic and jalapeno.
4. Remove the skillet from the oven and coat it with cooking spray. Pour in the batter, spreading evenly. Sprinkle cheese over the top. Bake the cornbread until golden brown and a knife inserted into the center comes out clean, 20 to 25 minutes. Serve warm.

TIPS & NOTES
- **Tip:** If you do not have an ovenproof skillet of the correct size, use an 8-by-8-inch glass baking dish. Do not preheat the empty baking dish in the oven before filling it.

NUTRITION

Per serving: 138 calories; 4 g fat (2 g sat, 1 g mono); 70 mg cholesterol; 20 g carbohydrates; 6 g protein; 1 g fiber; 319 mg sodium; 91 mg potassium.
Carbohydrate Servings: 1
Exchanges: 1 starch, 1 fat

Day 27
BREAKFAST

Morning Smoothie
Whole-wheat toast (1 slice)
Plum spread

LUNCH

Skim milk (1 cup)
Fillet of Sole with Spinach & Tomatoes or Tofu with Tomato-Mushroom Sauce
Whole-wheat pita bread (1 medium pita)

SNACK

Apple (1 cup, quartered)
Fat-free cheese (1 slice)

DINNER

Penne with Tomato & Sweet Pepper Sauce (Penne Saporite "Il Frantoio")
Really Low-Fat Garlic Bread or Herbed Potato Bread
The Diet House Salad
Strawberry Fool

DAY 27 RECIPES

Morning Smoothie

INGREDIENTS
- 1 1/4 cups orange juice, preferably calcium-fortified
- 1 banana
- 1 1/4 cups frozen berries, such as raspberries, blackberries, blueberries and/or strawberries
- 1/2 cup low-fat silken tofu, or low-fat plain yogurt
- 1 tablespoon sugar, or Splenda Granular (optional)

PREPARATION
1. Combine orange juice, banana, berries, tofu (or yogurt) and sugar (or Splenda), if using, in a blender; cover and blend until creamy. Serve immediately.

NUTRITION
Per serving: 139 calories; 2 g fat (0 g sat, 0 g mono); 0 mg cholesterol; 33 g carbohydrates; 0 g added sugars; 4 g protein; 4 g fiber; 19 mg sodium; 421 mg potassium.
Nutrition Bonus: Vitamin C (110% daily value), Fiber (16% dv).
Carbohydrate Servings: 2
Exchanges: 2 fruit, 1/2 low-fat milk

Plum spread

INGREDIENTS
- 5 pounds plums, pitted and sliced (14-15 cups)
- 3 Granny Smith apples, washed and quartered (not cored)
- 1/4 cup white grape juice, or other fruit juice
- 2 tablespoons lemon juice
- 3/4 cup sugar, or Splenda Granular
- 1/4 teaspoon ground cinnamon, or ginger (optional)

PREPARATION
1. Place a plate in the freezer for testing consistency later.
2. Combine plums, apples, grape juice (or fruit juice) and lemon juice in a large, heavy-bottomed, nonreactive Dutch oven. Bring to a boil over medium-high heat, stirring. Cover and boil gently, stirring occasionally, until the fruit is softened and juicy, 15 to 20 minutes. Uncover and boil gently, stirring occasionally, until the fruit is completely soft, about 20 minutes. (Adjust heat as necessary to maintain a gentle boil.)
3. Pass the fruit through a food mill to remove the skins and apple seeds.
4. Return the strained fruit to the pot. Add sugar (or Splenda) and cinnamon (or ginger), if using. Cook over medium heat, stirring frequently, until a spoonful of jam dropped onto the chilled plate holds its shape, about 15 minutes longer. (See Tip.) Remove from heat and skim off any foam.

TIPS & NOTES
- **Make Ahead Tip**: Store in an airtight container in the refrigerator for up to 2 months. For longer storage, process in a boiling-water bath (for detailed instructions, refer to www.homecanning.com or call the Home Canner's Hotline at 800-240-3340).
- **To test the consistency of the spread:** Drop a dollop of cooked spread onto a chilled plate. Carefully run your finger through the dollop. If the track remains unfilled, the jam is done.

NUTRITION
Per tablespoon with sugar: 14 calories; 0 g fat (0 g sat, 0 g mono); 0 mg cholesterol; 4 g carbohydrates; 0 g protein; 0 g fiber; 0 mg sodium; 30 mg potassium.
Exchanges: free food
Nutrition Note: Per tablespoon with Splenda: 0 Carbohydrate Servings; 12 calories; 3 g carbohydrate.

Fillet of Sole with Spinach & Tomatoes

INGREDIENTS
- 12 cups spinach, (1 1/4 pounds), trimmed and washed thoroughly
- 2 cloves garlic, minced
- 1/4 teaspoon salt
- Freshly ground pepper to taste
- 1 pound Pacific sole fillets, divided into 4 portions (see Tip)
- 4 small plum tomatoes, sliced

PREPARATION
1. Preheat oven to 400°F.
2. Put spinach, with water still clinging to its leaves, into a large pot. Cover; steam the spinach over medium-high heat, stirring occasionally, until just wilted, about 5 minutes. Drain; when cool enough to handle, press out excess liquid. Chop and place in a small bowl. Stir in garlic. Season with salt and pepper.
3. To make a packet, lay two 20-inch sheets of foil on top of each other (the double layers will help protect the contents from burning); generously coat the top piece with cooking spray. Place one-quarter of the spinach mixture in the center of the foil. Lay a portion of sole over the spinach and arrange tomato slices over the sole. Season with salt and pepper.
4. Bring the short ends of the foil together, leaving enough room in the packet for steam to gather and cook the food. Fold the foil over and pinch to seal. Pinch seams together along the sides. Make sure all the seams are tightly sealed to keep steam from escaping. Repeat with more foil, cooking spray and the remaining ingredients.
5. Place the packets on a baking sheet. Bake the packets until the fish is cooked through and the vegetables are just tender, 10 to 12 minutes. To serve, carefully open both ends of the packets and allow the steam to escape. Use a spatula to slide the contents onto plates.

TIPS & NOTES
- **Tip:** A number of flatfish are marketed as sole or flounder. Eco-friendly choices include U.S. and Canadian Pacific-caught English, Dover and petrale sole as well as sand dabs and flounder, according to the Monterey Bay Aquarium's Seafood Watch program. Pacific halibut is a good option if you can't find Pacific sole or flounder.

NUTRITION
Per serving: 138 calories; 2 g fat (0 g sat, 0 g mono); 53 mg cholesterol; 8 g carbohydrates; 0 g added sugars; 24 g protein; 4 g fiber; 343 mg sodium; 1213 mg potassium.

Nutrition Bonus: Vitamin A (280% daily value), Vitamin C (80% dv), Folate (73% dv), Potassium (35% dv), Iron (25% dv), Calcium (15% dv).
Carbohydrate Servings: 1/2
Exchanges: 1 1/2 vegetable, 3 lean meat

Tofu with Tomato-Mushroom Sauce

INGREDIENTS
- 14 ounces extra-firm tofu, preferably water-packed
- 2 teaspoons extra-virgin olive oil
- 2 medium tomatoes, coarsely chopped (about 1 1/2 cups)
- 1 1/2 cups sliced mushrooms, (4 ounces)
- 2 tablespoons prepared pesto
- 2 tablespoons crumbled feta cheese

PREPARATION

1. Drain and rinse tofu; pat dry. Slice the block crosswise into eight 1/2-inch-thick slabs. Coarsely crumble each slice into smaller, uneven pieces.
2. Heat oil in a large nonstick skillet over high heat. Add tofu and cook in a single layer, without stirring, until the pieces begin to turn golden brown on the bottom, about 5 minutes. Then gently stir and continue cooking, stirring occasionally, until all sides are golden brown, 5 to 7 minutes more.
3. Add tomatoes and mushrooms and cook, stirring, until the vegetables are just cooked, 1 to 2 minutes more. Remove from the heat and stir in pesto and feta.

NUTRITION
Per serving: 136 calories; 11 g fat (3 g sat, 5 g mono); 7 mg cholesterol; 6 g carbohydrates; 0 g added sugars; 12 g protein; 2 g fiber; 128 mg sodium; 415 mg potassium.
Nutrition Bonus: Calcium (16% daily value), Folate (15% dv).
Carbohydrate Servings: 1/2
Exchanges: 1 vegetable, 1 medium-fat meat, 1 fat (mono)

Penne with Tomato & Sweet Pepper Sauce (Penne Saporite "Il Frantoio")

INGREDIENTS
- 2 tablespoons extra-virgin olive oil
- 1 small onion, very finely chopped
- 2 large cloves garlic, very finely chopped
- 1/4 teaspoon crushed red pepper, or to taste
- 1 small yellow or red bell pepper, cored and diced
- 1 pound ripe plum tomatoes, peeled, seeded and chopped (5-6 tomatoes), or one 14-ounce can plum tomatoes, drained and chopped

- Salt to taste
- 3-4 tablespoons reduced-sodium chicken broth or water
- Freshly ground pepper to taste
- 1 pound whole-wheat penne

PREPARATION

1. Heat oil in a large skillet over medium-low heat. Add onions and cook, stirring, until soft, sweet and slightly caramelized, about 10 minutes. Add garlic and crushed red pepper and cook, stirring, for 1 minute to release their fragrance. Add bell peppers, tomatoes and salt. Cover, adjust heat to maintain a simmer, and stew, stirring occasionally, until the vegetables are very soft, about 15 minutes.
2. Transfer the mixture to a food processor or blender and puree, adding broth or water as needed to make a smooth sauce. Return the sauce to the pan. Reheat gently; taste and season with salt and black pepper. Keep warm.
3. Meanwhile, cook penne in a large pot of boiling salted water until al dente, 8 to 10 minutes. Drain, then transfer to a warm bowl. Add sauce and toss. Serve immediately on warm plates.

NUTRITION
Per serving: 262 calories; 5 g fat (1 g sat, 3 g mono); 0 mg cholesterol; 46 g carbohydrates; 0 g added sugars; 8 g protein; 6 g fiber; 53 mg sodium; 394 mg potassium.
Nutrition Bonus: Vitamin C (33% daily value), Vitamin A (16% dv).
Carbohydrate Servings: 2 1/2

Really Low-Fat Garlic Bread

INGREDIENTS
- 4 large cloves garlic
- 1 teaspoon extra-virgin olive oil
- 1/4 teaspoon salt
- 1/2 baguette, cut in half lengthwise

PREPARATION
1. Preheat oven to 450°F.
2. Place garlic in a small saucepan with enough cold water to cover and bring to a simmer over low heat. Cook 3 minutes and drain.
3. Mash the cooked garlic, oil and salt in a small bowl with the back of a spoon until a smooth paste forms. Spread the mixture over the cut surfaces of the bread.

4. Place the bread on a baking sheet and bake until the bread begins to brown around the edges, 4 to 6 minutes. Slice and serve.

NUTRITION
Per serving: 113 calories; 2 g fat (0 g sat, 1 g mono); 0 mg cholesterol; 22 g carbohydrates; 0 g added sugars; 6 g protein; 4 g fiber; 338 mg sodium; 12 mg potassium.
Carbohydrate Servings: 1 1/2
Exchanges: 1 1/2 starch, 1/2 fat

Herbed Potato Bread

INGREDIENTS
BREAD
- 1 all-purpose potato, (6 ounces), peeled and halved
- 1 tablespoon extra-virgin olive oil
- 1/2 teaspoon sugar
- 2 tablespoons lukewarm water
- 1 1/4 teaspoons active dry yeast
- 1 1/2 cups whole-wheat flour
- 1 tablespoon chopped fresh rosemary
- 1 tablespoon chopped fresh thyme
- 1 teaspoon chopped fresh sage
- 1 1/4 teaspoons salt
- 1 1/2-1 3/4 cups all-purpose flour
- Cornmeal, for dusting

GLAZE & DECORATION
- 6 fresh chives
- 6-8 sprigs fresh flat-leaf parsley
- 4-6 fresh sage leaves
- 1 egg white and 1 tablespoon water

PREPARATION

1. Place potato in a small saucepan and cover with water; bring to a boil. Reduce heat to medium-low, cover and cook until tender, 15 to 20 minutes. Drain, reserving 1 cup cooking liquid. Place the potato in a bowl and mash with a fork or potato masher. Drizzle with oil. Let mashed potato and reserved cooking liquid cool to lukewarm.
2. Dissolve sugar in water in a large bowl. Stir in yeast and let stand until foamy, about 5 minutes. Add the mashed potato and reserved cooking liquid. Gradually beat in whole-wheat flour. Beat for 1 minute. Stir in rosemary, thyme, sage and salt. Gradually beat in enough of the all-purpose flour until the dough is too stiff

to beat. Turn the dough out onto a lightly floured surface. Knead until smooth and elastic, adding just enough flour to prevent sticking, about 10 minutes. (Alternatively, use a stand-up mixer fitted with a dough hook to mix and knead the dough.)
3. Place the dough in a lightly oiled bowl. Turn to coat and cover with plastic wrap. Let rise until doubled in bulk, about 1 1/2 hours.
4. Coat a large baking sheet with cooking spray. Sprinkle with cornmeal. Punch the dough down. Turn out onto the work surface and knead several times. Divide dough in half and shape each piece into a ball. Place loaves several inches apart on the baking sheet. Cover with plastic wrap and let rise for 1 hour.
5. Half an hour before baking, place a baking stone or inverted baking sheet on the middle rack of the oven. Place a small baking pan on the rack below. Preheat oven to 450°F.
6. To decorate loaves: Place a large bowl of cold water beside the stove. Bring a large saucepan of water to a boil. Drop chives, parsley sprigs and sage leaves into the boiling water for a few seconds. Retrieve with tongs or a slotted spoon and drop into the cold water. Pat herbs dry.
7. Blend egg white and water with a fork in a small bowl; brush over the risen loaves. Arrange herb sprigs decoratively over the loaves. Brush again with the egg-white glaze.
8. Pour 1 cup water into the baking pan in the oven. Place the baking sheet on the baking stone (or inverted baking sheet) and bake the loaves for 20 minutes. Reduce oven temperature to 400° and bake until the loaves are golden and the bottoms sound hollow when tapped, 10 to 15 minutes. Transfer to a wire rack and let cool.

NUTRITION
Per slice: 101 calories; 1 g fat (0 g sat, 1 g mono); 0 mg cholesterol; 17 g carbohydrates; 4 g protein; 2 gfiber; 185 mg sodium; 57 mg potassium.
Carbohydrate Servings: 1
Exchanges: 1 1/3 starch

The Diet House Salad

INGREDIENTS
- 4 cups torn green leaf lettuce
- 1 cup sprouts
- 1 cup tomato wedges
- 1 cup peeled, sliced cucumber
- 1 cup shredded carrots
- 1/2 cup chopped radishes
- 1/2 cup Sesame Tamari Vinaigrette (recipe follows), or other dressing

PREPARATION
1. Toss lettuce, sprouts, tomato, cucumber, carrots and radishes in a large bowl with the dressing until the vegetables are coated.

NUTRITION

Per serving: 71 calories; 3 g fat (0 g sat, 1 g mono); 0 mg cholesterol; 11 g carbohydrates; 2 g protein; 3 gfiber; 334 mg sodium; 428 mg potassium.
Nutrition Bonus: Vitamin A (140% daily value), Vitamin C (30% dv), Folate (16% dv).
Carbohydrate Servings: 1
Exchanges: 2 vegetable, 1/2 fat

Strawberry Fool

INGREDIENTS
- 1/4 cup whipping cream
- 2 teaspoons sugar
- 1/8 teaspoon vanilla extract
- 1 quart fresh strawberries, hulled and finely chopped

PREPARATION
1. Chill a small bowl and the beaters of an electric mixer. Whip cream with chilled beaters until soft peaks form. Add sugar and vanilla and continue beating until the peaks are firm but not stiff. (Do not overbeat.) Fold in strawberries.

TIPS & NOTES
- **Make Ahead Tip**: Cover and refrigerate for up to 2 hours.

NUTRITION

Per serving: 98 calories; 5 g fat (3 g sat, 1 g mono); 17 mg cholesterol; 14 g carbohydrates; 1 g protein; 3 gfiber; 7 mg sodium; 235 mg potassium.
Nutrition Bonus: Vitamin C (141% daily value).
Carbohydrate Servings: 1
Exchanges: 1/2 fruit, 1 fat

DAY 28
BREAKFAST

Zucchini-Walnut Loaf
Skim milk (1 cup)
Grapefruit (1/2)

LUNCH

Chicken Potpieor Gnocchi with Tomatoes, Pancetta & Wilted Watercress
Skim milk (1 cup)

SNACK

Fat-free cheese (1 slice)

DINNER

Pizza-Style Meatloaf or Halibut with Herbs & Capers
Steamed broccoli (1/2 cup)
Quick-cooking barley (1 cup)
The Wedge
Apricot (1/2 cup, halves)

DAY 28 RECIPES

Zucchini-Walnut Loaf

INGREDIENTS
- 3/4 cup whole-wheat flour
- 3/4 cup all-purpose flour
- 1 teaspoon baking powder
- 1/4 teaspoon baking soda
- 1/4 teaspoon salt
- 1 teaspoon ground cinnamon
- 1/4 teaspoon ground nutmeg
- 2 large egg whites, at room temperature (see Tip)
- 1 cup sugar, or 1/2 cup
- 1/2 cup unsweetened applesauce
- 2 tablespoons canola oil
- 1/4 teaspoon lemon extract, (optional)
- 1 cup grated zucchini, lightly packed (about 8 ounces)
- 2 tablespoons chopped walnuts

PREPARATION
1. Preheat oven to 350°F. Coat 2 mini 6-by-3-inch loaf pans with cooking spray.
2. Whisk whole-wheat flour, all-purpose flour, baking powder, baking soda, salt, cinnamon and nutmeg in a large bowl.

3. Whisk egg whites, sugar (or Splenda), applesauce, oil and lemon extract (if using) in a medium bowl. Stir in zucchini.
4. Make a well in the dry ingredients; slowly, mix in the zucchini mixture with a rubber spatula. Fold in walnuts. Do not overmix. Transfer the batter to the prepared pans.
5. Bake the loaves until a toothpick comes out almost clean, 40 to 45 minutes. Cool in the pan on a wire rack for about 5 minutes, then turn out onto the rack to cool completely.

TIPS & NOTES
- **Tip:** To bring cold eggs to room temperature quickly: Place in a mixing bowl and set it in a larger bowl of warm water for a few minutes; the eggs will beat to a greater volume.

NUTRITION
Per slice: 118 calories; 3 g fat (0 g sat, 1 g mono); 0 mg cholesterol; 22 g carbohydrates; 2 g protein; 1 gfiber; 88 mg sodium; 37 mg potassium.
Carbohydrate Servings: 1 1/2
Exchanges: 1 1/2 starch

Chicken Potpie

INGREDIENTS
FILLING
- 3 teaspoons canola oil, divided
- 1 cup frozen pearl onions, thawed
- 1 cup peeled baby carrots
- 10 ounces cremini mushrooms, halved
- 2 1/2 cups reduced-sodium chicken broth, divided
- 1/4 cup cornstarch
- 2 1/2 cups diced cooked chicken, or turkey
- 1 cup frozen peas, thawed
- 1/4 cup reduced-fat sour cream
- 1/4 teaspoon salt
- Freshly ground pepper, to taste

BISCUIT TOPPING
- 3/4 cup whole-wheat pastry flour, (see Ingredient Note)
- 3/4 cup all-purpose flour
- 2 teaspoons sugar
- 1 1/4 teaspoons baking powder
- 1/2 teaspoon baking soda
- 1/2 teaspoon salt

- 1 teaspoon dried thyme
- 1 1/2 tablespoons cold butter, cut into small pieces
- 1 cup nonfat buttermilk, (see Tip)
- 1 tablespoon canola oil

PREPARATION
1. To prepare filling: Heat 1 teaspoon oil in a large skillet or Dutch oven over medium-high heat. Add onions and carrots; cook, stirring, until golden brown and tender, about 7 minutes. Transfer to a bowl. Heat the remaining 2 teaspoons oil in the pan over medium-high heat. Add mushrooms and cook, stirring often, until browned and their liquid has evaporated, 5 to 7 minutes. Return the onions and carrots to the pan. Add 2 cups broth and bring to a boil; reduce heat to a simmer. Mix cornstarch with the remaining 1/2 cup broth; add to the pan and cook, stirring, until the sauce thickens. Stir in chicken (or turkey), peas, sour cream, salt and pepper. Transfer the filling to a 2-quart baking dish.
2. To prepare biscuit topping & bake potpie: Preheat oven to 400°F. Whisk whole-wheat flour, all-purpose flour, sugar, baking powder, baking soda, salt and thyme in a large bowl. Using your fingertips or 2 knives, cut butter into the dry ingredients until crumbly. Add buttermilk and oil; stir until just combined. Drop the dough onto the filling in 6 even portions. Set the baking dish on a baking sheet.
3. Bake the potpie until the topping is golden and the filling is bubbling, 30 to 35 minutes. Let cool for 10 minutes before serving.

TIPS & NOTES

- **Ingredient Note:** Whole-wheat pastry flour is milled from soft wheat. It contains less gluten than regular whole-wheat flour and helps ensure a tender result in delicate baked goods while providing the nutritional benefits of whole grains. Available in large supermarkets and in natural-foods stores. Store in the freezer.
- **Tip:** No buttermilk? You can use buttermilk powder prepared according to package directions. Or make "sour milk": mix 1 tablespoon lemon juice or vinegar to 1 cup milk.

NUTRITION
Per serving: 403 calories; 12 g fat (4 g sat, 4 g mono); 64 mg cholesterol; 46 g carbohydrates; 29 g protein;4 g fiber; 667 mg sodium; 427 mg potassium.
Nutrition Bonus: Vitamin A (70% daily value), Fiber (16% dv).
Carbohydrate Servings: 2 1/2
Exchanges: 2 starch, 1 vegetable, 3 lean meat

Gnocchi with Tomatoes, Pancetta & Wilted Watercress

INGREDIENTS

- 2 ounces pancetta, chopped
- 3 cloves garlic, minced
- 2 large tomatoes, chopped
- 1/2 teaspoon sugar
- 1/4 teaspoon crushed red pepper
- 2 teaspoons red-wine vinegar
- 1/4 teaspoon salt
- 1 pound gnocchi, (see Shopping Tip)
- 4 ounces watercress, tough stems removed, coarsely chopped (6 cups packed)
- 1/3 cup freshly grated Parmesan cheese

PREPARATION

1. Put a large pan of water on to boil.
2. Cook pancetta in a large nonstick skillet over medium heat, stirring occasionally, until it begins to brown, 4 to 5 minutes. Add garlic and cook, stirring, for 30 seconds. Add tomatoes, sugar and crushed red pepper and cook, stirring, until the tomatoes are almost completely broken down, about 5 minutes. Stir in vinegar and salt. Remove from the heat.
3. Cook gnocchi in the boiling water until they float, 3 to 5 minutes or according to package directions. Place watercress in a colander and drain the gnocchi over the watercress, wilting it slightly. Add the gnocchi and watercress to the sauce in the pan; toss to combine. Serve immediately, with Parmesan.

TIPS & NOTES

- **Shopping Tip:** We like the texture of "shelf-stable" prepared gnocchi found in the Italian section of most supermarkets, but frozen and fresh refrigerated gnocchi also work well here.

NUTRITION

Per serving: 377 calories; 7 g fat (3 g sat, 1 g mono); 16 mg cholesterol; 63 g carbohydrates; 14 g protein; 3 g fiber; 686 mg sodium; 329 mg potassium.
Nutrition Bonus: Vitamin C (50% daily value), Vitamin A (45% dv), Calcium & Iron (15% dv).
Carbohydrate Servings: 4
Exchanges: 4 starch, 1 vegetable, 1 fat

Pizza-Style Meatloaf

INGREDIENTS

- 1 teaspoon extra-virgin olive oil

- 1 medium onion, sliced
- 1 red or yellow bell pepper, sliced
- 4 ounces mushrooms, sliced
- 1/4 cup chopped fresh basil
- 1 pound lean ground beef
- 1 clove garlic, minced
- 1/3 cup seasoned (Italian-style) breadcrumbs
- 1/3 cup low-fat milk and 1/2 teaspoon salt
- 1/2 cup prepared marinara sauce
- 1/4 cup shredded sharp Cheddar cheese

PREPARATION

1. Preheat oven to 400°F. Coat a 12-inch pizza pan with cooking spray and place it on a large baking sheet with sides.
2. Heat oil in a large skillet over medium heat. Add onion, bell pepper, mushrooms and basil; cook, stirring, until softened, about 10 minutes.
3. Meanwhile, combine beef, garlic, breadcrumbs, milk and salt in a large bowl. Mix well.
4. Transfer the meat mixture to the prepared pan. With dampened hands, pat into a 10-inch circle. Top with marinara sauce. Spoon the vegetable mixture over the sauce and sprinkle with cheese.
5. Bake until the meat is browned and the cheese has melted, about 30 minutes. Drain off any fat. Cut into wedges and serve.

TIPS & NOTES
- **Make Ahead Tip**: Equipment: Use a perforated pizza pan so excess fat drips away.

NUTRITION
Per serving: 195 calories; 8 g fat (3 g sat, 2 g mono); 53 mg cholesterol; 11 g carbohydrates; 20 g protein; 2 g fiber; 471 mg sodium; 414 mg potassium.
Nutrition Bonus: Vitamin C (48% daily value), Zinc (27% dv), Selenium (21% dv), Vitamin A (18% dv).
Carbohydrate Servings: 1
Exchanges: 1 other carbohydrate, 2 1/2 lean meat

Halibut with Herbs & Capers

INGREDIENTS
- 1/4 cup chopped onion
- 1/4 cup fresh parsley leaves
- 1 tablespoon fresh cilantro leaves

- 2 teaspoons freshly grated lemon zest
- 1 tablespoon lemon juice, juice
- 1 tablespoon chopped pitted green olives
- 2 teaspoons drained capers, rinsed
- 1 clove garlic, minced
- 1/8 teaspoon freshly ground pepper
- 2 tablespoons extra-virgin olive oil
- 1 1-pound halibut fillet, cut into 4 portions

PREPARATION
1. Place onion, parsley, cilantro, lemon zest, lemon juice, olives, capers, garlic and pepper in a food processor; pulse several times to chop. Add oil and process, scraping down the sides several times, until a pesto-like paste forms. Pat halibut with the herb paste. Cover and refrigerate for 30 minutes.
2. Preheat oven to 450°F. Coat a 7-by-11-inch baking dish with cooking spray. Arrange the halibut in the dish and spoon any extra herb mixture on top. Bake, uncovered, until the fish is opaque in the center, 15 to 20 minutes. Serve immediately.

NUTRITION
Per serving: 199 calories; 10 g fat (1 g sat, 6 g mono); 36 mg cholesterol; 2 g carbohydrates; 0 g added sugars; 24 g protein; 1 g fiber; 125 mg sodium; 557 mg potassium.
Nutrition Bonus: Selenium (60% daily value), Vitamin C (15% dv).
Exchanges: 3 very lean meat, 2 fat (mono)

The Wedge

INGREDIENTS
- 2 heart of romaine, quartered lengthwise and cores removed
- 1/4 cup chopped fresh chives
- 2 slices cooked bacon, crumbled
- 2 ounces crumbled blue cheese
- 1/2 cup Buttermilk Ranch Dressing, (recipe follows)

PREPARATION
1. Place 2 romaine quarters on each of 4 salad plates. Sprinkle with chives, bacon and blue cheese. Drizzle with Buttermilk Ranch Dressing.

NUTRITION

Per serving: 111 calories; 8 g fat (3 g sat, 2 g mono); 17 mg cholesterol; 5 g carbohydrates; 6 g protein; 1 gfiber; 481 mg sodium; 97 mg potassium.
Nutrition Bonus: Folate, calcium, potassium.
Exchanges: 1 vegetable, 1/2 high-fat meat

1500 CALORIE MEAL PLAN

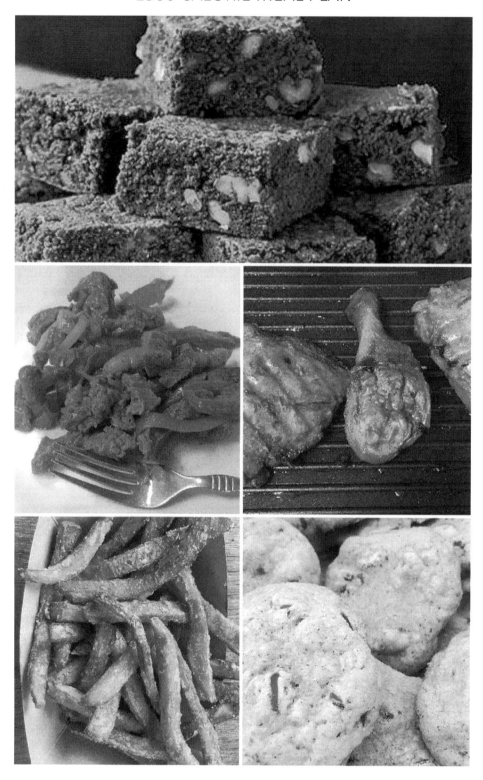

DAY 1
BREAKFAST
Morning Smoothie
Whole-wheat toast (1 slice)
Plum spread

LUNCH
Grape and Feta Mixed Green Special
Shrimp French Brisque or Roasted Cod, Tomatoes, Orange & Onions
Whole-wheat toast (1 slice)
Skim Milk

SNACK
Apple (1 cup, quartered)
Nonfat plain yogurt (8 oz.)

DINNER
Hot and Spicy Halibut
Barley & Wild Rice Pilaf
Green Beans with Toasted Nuts or Lemon Lovers' Asparagus
Chocolate Malted Ricotta

DAY 1 RECIPES

Morning Smoothie
INGREDIENTS
- 1 1/4 cups orange juice, preferably calcium-fortified
- 1 banana
- 1 1/4 cups frozen berries, such as raspberries, blackberries, blueberries and/or strawberries
- 1/2 cup low-fat silken tofu, or low-fat plain yogurt
- 1 tablespoon sugar, or Splenda Granular (optional)

PREPARATION
Combine orange juice, banana, berries, tofu (or yogurt) and sugar (or Splenda), if using, in a blender; cover and blend until creamy. Serve immediately.

NUTRITION

Per serving: 139 calories; 2 g fat (0 g sat, 0 g mono); 0 mg cholesterol; 33 g carbohydrates; 0 g added sugars; 4 g protein; 4 g fiber; 19 mg sodium; 421 mg potassium.

Nutrition Bonus: Vitamin C (110% daily value), Fiber (16% dv).
Carbohydrate Servings: 2
Exchanges: 2 fruit, 1/2 low-fat milk

Plum spread

INGREDIENTS
- 5 pounds plums, pitted and sliced (14-15 cups)
- 3 Granny Smith apples, washed and quartered (not cored)
- 1/4 cup white grape juice, or other fruit juice
- 2 tablespoons lemon juice
- 3/4 cup sugar, or Splenda Granular
- 1/4 teaspoon ground cinnamon, or ginger (optional)

PREPARATION
1. Place a plate in the freezer for testing consistency later.
2. Combine plums, apples, grape juice (or fruit juice) and lemon juice in a large, heavy-bottomed, nonreactive Dutch oven. Bring to a boil over medium-high heat, stirring. Cover and boil gently, stirring occasionally, until the fruit is softened and juicy, 15 to 20 minutes. Uncover and boil gently, stirring occasionally, until the fruit is completely soft, about 20 minutes. (Adjust heat as necessary to maintain a gentle boil.)
3. Pass the fruit through a food mill to remove the skins and apple seeds.
4. Return the strained fruit to the pot. Add sugar (or Splenda) and cinnamon (or ginger), if using. Cook over medium heat, stirring frequently, until a spoonful of jam dropped onto the chilled plate holds its shape, about 15 minutes longer. (See Tip.) Remove from heat and skim off any foam.

TIPS & NOTES
- **Make Ahead Tip**: Store in an airtight container in the refrigerator for up to 2 months.
- **To test the consistency of the spread:** Drop a dollop of cooked spread onto a chilled plate. Carefully run your finger through the dollop. If the track remains unfilled, the jam is done.

NUTRITION

Per tablespoon with sugar: 14 calories; 0 g fat (0 g sat, 0 g mono); 0 mg cholesterol; 4 g carbohydrates; 0 g protein; 0 g fiber; 0 mg sodium; 30 mg potassium.
Exchanges: free food
Nutrition Note: Per tablespoon with Splenda: 0 Carbohydrate Servings; 12 calories; 3 g carbohydrate.

Grape and Feta Mixed Green Special

INGREDIENTS
DRESSING
- 1/4 cup extra-virgin olive oil
- 2 tablespoons red-wine vinegar
- 1/4 teaspoon salt, or to taste
- Freshly ground pepper, to taste

SALAD
- 8 cups mesclun salad greens, (5 ounces)
- 1 head radicchio, thinly sliced
- 2 cups halved seedless grapes, (about 1 pound), preferably red and green
- 3/4 cup crumbled feta, or blue cheese

PREPARATION
1. To prepare dressing: Whisk (or shake) oil, vinegar, salt and pepper in a small bowl (or jar) until blended.
2. To prepare salad: Just before serving, toss greens and radicchio in a large bowl. Drizzle the dressing on top and toss to coat. Divide the salad among 8 plates. Scatter grapes and cheese over each salad; serve immediately.

TIPS & NOTES
- **Make Ahead Tip**: The dressing will keep, covered, in the refrigerator for up to 2 days.

NUTRITION

Per serving: 133 calories; 10 g fat (3 g sat, 6 g mono); 13 mg cholesterol; 9 g carbohydrates; 3 g protein; 1 g fiber; 239 mg sodium; 183 mg potassium.
Nutrition Bonus: Vitamin C (15% daily value), Folate (9% dv).
Carbohydrate Servings: 1/2
Exchanges: 1/2 fruit, 1 vegetable, 2 fat

Shrimp French Brisque

INGREDIENTS

- 12 ounces shrimp (30-40 per pound), shell-on
- 1 onion, chopped, divided
- 1 carrot, peeled and sliced
- 1 stalk celery (with leaves), sliced
- 1/2 cup dry white wine
- 1/2 teaspoon black peppercorns
- 1 bay leaf
- 3 cups water
- 1 tablespoon extra-virgin olive oil
- 4 ounces mushrooms, wiped clean and sliced (about 1 1/2 cups)
- 1/2 green bell pepper, chopped
- 1/4 cup chopped scallions
- 2 tablespoons chopped fresh parsley
- 1/4 cup all-purpose flour
- 1 1/2 cups low-fat milk
- 1/4 cup reduced-fat sour cream
- 1/4 cup dry sherry
- 1 tablespoon lemon juice
- 1/4 teaspoon salt
- Freshly ground pepper to taste
- Dash of hot sauce

PREPARATION

1. Peel and devein shrimp, reserving the shells. Cut the shrimp into 3/4-inch pieces; cover and refrigerate.
2. Combine the shrimp shells with about half the onion, all the carrot, celery, wine, peppercorns and bay leaf in a large heavy saucepan. Add water and simmer over low heat for about 30 minutes. Strain through a sieve, pressing on the solids to extract all the juices; discard the solids. Measure the shrimp stock and add water, if necessary, to make 1 1/2 cups.
3. Heat oil in the same pan over medium heat. Add mushrooms, bell pepper, scallions, parsley and the remaining onion. Cook, stirring, until the mushrooms are soft, about 5 minutes. Sprinkle with flour and cook, stirring constantly, until it starts to turn golden, 2 to 3 minutes. Slowly stir in milk and the shrimp stock. Cook, stirring to loosen any flour sticking to the bottom of the pot, until the soup returns to a simmer and thickens, about 5 minutes. Add the reserved shrimp and cook until they turn opaque in the center, about 2 minutes more. Add sour cream, sherry and lemon juice; stir over low heat until heated through;do not let it come to a boil. Taste and adjust seasonings with salt, pepper and hot sauce.

TIPS & NOTES
- **Make Ahead Tip**: Cover and refrigerate for up to 1 day.

NUTRITION
Per serving: 163 calories; 5 g fat (2 g sat, 2 g mono); 92 mg cholesterol; 12 g carbohydrates; 13 g protein; 1 g fiber; 241 mg sodium; 255 mg potassium.
Nutrition Bonus: Selenium (30% daily value), Vitamin A (26% dv), Vitamin C (24% dv).
Carbohydrate Servings: 1
Exchanges: 1 starch; 2 very lean meat; 1 fat

Roasted Cod, Tomatoes, Orange & Onions

INGREDIENTS
- 1 pound ripe but firm small round or plum tomatoes, cut into 1/2-inch-thick wedges
- 2 medium yellow onions, cut into 1/4-inch-thick wedges
- 1 tablespoon finely slivered orange zest (see Tips)
- 1 tablespoon extra-virgin olive oil
- 1 tablespoon chopped fresh thyme leaves, plus sprigs for garnish
- 1/2 teaspoon kosher salt, divided
- Freshly ground pepper, to taste
- 1 pound boneless, skinless cod (see Tips) or other thick-cut, firm-fleshed fish, cut into 4 equal portions

PREPARATION
1. Preheat oven to 400°F.
2. Combine tomatoes, onions, orange zest, oil and chopped thyme in a 3-quart glass or ceramic baking dish. Sprinkle with 1/4 teaspoon salt and pepper; stir to combine.
3. Roast, stirring occasionally, until the onions are golden and brown on the edges, about 45 minutes. Remove from the oven. Increase oven temperature to 450°F.
4. Push the vegetables aside, add fish and season with the remaining 1/4 teaspoon salt and pepper; spoon the vegetables over the fish.
5. Return the baking dish to the oven and bake until the fish is opaque in the center, about 10 to 12 minutes. To serve, divide the fish and vegetables among 4 plates and garnish with thyme sprigs.

TIPS & NOTES
- **Tip:** Using a vegetable peeler, remove 3 or 4 pieces of zest from a large orange. Stack the pieces on top of each other and slice into 1/8-inch-wide strips.
- **Tip:** Overfishing and trawling have drastically reduced the number of cod in the U.S. and Canadian Atlantic Ocean and destroyed its sea floor. For sustainably

fished cod, choose U.S. Pacific cod or Atlantic cod from Iceland and the northeast Arctic.

NUTRITION
Per serving: 160 calories; 5 g fat (1 g sat, 3 g mono); 43 mg cholesterol; 11 g carbohydrates; 0 g added sugars; 20 g protein; 2 g fiber; 308 mg sodium; 528 mg potassium.
Nutrition Bonus: Vitamin C (60% daily value), Vitamin A (16% dv), Potassium (15% dv).
Carbohydrate Servings: 1
Exchanges: 1 1/2 vegetable, 3 very lean meat, 1 fat

Hot and Spicy Halibut

INGREDIENTS
- 1 1/4 pounds halibut, striped bass or tilapia fillet, cut into 4 portions
- 1 teaspoon ground cumin, divided
- 1/4 teaspoon salt
- Freshly ground pepper, to taste
- 1 10-ounce can diced tomatoes with green chiles
- 1/4 cup sliced green olives with pimientos
- 2 tablespoons chopped fresh cilantro
- 1 teaspoon extra-virgin olive oil

PREPARATION
1. Preheat oven to 450°F. Coat a baking sheet with cooking spray. Arrange fish on baking sheet. Season with 1/2 teaspoon cumin, salt and pepper.
2. Combine tomatoes, olives, cilantro, oil and the remaining 1/2 teaspoon cumin in a small bowl. Spoon over the fish.
3. Bake the fish until flaky and opaque in the center, 12 to 15 minutes. Serve immediately.

NUTRITION
Per serving: 188 calories; 7 g fat (1 g sat, 4 g mono); 45 mg cholesterol; 4 g carbohydrates; 30 g protein; 1 g fiber; 758 mg sodium; 638 mg potassium.
Nutrition Bonus: Potassium (18% daily value).
Exchanges: 4 very lean meat, 1 fat (mono)

Barley & Wild Rice Pilaf

INGREDIENTS
- 2 teaspoons extra-virgin olive oil
- 1 medium onion, finely chopped
- 1/2 cup wild rice, rinsed

- 1/2 cup pearl barley
- 3 cups reduced-sodium chicken broth, or vegetable broth
- 1/3 cup pine nuts
- 1 cup pomegranate seeds, (1 large fruit; see Tip)
- 2 teaspoons freshly grated lemon zest
- 2 tablespoons chopped flat-leaf parsley

PREPARATION
1. Heat oil in a large saucepan over medium heat. Add onion and cook, stirring often, until softened. Add wild rice and barley; stir for a few seconds. Add broth and bring to a simmer. Reduce heat to low, cover and simmer until the wild rice and barley are tender and most of the liquid has been absorbed, 45 to 50 minutes.
2. Meanwhile, toast pine nuts in a small, dry skillet over medium-low heat, stirring constantly, until light golden and fragrant, 2 to 3 minutes. Transfer to a small bowl to cool.
3. Add pomegranate seeds, lemon zest, parsley and the toasted pine nuts to the pilaf; fluff with a fork. Serve hot.

TIPS & NOTES
- **Make Ahead Tip**: Prepare through Step 2. Cover and refrigerate for up to 2 days. To reheat, place in a baking dish, add 1/4 cup water and cover. Microwave on High for 10 to 15 minutes or bake at 350°F or 25 to 30 minutes.
- **Tip:** To seed a pomegranate and avoid the enduring stains of pomegranate juice, work under water. Fill a large bowl with water. Hold the pomegranate in the water and slice off the crown. Lightly score the fruit into quarters, from crown to stem end. Keeping the fruit under water, break it apart, gently separating the plump seeds from the outer skin and white pith. The seeds will drop to the bottom of the bowl and the pith will float to the surface. Discard the pith. Pour the seeds into a colander. Rinse and pat dry. The seeds can be frozen in an airtight container or sealable bag for up to 3 months.

NUTRITION
Per serving: 209 calories; 7 g fat (1 g sat, 3 g mono); 3 mg cholesterol; 31 g carbohydrates; 0 g added sugars; 7 g protein; 4 g fiber; 75 mg sodium; 250 mg potassium.
Nutrition Bonus: Magnesium (15% dv)
Carbohydrate Servings: 2
Exchanges: 2 starch, 1 fat

Green Beans with Toasted Nuts

INGREDIENTS
- 1 pound green beans, stem ends trimmed
- 2 teaspoons extra-virgin olive oil
- 2 tablespoons chopped peeled hazelnuts, or walnuts
- 1/4 teaspoon salt
- Freshly ground pepper, to taste

PREPARATION
1. Cook beans in a large pot of boiling salted water until just tender, 5 to 7 minutes. Drain.
2. Heat oil in a large nonstick skillet over low heat. Add nuts and cook, stirring, until golden, about 1 minute. Return the reserved beans to the pot and toss to coat. Season with salt and pepper.

NUTRITION
Per serving: 104 calories; 5 g fat (1 g sat, 3 g mono); 0 mg cholesterol; 9 g carbohydrates; 0 g added sugars; 3 g protein; 4 g fiber; 152 mg sodium; 261 mg potassium.
Nutrition Bonus: Fiber (28% daily value), Vitamin C (22% dv).
Exchanges: 1 vegetable, 1 fat (mono)

Lemon Lovers' Asparagus

INGREDIENTS
- 2 bunches asparagus, tough ends trimmed
- 2 lemons, thinly sliced
- 2 tablespoons extra-virgin olive oil
- 4 teaspoons chopped fresh oregano or 1 teaspoon dried
- 1/2 teaspoon salt
- 1/2 teaspoon freshly ground pepper

PREPARATION
1. Preheat oven to 450°F.
2. Toss asparagus, lemon slices, oil, oregano, salt and pepper on a large rimmed baking sheet. Roast, shaking the pan occasionally to toss, until the asparagus is tender-crisp, 13 to 15 minutes.

NUTRITION

Per serving: 91 calories; 7 g fat (1 g sat, 5 g mono); 0 mg cholesterol; 9 g carbohydrates; 0 g added sugars;2 g protein; 4 g fiber; 302 mg sodium; 241 mg potassium.
Nutrition Bonus: Vitamin C (90% daily value), Folate (42% dv), Vitamin A (25% dv).
Carbohydrate Servings: 1/2
Exchanges: 1 vegetable, 1/2 fruit, 1 1/2 fat

Chocolate Malted Ricotta

INGREDIENTS
- 1/4 cup part-skim ricotta
- 1 tablespoon cocoa powder
- 1 teaspoon malted-milk powder

PREPARATION
1. Combine ricotta with hot cocoa mix and malted-milk powder.

NUTRITION

Per serving: 128 calories; 6 g fat (4 g sat, 2 g mono); 21 mg cholesterol; 11 g carbohydrates; 9 g protein; 2 g fiber; 107 mg sodium; 212 mg potassium.
Carbohydrate Servings: 1
Exchanges: 1 1/2 medium-fat meat, 1 carbohydrate

DAY 2
BREAKFAST
Tofu Scrambled Egg
Salsa Cornbread
Strawberries (1 cup)
LUNCH
Spicy Red Lentil Soup
Mixed Greens with Berries & Honey-Glazed Hazelnuts or Raspberry, Avocado & Mango Salad
Wasa crispbread (2 crackers)
Skim milk (1 cup)
SNACK
Carrot Sticks (1/2 cup)
Fat Free Cheese slice
DINNER
Turkey Cutlets with Sage & Lemon or Grilled Salmon with Mustard & Herbs
Glazed Mini Carrots

Spring Green Salad with Rouille Dressing
Steamed broccoli (1/2 cup)
Buttermilk-Herb Mashed Potatoes
Dark Fudgy Brownies

DAY 2 RECIPES

Tofu Scrambled Egg

INGREDIENTS
- 1 large egg
- 1/2 teaspoon dried tarragon
- Dash of hot sauce, such as
- Pinch of salt
- Freshly ground pepper, to taste
- 1 teaspoon extra-virgin olive oil, or canola oil
- 2 tablespoons crumbled tofu, (silken or regular)

PREPARATION
1. Blend egg, tarragon, hot sauce, salt and pepper in a small bowl with a fork. Heat oil in a small nonstick skillet over medium-low heat. Add tofu and cook, stirring, until warmed through, 20 to 30 seconds. Add egg mixture and stir until the egg is set, but still creamy, 20 to 30 seconds. Serve immediately.

NUTRITION
Per serving: 140 calories; 11 g fat (2 g sat, 6 g mono); 212 mg cholesterol; 2 g carbohydrates; 0 g added sugars; 9 g protein; 1 g fiber; 230 mg sodium; 93 mg potassium.
Nutrition Bonus: Selenium (23% daily value).
Exchanges: 1 medium-fat meat. 1 fat (mono)

Salsa Cornbread

INGREDIENTS

- 1 cup all-purpose flour
- 1/2 cup whole-wheat flour
- 1/2 cup cornmeal
- 2 teaspoons baking powder
- 1/2 teaspoon salt
- Freshly ground pepper, to taste
- 3 large eggs, lightly beaten
- 1/2 cup buttermilk, or equivalent buttermilk powder

- 1 tablespoon butter, melted
- 1 tablespoon honey
- 1/2 cup drained canned corn kernels
- 1 small onion, diced
- 1/2 cup chopped tomato
- 1 clove garlic, minced
- 1 jalapeno pepper, seeded and minced
- 1/2 cup grated Cheddar cheese

PREPARATION
1. Preheat oven to 425° F. Place a 9-inch cast-iron skillet (or similar ovenproof skillet, see Tip) in the oven to heat.
2. Whisk all-purpose flour, whole-wheat flour, cornmeal, baking powder, salt and pepper in a large mixing bowl.
3. Whisk eggs, buttermilk, butter and honey in a medium bowl. Add the egg mixture to the dry ingredients; mix with a rubber spatula. Stir in corn, onion, tomato, garlic and jalapeno.
4. Remove the skillet from the oven and coat it with cooking spray. Pour in the batter, spreading evenly. Sprinkle cheese over the top. Bake the cornbread until golden brown and a knife inserted into the center comes out clean, 20 to 25 minutes. Serve warm.

TIPS & NOTES
- **Tip:** If you do not have an ovenproof skillet of the correct size, use an 8-by-8-inch glass baking dish. Do not preheat the empty baking dish in the oven before filling it.

NUTRITION

Per serving: 138 calories; 4 g fat (2 g sat, 1 g mono); 70 mg cholesterol; 20 g carbohydrates; 6 g protein; 1 g fiber; 319 mg sodium; 91 mg potassium.
Carbohydrate Servings: 1
Exchanges: 1 starch, 1 fat

Spicy Red Lentil Soup

INGREDIENTS
- 6 teaspoons extra-virgin olive oil, divided
- 2 onions, chopped (1 1/2 cups)
- 3 cloves garlic, minced
- 2 teaspoons ground cumin
- 8 cups reduced-sodium chicken broth, or vegetable broth

- 1 1/2 cups red lentils, rinsed (see Tip)
- 1/3 cup bulgur
- 2 tablespoons tomato paste
- 1 bay leaf
- 3 tablespoons lemon juice
- Freshly ground pepper to taste
- 1 teaspoon paprika
- 1 teaspoon cayenne pepper

PREPARATION
1. Heat 2 teaspoons oil in a soup pot or Dutch oven over medium heat. Add onions and cook, stirring, until softened, 3 to 5 minutes. Add garlic and cumin; cook for 1 minute. Add broth, lentils, bulgur, tomato paste and bay leaf; bring to a simmer, stirring occasionally. Cover and cook over low heat until the lentils and bulgur are very tender, 25 to 30 minutes. Discard the bay leaf.
2. Ladle about 4 cups of the soup into a food processor and puree. Return the pureed soup to the soup pot and heat through. Stir in lemon juice and season with pepper.
3. Just before serving, ladle the soup into bowls. Heat the remaining 4 teaspoons oil in a small skillet and stir in paprika and cayenne. Drizzle about 1/2 teaspoon of the sizzling spice mixture over each bowlful and serve immediately.

TIPS & NOTES
- **Make Ahead Tip**: Prepare through Step 2. Cover and refrigerate for up to 2 days or freeze for up to 2 months.
- **Tip:** You can replace red lentils with brown lentils; add 1/2 cup water and simmer 40 to 45 minutes.

NUTRITION
Per serving: 218 calories; 5 g fat (1 g sat, 3 g mono); 5 mg cholesterol; 31 g carbohydrates; 0 g added sugars; 15 g protein; 7 g fiber; 151 mg sodium; 406 mg potassium.
Nutrition Bonus: Fiber (29% daily value), Iron (15% dv).
Carbohydrate Servings: 2
Exchanges: 1 1/2 starch, 1 vegetable, 1 lean meat

Mixed Greens with Berries & Honey-Glazed Hazelnuts
INGREDIENTS
NUTS
- 1 teaspoon extra-virgin olive oil

- 1 teaspoon honey
- 1/4 cup chopped hazelnuts, or walnuts

DRESSING
- 1/3 cup raspberries, blackberries and/or blueberries
- 2 tablespoons extra-virgin olive oil
- 1 tablespoon balsamic vinegar
- 1 tablespoon water
- 1 teaspoon Dijon mustard
- 1 small clove garlic, crushed and peeled
- 1/2 teaspoon honey
- 1/8 teaspoon salt, or to taste
- Freshly ground pepper, to taste
- 2 tablespoons finely chopped shallots

SALAD
- 10 cups mesclun salad greens, (about 8 ounces)
- 1 cup blackberries, raspberries and/or blueberries
- 1/2 cup crumbled feta, or goat cheese (4 ounces)

PREPARATION
1. To prepare nuts: Preheat oven to 350°F. Coat a small baking dish with cooking spray. Combine oil and honey in a small bowl. Add nuts and toss to coat. Transfer to the prepared baking dish and bake, stirring from time to time, until golden, 10 to 14 minutes. Let cool completely.
2. To prepare dressing: Combine berries, oil, vinegar, water, mustard, garlic, honey, salt and pepper in a blender or food processor. Blend until smooth. Transfer to a small bowl and stir in shallots.
3. To prepare salad: Just before serving, place greens in a large bowl. Drizzle the dressing over the greens and toss to coat. Divide the salad among 4 plates. Scatter berries, cheese and the glazed nuts over each salad; serve immediately.

TIPS & NOTES
- **Make Ahead Tip**: Cover and refrigerate the dressing (Step 2) for up to 2 days.

NUTRITION
Per serving: 232 calories; 17 g fat (4 g sat, 10 g mono); 17 mg cholesterol; 15 g carbohydrates; 7 g protein; 6 g fiber; 349 mg sodium; 596 mg potassium.
Nutrition Bonus: Vitamin A (80% daily value), Vitamin C (60% dv), Calcium (20% dv).
Carbohydrate Servings: 1/2
Exchanges: 2 vegetable, 1 medium-fat meat, 2 fat

Raspberry, Avocado & Mango Salad

INGREDIENTS

- 1 1/2 cups fresh raspberries, divided
- 1/4 cup extra-virgin olive oil
- 1/4 cup red-wine vinegar
- 1 small clove garlic, coarsely chopped
- 1/4 teaspoon kosher salt
- 1/8 teaspoon freshly ground pepper
- 8 cups mixed salad greens
- 1 ripe mango, diced (see Tip)
- 1 small ripe avocado, diced
- 1/2 cup thinly sliced red onion
- 1/4 cup toasted chopped hazelnuts, or sliced almonds (see Tip), optional

PREPARATION

1. Puree 1/2 cup raspberries, oil, vinegar, garlic, salt and pepper in a blender until combined.
2. Combine greens, mango, avocado and onion in a large bowl. Pour the dressing on top and gently toss to coat. Divide the salad among 5 salad plates. Top each with the remaining raspberries and sprinkle with nuts, if using.

TIPS & NOTES

- **Tips:** To dice a mango:
- 1. Slice both ends off the mango, revealing the long, slender seed inside. Set the fruit upright on a work surface and remove the skin with a sharp knife.
- 2. With the seed perpendicular to you, slice the fruit from both sides of the seed, yielding two large pieces.
- 3. Turn the seed parallel to you and slice the two smaller pieces of fruit from each side.
- 4. Cut the fruit into the desired shape.
- To toast chopped or sliced nuts, heat a small dry skillet over medium-low heat. Add nuts and cook, stirring, until lightly browned and fragrant, 2 to 3 minutes.

NUTRITION

Per serving: 229 calories; 16 g fat (2 g sat, 12 g mono); 0 mg cholesterol; 21 g carbohydrates; 3 g protein; 8 g fiber; 82 mg sodium; 613 mg potassium.
Nutrition Bonus: Vitamin C (70% daily value), Vitamin A (60% dv), Folate (36% dv), Potassium (16% dv).
Carbohydrate Servings: 1
Exchanges: 1/2 fruit, 2 vegetable, 3 fat

Turkey Cutlets with Sage & Lemon

INGREDIENTS

- 3 tablespoons all-purpose
- 1 pound turkey breast cutlets
- 1/4 teaspoon salt
- Freshly ground pepper, to taste
- 3 teaspoons extra-virgin olive oil, divided
- 2 cloves garlic, minced
- 2 teaspoons chopped fresh sage
- 1/4 cup dry white wine
- 3/4 cup reduced-sodium chicken broth
- 1 teaspoon lemon juice
- 1 teaspoon butter

PREPARATION

1. Spread flour on a large plate. Cut several small slits in outer edges of the turkey to prevent curling. Pat dry with paper towels and season with salt and pepper. Dredge lightly in flour. Discard any remaining flour.
2. Heat 1 teaspoon oil in a large nonstick skillet over medium-high heat. Add half the turkey and cook until golden outside and no longer pink inside, 1 to 2 minutes per side. Transfer to a platter and tent with foil to keep warm. Saute the remaining turkey in another 1 teaspoon oil until golden; transfer to platter.
3. Add the remaining 1 teaspoon oil to the pan. Add garlic and sage; cook, stirring, until fragrant, about 1 minute. Add wine and cook, scraping up any browned bits, until reduced by half, about 1 minute. Add broth and cook until the liquid is reduced by half, 4 to 5 minutes. Stir in lemon juice and any juices accumulated from the turkey and simmer for 1 minute more. Remove from heat and swirl in butter. Serve, spooning the sauce over the turkey.

NUTRITION
Per serving: 205 calories; 5 g fat (1 g sat, 3 g mono); 48 mg cholesterol; 6 g carbohydrates; 0 g added sugars; 29 g protein; 0 g fiber; 273 mg sodium; 358 mg potassium.
Nutrition Bonus: Selenium (47% daily value).
Exchanges: 4 very lean meat, 1 fat

Grilled Salmon with Mustard & Herbs

INGREDIENTS

- 2 lemons, thinly sliced, plus 1 lemon cut into wedges for garnish
- 20-30 sprigs mixed fresh herbs, plus 2 tablespoons chopped, divided

- 1 clove garlic
- 1/4 teaspoon salt
- 1 tablespoon Dijon mustard
- 1 pound center-cut salmon, skinned (see Tip)

PREPARATION
1. Preheat grill to medium-high.
2. Lay two 9-inch pieces of heavy-duty foil on top of each other and place on a rimless baking sheet. Arrange lemon slices in two layers in the center of the foil. Spread herb sprigs over the lemons. With the side of a chef's knife, mash garlic with salt to form a paste. Transfer to a small dish and stir in mustard and the remaining 2 tablespoons chopped herbs. Spread the mixture over both sides of the salmon. Place the salmon on the herb sprigs.
3. Slide the foil and salmon off the baking sheet onto the grill without disturbing the salmon-lemon stack. Cover the grill; cook until the salmon is opaque in the center, 18 to 24 minutes. Wearing oven mitts, carefully transfer foil and salmon back onto the baking sheet. Cut the salmon into 4 portions and serve with lemon wedges (discard herb sprigs and lemon slices).

TIPS & NOTES
- **Tip:** How to skin a salmon fillet: Place skin-side down. Starting at the tail end, slip a long knife between the fish flesh and the skin, holding down firmly with your other hand. Gently push the blade along at a 30° angle, separating the fillet from the skin without cutting through either.

NUTRITION
Per serving: 212 calories; 12 g fat (2 g sat, 4 g mono); 67 mg cholesterol; 1 g carbohydrates; 0 g added sugars; 23 g protein; 0 g fiber; 261 mg sodium; 428 mg potassium.
Nutrition Bonus: Vitamin C (17% daily value), Omega-3s.
Carbohydrate Servings: 0
Exchanges: 3 lean meat

Glazed Mini Carrots

INGREDIENTS
- 3 cups mini carrots, (1 pound)
- 1/3 cup water
- 1 tablespoon honey
- 2 teaspoons butter
- 1/4 teaspoon salt, or to taste
- 1 tablespoon lemon juice

- Freshly ground pepper, to taste
- 2 tablespoons chopped fresh parsley

PREPARATION
1. Combine carrots, water, honey, butter and salt in a large skillet. Bring to a simmer over medium-high heat. Cover and cook until tender, 5 to 7 minutes. Uncover and cook, stirring often, until the liquid is a syrupy glaze, 1 to 2 minutes. Stir in lemon juice and pepper. Sprinkle with parsley and serve.

NUTRITION
Per serving: 74 calories; 2 g fat (1 g sat, 1 g mono); 5 mg cholesterol; 14 g carbohydrates; 1 g protein; 2 gfiber; 236 mg sodium; 287 mg potassium.
Nutrition Bonus: Vitamin A (320% daily value), Vitamin C (23% dv).
Carbohydrate Servings: 1
Exchanges: 1 vegetable, 1/2 fat

Spring Green Salad with Rouille Dressing

INGREDIENTS
- 1/3 cup chopped hazelnuts
- 1/2 cup jarred pimiento peppers, rinsed
- 1/2 teaspoon chopped garlic
- 2 tablespoons water
- 1 1/2 tablespoons white balsamic vinegar, (see Note)
- 1/2 teaspoon salt
- 1/2 teaspoon freshly ground pepper
- 1 large cucumber, peeled, halved, seeded and cut into thin half-moons
- 2 stalks celery, thinly sliced
- 4 cups romaine lettuce, cut or torn into bite-size pieces (about 6 ounces)
- 1 cup baby spinach leaves
- 24 leaves fresh basil, chopped

PREPARATION

1. Toast hazelnuts in a small dry skillet over medium heat, stirring often, until lightly browned, about 4 minutes. Transfer to a food processor and let cool for 5 minutes. Add pimientos, garlic, water, vinegar, salt and pepper. Process until smooth.
2. Combine cucumber, celery, romaine, spinach and basil in a salad bowl. Add the dressing, toss gently, and serve.

TIPS & NOTES
- **Note:** White balsamic vinegar is unaged balsamic made from Italian white wine grapes and grape musts (unfermented crushed grapes). Its mild flavor and clear color make it ideal for salad dressing.

NUTRITION
Per serving: 64 calories; 4 g fat (0 g sat, 3 g mono); 0 mg cholesterol; 7 g carbohydrates; 0 g added sugars;3 g protein; 2 g fiber; 362 mg sodium; 243 mg potassium.
Nutrition Bonus: Vitamin A (60% daily value), Vitamin C (20% dv), Folate (18% dv).
Carbohydrate Servings: 1/2
Exchanges: 1 vegetable, 1/2 fat

Buttermilk-Herb Mashed Potatoes

INGREDIENTS
1 large Yukon Gold potato, peeled and cut into chunks
1 clove garlic, peeled
1 teaspoon butter
2 tablespoons nonfat buttermilk
1 1/2 teaspoons chopped fresh herbs
Salt & freshly ground pepper, to taste

PREPARATION
1. Place potato in a small saucepan and cover with water. Add garlic. Bring to a boil; cook until the potato is tender. Drain; add butter and buttermilk, and mash with a potato masher to the desired consistency. Stir in herbs. Season with salt and freshly ground pepper.

NUTRITION
Per serving: 85 calories; 2 g fat (1 g sat, 0 g mono); 5 mg cholesterol; 14 g carbohydrates; 0 g added sugars; 2 g protein; 1 g fiber; 87 mg sodium; 416 mg potassium.
Carbohydrate Servings: 1
Exchanges: 1 starch

Dark Fudgy Brownies

INGREDIENTS
- 3/4 cup all-purpose flour
- 2/3 cup confectioners' sugar
- 3 tablespoons unsweetened cocoa powder, American-style or Dutch-process
- 3 ounces semisweet or bittersweet chocolate (50-72% cacao), coarsely chopped, plus 2 1/2 ounces chopped into mini chip-size pieces, divided

- 1 1/2 tablespoons canola oil
- 1/4 cup granulated sugar
- 1 1/2 tablespoons light corn syrup, blended with 3 tablespoons lukewarm water
- 2 teaspoons vanilla extract
- 1/8 teaspoon salt
- 1 large egg
- 1/3 cup chopped toasted walnuts, (see Tip), optional

PREPARATION
1. Position rack in center of oven; preheat to 350°F. Line an 8-inch-square baking pan with foil, letting it overhang on two opposing sides. Coat with cooking spray.
2. Sift flour, confectioners' sugar and cocoa together into a small bowl. Combine the 3 ounces coarsely chopped chocolate and oil in a heavy medium saucepan; place over the lowest heat, stirring, until just melted and smooth, being very careful the chocolate does not overheat. Remove from the heat and stir in granulated sugar, corn syrup mixture, vanilla and salt until the sugar dissolves.
3. Vigorously stir in egg until smoothly incorporated. Gently stir in the dry ingredients. Fold in the walnuts (if using) and the remaining 2 1/2 ounces chopped chocolate just until well blended. Turn out the batter into the pan, spreading evenly.
4. Bake the brownies until almost firm in the center and a toothpick inserted comes out with some moist batter clinging to it, 20 to 24 minutes. Let cool completely on a wire rack, about 2 1/2 hours.
5. Using the overhanging foil as handles, carefully lift the brownie slab from the pan. Peel the foil from the bottom; set the slab right-side up on a cutting board. Using a large, sharp knife, trim off any dry edges. Mark and then cut the slab crosswise into fifths and lengthwise into fourths. Wipe the blade with a damp cloth between cuts.

TIPS & NOTES
- **Make Ahead Tip**: Store in an airtight container for up to 3 days or in the freezer for up to 2 weeks.
- **Tip:** To toast chopped nuts: Cook in a small dry skillet over medium-low heat, stirring constantly, until fragrant and lightly browned, 2 to 4 minutes.

NUTRITION
Per brownie: 86 calories; 3 g fat (1 g sat, 1 g mono); 11 mg cholesterol; 15 g carbohydrates; 2 g protein; 0 gfiber; 19 mg sodium; 25 mg potassium.
Carbohydrate Servings: 1
Exchanges: 1 other carbohydrate

DAY 3
BREAKFAST

Cranberry Muesli
Skim milk (1 cup)

LUNCH

Pasta & Bean Soup or Grilled Shrimp Remoulade
Spinach, Avocado & Mango Salad
Whole-wheat toast (1 slice)
Skim milk (1 cup)

SNACK

Berry Frozen Yogurt

DINNER

Curry-Roasted Shrimp with Oranges or Slow-Cooker Braised Pork with Salsa
Brown rice (1 cup)
Sesame Green Beans
Raspberries (1 cup)

DAY 3 RECIPES

Cranberry Muesli

INGREDIENTS

- 1/2 cup low-fat plain yogurt
- 1/2 cup unsweetened or fruit-juice-sweetened cranberry juice
- 6 tablespoons old-fashioned rolled oats, (not quick-cooking or steel-cut)
- 2 tablespoons dried cranberries
- 1 tablespoon unsalted sunflower seeds
- 1 tablespoon wheat germ
- 2 teaspoons honey
- 1/4 teaspoon vanilla extract
- 1/8 teaspoon salt

PREPARATION

1. Combine yogurt, juice, oats, cranberries, sunflower seeds, wheat germ, honey, vanilla and salt in a medium bowl; cover and refrigerate for at least 8 hours and up to 1 day.

TIPS & NOTES

- **Make Ahead Tip**: Cover and refrigerate for up to 1 day.

NUTRITION

Per serving: 209 calories; 4 g fat (1 g sat, 1 g mono); 4 mg cholesterol; 37 g carbohydrates; 8 g protein; 3 gfiber; 190 mg sodium; 266 mg potassium.

Nutrition Bonus: Calcium (15% daily value)

Carbohydrate Servings: 2 1/2

Exchanges: 1 starch, 1 fruit, 1/2 other carbohydrate, 1/2 fat

Pasta & Bean Soup

INGREDIENTS

- 4 14-ounce cans reduced-sodium chicken broth
- 6 cloves garlic, crushed and peeled
- 4 4-inch sprigs fresh rosemary, or 1 tablespoon dried
- 1/8-1/4 teaspoon crushed red pepper
- 1 15-1/2-ounce or 19-ounce can cannellini, (white kidney) beans, rinsed, divided
- 1 14-1/2-ounce can diced tomatoes
- 1 cup medium pasta shells, or orecchiette
- 2 cups individually quick-frozen spinach, (6 ounces) (see Ingredient note)
- 6 teaspoons extra-virgin olive oil, (optional)
- 6 tablespoons freshly grated Parmesan cheese

PREPARATION

1. Combine broth, garlic, rosemary and crushed red pepper in a 4- to 6-quart Dutch oven or soup pot; bring to a simmer. Partially cover and simmer over medium-low heat for 20 minutes to intensify flavor. Meanwhile, mash 1 cup beans in a small bowl.

2. Scoop garlic cloves and rosemary from the broth with a slotted spoon (or pass the soup through a strainer and return to the pot). Add mashed and whole beans to the broth, along with tomatoes; return to a simmer. Stir in pasta, cover and cook over medium heat, stirring occasionally, until the pasta is just tender, 10 to 12 minutes.

3. Stir in spinach, cover and cook just until the spinach has thawed, 2 to 3 minutes. Ladle the soup into bowls and garnish each serving with a drizzle of oil, if desired, and a sprinkling of Parmesan. Variation: Substitute chickpeas (garbanzo beans) for the cannellini beans; use a food processor to puree them.

TIPS & NOTES

- **Ingredient Note:** Individually quick-frozen (IQF) spinach is sold in convenient plastic bags. If you have a 10-ounce box of spinach on hand, use just over half of it and cook according to package directions before adding to the soup in Step 3.

NUTRITION

Per serving: 133 calories; 2 g fat (1 g sat, 0 g mono); 6 mg cholesterol; 21 g carbohydrates; 9 g protein; 4 gfiber; 356 mg sodium; 29 mg potassium.

Nutrition Bonus: Vitamin A (35% daily value), Fiber (16% dv).

Carbohydrate Servings: 1

Exchanges: 1 1/ 2 starch, 1 vegetable, 1 lean meat

Spinach, Avocado & Mango Salad

INGREDIENTS

DRESSING

- 1/3 cup orange juice

- 1 tablespoon red-wine vinegar
- 2 tablespoons hazelnut oil, almond oil or canola oil
- 1 teaspoon Dijon mustard
- 1/4 teaspoon salt, or to taste
- Freshly ground pepper, to taste

SALAD

- 10 cups baby spinach leaves, (about 8 ounces)
- 1 1/2 cups radicchio, torn into bite-size pieces
- 8-12 small red radishes, (1 bunch), sliced
- 1 small ripe mango, sliced and 1 medium avocado, sliced

PREPARATION

1. To prepare dressing: Whisk juice, vinegar, oil, mustard, salt and pepper in a bowl.

2. To prepare salad: Just before serving, combine spinach, radicchio, radishes and mango in a large bowl. Add the dressing; toss to coat. Garnish each serving with avocado slices.

NUTRITION

Per serving: 210 calories; 14 g fat (2 g sat, 2 g mono); 0 mg cholesterol; 10 g carbohydrates; 3 g protein; 6 g fiber; 258 mg sodium; 479 mg potassium.

Nutrition Bonus: Vitamin C (70% daily value), Vitamin A (40% dv), Fiber (26% dv).

Carbohydrate Servings: 1

Exchanges: 3 vegetable, 3 fat (mono)

Berry Frozen Yogurt

INGREDIENTS

- 3 cups fresh or frozen and partially thawed blackberries, or raspberries or a mixture of blackberries, raspberries and blueberries (see Tip)

- 6 tablespoons sugar
- 1 tablespoon lemon juice
- 3/4 cup low-fat plain yogurt

PREPARATION

1. Combine berries, sugar and lemon juice in a food processor; process until smooth. Add yogurt and pulse until mixed in. If using fresh berries, transfer the mixture to a medium bowl, cover and refrigerate until chilled, about 1 hour.

2. Transfer the berry mixture to an ice cream maker and freeze according to manufacturer's directions. (Alternatively, freeze the mixture in a shallow metal pan until solid, about 6 hours. Break into chunks and process in a food processor until smooth and creamy.) Serve immediately or transfer to a storage container and let harden in the freezer for 1 to 1 1/2 hours. Serve in chilled dishes.

TIPS & NOTES

- **Make Ahead Tip**: Store in an airtight container in the freezer for up to 1 week. Let soften in the refrigerator for 1/2 hour before serving. | Equipment: Ice cream maker or food processor
- **Tip:** To freeze fresh berries: Wash berries and pat dry. Spread in a single layer on a tray, cover with plastic wrap and freeze until solid. Pack frozen fruit into ziplock bags, taking care to remove air from the bags. Freeze for up to 1 year.

NUTRITION

Per serving: 106 calories; 1 g fat (0 g sat, 0 g mono); 2 mg cholesterol; 22 g carbohydrates; 3 g protein; 4 gfiber; 22 mg sodium; 192 mg potassium.

Nutrition Bonus: Vitamin C (28% daily value), Fiber (16% dv).

Carbohydrate Servings: 1 1/2

Exchanges: 1 1/2 fruit

Curry-Roasted Shrimp with Oranges

INGREDIENTS

- 2 large seedless oranges
- 1/2 teaspoon kosher salt, divided
- 1 1/2 pounds shrimp, (30-40 per pound), peeled and deveined
- 1 tablespoon extra-virgin olive oil
- 1 tablespoon curry powder, preferably Madras (see Note)
- 1/2 teaspoon freshly ground pepper

PREPARATION

1. Preheat oven to 400°F. Line a baking sheet (with sides) with parchment paper. Finely grate the zest of 1 orange; set aside. Using a sharp knife, peel both oranges, removing all the bitter white pith. Thinly slice the oranges crosswise, then cut the slices into quarters. Spread the orange slices on the prepared baking sheet and sprinkle with 1/4 teaspoon salt. Roast until the oranges are slightly dry, about 12 minutes.

2. Meanwhile, toss shrimp with oil, curry powder, pepper, the orange zest and the remaining 1/4 teaspoon salt in a large bowl. Transfer the shrimp to the baking sheet with the oranges and roast until pink and curled, about 6 minutes. Divide the oranges and the shrimp among 4 plates and serve.

TIPS & NOTES

- **Make Ahead Tip**: Refrigerate for up to 4 days. Reheat before serving.
- **Note:** Madras curry powder is made with a hotter blend of spices than standard curry powder.

NUTRITION

Per serving: 253 calories; 7 g fat (1 g sat, 3 g mono); 259 mg cholesterol; 13 g carbohydrates; 0 g added sugars; 35 g protein; 4 g fiber; 548 mg sodium; 338 mg potassium.

Nutrition Bonus: Selenium (93% daily value), Vitamin C (70% dv).

Carbohydrate Servings: 1

Exchanges: 1 fruit, 5 very lean meat, 1 fat (mono)

Slow-Cooker Braised Pork with Salsa

INGREDIENTS

- 3 pounds boneless pork shoulder, or butt
- 1 1/2 cups prepared tomatillo salsa, (see Ingredient Note)
- 1 3/4 cups reduced-sodium chicken broth
- 1 medium onion, thinly sliced
- 1 teaspoon cumin seeds, or ground cumin
- 3 plum tomatoes, (1/2 pound), thinly sliced
- 1/2 cup chopped fresh cilantro, divided
- 1/2 cup reduced-fat sour cream

PREPARATION

1. Trim and discard pork surface fat. Cut meat apart following layers of fat around muscles; trim and discard fat. Cut into 2-inch chunks and rinse with cold water. Place in a 5- or 6-quart slow cooker. Turn heat to high.
2. Combine salsa, broth, onion and cumin seeds in a saucepan and bring to a boil over high heat. Pour over the meat. Add tomatoes and mix gently. Put the lid on and cook until the meat is pull-apart tender, 6 to 7 hours.
3. With a slotted spoon, transfer the pork to a large bowl; cover and keep warm. Pour the sauce and vegetables into a large skillet; skim fat. Bring to a boil over high heat. Boil, skimming froth from time to time, for about 20 minutes, to intensify flavors and thicken slightly. Add the pork and 1/4 cup cilantro; heat through.
4. To serve, ladle into bowls and garnish each serving with a dollop of sour cream and a sprinkling of the remaining 1/4 cup cilantro. Oven method: Total: 3 hours Preheat oven to 350°F. Combine pork, salsa, 1/2 cup chicken broth, onion, cumin

seeds and tomatoes in a 9-by-13-inch baking dish; cover snugly with foil. Bake until the pork is pull-apart tender, about 2 1/4 hours. Skim fat. Uncover and bake until the meat begins to brown, about 15 minutes more. Stir in 1/4 cup cilantro. Ladle into bowls, garnish with sour cream and remaining cilantro.

TIPS & NOTES

- **Make Ahead Tip**: Cover and refrigerate for up to 2 days or freeze for up to 3 months. Reheat on the stovetop, in a microwave or in the oven.
- **Ingredient Note:** Tomatillo salsa (sometimes labeled salsa verde or green salsa) is a blend of green chiles, onions and tomatillos. It is sold in supermarkets.For easy cleanup, try a slow-cooker liner. These heat-resistant, disposable liners fit neatly inside the insert and help prevent food from sticking to the bottom and sides of your slow cooker.

NUTRITION

Per serving: 276 calories; 15 g fat (6 g sat, 7 g mono); 104 mg cholesterol; 6 g carbohydrates; 27 g protein;1 g fiber; 211 mg sodium; 413 mg potassium.

Nutrition Bonus: Zinc (27% daily value), Potassium (24% dv).

Carbohydrate Servings: 2

Exchanges: 1 vegetable, 4 lean meat

Sesame Green Beans

INGREDIENTS

- 1 pound green beans, trimmed
- 2 teaspoons extra-virgin olive oil
- 2 teaspoons toasted sesame seeds, (see Tip)
- 1 teaspoon sesame oil
- Salt & freshly ground pepper, to taste

PREPARATION

1. Preheat oven to 500°F.

2. Toss green beans with olive oil. Spread in an even layer on a rimmed baking sheet. Roast, turning once halfway through cooking, until tender and beginning to brown, about 10 minutes. Toss with sesame seeds, sesame oil, salt and pepper.

TIPS & NOTES

- **Tip:** To toast sesame seeds: Place in a small dry skillet and cook over medium-low heat, stirring constantly, until fragrant and lightly browned, 2 to 4 minutes.

NUTRITION

Per serving: 67 calories; 4 g fat (1 g sat, 3 g mono); 0 mg cholesterol; 7 g carbohydrates; 0 g added sugars;2 g protein; 4 g fiber; 73 mg sodium; 280 mg potassium.

Nutrition Bonus: Vitamin C (15% daily value).

Carbohydrate Servings: 1/2

Exchanges: 1 vegetable

DAY 4
BREAKFAST
Apricot Smoothie
Whole-wheat toast (1 slice)
Roasted Apple Butter
LUNCH
Lettuce Wraps with Spiced Pork or Mediterranean Tuna Panini
Sweet & Tangy Watermelon Salad
Skim milk (1 cup)
SNACK
Carrot sticks (1 cup)
Feta & Herb Dip or Creamy Dill Sauce
DINNER
Chicken Breasts with Roasted Lemons

Arugula-Mushroom Salad
Baked potato (1 medium)
Fat-free cheese slice
Almond Cream with Strawberries

DAY 4 RECIPES

Apricot Smoothie

INGREDIENTS
- 1 cup canned apricot halves in light syrup
- 6 ice cubes
- 1 cup nonfat plain yogurt
- 3 tablespoons sugar

PREPARATION
1. Blend apricot halves, ice cubes, yogurt and sugar in a blender until frothy.

NUTRITION
Per serving: 202 calories; 0 g fat (0 g sat, 0 g mono); 3 mg cholesterol; 49 g carbohydrates; 6 g protein; 2 gfiber; 74 mg sodium; 175 mg potassium.
Carbohydrate Servings: 3
Exchanges: 1 1/2 fruit, 1/2 fat-free milk, 1 other carbohydrate

Roasted Apple Butter

INGREDIENTS
- 8 medium McIntosh apples, (2 3/4 pounds), peeled, cored and quartered
- 2 cups unsweetened apple juice

PREPARATION
1. Preheat oven to 450°F. Arrange apples in a large roasting pan. Pour apple juice over the apples. Bake until tender and lightly browned, about 30 minutes. Using a fork or potato masher, thoroughly mash the apples in the roasting pan.
2. Reduce oven temperature to 350°. Bake the apple puree, stirring occasionally, until very thick and deeply browned, 1 1/2 to 1 3/4 hours. Scrape into a bowl and let cool.

TIPS & NOTES
- **Make Ahead Tip**: Store in an airtight container in the refrigerator for up to 2 weeks or freeze for up to 6 months.

NUTRITION

Per tablespoon: 27 calories; 0 g fat (0 g sat, 0 g mono); 0 mg cholesterol; 7 g carbohydrates; 0 g protein; 1 g fiber; 0 mg sodium; 18 mg potassium.
Carbohydrate Servings: 1/2
Exchanges: 1/2 fruit

Lettuce Wraps with Spiced Pork

INGREDIENTS
SAUCE
- 2 tablespoons oyster sauce
- 2 tablespoons water
- 1 tablespoon hoisin sauce
- 1 tablespoon rice vinegar
- 1 tablespoon dry sherry, or rice wine
- 2 teaspoons cornstarch
- 1 teaspoon brown sugar
- 1 teaspoon reduced-sodium soy sauce
- 1 teaspoon sesame oil

STIR-FRY
- 3 teaspoons canola oil, divided
- 1 pound thin center-cut boneless pork chops, trimmed of fat and cut into thin julienne strips
- 2 cloves garlic, minced
- 1 tablespoon minced fresh ginger
- 1 8-ounce can sliced water chestnuts, rinsed and coarsely chopped
- 1 8-ounce can sliced bamboo shoots, rinsed and coarsely chopped
- 8 ounces shiitake mushrooms, stemmed, cut into julienne strips
- 4 scallions, greens only, sliced
- 1 head iceberg lettuce, leaves separated

PREPARATION
1. To prepare sauce: Combine oyster sauce, water, hoisin sauce, vinegar, sherry (or rice wine), cornstarch, brown sugar, soy sauce and sesame oil in a small bowl.
2. To prepare stir-fry: Heat 2 teaspoons canola oil over medium-high heat in a large nonstick skillet or wok. Add pork; cook, stirring constantly, until no longer pink, about 4 minutes. Transfer to a plate. Wipe out the pan.
3. Add remaining 1 teaspoon oil, garlic and ginger; cook, stirring constantly, until fragrant, 30 seconds. Add water chestnuts, bamboo shoots and mushrooms; cook, stirring often, until the mushrooms have softened, about 4 minutes. Return the pork to the pan and add the sauce. Cook, stirring constantly, until a

thick glossy sauce has formed, about 1 minute. Serve sprinkled with scallions and wrapped in lettuce leaves.

TIPS & NOTES
- **Make Ahead Tip**: The sauce will keep, covered, in the refrigerator for up to 2 days.

NUTRITION

Per serving: 350 calories; 16 g fat (5 g sat, 8 g mono); 59 mg cholesterol; 29 g carbohydrates; 25 g protein;7 g fiber; 810 mg sodium; 675 mg potassium.
Nutrition Bonus: Vitamin C (20% daily value), Iron (15% dv).
Carbohydrate Servings: 1
Exchanges: 1/2 other carbohydrate, 2 vegetable, 3 medium-fat meat

Mediterranean Tuna Panini

INGREDIENTS
- 2 6-ounce cans chunk light tuna, drained (see Note)
- 1 plum tomato, chopped
- 1/4 cup crumbled feta cheese
- 2 tablespoons chopped marinated artichoke hearts
- 2 tablespoons minced red onion
- 1 tablespoon chopped pitted kalamata olives
- 1 teaspoon capers, rinsed and chopped
- 1 teaspoon lemon juice
- Freshly ground pepper, to taste
- 8 slices whole-wheat bread
- 2 teaspoons canola oil

PREPARATION
1. Have four 15-ounce cans and a medium skillet (not nonstick) ready by the stove.
2. Place tuna in a medium bowl and flake with a fork. Add tomato, feta, artichokes, onion, olives, capers, lemon juice and pepper; stir to combine. Divide the tuna mixture among 4 slices of bread (about 1/2 cup each). Top with the remaining bread.
3. Heat 1 teaspoon canola oil in a large nonstick skillet over medium heat. Place 2 panini in the pan. Place the medium skillet on top of the panini, then weigh it down with the cans. Cook the panini until golden on one side, about 2 minutes. Reduce the heat to medium-low, flip the panini, replace the top skillet and cans, and cook until the second side is golden, 1 to 3 minutes more. Repeat with another 1 teaspoon oil and the remaining panini.

TIPS & NOTES

- **Note:** Chunk light tuna, which comes from the smaller skipjack or yellowfin, has less mercury than canned white albacore tuna. The FDA/EPA advises that women who are or might become pregnant, nursing mothers and young children consume no more than 6 ounces of albacore a week; up to 12 ounces of canned light tuna is considered safe.

NUTRITION

Per serving: 336 calories; 6 g fat (2 g sat, 3 g mono); 61 mg cholesterol; 35 g carbohydrates; 3 g added sugars; 34 g protein; 5 g fiber; 543 mg sodium; 52 mg potassium.
Nutrition Bonus: Fiber (20% daily value), Calcium & Iron (15% dv), omega-3s.
Carbohydrate Servings: 2
Exchanges: 2 starch, 3 very lean meat

Sweet & Tangy Watermelon Salad

INGREDIENTS

- 2 tablespoons rice vinegar
- 2 1/2 teaspoons sugar
- 2 cups diced seeded watermelon
- 2 cups diced cucumber
- 1/2 cup chopped fresh cilantro
- 1/4 cup unsalted dry-roasted peanuts, toasted (see Tip) and coarsely chopped

PREPARATION

1. Stir together vinegar and sugar in a medium bowl until the sugar almost dissolves. Add watermelon, cucumber and cilantro; toss gently to combine. Just before serving, sprinkle with peanuts.

TIPS & NOTES

- **Tip:** To toast nuts:
- Heat a small dry skillet over medium-low heat. Add nuts and cook, stirring, until lightly browned and fragrant, 2 to 3 minutes. Transfer to a bowl to cool.

NUTRITION

Per serving: 63 calories; 3 g fat (0 g sat, 2 g mono); 0 mg cholesterol; 8 g carbohydrates; 2 g protein; 1 gfiber; 3 mg sodium; 164 mg potassium.
Carbohydrate Servings: 1/2
Exchanges: 1/2 fruit, 1/2 vegetable, 1/2 fat

Feta & Herb Dip

INGREDIENTS
- 1 15-ounce can white beans, rinsed
- 3/4 cup nonfat plain yogurt
- 1/2 cup crumbled feta cheese
- 1 tablespoon lemon juice
- 1 teaspoon garlic salt
- 1 teaspoon freshly ground pepper
- 1/4 cup chopped fresh parsley
- 1/4 cup chopped fresh dill
- 1/4 cup chopped fresh mint
- 1/4 cup chopped fresh chives

PREPARATION
1. Place beans, yogurt, feta, lemon juice, garlic salt and pepper in a food processor and puree until smooth. Add herbs; puree until incorporated. Chill until ready to serve.

TIPS & NOTES
- **Make Ahead Tip**: Cover and refrigerate for up to 2 days.

NUTRITION
Per serving: 32 calories; 1 g fat (1 g sat, 0 g mono); 4 mg cholesterol; 5 g carbohydrates; 0 g added sugars; 2 g protein; 1 g fiber; 167 mg sodium; 77 mg potassium.
Nutrition Bonus: Calcium, protein, fiber, folate.
Exchanges: 1/2 starch, 1/2 very lean meat

Creamy Dill Sauce

INGREDIENTS
- 1/4 cup reduced-fat mayonnaise
- 1/4 cup nonfat plain yogurt
- 2 scallions, thinly sliced
- 1 tablespoon lemon juice
- 1 tablespoon finely chopped fresh dill, or parsley
- Freshly ground pepper, to taste

PREPARATION
1. Combine mayonnaise, yogurt, scallions, lemon juice, dill (or parsley) and pepper in a small bowl and mix well.

TIPS & NOTES
- **Make Ahead Tip**: Cover and refrigerate for up to 2 days.

NUTRITION
Per tablespoon: 28 calories; 2 g fat (0 g sat, 0 g mono); 2 mg cholesterol; 2 g carbohydrates; 0 g protein; 0 g fiber; 50 mg sodium; 13 mg potassium.
Exchanges: free food

Chicken Breasts with Roasted Lemons

INGREDIENTS
ROASTED LEMONS
- 3 medium lemons, thinly sliced and seeded
- 1 teaspoon extra-virgin olive oil
- 1/8 teaspoon salt

CHICKEN
- 4 boneless, skinless chicken breast halves, (about 1 pound total), trimmed
- 1/8 teaspoon salt
- Freshly ground pepper, to taste
- 1/4 cup all-purpose flour
- 2 teaspoons extra-virgin olive oil
- 1 1/4 cups reduced-sodium chicken broth
- 2 tablespoons drained capers, rinsed and 2 teaspoons butter
- 3 tablespoons chopped fresh parsley, divided

PREPARATION
1. To prepare roasted lemons: Preheat oven to 325°F. Line a baking sheet with parchment paper. Arrange lemon slices in a single layer on it. Brush the lemon slices with 1 tablespoon oil and sprinkle with 1/8 teaspoon salt. Roast the lemons until slightly dry and beginning to brown around the edges, 25 to 30 minutes.
2. Meanwhile, prepare chicken: Cover chicken with plastic wrap and pound with a rolling pin or heavy skillet until flattened to about 1/2 inch thick. Sprinkle the chicken with 1/8 teaspoon salt and pepper. Place flour in a shallow dish and dredge the chicken to coat both sides; shake off excess (discard remaining flour).
3. Heat 2 teaspoons oil in a large nonstick skillet over medium-high heat. Add the chicken and cook until golden brown, 2 to 3 minutes per side. Add broth and bring to a boil, scraping up any browned bits. Stir in capers. Boil until the liquid is reduced to syrup consistency, 5 to 8 minutes, turning the chicken halfway. Add the roasted lemons, butter, 2 tablespoons parsley and more pepper, if desired; simmer until the butter melts and the chicken is cooked through, about 2 minutes. Transfer to a platter. Sprinkle with the remaining 1 tablespoon parsley and serve.

TIPS & NOTES
- **Make Ahead Tip**: Cover and refrigerate the roasted lemons (Step 1) for up to 2 days.

NUTRITION
Per serving: 219 calories; 7 g fat (2 g sat, 3 g mono); 72 mg cholesterol; 6 g carbohydrates; 0 g added sugars; 28 g protein; 1 g fiber; 396 mg sodium; 376 mg potassium.
Nutrition Bonus: Vitamin C (40% daily value).
Carbohydrate Servings: 1/2
Exchanges: 1/2 fruit, 4 very lean meat, 1 fat

Arugula-Mushroom Salad

INGREDIENTS
- 1 clove garlic, peeled
- 1/4 teaspoon salt
- 1 tablespoon lemon juice
- 1 tablespoon reduced-fat mayonnaise
- 1 tablespoon extra-virgin olive oil
- 1 tablespoon chopped fresh parsley
- Freshly ground pepper, to taste
- 6 cups arugula leaves
- 2 cups sliced mushrooms

PREPARATION

1. Place garlic on a cutting board and crush. Sprinkle with salt and use the flat of a chefs knife blade to mash the garlic to a paste; transfer to a serving bowl. Whisk in lemon juice, mayonnaise, oil and parsley. Season with pepper. Add arugula and mushrooms; toss to coat with the dressing.

NUTRITION
Per serving: 62 calories; 4 g fat (1 g sat, 3 g mono); 1 mg cholesterol; 3 g carbohydrates; 0 g added sugars;2 g protein; 1 g fiber; 188 mg sodium; 235 mg potassium.
Nutrition Bonus: Vitamin C (15% daily value).
Exchanges: 1 vegetable, 1 fat (mono)

Almond Cream with Strawberries

INGREDIENTS
- 1/4 cup slivered almonds
- 2 cups strawberries, rinsed
- 1 cup part-skim ricotta
- 2 tablespoons sugar or Splenda Granular
- 1/4 teaspoon almond extract

PREPARATION
1. Toast almonds in a small dry skillet over medium-low heat, stirring constantly, until golden and fragrant, 2 to 3 minutes. Transfer to a plate to cool.
2. Hull strawberries, slice and divide among 4 dessert plates. Mix ricotta with sugar (or Splenda) and almond extract until smooth. Spoon over the berries and sprinkle with the toasted almonds.

NUTRITION
Per serving: 189 calories; 9 g fat (3 g sat, 4 g mono); 19 mg cholesterol; 16 g carbohydrates; 9 g protein; 2 g fiber; 78 mg sodium; 237 mg potassium.
Nutrition Bonus: Vitamin C (82% daily value), Calcium (19% dv).
Carbohydrate Servings: 1
Exchanges: 1 fruit, 1 medium-fat meat
Nutrition Note: Per serving with Splenda: 1; 168 calories, 12 g carbohydrate

DAY 5
BREAKFAST

Baked Asparagus & Cheese Frittata
Skim milk (1 cup)
Apple (1 cup, quartered)

LUNCH

Broccoli-Cheese Chowder
Chicken Tabbouleh or Cuban-Style Pork & Rice
Skim milk (1 cup)

SNACK

Orange (1 large)

DINNER

Grilled Pork Tenderloin with Mustard, Rosemary & Apple Marinade
    or Roasted Cod with Warm Tomato-Olive-Caper Tapenade
Salad of Boston Lettuce with Creamy Orange-Shallot Dressing
Brown Rice (1 cup)
Smashed Spiced Sweet Potatoes

DAY 5 RECIPES

Baked Asparagus & Cheese Frittata

INGREDIENTS
- 2 tablespoons fine dry breadcrumbs
- 1 pound thin asparagus
- 1 1/2 teaspoons extra-virgin olive oil
- 2 onions, chopped
- 1 red bell pepper, chopped
- 2 cloves garlic, minced
- 1/2 teaspoon salt, divided
- 1/2 cup water
- Freshly ground pepper, to taste
- 4 large eggs and 2 large egg whites
- 1 cup part-skim ricotta cheese
- 1 tablespoon chopped fresh parsley
- 1/2 cup shredded Gruyère cheese

PREPARATION

1. Preheat oven to 325°F. Coat a 10-inch pie pan or ceramic quiche dish with cooking spray. Sprinkle with breadcrumbs, tapping out the excess.
2. Snap tough ends off asparagus. Slice off the top 2 inches of the tips and reserve. Cut the stalks into 1/2-inch-long slices.
3. Heat oil in a large nonstick skillet over medium-high heat. Add onions, bell pepper, garlic and 1/4 teaspoon salt; cook, stirring, until softened, 5 to 7 minutes.
4. Add water and the asparagus stalks to the skillet. Cook, stirring, until the asparagus is tender and the liquid has evaporated, about 7 minutes (the mixture should be very dry). Season with salt and pepper. Arrange the vegetables in an even layer in the prepared pan.
5. Whisk eggs and egg whites in a large bowl. Add ricotta, parsley, the remaining 1/4 teaspoon salt and pepper; whisk to blend. Pour the egg mixture over the vegetables, gently shaking the pan to distribute. Scatter the reserved asparagus tips over the top and sprinkle with Gruyère.
6. Bake the frittata until a knife inserted in the center comes out clean, about 35 minutes. Let stand for 5 minutes before serving.

NUTRITION
Per serving: 195 calories; 11 g fat (5 g sat, 4 g mono); 164 mg cholesterol; 10 g carbohydrates; 15 gprotein; 2 g fiber; 357 mg sodium; 310 mg potassium.
Nutrition Bonus: Vitamin C (70% daily value), Vitamin A (30% dv).

Carbohydrate Servings: 1/2
Exchanges: 2 vegetable, 1 medium-fat meat, 1/2 high-fat meat

Broccoli-Cheese Chowder

INGREDIENTS
- 1 tablespoon extra-virgin olive oil
- 1 large onion, chopped
- 1 large carrot, diced
- 2 stalks celery, diced
- 1 large potato, peeled and diced
- 2 cloves garlic, minced
- 1 tablespoon all-purpose flour
- 1/2 teaspoon dry mustard
- 1/8 teaspoon cayenne pepper
- 2 14-ounce cans vegetable broth, or reduced-sodium chicken broth
- 8 ounces broccoli crowns, (see Ingredient Note), cut into 1-inch pieces, stems and florets separated
- 1 cup shredded reduced-fat Cheddar cheese
- 1/2 cup reduced-fat sour cream
- 1/8 teaspoon salt

PREPARATION
1. Heat oil in a Dutch oven or large saucepan over medium-high heat. Add onion, carrot and celery; cook, stirring often, until the onion and celery soften, 5 to 6 minutes. Add potato and garlic; cook, stirring, for 2 minutes. Stir in flour, dry mustard and cayenne; cook, stirring often, for 2 minutes.
2. Add broth and broccoli stems; bring to a boil. Cover and reduce heat to medium. Simmer, stirring occasionally, for 10 minutes. Stir in florets; simmer, covered, until the broccoli is tender, about 10 minutes more. Transfer 2 cups of the chowder to a bowl and mash; return to the pan.
3. Stir in Cheddar and sour cream; cook over medium heat, stirring, until the cheese is melted and the chowder is heated through, about 2 minutes. Season with salt.

TIPS & NOTES
- **Make Ahead Tip**: Prepare through Step 2. Cover and refrigerate for up to 2 days or freeze for up to 2 months.
- **Ingredient note:** Most supermarkets sell broccoli crowns, which are the tops of the bunches, with the stalks cut off. Although crowns are more expensive than entire bunches, they are convenient and there is considerably less waste.

NUTRITION

Per serving: 205 calories; 9 g fat (4 g sat, 3 g mono); 21 mg cholesterol; 23 g carbohydrates; 9 g protein; 4 g fiber; 508 mg sodium; 436 mg potassium.
Nutrition Bonus: Vitamin C (61% daily value), Vitamin A (64% dv), Calcium (34% dv).
Carbohydrate Servings: 1 1/2
Exchanges: 1 starch, 1 vegetable, 1 high-fat meat

Chicken Tabbouleh

INGREDIENTS
- 3 cups water
- 1 cup bulgur
- 3 cups cubed skinless cooked chicken, (1-inch cubes)
- 1 cup chopped fresh parsley
- 1 cup chopped scallions
- 1/3 cup currants
- 1/4 cup frozen orange juice concentrate
- 2 tablespoons lemon juice
- 1 tablespoon extra-virgin olive oil
- 1 teaspoon ground cumin
- 1/4 teaspoon cayenne pepper, or to taste
- 1/4 teaspoon salt
- Freshly ground pepper, to taste

PREPARATION
1. Bring water to a boil in a large saucepan. Add bulgur and remove from the heat. Let stand until most of the water is absorbed, 20 to 30 minutes.
2. Drain bulgur well, squeezing out excess moisture. Transfer to a large bowl. Add chicken, parsley, scallions and currants.
3. Whisk orange juice concentrate, lemon juice, oil, cumin and cayenne in a small bowl until blended. Toss with the bulgur mixture. Season with salt and pepper and serve.

TIPS & NOTES
- **To poach chicken breasts:** Place boneless, skinless chicken breasts in a medium skillet or saucepan and add lightly salted water to cover; bring to a boil. Cover, reduce heat to low and simmer gently until chicken is cooked through and no longer pink in the middle, 10 to 12 minutes.
- **Ingredient note:** Bulgur is made by parboiling, drying and coarsely grinding or cracking wheat berries. Don't confuse bulgur with cracked wheat, which is simply that cracked wheat. Since the parboiling step is skipped, cracked wheat must be cooked for up to an hour whereas bulgur simply needs a quick soak in

hot water for most uses. Look for it in the natural-foods section of large supermarkets, near other grains, or online at kalustyans.com, lebaneseproducts.com.

NUTRITION
Per serving: 260 calories; 5 g fat (1 g sat, 3 g mono); 60 mg cholesterol; 31 g carbohydrates; 0 g added sugars; 26 g protein; 6 g fiber; 166 mg sodium; 536 mg potassium.
Nutrition Bonus: Vitamin C (60% daily value), Fiber (24% dv), Potassium (15% dv).
Carbohydrate Servings: 1 1/2
Exchanges: 2 starch, 3 very lean meat

Cuban-Style Pork & Rice

INGREDIENTS
- 1/4 cup paprika
- 1/4 cup lime juice
- 3 tablespoons extra-virgin olive oil, divided
- 2 tablespoons rum, (optional)
- 2 teaspoons minced garlic, plus 2 tablespoons chopped garlic, divided
- 2 teaspoons fresh oregano, chopped
- 1 teaspoon kosher salt
- 1 teaspoon freshly ground pepper
- 1/2 teaspoon ground cumin, cumin
- 1 1/2 pounds boneless pork chops, (3/4-1 inch thick), trimmed, cut into cubes
- 2 cups onion, chopped
- 2 cups arborio rice, or short-grain brown rice
- 2 14-ounce cans reduced-sodium chicken broth
- 1 cup canned diced tomatoes
- 2 tablespoons capers, rinsed
- 1/4 teaspoon saffron threads, (see Note)
- 16 large raw shrimp, (21-25 per pound), peeled and deveined (optional)
- 2 cups frozen artichoke hearts, thawed, or cooked green beans, fresh or frozen, thawed
- 1/2 cup roasted red peppers, cut into strips

PREPARATION
1. Combine paprika, lime juice, 2 tablespoons oil, rum (if using), 2 teaspoons minced garlic, oregano, salt, pepper and cumin in a medium bowl, stirring to make a homogeneous paste. Add pork and stir to coat.

2. Heat the remaining 1 tablespoon oil in a Dutch oven over medium-high heat. Add the pork, leaving any excess spice mixture in the bowl to add later. Cook the pork, stirring, until just cooked on the outside and the spices are very fragrant, 2 to 3 minutes. Transfer the pork to a plate.
3. Add onion and the remaining 2 tablespoons garlic to the pan and cook, stirring often, until the onion is softened, 4 to 5 minutes. Add rice and cook, stirring, until well coated with the onion mixture. Stir in broth, tomatoes, capers, saffron and any remaining spice mixture. (If using brown rice, also add 3/4 cup water now.) Bring to a boil, then reduce to a low simmer; cook, stirring occasionally, 15 minutes for arborio, 30 minutes for brown rice.
4. Preheat oven to 350°F.
5. Stir shrimp (if using) and artichokes (or green beans) into the rice. Cover and bake for 20 minutes. Stir in the pork and any accumulated juices from the plate; scatter roasted peppers on top.
Cover and continue baking until the rice is tender and the liquid has been absorbed (if you've added shrimp, they should be opaque and pink), 10 to 15 minutes more.

TIPS & NOTES
- **Note:** Saffron is the dried stigma of a saffron crocus. It contributes a pungent flavor and intense yellow color to classic dishes like paella. Saffron is sold in threads and powdered form.

NUTRITION
Per serving: 257 calories; 9 g fat (2 g sat, 5 g mono); 40 mg cholesterol; 26 g carbohydrates; 19 g protein; 5 g fiber; 257 mg sodium; 414 mg potassium.
Nutrition Bonus: Vitamin A (40% daily value), Vitamin C (35% dv), Selenium (32% dv), Folate (17% dv).
Carbohydrate Servings: 1 1/2
Exchanges: 1 starch, 1 vegetable, 2 lean meat, 1 fat

Grilled Pork Tenderloin with Mustard, Rosemary & Apple Marinade

INGREDIENTS
- 1/4 cup frozen apple juice concentrate
- 2 tablespoons plus 1 1/2 teaspoons Dijon mustard
- 2 tablespoons extra-virgin olive oil, divided
- 2 tablespoons chopped fresh rosemary, or thyme
- 4 cloves garlic, minced
- 1 teaspoon crushed peppercorns
- 2 12-ounce pork tenderloins, trimmed of fat
- 1 tablespoon minced shallot

- 3 tablespoons port, or brewed black tea
- 2 tablespoons balsamic vinegar
- 1/4 teaspoon salt, or to taste
- Freshly ground pepper, to taste

PREPARATION
1. Whisk apple juice concentrate, 2 tablespoons mustard, 1 tablespoon oil, rosemary (or thyme), garlic and peppercorns in a small bowl. Reserve 3 tablespoons marinade for basting. Place
- tenderloins in a shallow glass dish and pour the remaining marinade over them, turning to coat. Cover and marinate in the refrigerator for at least 20 minutes or for up to 2 hours, turning several times.
2. Heat a grill or broiler.
3. Combine shallot, port (or tea), vinegar, salt, pepper and the remaining 1 1/2 teaspoons mustard and 1 tablespoon oil in a small bowl or a jar with a tight-fitting lid; whisk or shake until blended. Set aside.
4. Grill or broil the tenderloins, turning several times and basting the browned sides with the reserved marinade, until just cooked through, 15 to 20 minutes. (An instant-read thermometer inserted in the center should register 155°F. The temperature will increase to 160° during resting.)
5. Transfer the tenderloins to a clean cutting board, tent with foil and let them rest for about 5 minutes before carving them into 1/2-inch-thick slices. Arrange the pork slices on plates and drizzle with the shallot dressing. Serve immediately.

TIPS & NOTES
- **Make Ahead Tip**: The pork can be marinated (Step 1) for up to 2 hours.

NUTRITION
Per serving: 165 calories; 5 g fat (1 g sat, 2 g mono); 63 mg cholesterol; 5 g carbohydrates; 0 g added sugars; 23 g protein; 0 g fiber; 186 mg sodium; 397 mg potassium.
Nutrition Bonus: Vitamin C (20% daily value).
Carbohydrate Servings: 1/2
Exchanges: 1/2 other carbohydrate, 3 lean meat

Roasted Cod with Warm Tomato-Olive-Caper Tapenade

INGREDIENTS
- 1 pound cod fillet (see Tip)
- 3 teaspoons extra-virgin olive oil, divided
- 1/4 teaspoon freshly ground pepper
- 1 tablespoon minced shallot

- 1 cup halved cherry tomatoes
- 1/4 cup chopped cured olives
- 1 tablespoon capers, rinsed and chopped
- 1 1/2 teaspoons chopped fresh oregano
- 1 teaspoon balsamic vinegar

PREPARATION
1. Preheat oven to 450°F. Coat a baking sheet with cooking spray.
2. Rub cod with 2 teaspoons oil. Sprinkle with pepper. Place on the prepared baking sheet. Transfer to the oven and roast until the fish flakes easily with a fork, 15 to 20 minutes, depending on the thickness of the fillet.
3. Meanwhile, heat the remaining 1 teaspoon oil in a small skillet over medium heat. Add shallot and cook, stirring, until beginning to soften, about 20 seconds. Add tomatoes and cook, stirring, until softened, about 1 1/2 minutes. Add olives and capers; cook, stirring, for 30 seconds more. Stir in oregano and vinegar; remove from heat. Spoon the tapenade over the cod to serve.

TIPS & NOTES
- **Tip:** Overfishing and trawling have drastically reduced the number of cod in the U.S. and Canadian Atlantic Ocean and destroyed its sea floor. For sustainably fished cod, choose U.S. Pacific cod or Atlantic cod from Iceland and the northeast Arctic. For more information, visit Monterey Bay Aquarium Seafood Watch at seafoodwatch.org.

NUTRITION
Per serving: 151 calories; 8 g fat (1 g sat, 6 g mono); 45 mg cholesterol; 4 g carbohydrates; 0 g added sugars; 15 g protein; 1 g fiber; 602 mg sodium; 335 mg potassium.
Carbohydrate Servings: 0
Exchanges: 3 lean meat, 1.5 fat (mono)

Salad of Boston Lettuce with Creamy Orange-Shallot Dressing
INGREDIENTS
DRESSING
- 1/4 cup reduced-fat mayonnaise
- 1/2 teaspoon Dijon mustard
- 1/4 cup orange juice
- 2 teaspoons finely chopped shallot
- Freshly ground pepper, to taste

SALAD
- 1 large head Boston lettuce, torn into bite-size pieces (5 cups)

- 1 cup julienned or grated carrot, (1 carrot)
- 1 cup cherry or grape tomatoes, rinsed and cut in half
- 2 tablespoons snipped fresh tarragon, or chives (optional)

PREPARATION
1. To prepare dressing: Whisk mayonnaise and mustard in a small bowl. Slowly whisk in orange juice until smooth. Stir in shallot. Season with pepper.
2. To prepare salad: Divide lettuce among 4 plates and scatter carrot and tomatoes on top. Drizzle the dressing over the salads and sprinkle with tarragon (or chives), if desired. Serve immediately.

NUTRITION
Per serving: 64 calories; 1 g fat (0 g sat, 0 g mono); 0 mg cholesterol; 12 g carbohydrates; 1 g added sugars; 2 g protein; 2 g fiber; 182 mg sodium; 386 mg potassium.
Nutrition Bonus: Vitamin A (120% daily value), Vitamin C (30% dv), Folate (16% dv).
Carbohydrate Servings: 1
Exchanges: 2 vegetable

Smashed Spiced Sweet Potatoes

INGREDIENTS
- 4 pounds sweet potatoes, (4-5 large)
- 2 tablespoons butter
- 2 tablespoons pure maple syrup
- 1 tablespoon chili powder
- 2 teaspoons cumin seeds, toasted and ground (see Tip)
- 1 teaspoon ground ginger
- 1 teaspoon salt
- 1/2 teaspoon freshly ground pepper

PREPARATION
1. Preheat oven to 350 degrees F. Pierce each sweet potato in several places with a fork. Place directly on the oven rack and roast until soft, 45 minutes to 1 hour. Transfer to a cutting board; let stand until cool enough to handle, about 10 minutes. Slip off the skins and cut the sweet potatoes into 1-inch slices; transfer to a large bowl. Add butter. Smash the sweet potatoes with a potato masher or fork until fluffy but some lumps remain. Add maple syrup, chili powder, ground cumin, ginger, salt and pepper; stir to combine.

TIPS & NOTES
- **Tip:** Toast cumin seeds in a small skillet over medium heat, stirring occasionally, until fragrant, about 2 minutes. Transfer to a plate to cool. Grind in a spice mill or blender into a fine powder.

NUTRITION
Per serving: 113 calories; 2 g fat (1 g sat, 1 g mono); 5 mg cholesterol; 22 g carbohydrates; 2 g protein; 3 gfiber; 243 mg sodium; 468 mg potassium.
Nutrition Bonus: Vitamin A (360% daily value), Vitamin C (30% dv).
Carbohydrate Servings: 1 1/2
Exchanges: 1.5 starch

DAY 6
BREAKFAST
Jam-Filled Almond Muffins or Blueberry-Ricotta Pancakes
Skim milk (1 cup)
Banana (1 cup)
LUNCH
The Taco
Calabacitas
Fat-free cheese (1 slice)
SNACK
Nonfat plain yogurt (8 oz.)
Strawberries (1 cup)
DINNER
Sloppy Joes
Steamed broccoli (1/2 cup)
Vinegary Coleslaw
Plum Fool or Farmer's Cheese & Strawberries

DAY 6 RECIPES

Jam-Filled Almond Muffins
INGREDIENTS
- 1 1/4 cups whole-wheat flour
- 1 cup all-purpose flour
- 1 1/2 teaspoons baking powder
- 1/2 teaspoon baking soda
- 1/4 teaspoon salt

- 2 large eggs
- 1/2 cup packed light brown sugar
- 1 cup buttermilk, (see Tip)
- 1/4 cup orange juice
- 1/4 cup canola oil
- 1 teaspoon vanilla extract
- 1/3 cup blackberry, blueberry, raspberry or cherry jam
- 1/4 teaspoon almond extract
- 1/2 cup sliced almonds
- 1 tablespoon granulated sugar

PREPARATION
1. Preheat oven to 400°F. Coat 12 muffin cups with cooking spray.
2. Whisk whole-wheat flour, all-purpose flour, baking powder, baking soda and salt in a large bowl.
3. Whisk eggs and brown sugar in a medium bowl until smooth. Add buttermilk, orange juice, oil and vanilla; whisk to blend. Add to the dry ingredients and mix with a rubber spatula just until moistened.
4. Scoop half the batter into the prepared pan. Mix jam and almond extract; drop a generous teaspoonful into the center of each muffin. Spoon on the remaining batter, filling each muffin cup completely. Sprinkle with almonds, then sugar.
5. Bake the muffins until the tops are golden brown and spring back when touched lightly, 15 to 25 minutes. Loosen edges and turn muffins out onto a wire rack to cool slightly before serving.

TIPS & NOTES
- **Tip:** You can use buttermilk powder in place of fresh buttermilk. Or make "sour milk": mix 1 tablespoon lemon juice or vinegar to 1 cup milk.

NUTRITION
Per muffin: 229 calories; 8 g fat (1 g sat, 4 g mono); 36 mg cholesterol; 33 g carbohydrates; 6 g protein; 2 gfiber; 182 mg sodium; 77 mg potassium.
Carbohydrate Servings: 2
Exchanges: 2 starch, 1 fat

Blueberry-Ricotta Pancakes
INGREDIENTS
- 1/2 cup whole-wheat pastry flour (see Source)
- 1/4 cup plus 2 tablespoons all-purpose flour
- 1 teaspoon sugar
- 1 teaspoon baking powder

- 1/4 teaspoon baking soda
- 1/2 teaspoon freshly grated nutmeg
- 3/4 cup part-skim ricotta cheese
- 1 large egg
- 1 large egg white
- 1/2 cup nonfat buttermilk (see Tip)
- 1 teaspoon freshly grated lemon zest
- 1 tablespoon lemon juice
- 2 teaspoons canola oil, divided
- 3/4 cup fresh or frozen (not thawed) blueberries

PREPARATION
1. Whisk whole-wheat flour, all-purpose flour, sugar, baking powder, baking soda and nutmeg in a small bowl. Whisk ricotta, egg, egg white, buttermilk, lemon zest and juice in a large bowl until smooth. Stir the dry ingredients into the wet ingredients until just combined.
2. Brush a large nonstick skillet with 1/2 teaspoon oil and place over medium heat until hot. Using a generous 1/4 cup of batter for each pancake, pour the batter for 2 pancakes into the pan, sprinkle blueberries on each pancake and cook until the edges are dry and bubbles begin to form, about 2 minutes. Flip the pancakes and cook until golden brown, about 2 minutes more. Repeat with the remaining oil, batter and berries, adjusting the heat as necessary to prevent burning.

TIPS & NOTES
- **Source:** Look for whole-wheat pastry flour in the natural-foods section of large supermarkets and natural-foods stores.
- **Tip:** No buttermilk? Mix 1 tablespoon lemon juice into 1 cup milk.

NUTRITION
Per serving: 238 calories; 8 g fat (3 g sat, 3 g mono); 68 mg cholesterol; 30 g carbohydrates; 12 g protein; 3 g fiber; 334 mg sodium; 128 mg potassium.
Nutrition Bonus: Calcium (16% daily value).
Carbohydrate Servings: 2
Exchanges: 2 starch, 1 medium-fat meat

The Taco

INGREDIENTS
HOMEMADE TACO SHELLS
- 12 6-inch corn tortillas
- Canola oil cooking spray
- 3/4 teaspoon chili powder, divided

- 1/4 teaspoon salt, divided

TACO MEAT
- 8 ounces 93%-lean ground beef
- 8 ounces 99%-lean ground turkey breast
- 1/2 cup chopped onion
- 1 10-ounce can diced tomatoes with green chiles, preferably Rotel brand (see Tip), or 1 1/4 cups petite-diced tomatoes
- 1/2 teaspoon ground cumin
- 1/2 teaspoon ground chipotle chile or 1 teaspoon chili powder
- 1/2 teaspoon dried oregano

TOPPINGS
- 3 cups shredded romaine lettuce
- 3/4 cup shredded reduced-fat Cheddar cheese
- 3/4 cup diced tomatoes
- 3/4 cup prepared salsa
- 1/4 cup diced red onion

PREPARATION
1. To prepare taco shells: Preheat oven to 375°F.
2. Working with 6 tortillas at a time, wrap in a barely damp cloth or paper towel and microwave on High until steamed, about 30 seconds. Lay the tortillas on a clean work surface and coat both sides with cooking spray; sprinkle a little chili powder and salt on one side. Carefully drape each tortilla over two bars of the oven rack. Bake until crispy, 7 to 10 minutes. Repeat with the remaining 6 tortillas.
3. To prepare taco meat: Place beef, turkey and onion in a large nonstick skillet over medium heat. Cook, breaking up the meat with a wooden spoon, until cooked through, about 10 minutes. Transfer to a colander to drain off fat. Wipe out the pan. Return the meat to the pan and add tomatoes, cumin, ground chipotle (or chili powder) and oregano. Cook over medium heat, stirring occasionally, until most of the liquid has evaporated, 3 to 6 minutes.
4. To assemble tacos: Fill each shell with a generous 3 tablespoons taco meat, 1/4 cup lettuce, 1 tablespoon each cheese, tomato and salsa and 1 teaspoon onion.

TIPS & NOTES
- **Make Ahead Tip**: Store taco shells in an airtight container for up to 2 days. Reheat at 375°F for 1 to 2 minutes before serving. Cover and refrigerate taco meat for up to 1 day. Reheat just before serving.
- **Tip:** Look for Rotel brand diced tomatoes with green chiles original or mild, depending on your spice preference and set the heat level with either ground chipotle chile (adds smoky heat) or chili powder (adds rich chili taste without extra spice).

NUTRITION

Per serving: 252 calories; 5 g fat (1 g sat, 1 g mono); 38 mg cholesterol; 30 g carbohydrates; 0 g added sugars; 24 g protein; 5 g fiber; 576 mg sodium; 254 mg potassium.
Nutrition Bonus: Vitamin A (49% daily value), Vitamin C & Zinc (17% dv)
Carbohydrate Servings: 2
Exchanges: 1 1/2 starch, 1 vegetable, 3 lean meat

Calabacitas

INGREDIENTS
- 1 tablespoon extra-virgin olive oil
- 1 medium onion, chopped
- 1 poblano or Anaheim chile pepper, seeded and diced
- 2 cups diced zucchini
- 2 cups diced summer squash
- 1/2 teaspoon salt
- 2 tablespoons chopped fresh cilantro, (optional)

PREPARATION
1. Heat oil in a large nonstick skillet over medium heat. Add onion and chile; cook, stirring, until soft, about 4 minutes. Add zucchini, summer squash and salt; cover and cook, stirring once or twice, until tender, about 3 minutes. Remove from the heat and stir in cilantro (if using).

NUTRITION
Per serving: 40 calories; 2 g fat (0 g sat, 2 g mono); 0 mg cholesterol; 4 g carbohydrates; 0 g added sugars;1 g protein; 1 g fiber; 199 mg sodium; 201 mg potassium.
Nutrition Bonus: Vitamin C (30% dv).
Exchanges: 1 vegetable, 1/2 fat

Sloppy Joes

INGREDIENTS
- 12 ounces 90%-lean ground beef
- 1 large onion, finely diced
- 2 cups finely chopped cremini mushrooms, (about 4 ounces)
- 5 plum tomatoes, diced
- 2 tablespoons all-purpose flour
- 1/2 cup water
- 1/4 cup cider vinegar
- 1/4 cup chili sauce, such as Heinz

- 1/4 cup ketchup
- 8 whole-wheat hamburger buns, toasted if desired

PREPARATION
1. Crumble beef into a large nonstick skillet; cook over medium heat until it starts to sizzle, about 1 minute. Add onion and mushrooms and cook, stirring occasionally, breaking up the meat with a wooden spoon, until the vegetables are soft and the moisture has evaporated, 8 to 10 minutes.
2. Add tomatoes and flour; stir to combine. Stir in water, vinegar, chili sauce and ketchup and bring to a simmer, stirring often. Reduce heat to a low simmer and cook, stirring occasionally, until the sauce is thickened and the onion is very tender, 8 to 10 minutes. Serve warm on buns.

TIPS & NOTES
- **Make Ahead Tip**: The filling will keep in the freezer for up to 1 month.

NUTRITION
Per serving: 233 calories; 6 g fat (2 g sat, 2 g mono); 28 mg cholesterol; 31 g carbohydrates; 14 g protein; 5 g fiber; 436 mg sodium; 504 mg potassium.
Nutrition Bonus: Zinc (20% daily value), Vitamin C (15% dv).
Carbohydrate Servings: 2
Exchanges: 2 starch, 1 1/2 very lean meat

Vinegary Coleslaw

INGREDIENTS
- 2 tablespoons white-wine vinegar
- 1 tablespoon canola oil
- 1 teaspoon sugar
- 1 teaspoon Dijon mustard
- Pinch of celery seed
- Pinch of salt
- 1 1/2 cups shredded cabbage
- 1 carrot, peeled and grated
- 1/4 cup slivered red onion

PREPARATION
1. Whisk vinegar, oil, sugar, mustard, celery seed and salt in a medium bowl. Add cabbage, carrot and onion and toss to coat.

NUTRITION
Per serving: 101 calories; 7 g fat (1 g sat, 4 g mono); 0 mg cholesterol; 9 g carbohydrates; 2 g added sugars; 1 g protein; 2 g fiber; 138 mg sodium; 248 mg potassium.
Nutrition Bonus: Vitamin A (100% daily value), Vitamin C (35% dv).
Carbohydrate Servings: 1
Exchanges: 1 vegetable, 1 1/2 fat

Plum Fool

INGREDIENTS
- 1 pound plums, pitted and sliced (about 2 1/2 cups)
- 1/4-1/2 cup sugar, or Splenda Granular
- 1/2 teaspoon grated fresh ginger
- 1/2 teaspoon ground cinnamon
- 1 1/2 cups low-fat vanilla yogurt
- 1/3 cup whipping cream

PREPARATION
1. Set aside a few plum slices for garnish. Combine the remaining plum slices, 1/4 cup sugar (or Splenda), ginger and cinnamon in a small heavy saucepan. Bring to a simmer, stirring, over medium heat. Cook until the mixture has softened into a chunky puree, 15 to 20 minutes. Taste and add more sugar (or Splenda), if desired. Transfer to a bowl and chill until cool, about 1 hour.
2. Meanwhile, set a fine-mesh stainless-steel sieve over a bowl. Spoon in yogurt and let drain in the refrigerator until reduced to 1 cup, about 1 hour.
3. Whip cream to soft peaks in a chilled bowl. Gently fold in the drained yogurt with a rubber spatula. Fold this mixture into the fruit puree, leaving distinct swirls. Spoon into 6 dessert dishes and cover with plastic wrap. Refrigerate for at least 1 hour or up to 2 days. Garnish with the reserved plum slices before serving.

NUTRITION
Per serving: 156 calories; 5 g fat (3 g sat, 2 g mono); 18 mg cholesterol; 25 g carbohydrates; 4 g protein; 1 g fiber; 45 mg sodium; 259 mg potassium.
Nutrition Bonus: Calcium (12% daily value), Vitamin C (12% dv).
Carbohydrate Servings: 1 1/2
Exchanges: 11/2 fruit, 1 fat
Nutrition Note: Per serving with Splenda: 1 Carbohydrate Serving, 128 calories, 18 g carbohydrate.

Farmer's Cheese & Strawberries

INGREDIENTS
- 1 cup sliced fresh strawberries
- 1/4 cup farmer's cheese

PREPARATION
1. Top strawberries with cheese.

NUTRITION
Per serving: 153 calories; 5 g fat (3 g sat, 0 g mono); 20 mg cholesterol; 13 g carbohydrates; 11 g protein; 3 g fiber; 242 mg sodium; 254 mg potassium.
Nutrition Bonus: Vitamin C (160% daily value).
Carbohydrate Servings: 1
Exchanges: 1 fat

DAY 7
BREAKFAST

Crustless Crab Quiche
Strawberries (1 cup)
Whole-wheat toast (1 slice)

LUNCH

Curried Corn Bisque or Lebanese Potato Salad
Asian Slaw with Tofu & Shiitake Mushrooms
Skim milk (1 cup)
Apple (1 cup, quartered)

SNACK

Apricot-Almond Bars with Chocolate
Skim milk (1 cup)

DINNER

Tofu with Peanut-Ginger Sauce or Tandoori Chicken
Brown rice (1/2 cup, cooked)
Spinach Salad with Black Olive Vinaigrette
Raspberries (1/2 cup)

DAY 7 RECIPES

Crustless Crab Quiche

INGREDIENTS
- 2 teaspoons extra-virgin olive oil, divided
- 1 onion, chopped
- 1 red bell pepper, chopped

- 12 ounces mushrooms, wiped clean and sliced (about 4 1/2 cups)
- 2 large eggs
- 2 large egg whites
- 1 1/2 cups low-fat cottage cheese
- 1/2 cup low-fat plain yogurt
- 1/4 cup all-purpose flour
- 1/4 cup freshly grated Parmesan cheese
- 1/4 teaspoon cayenne pepper
- 1/4 teaspoon salt
- 1/4 teaspoon freshly ground pepper
- 8 ounces cooked lump crabmeat, (fresh or frozen and thawed), drained and picked over (about 1 cup)
- 1/2 cup grated sharp Cheddar cheese, (2 ounces)
- 1/4 cup chopped scallions

PREPARATION
1. Preheat oven to 350°F. Coat a 10-inch pie pan or ceramic quiche dish with cooking spray.
2. Heat 1 teaspoon oil in large nonstick skillet over medium-high heat. Add onion and bell pepper; cook, stirring, until softened, about 5 minutes; transfer to a large bowl. Add the remaining 1 teaspoon oil to the skillet and heat over high heat. Add mushrooms and cook, stirring, until they have softened and most of their liquid has evaporated, 5 to 7 minutes. Add to the bowl with the onion mixture.
3. Place eggs, egg whites, cottage cheese, yogurt, flour, Parmesan, cayenne, salt and pepper in a food processor or blender; blend until smooth. Add to the vegetable mixture, along with crab, Cheddar and scallions; mix with a rubber spatula. Pour into the prepared baking dish.
4. Bake the quiche until a knife inserted in the center comes out clean, 40 to 50 minutes. Let stand for 5 minutes before serving.

NUTRITION
Per serving: 225 calories; 10 g fat (4 g sat, 3 g mono); 122 mg cholesterol; 14 g carbohydrates; 27 gprotein; 2 g fiber; 661 mg sodium; 355 mg potassium.
Nutrition Bonus: Vitamin C (70% daily value), Calcium (25% dv), Vitamin A (20% dv).
Carbohydrate Servings: 1
Exchanges: 2 1/2 vegetable, 1 1/2 very lean meat, 1 high-fat meat

Curried Corn Bisque

INGREDIENTS
- 2 teaspoons canola oil
- 1 cup fresh or frozen chopped onions
- 1 tablespoon curry powder
- 1/2 teaspoon hot sauce, or to taste
- 1/4 teaspoon salt, or to taste
- 1/4 teaspoon freshly ground pepper
- 2 16-ounce packages frozen corn, or 3 10-ounce boxes
- 2 cups reduced-sodium chicken broth
- 2 cups water
- 1 cup "lite" coconut milk, (see Ingredient note)

PREPARATION
1. Heat oil in a large saucepan over medium-high heat. Add onions and cook, stirring occasionally, until soft, about 3 minutes. Add curry powder, hot sauce, salt and pepper and stir to coat the onions. Stir in corn, broth and water; increase the heat to high and bring the mixture to a boil. Remove from the heat and puree in a blender or food processor (in batches, if necessary) into a homogeneous mixture that still has some texture. Pour the soup into a clean pot, add coconut milk and heat through. Serve hot or cold. Make Curried Sweet Pea Bisque by substituting frozen peas for the corn.

TIPS & NOTES
- **Make Ahead Tip**: Cover and refrigerate for up to 2 days or freeze for up to 2 months.
- **Ingredient Note:** Look for reduced-fat coconut milk (labeled "lite") in the Asian section of your market.

NUTRITION

Per serving: 138 calories; 4 g fat (2 g sat, 1 g mono); 1 mg cholesterol; 24 g carbohydrates; 0 g added sugars; 5 g protein; 3 g fiber; 121 mg sodium; 291 mg potassium.
Nutrition Bonus: Fiber (13% daily value).

Carbohydrate Servings: 1 1/2
Exchanges: 1 1/2 starch, 1 fat

Lebanese Potato Salad

INGREDIENTS
- 2 pounds russet potatoes, (about 3 medium)
- 1/4 cup lemon juice
- 3 tablespoons extra-virgin olive oil
- 1/2 teaspoon salt
- Freshly ground pepper, to taste
- 4 scallions, thinly sliced
- 1/4 cup chopped fresh mint

PREPARATION
1. Place potatoes in a large saucepan or Dutch oven and cover with lightly salted water. Bring to a boil and cook until tender, 25 to 30 minutes. Drain and rinse with cold water. Transfer to a cutting board. Let cool for 20 minutes. Cut the cooled potatoes into 1/2-inch pieces.
2. Whisk lemon juice, oil, salt and pepper in a large bowl. Add the potatoes and toss to coat.
3. Just before serving, add scallions and mint to the salad and toss gently.

TIPS & NOTES
- **Make Ahead Tip**: Prepare through Step 2; cover and refrigerate for up to 2 days. Add additional lemon juice and/or salt to taste.

NUTRITION
Per serving: 143 calories; 5 g fat (1 g sat, 4 g mono); 0 mg cholesterol; 22 g carbohydrates; 0 g added sugars; 3 g protein; 2 g fiber; 153 mg sodium; 516 mg potassium.
Nutrition Bonus: Vitamin C (20% daily value), Potassium (15% dv).
Carbohydrate Servings: 1 1/2
Exchanges: 1 1/2 starch, 1 fat

Asian Slaw with Tofu & Shiitake Mushrooms

INGREDIENTS
- 1/4 cup reduced-sodium soy sauce
- 2 1/2 tablespoons lemon juice
- 1 teaspoon wasabi powder, (see Note)
- 1 clove garlic, minced
- 12 ounces firm silken tofu, drained and cut into 1/2-inch cubes
- 4 cups lightly packed shredded napa cabbage, (see Ingredient note)
- 2 cups lightly packed shredded bok choy, (see Ingredient note)
- 2 tablespoons canola oil and 2 teaspoons sesame oil
- 2 cups sliced shiitake mushroom caps

PREPARATION

1. Whisk soy sauce, lemon juice, wasabi powder and garlic in a medium bowl. Gently stir in tofu. Cover and marinate in the refrigerator for 15 minutes, stirring occasionally.
2. Place cabbage and bok choy in a large serving bowl.
3. Drain the tofu, reserving the marinade. Heat canola oil in a large skillet or wok over medium-high heat. Add mushrooms and sesame oil; cook, stirring often, for 2 minutes. Add the tofu; cook, stirring often, until the tofu is lightly browned, about 4 minutes.
4. Spoon the tofu mixture over cabbage. Add the reserved marinade to the pan and bring to a boil, stirring. Pour the hot marinade over the salad and toss gently to coat. Serve immediately.

TIPS & NOTES

- **Note:** Wasabi, a fiery condiment similar to horseradish, is made from the root of an Asian plant. It is available, as both a paste and a powder, in specialty stores and Asian markets.
- **Ingredient Notes:** Look for heads of napa that are tight, without any browned leaves.
- The best bok choy has large dark green leaves and small white stems. More leaf and less stem makes for a less bitter taste.

NUTRITION

Per serving: 178 calories; 12 g fat (1 g sat, 6 g mono); 0 mg cholesterol; 11 g carbohydrates; 0 g added sugars; 9 g protein; 2 g fiber; 598 mg sodium; 330 mg potassium.
Nutrition Bonus: Vitamin C (63% daily value), Selenium (27% dv).
Carbohydrate Servings: 1/2
Exchanges: 2 vegetable, 1 medium-fat meat, 2 fat (mono)

Apricot-Almond Bars with Chocolate

INGREDIENTS
- 1 cup dried apricots, divided
- 1/2 cup water
- 3/4 cup whole-wheat pastry flour
- 1/2 teaspoon baking powder
- 1/4 teaspoon baking soda
- 1/4 teaspoon salt
- 1 large egg
- 1 large egg white
- 1/4 cup canola oil

- 2 tablespoons honey
- 1 teaspoon vanilla extract
- 3/4 cup chopped bittersweet chocolate, (6 ounces) or semisweet chocolate chips, divided
- 1/4 cup sliced almonds

PREPARATION

1. Preheat oven to 350°F. Coat a 7-by-11-inch baking pan with cooking spray.
2. Combine 1/2 cup dried apricots and water in a small saucepan; bring to a simmer over medium heat. Cover and cook for 2 minutes. Remove from heat and set aside to cool. Coarsely chop the remaining 1/2 cup apricots.
3. Whisk flour, baking powder, baking soda and salt in a medium bowl.
4. Puree the cooked apricots and any remaining cooking liquid in a food processor. Add egg, egg white, oil, honey and vanilla; process until smooth. Add the flour mixture, 1/2 cup chocolate and the chopped apricots; pulse just until combined. Scrape the batter into the prepared pan, spreading evenly. Sprinkle with almonds.
5. Bake the bars until lightly browned and a toothpick inserted in the center comes out clean, 20 to 25 minutes. Let them cool in the pan on a wire rack.
6. Melt the remaining 1/4 cup chocolate in a double boiler over barely simmering water or in the microwave on Medium for 30 to 60 seconds. Spoon the chocolate into a sealable plastic bag, cut off the tip of one corner and drizzle the melted chocolate over the cooled bars. Let stand for about 10 minutes before cutting into bars.

TIPS & NOTES
- **Make Ahead Tip**: Store in an airtight container for up to 2 days or freeze for longer storage.

NUTRITION
Per serving: 75 calories; 5 g fat (1 g sat, 2 g mono); 9 mg cholesterol; 10 g carbohydrates; 1 g protein; 1 gfiber; 51 mg sodium; 6 mg potassium.
Carbohydrate Servings: 1/2
Exchanges: 1 other carbohydrate, 1/2 fat

Tofu with Peanut-Ginger Sauce

INGREDIENTS
SAUCE
- 5 tablespoons water
- 4 tablespoons smooth natural peanut butter

- 1 tablespoon rice vinegar, (see Ingredient note) or white vinegar
- 2 teaspoons reduced-sodium soy sauce
- 2 teaspoons honey
- 2 teaspoons minced ginger
- 2 cloves garlic, minced

TOFU & VEGETABLES
- 14 ounces extra-firm tofu, preferably water-packed
- 2 teaspoons extra-virgin olive oil
- 4 cups baby spinach, (6 ounces)
- 1 1/2 cups sliced mushrooms, (4 ounces)
- 4 scallions, sliced (1 cup)

PREPARATION
1. To prepare sauce: Whisk water, peanut butter, rice vinegar (or white vinegar), soy sauce, honey, ginger and garlic in a small bowl.
2. To prepare tofu: Drain and rinse tofu; pat dry. Slice the block crosswise into eight 1/2-inch-thick slabs. Coarsely crumble each slice into smaller, uneven pieces.
3. Heat oil in a large nonstick skillet over high heat. Add tofu and cook in a single layer, without stirring, until the pieces begin to turn golden brown on the bottom, about 5 minutes. Then gently stir and continue cooking, stirring occasionally, until all sides are golden brown, 5 to 7 minutes more.
4. Add spinach, mushrooms, scallions and the peanut sauce and cook, stirring, until the vegetables are just cooked, 1 to 2 minutes more.

TIPS & NOTES
- **Ingredient Note:** Rice vinegar (or rice-wine vinegar) is mild, slightly sweet vinegar made from fermented rice. Find it in the Asian section of supermarkets and specialty stores.

NUTRITION

Per serving: 221 calories; 14 g fat (2 g sat, 3 g mono); 0 mg cholesterol; 15 g carbohydrates; 3 g added sugars; 12 g protein; 4 g fiber; 231 mg sodium; 262 mg potassium.
Nutrition Bonus: Calcium (16% daily value), Iron (16% dv).
Carbohydrate Servings: 1
Exchanges: 2 vegetable, 2 medium-fat meat

Tandoori Chicken

INGREDIENTS
- 1 cup nonfat plain yogurt
- 1 small onion, minced
- 2 cloves garlic, minced
- 1 1/2 tablespoons lemon juice
- 1 teaspoon chopped fresh cilantro
- 1/2 teaspoon paprika
- 1/2 teaspoon ground cumin
- 1/2 teaspoon ground turmeric
- 1/2 teaspoon ground ginger
- 1/2 teaspoon salt, or to taste
- 1/4 teaspoon freshly ground pepper
- 1/4 teaspoon ground cinnamon
- Pinch of ground cloves
- 4 bone-in chicken thighs, (about 1 1/2 pounds), skinned and trimmed of fat

PREPARATION
1. Stir together yogurt, onion and garlic in a shallow glass dish. Add lemon juice, cilantro, paprika, cumin, turmeric, ginger, salt, pepper, cinnamon and cloves. Add chicken and coat well. Cover and marinate in the refrigerator for at least 2 hours or overnight.
2. Preheat oven to 500°F. Coat a wire rack with cooking spray and set it over a foil-covered baking sheet. Place the chicken on the prepared rack.
3. Bake the chicken until browned and no trace of pink remains in the center, 25 to 30 minutes. Serve hot.

TIPS & NOTES
- **Make Ahead Tip**: Marinate the chicken (Step 1) overnight.

NUTRITION
Per serving: 227 calories; 10 g fat (3 g sat, 4 g mono); 87 mg cholesterol; 8 g carbohydrates; 0 g added sugars; 27 g protein; 1 g fiber; 398 mg sodium; 224 mg potassium.
Nutrition Bonus: Selenium (24% daily value), Zinc (18% dv).

Carbohydrate Servings: 1/2
Exchanges: 1/2 other carbohydrate, 4 lean meat

Spinach Salad with Black Olive Vinaigrette

INGREDIENTS
- 3 tablespoons extra-virgin olive oil
- 1 1/2 tablespoons red-wine vinegar, or lemon juice
- 6 pitted Kalamata olives, finely chopped
- 1/4 teaspoon salt
- Freshly ground pepper, to taste
- 6 cups torn spinach leaves
- 1/2 cucumber, seeded and sliced
- 1/2 red onion, thinly sliced

PREPARATION
1. Whisk oil, vinegar (or lemon juice) and olives in a salad bowl. Season with salt and pepper. Add spinach, cucumbers and onions; toss well. Serve immediately.

NUTRITION
Per serving: 128 calories; 12 g fat (2 g sat, 9 g mono); 0 mg cholesterol; 3 g carbohydrates; 2 g protein; 1 gfiber; 271 mg sodium; 284 mg potassium.
Nutrition Bonus: Vitamin A (80% daily value), Folate (22% dv), Vitamin C (20% dv).
Exchanges: 1 vegetable, 2 fat

DAY 8
BREAKFAST

Overnight Oatmeal or Spiced Creamy Wheat with Cashews
Apricot (1 cup, halves)
Skim milk (1 cup)

LUNCH

Chicken, Escarole & Rice Soup
Strawberry, Melon & Avocado Salad
Whole-wheat toast (1 slice)

SNACK

Skim Milk
Banana (1 cup)

DINNER

Southwestern Steak & Peppers
Oven "Fries" or Roasted Corn with Basil-Shallot Vinaigrette
Steamed broccoli (1 cup)
Mocha-Almond Biscotti

DAY 8 RECIPES

Overnight Oatmeal

INGREDIENTS
- 8 cups water
- 2 cups steel-cut oats, (see Ingredient note)
- 1/3 cup dried cranberries
- 1/3 cup dried apricots, chopped
- 1/4 teaspoon salt, or to taste

PREPARATION
1. Combine water, oats, dried cranberries, dried apricots and salt in a 5- or 6-quart slow cooker. Turn heat to low. Put the lid on and cook until the oats are tender and the porridge is creamy, 7 to 8 hours. Stovetop Variation Halve the above recipe to accommodate the size of most double boilers: Combine 4 cups water, 1 cup steel-cut oats, 3 tablespoons dried cranberries, 3 tablespoons dried apricots and 1/8 teaspoon salt in the top of a double boiler. Cover and cook over boiling water for about 1 1/2 hours, checking the water level in the bottom of the double boiler from time to time.

TIPS & NOTES
- **Ingredient Note:** Steel-cut oats, sometimes labeled "Irish oatmeal," look like small pebbles. They are toasted oat groats for which the oat kernel that has been removed from the husk that have been cut in 2 or 3 pieces. Do not substitute regular rolled oats, which have a shorter cooking time, in the slow-cooker oatmeal recipe.
- For easy cleanup, try a slow-cooker liner. These heat-resistant, disposable liners fit neatly inside the insert and help prevent food from sticking to the bottom and sides of your slow cooker.

NUTRITION

Per serving: 193 calories; 3 g fat (0 g sat, 1 g mono); 0 mg cholesterol; 34 g carbohydrates; 0 g added sugars; 6 g protein; 9 g fiber; 77 mg sodium; 195 mg potassium.
Nutrition Bonus: Fiber (36% daily value).
Carbohydrate Servings: 2
Exchanges: 2 starch, 1/2 fruit

Spiced Creamy Wheat with Cashews

INGREDIENTS
- 2 tablespoons canola oil
- 1 teaspoon black or yellow mustard seeds
- 1/4 cup cashews, chopped (1 1/4 ounces)
- 1/4 cup dried yellow split peas, (chana dal)
- 1 small onion, finely chopped (1/2 cup)
- 1 tablespoon finely chopped fresh ginger
- 3 cups water
- 2 medium red potatoes, peeled and cut into 1/4-inch dice
- 1 cup frozen green peas
- 2-3 fresh Thai, serrano or cayenne chiles, seeded and finely chopped
- 1 teaspoon salt
- 1/2 teaspoon ground turmeric
- 1 cup wheat cereal, (farina), such as Cream of Wheat (not instant)
- 1 medium tomato, chopped (3/4 cup)
- 2 tablespoons chopped fresh cilantro

PREPARATION
1. Heat oil and mustard seeds in a medium saucepan over medium-high heat. Once seeds begin to pop, cover the pan and wait until the popping stops. Add cashews and yellow split peas; stir-fry until golden brown, about 30 seconds. Add onion and ginger; stir-fry until the onion is golden brown, 2 to 3 minutes.
2. Stir in water, potatoes, peas, chiles, salt and turmeric; bring to a boil. Reduce heat to medium-low, cover and simmer until the potatoes are tender, 5 to 6 minutes. Stir in wheat cereal; simmer, covered, until all the water is absorbed, 3 to 4 minutes. Stir in tomato and cilantro. Cover and simmer until the tomato is warm, 1 to 2 minutes. Serve.

NUTRITION
Per serving: 199 calories; 6 g fat (1 g sat, 3 g mono); 0 mg cholesterol; 28 g carbohydrates; 0 g added sugars; 6 g protein; 5 g fiber; 322 mg sodium; 313 mg potassium.
Nutrition Bonus: Iron (40% daily value), Vitamin C (20% dv).
Carbohydrate Servings: 2
Exchanges: 2 starch, 1 fat

Chicken, Escarole & Rice Soup

INGREDIENTS
- 1 tablespoon extra-virgin olive oil
- 1 large onion, chopped

- 2 cloves garlic, minced
- 1 head escarole, trimmed and thinly sliced
- 3 14-ounce cans reduced-sodium chicken broth
- 1 14-ounce can diced tomatoes
- 1/2 cup long-grain white rice
- 1 pound boneless, skinless chicken breasts, trimmed and cut into 1/2-inch pieces
- Freshly ground pepper, to taste
- 6 tablespoons freshly grated Romano or Parmesan cheese

PREPARATION
1. Heat oil in a large pot over medium-high heat. Add onion and garlic; cook, stirring frequently, until they soften and begin to brown, 5 to 7 minutes. Add escarole and cook, stirring occasionally, until wilted, 2 to 3 minutes. Add broth, tomatoes and rice; bring to a boil. Reduce heat to low, cover and simmer until the rice is almost tender, 12 to 15 minutes.
2. Add chicken and simmer until it is no longer pink in the center and the rice is tender, about 5 minutes. Season with pepper. Serve hot, sprinkled with Romano (or Parmesan).

TIPS & NOTES
- **Make Ahead Tip**: Cover and refrigerate for up to 2 days or freeze for up to 2 months.

NUTRITION

Per serving: 157 calories; 4 g fat (1 g sat, 2 g mono); 30 mg cholesterol; 15 g carbohydrates; 16 g protein; 2 g fiber; 166 mg sodium; 337 mg potassium.
Nutrition Bonus: Folate (21% daily value), Vitamin A (20% dv).
Carbohydrate Servings: 1
Exchanges: 1 starch, 1 1/2 lean meat

Strawberry, Melon & Avocado Salad

INGREDIENTS
- 1/4 cup honey
- 2 tablespoons sherry vinegar, or red-wine vinegar
- 2 tablespoons finely chopped fresh mint
- 1/4 teaspoon freshly ground pepper
- Pinch of salt
- 4 cups baby spinach
- 1 small avocado, (4-5 ounces), peeled, pitted and cut into 16 slices

- 16 thin slices cantaloupe, (about 1/2 small cantaloupe), rind removed
- 2 teaspoons sesame seeds, toasted (see Tip)

PREPARATION
1. Whisk honey, vinegar, mint, pepper and salt in a small bowl.
2. Divide spinach among 4 salad plates. Arrange alternating slices of avocado and cantaloupe in a fan on top of the spinach. Top each salad with strawberries, drizzle with dressing and sprinkle with sesame seeds.

TIPS & NOTES
- **Make Ahead Tip**: The dressing will keep, covered, in the refrigerator for up to 1 day.
- **Tip:** To toast sesame seeds, heat a small dry skillet over low heat. Add sesame seeds and stir constantly until golden and fragrant, about 2 minutes. Transfer to a small bowl and let cool.

NUTRITION
Per serving: 202 calories; 8 g fat (1 g sat, 1 g mono); 0 mg cholesterol; 24 g carbohydrates; 3 g protein; 7 gfiber; 90 mg sodium; 503 mg potassium.
Nutrition Bonus: Vitamin C (100% daily value), Vitamin A (60% dv), Folate (18% dv).
Carbohydrate Servings: 2
Exchanges: 1 vegetable, 2 fruit, 1 1/2 fat (mono)

Southwestern Steak & Peppers

INGREDIENTS
- 1/2 teaspoon ground cumin
- 1/2 teaspoon ground coriander
- 1/2 teaspoon chili powder
- 1/4 teaspoon salt, or to taste
- 3/4 teaspoon coarsely ground pepper, plus more to taste
- 1 pound boneless top sirloin steak, trimmed of fat
- 3 cloves garlic, peeled, 1 halved and 2 minced
- 3 teaspoons canola oil, or extra-virgin olive oil, divided
- 2 red bell peppers, thinly sliced
- 1 medium white onion, halved lengthwise and thinly sliced
- 1 teaspoon brown sugar
- 1/2 cup brewed coffee, or prepared instant coffee
- 1/4 cup balsamic vinegar
- 4 cups watercress sprigs

PREPARATION
1. Mix cumin, coriander, chili powder, salt and 3/4 teaspoon pepper in a small bowl. Rub steak with the cut garlic. Rub the spice mix all over the steak.
2. Heat 2 teaspoons oil in a large heavy skillet, preferably cast iron, over medium-high heat. Add the steak and cook to desired doneness, 4 to 6 minutes per side for medium-rare. Transfer to a cutting board and let rest.
3. Add remaining 1 teaspoon oil to the skillet. Add bell peppers and onion; cook, stirring often, until softened, about 4 minutes. Add minced garlic and brown sugar; cook, stirring often, for 1 minute. Add coffee, vinegar and any accumulated meat juices; cook for 3 minutes to intensify flavor. Season with pepper.
4. To serve, mound 1 cup watercress on each plate. Top with the sauteed peppers and onion. Slice the steak thinly across the grain and arrange on the vegetables. Pour the sauce from the pan over the steak. Serve immediately.

NUTRITION
Per serving: 226 calories; 12 g fat (3 g sat, 5 g mono); 60 mg cholesterol; 12 g carbohydrates; 1 g added sugars; 26 g protein; 3 g fiber; 216 mg sodium; 606 mg potassium.
Nutrition Bonus: Vitamin C (210% daily value), Vitamin A (60% dv), Iron (25% dv).
Carbohydrate Servings: 1
Exchanges: 2 vegetable, 3 lean meat

Oven "Fries"

INGREDIENTS
- 2 large Yukon Gold potatoes, cut into wedges
- 4 teaspoons extra-virgin olive oil
- 1/2 teaspoon salt
- 1/2 teaspoon dried thyme, (optional)

PREPARATION
1. Preheat oven to 450°F.
2. Toss potato wedges with oil, salt and thyme (if using). Spread the wedges out on a rimmed baking sheet.
3. Bake until browned and tender, turning once, about 20 minutes total.

NUTRITION
Per serving: 102 calories; 5 g fat (1 g sat, 4 g mono); 0 mg cholesterol; 13 g carbohydrates; 0 g added sugars; 2 g protein; 1 g fiber; 291 mg sodium; 405 mg potassium.
Carbohydrate Servings: 1
Exchanges: 1 starch, 1 fat

Roasted Corn with Basil-Shallot Vinaigrette

INGREDIENTS
- 3 cups fresh corn kernels
- 2 tablespoons extra-virgin olive oil

- 1/4 cup chopped fresh basil
- 1 tablespoon minced shallot
- 1 tablespoon red-wine vinegar
- 1/4 teaspoon salt
- Freshly ground pepper, to taste

PREPARATION
1. Preheat oven to 450°F. Toss corn and oil to coat and spread out on a large baking sheet. Bake, stirring once, until some kernels begin to brown, about 20 minutes. Combine basil, shallot, vinegar, salt and pepper in a medium bowl. Add the corn; toss to coat. Serve warm or cold.

TIPS & NOTES
- **Make Ahead Tip**: Cover and refrigerate for up to 1 day.

NUTRITION
Per serving: 165 calories; 8 g fat (1 g sat, 6 g mono); 0 mg cholesterol; 23 g carbohydrates; 0 g added sugars; 4 g protein; 3 g fiber; 163 mg sodium; 332 mg potassium.
Nutrition Bonus: Vitamin C (15% daily value).
Carbohydrate Servings: 1 1/2
Exchanges: 1 1/2 starch, 1 1/2 fat

Mocha-Almond Biscotti

INGREDIENTS
- 1/2 cup whole unblanched almonds
- 2 cups all-purpose flour
- 1 cup sugar
- 1 teaspoon baking powder
- 1/2 teaspoon baking soda
- 1/4 teaspoon salt
- 2 large eggs
- 2 large egg whites
- 1 teaspoon vanilla extract
- 1 tablespoon unsweetened cocoa powder
- 2 teaspoons instant coffee powder

- 4 teaspoons water
- 1 ounce unsweetened chocolate, melted
- 1/2 teaspoon almond extract

PREPARATION

1. Preheat oven to 325°F. Lightly oil a baking sheet or coat it with nonstick cooking spray.
2. Spread almonds on a second baking sheet and bake for 12 to 14 minutes, or until lightly toasted.
3. Stir together flour, sugar, baking powder, baking soda and salt in a large bowl. Whisk together eggs, egg whites and vanilla in a small bowl and add to the dry ingredients; mix just until smooth.
4. Combine cocoa, instant coffee and water in a small bowl. Divide the dough in half. Add the cocoa mixture and melted chocolate to one half. Mix just until incorporated. Stir almond extract and the almonds into the other half.
5. Place half of the almond dough on a well-floured work surface. Pat into a 4-by-8-inch rectangle. Top with half of the chocolate dough. Roll up into a cylinder, then roll the cylinder back and forth to form a 14-by-1 1/2 inch log. Repeat with the remaining doughs. Place the logs on a prepared baking sheet. Bake until firm to the touch, 20 to 25 minutes. Transfer the logs to a rack to cool. Reduce the oven temperature to 300°F.
6. Cut the logs diagonally into 1/2-inch-thick slices. Stand the slices upright on the baking sheet and bake for 40 minutes. Let cool before storing.

NUTRITION
Per biscotti: 50 calories; 1 g fat (0 g sat, 1 g mono); 9 mg cholesterol; 8 g carbohydrates; 1 g protein; 0 gfiber; 42 mg sodium; 18 mg potassium.
Carbohydrate Servings: 1/2
Exchanges: 1/2 carbohydrate

DAY 9
BREAKFAST

Nonfat plain yogurt (8 oz.)
Whole-wheat toast (1 slice)
Pear Butter
LUNCH

Creamy Tomato Bisque with Mozzarella Crostini
Tuna & White Bean Salad
Skim milk (1 cup)
Whole-wheat pita bread (1 medium pita)

SNACK

Chewy Chocolate Brownies or Outrageous Macaroons
Blueberries (1 cup)

DINNER

Korean-Style Steak & Lettuce Wraps or Wok-Seared Chicken Tenders with Asparagus & Pistachios
Shredded carrots (1 cup)
Cucumber Salad
Strawberry-Rhubarb Tart

DAY 9 RECIPES

Pear Butter

INGREDIENTS

- 4 ripe but firm Bartlett pears, (1-1 1/4 pounds), peeled, cored and cut into 1-inch chunks
- 3/4 cup pear nectar

PREPARATION

1. Place pears and pear nectar in a heavy medium saucepan; bring to a simmer. Cover and simmer over medium-low heat, stirring occasionally, until the pears are very tender, 30 to 35 minutes. Cooking time will vary depending on the ripeness of the pears.
2. Mash the pears with a potato masher. Cook, uncovered, over medium-low heat, stirring often, until the puree has cooked down to a thick mass (somewhat thicker than applesauce), 20 to 30 minutes. Stir almost constantly toward the end of cooking. Scrape the pear butter into a bowl or storage container and let cool.

TIPS & NOTES

- **Make Ahead Tip**: Store in an airtight container in the refrigerator for up to 2 weeks or freeze for up to 6 months.

NUTRITION
Per tablespoon: 22 calories; 0 g fat (0 g sat, 0 g mono); 0 mg cholesterol; 6 g carbohydrates; 0 g protein; 1 g fiber; 1 mg sodium; 33 mg potassium.
Carbohydrate Servings: 1/2
Exchanges: 1/2 fruit

Creamy Tomato Bisque with Mozzarella Crostini

INGREDIENTS
- 2 tablespoons extra-virgin olive oil
- 1 large onion, chopped
- 4 cloves garlic, crushed and peeled
- 1 14-ounce can reduced-sodium chicken broth
- 2 cups water
- 1/4 cup white rice
- 1 28-ounce can crushed tomatoes
- 1/2 cup silken tofu
- 1 tablespoon rice vinegar
- 6 3/4-inch-thick slices baguette, preferably whole-grain
- 3 tablespoons shredded part-skim mozzarella cheese

PREPARATION
1. Heat oil in a Dutch oven over medium heat. Add onion and garlic and cook, stirring occasionally, until beginning to soften, about 3 minutes. Stir in broth, water and rice; bring to a boil. Reduce heat to a simmer and cook, stirring occasionally, until the rice is very tender, about 15 minutes.
2. Preheat oven to 450°F.
3. Stir tomatoes, tofu and vinegar into the soup. Remove from the heat and puree, in batches, in a blender. (Use caution when pureeing hot liquids.) Return the soup to the pot and reheat over medium-high heat, stirring often.
4. Meanwhile, top slices of baguette with mozzarella and place on a baking sheet. Bake until the cheese is melted and bubbly, about 5 minutes. Ladle soup into bowls and top each serving with a cheesy crostini.

TIPS & NOTES
- **Make Ahead Tip**: Prepare the soup (Steps 1 & 3), cover and refrigerate for up to 2 days. When ready to serve, make crostini and reheat the soup (Steps 2 & 4).

NUTRITION
Per serving: 218 calories; 8 g fat (1 g sat, 4 g mono); 3 mg cholesterol; 31 g carbohydrates; 8 g protein; 4 gfiber; 355 mg sodium; 478 mg potassium.
Nutrition Bonus: Vitamin C (25% daily value), Vitamin ∧ (20% dv), Iron (15% dv).
Carbohydrate Servings: 2
Exchanges: 1 starch, 1 vegetable, 1 medium-fat meat

Tuna & White Bean Salad

INGREDIENTS
- 3 tablespoons lemon juice
- 2 tablespoons extra-virgin olive oil

- 1 clove garlic, minced
- 1/8 teaspoon salt
- Freshly ground pepper, to taste
- 1 19-ounce can cannellini (white kidney) beans, rinsed
- 1 6-ounce can chunk light tuna in water, drained and flaked (see Note)
- 1/4 cup chopped red onion
- 3 tablespoons chopped fresh parsley
- 3 tablespoons chopped fresh basil

PREPARATION
1. Whisk lemon juice, oil, garlic, salt and pepper in a medium bowl. Add beans, tuna, onion, parsley and basil; toss to coat well.

TIPS & NOTES
- **Make Ahead Tip**: Cover and refrigerate for up to 2 days.
- **Note:** Chunk light tuna, which comes from the smaller skipjack or yellowfin, has less mercury than canned white albacore tuna. The FDA/EPA advises that women who are or might become pregnant, nursing mothers and young children consume no more than 6 ounces of albacore a week; up to 12 ounces of canned light tuna is considered safe.

NUTRITION
Per serving: 226 calories; 8 g fat (1 g sat, 5 g mono); 13 mg cholesterol; 21 g carbohydrates; 0 g added sugars; 16 g protein; 6 g fiber; 498 mg sodium; 157 mg potassium.
Nutrition Bonus: Fiber (24% daily value), Iron (16% dv), Vitamin C (15% dv).
Carbohydrate Servings: 1
Exchanges: 1 starch, 2 very lean meat, 1 fat (mono)

Chewy Chocolate Brownies

INGREDIENTS
- 16 whole chocolate graham crackers, (8 ounces) (see Ingredient notes)
- 2 tablespoons unsweetened cocoa powder
- 1/4 teaspoon salt
- 2 large eggs and 1 large egg white
- 1/3 cup packed light brown sugar, or 3 tablespoons
- 1/3 cup granulated sugar, or 3 tablespoons
- 2 teaspoons instant coffee granules
- 2 teaspoons vanilla extract
- 2/3 cup chopped pitted dates
- 1/4 cup semisweet chocolate chips

PREPARATION
1. Preheat oven to 300°F. Coat an 8-by-11 1/2-inch baking dish with cooking spray.
2. Pulse graham crackers into crumbs in a food processor or place in a large plastic bag and crush with a rolling pin. You should have about 2 cups crumbs. Transfer to a small bowl; add cocoa and salt and mix well.
3. Combine eggs, egg white, brown sugar (or Splenda) and granulated sugar (or Splenda) in a large bowl. Beat with an electric mixer at high speed until thickened, about 2 minutes. Blend in coffee granules and vanilla. Gently fold in dates, chocolate chips and the reserved crumb mixture. Scrape the batter into the prepared baking dish, spreading evenly.
4. Bake the brownies until the top springs back when lightly touched, 25 to 30 minutes. Let cool completely in the pan on a wire rack before cutting.

TIPS & NOTES
- **Make Ahead Tip**: Store in an airtight container for up to 3 days or freeze for longer storage.
- **Ingredient Notes:** To avoid trans-fatty acids, look for brands of graham crackers that do not contain partially hydrogenated canola oil, such as Mi-Del chocolate snaps or Barbara's Chocolate Go-Go Grahams.
- **Substituting with Splenda:** In the test Kitchen, sucralose is the only alternative sweetener we test with when we feel the option is appropriate. For nonbaking recipes, we use Splenda Granular (boxed, not in a packet). For baking, we use Splenda Sugar Blend for Baking, a mix of sugar and sucralose. It can be substituted in recipes (1/2 cup of the blend for each 1 cup of sugar) to reduce sugar calories by half while maintaining some of the baking properties of sugar. If you make a similar blend with half sugar and half Splenda Granular, substitute this homemade mixture cup for cup.
- When choosing any low- or no-calorie sweetener, be sure to check the label to make sure it is suitable for your intended use.
- Easy cleanup: Dessert pans can be a headache to clean. Skip the soaking and scrubbing by lining your pan with parchment paper before you bake.

NUTRITION
Per brownie: 93 calories; 2 g fat (0 g sat, 0 g mono); 18 mg cholesterol; 15 g carbohydrates; 2 g protein; 1 gfiber; 72 mg sodium; 60 mg potassium.
Carbohydrate Servings: 1
Exchanges: 1 other carbohydrate

Outrageous Macaroons

INGREDIENTS
OUTRAGEOUS MACAROONS
- 1 14-ounce can nonfat sweetened condensed milk
- 1 teaspoon almond extract
- 2 cups sliced almonds
- 2 cups coconut flakes, preferably unsweetened
- 1/2 cup dried cranberries
- 1/2 cup chopped shelled pistachios
- 2 large egg whites
- 1/4 teaspoon salt

GARNISH (OPTIONAL)
- 3/4 cup bittersweet or semisweet chocolate chips
- 1/4 cup dried cranberries
- 1/4 cup chopped shelled pistachios

PREPARATION
1. Position racks in upper and lower thirds of oven; preheat to 325°F. Line 2 large baking sheets with parchment paper or silicone baking mats.
2. Whisk condensed milk and almond extract in a large bowl until combined. Pulse almonds in a food processor (about 10 quick pulses) until broken into small pieces. Stir the almonds, coconut, 1/2 cup cranberries and 1/2 cup pistachios into the condensed milk mixture.
3. Beat egg whites and salt in a medium bowl with an electric mixer on medium-high speed until soft peaks form, about 1 minute. Fold 1/2 cup of the egg whites into the coconut mixture. Add the remaining egg whites, gently folding into the mixture until just combined. Drop 1 teaspoon of dough onto a prepared baking sheet and top with another teaspoon of dough, making a double-tall macaroon. Repeat with the remaining batter, spacing the macaroons 1 inch apart.
4. Bake the macaroons, switching the pans back to front and top to bottom halfway through, until the coconut is lightly golden, 18 to 22 minutes (sweetened coconut will brown faster than unsweetened). Let cool on the pans on a wire rack until cool to the touch, 30 minutes.
5. Optional garnish: Place 1/2 cup chocolate chips in a microwave-safe bowl and melt in the microwave on Medium in 30-second bursts, stirring after each burst to ensure even melting, until completely melted. (Alternatively, melt the chocolate in a double boiler over hot water, stirring constantly.) Stir the remaining 1/4 cup chips into the melted chocolate until smooth. Drizzle or spoon the melted chocolate over the top of each cooled macaroon; sprinkle with

cranberries and pistachios. Let the chocolate dry completely before storing or packing.

TIPS & NOTES
- **Make Ahead Tip**: These macaroons are best eaten fresh, but will keep for up to 5 days at room temperature.
- **Storage smarts**: To extend the life of your baked goods, store them in an airtight container in a single layer or between layers of parchment paper to prevent sticking.

NUTRITION
Per cookie (with garnish): 85 calories; 4 g fat (2 g sat, 1 g mono); 0 mg cholesterol; 7 g carbohydrates; 2 gprotein; 1 g fiber; 21 mg sodium; 81 mg potassium.
Carbohydrate Servings: 1/2
Exchanges: 1/2 other carbohydrate, 1 fat
Nutrition Note: Per cookie (without garnish): 69 calories; 4 g fat (2 g sat, 1 g mono); 0 mg cholesterol; 7 g carbohydrate; 2 g protein; 1 g fiber; 21 mg sodium.

Korean-Style Steak & Lettuce Wraps

INGREDIENTS
- 1 pound flank steak
- 1/4 teaspoon salt
- 1/4 teaspoon freshly ground pepper
- 1 cup diced peeled cucumber
- 6 cherry tomatoes, halved
- 1/4 cup thinly sliced shallot
- 1 tablespoon finely chopped fresh mint
- 1 tablespoon finely chopped fresh basil
- 1 tablespoon finely chopped fresh cilantro
- 1 tablespoon brown sugar
- 2 tablespoons reduced-sodium soy sauce
- 2 tablespoons lime juice
- 1/2 teaspoon crushed red pepper
- 1 head Bibb lettuce, leaves separated

PREPARATION
1. Preheat grill to medium-high.
2. Sprinkle steak with salt and pepper. Oil the grill rack (see Tip). Grill the steak for 6 to 8 minutes per side for medium. Transfer to a cutting board and let rest for 5 minutes. Cut across the grain into thin slices.
3. Combine the sliced steak, cucumber, tomatoes, shallot, mint, basil and cilantro in a large bowl. Mix sugar, soy sauce, lime juice and crushed red pepper in a

small bowl. Drizzle over the steak mixture; toss well to coat. To serve, spoon a portion of the steak mixture into a lettuce leaf and roll into a "wrap."

TIPS & NOTES
- **Make Ahead Tip**: The steak mixture will keep, covered, in the refrigerator for up to 1 day.
- **To oil a grill rack**: Oil a folded paper towel, hold it with tongs and rub it over the rack. Do not use cooking spray on a hot grill.

NUTRITION

Per serving: 199 calories; 7 g fat (3 g sat, 3 g mono); 45 mg cholesterol; 9 g carbohydrates; 3 g added sugars; 24 g protein; 1 g fiber; 465 mg sodium; 542 mg potassium.
Nutrition Bonus: Vitamin A (35% daily value), Vitamin C (20% dv), Iron (15% dv).
Carbohydrate Servings: 1/2
Exchanges: 1 1/2 vegetable, 3 lean meat

Wok-Seared Chicken Tenders with Asparagus & Pistachios

INGREDIENTS
- 1 tablespoon toasted sesame oil
- 1 1/2 pounds fresh asparagus, tough ends trimmed, cut into 1-inch pieces
- 1 pound chicken tenders, (see Ingredient Note), cut into bite-size pieces
- 4 scallions, trimmed and cut into 1-inch pieces
- 2 tablespoons minced fresh ginger
- 1 tablespoon oyster-flavored sauce
- 1 teaspoon chile-garlic sauce, (see Ingredient Note)
- 1/4 cup shelled salted pistachios, coarsely chopped

PREPARATION

1. Heat oil in a wok or large skillet over high heat. Add asparagus; cook, stirring, for 2 minutes. Add chicken; cook, stirring, for 4 minutes. Stir in scallions, ginger, oyster sauce and chile-garlic sauce; cook, stirring, until the chicken is juicy and just cooked through, 1 to 2 minutes more. Stir in pistachios and serve immediately.

TIPS & NOTES
- **Ingredient Notes:** Chicken tenders, virtually fat-free, are a strip of rib meat typically found attached to the underside of the chicken breast, but they can

also be purchased separately. Four 1-ounce tenders will yield a 3-ounce cooked portion. Tenders are perfect for quick stir-fries, chicken satay or kid-friendly breaded "chicken fingers."
- Chile-garlic sauce is a blend of ground red chiles, garlic and vinegar and is commonly used to add heat and flavor to Asian soups, sauces and stir-fries. It can be found in the Asian-food section of large supermarkets. It will keep in the refrigerator for up to 1 year.

NUTRITION

Per serving: 208 calories; 8 g fat (1 g sat, 3 g mono); 67 mg cholesterol; 7 g carbohydrates; 0 g added sugars; 30 g protein; 3 g fiber; 175 mg sodium; 326 mg potassium.
Nutrition Bonus: Folate (35% daily value), Vitamin A (20% dv), Vitamin C (15% dv).
Carbohydrate Servings: 1/2
Exchanges: 1 vegetable , 4 very lean meat, 1 fat

Cucumber Salad

INGREDIENTS
- 2 cucumbers, peeled, seeded and cut crosswise into 1/4-inch slices
- 1 tablespoon rice-wine vinegar, or distilled white vinegar
- 1/4 teaspoon sugar
- Cayenne pepper, to taste
- Salt & freshly ground pepper, to taste

PREPARATION

1. Whisk together vinegar, sugar and a pinch of cayenne pepper. Season with salt and pepper. Add cucumbers and toss to coat. Chill until ready to serve.

NUTRITION
Per serving: 24 calories; 0 g fat (0 g sat, 0 g mono); 0 mg cholesterol; 6 g carbohydrates; 0 g added sugars;1 g protein; 1 g fiber; 145 mg sodium; 222 mg potassium.
Carbohydrate Servings: 1/2
Exchanges: 1 vegetable

Strawberry-Rhubarb Tart

INGREDIENTS
FILLING
- 2 cups diced fresh or frozen rhubarb
- 3 cups fresh strawberries, sliced, divided
- 1/4 cup sugar, or Splenda Granular (see Ingredient note)

- 1/2 teaspoon freshly grated lemon zest
- 1 1/2 tablespoons cornstarch
- 1 tablespoon cold water
- 3 tablespoons red currant jelly

CRUST
- 1/2 cup old-fashioned rolled oats
- 3 tablespoons 1% milk
- 1/2 teaspoon vanilla extract
- 2/3 cup all-purpose flour
- 1/4 cup sugar
- 1 teaspoon freshly grated lemon zest
- 3/4 teaspoon baking powder
- 1/4 teaspoon salt
- 2 tablespoons canola oil

PREPARATION
1. To prepare filling: Combine rhubarb, 1 cup strawberries, sugar (or Splenda) and lemon zest in a large nonreactive saucepan. Let stand for 20 minutes (35 minutes if rhubarb is frozen). Bring to a simmer over medium-low heat. Cook, stirring often, until the rhubarb is tender but still holds its shape, 5 to 8 minutes.
2. Meanwhile, stir cornstarch and water in a small bowl until smooth. Stir into the simmering fruit. Cook, stirring constantly, until the mixture is clear and very thick, about 1 minute. Transfer to a bowl.
Place a piece of plastic wrap directly on the surface and refrigerate until chilled.
3. To prepare crust & assemble tart: Preheat oven to 350°F. Coat a 9-inch tart pan with a removable bottom with cooking spray.
4. Spread oats in a small baking dish and bake, stirring occasionally, until toasted, 10 to 15 minutes. Let cool. Place the oats in a food processor and process until finely ground.
5. Combine milk and vanilla in a small bowl. Whisk the ground oats, flour, sugar, lemon zest, baking powder and salt in a large bowl. Drizzle oil onto the dry ingredients and stir with a fork or your fingers until crumbly. Use a fork to stir in the milk mixture, 1 tablespoon at a time, until the dough just comes together.
6. Turn the dough out onto a floured work surface and knead 7 to 8 times. Roll the dough out to an 11-inch circle, dusting with flour if necessary. Transfer to the prepared pan, pressing to fit. Trim the edges.
7. Line the tart shell with a piece of foil or parchment paper and fill with pie weights or dried beans. Bake the tart shell until set, 10 to 12 minutes. Remove weights and foil or paper and bake until lightly browned, 8 to 12 minutes more. Cool in the pan on a wire rack.
8. Shortly before serving, spread the strawberry-rhubarb filling evenly into the tart shell. Arrange the remaining 2 cups strawberries decoratively over the filling.

9. Heat jelly in a small saucepan over low heat, stirring constantly. With a pastry brush, glaze the strawberries with the jelly.

TIPS & NOTES
- **Make Ahead Tip**: Cover and refrigerate the filling (Steps 1-2) for up to 2 days. Loosely cover the crust (Steps 3-7) with foil and store at room temperature for up to 1 day.
- **Ingredient Note:** In the test Kitchen, sucralose is the only alternative sweetener we test with when we feel the option is appropriate. For nonbaking recipes, we use Splenda Granular (boxed, not in a packet). For baking, we use Splenda Sugar Blend for Baking, a mix of sugar and sucralose. It can be substituted in recipes (1/2 cup of the blend for each 1 cup of sugar) to reduce
sugar calories by half while maintaining some of the baking properties of sugar. If you make a similar blend with half sugar and half Splenda Granular, substitute this homemade mixture cup for cup.
- When choosing any low- or no-calorie sweetener, be sure to check the label to make sure it is suitable for your intended use.

NUTRITION
Per serving: 185 calories; 4 g fat (0 g sat, 2 g mono); 0 mg cholesterol; 30 g carbohydrates; 3 g protein; 3 gfiber; 115 mg sodium; 211 mg potassium.
Nutrition Bonus: Vitamin C (66% daily value).
Carbohydrate Servings: 2 1/2
Exchanges: 21/2 other carbohydrate, 1 fat

DAY 10
BREAKFAST
Eggs Baked Over a Spicy Vegetable Ragout
Skim milk (1 cup)
LUNCH
Asian Chicken Salad
Roasted Tomato Soup or Watermelon Gazpacho
Skim milk (1 cup)
SNACK
Melon (1 cup cubed)
DINNER
Grilled Lamb with Fresh Mint Chutney or Pork Roast with Walnut-Pomegranate Filling
Green Beans with Poppy Seed Dressing
Whole-wheat couscous (1 cup, cooked)
Orange Slices with Warm Raspberries

DAY 10 RECIPES

Eggs Baked Over a Spicy Vegetable Ragout

INGREDIENTS
- 3 teaspoons extra-virgin olive oil, divided
- 1 small eggplant, cut into 1/2-inch cubes
- 1 medium onion, chopped
- 1 large red bell pepper, diced
- 6 cloves garlic, minced
- 2 teaspoons ground cumin
- 1/8-1/4 teaspoon hot sauce, such as Hot pepper
- 1 medium summer squash, halved lengthwise and thinly sliced
- 1 14-ounce can diced tomatoes
- 1/4 cup water
- 3 tablespoons chopped fresh parsley, divided
- 1/8 teaspoon salt
- Freshly ground pepper to taste
- 4 large large eggs

PREPARATION

1. Preheat oven to 400°F. Coat a shallow 2-quart baking dish with cooking spray.
2. Heat 2 teaspoons oil in a large nonstick skillet over medium-high heat. Add eggplant and cook, stirring frequently, until browned and softened, 5 to 7 minutes. Transfer to a plate.
3. Heat the remaining 1 teaspoon oil in a Dutch oven or large deep sauté pan on medium heat. Add onion and cook, stirring occasionally, until softened, 3 to 5 minutes. Add bell pepper and cook, stirring occasionally, until softened, 3 to 5 minutes. Add garlic, cumin and hot sauce and cook until fragrant, 15 to 30 seconds. Stir in squash, tomatoes, water and the eggplant. Cover and simmer for 10 minutes. Stir in 2 tablespoons parsley, salt and pepper.
4. Spread the vegetable ragout in the prepared baking dish. Make 4 shallow wells in the ragout and gently crack 1 egg into each well, being careful not to break yolks.
5. Bake, uncovered, until the eggs are barely set, 10 to 12 minutes. (Caution: Eggs can overcook very quickly. Check them often and remove from the oven when they still look a little underdone; they will continue to cook in the hot ragout. If the baking dish is ceramic, the cooking time will be closer to 12 minutes. A glass dish will cook eggs much faster.) Sprinkle with the remaining 1 tablespoon parsley. Serve immediately.

TIPS & NOTES
- **Make Ahead Tip**: Prepare through Step 3, cover and refrigerate for up to 2 days. Reheat before continuing.

NUTRITION
Per serving: 201 calories; 9 g fat (2 g sat, 5 g mono); 212 mg cholesterol; 23 g carbohydrates; 0 g added sugars; 10 g protein; 6 g fiber; 282 mg sodium; 471 mg potassium.
Nutrition Bonus: Vitamin C (170% daily value), Vitamin A (45% dv), Fiber (24% dv), Folate (17% dv), Iron (15% dv).
Carbohydrate Servings: 1
Exchanges: 4 vegetable; 1 medium-fat meat; 1/2 fat (mono)

Asian Chicken Salad

INGREDIENTS
DRESSING
- 1/4 cup reduced-sodium soy sauce
- 3 tablespoons rice-wine vinegar
- 1 1/2 tablespoons brown sugar
- 1 1/2 teaspoons sesame oil
- 1 1/2 teaspoons chile-garlic sauce, (see Ingredient notes)
- 3 tablespoons canola oil
- 1 tablespoon minced fresh ginger
- 2 cloves garlic, minced
- 1 tablespoon tahini paste
- 3/4 cup reduced-sodium chicken broth, or reserved chicken-poaching liquid

SALAD
- 2 tablespoons sesame seeds
- 8 cups shredded napa cabbage, (1 small head; see Ingredient notes)
- 1 1/2 cups grated carrots, (2-3 medium)
- 5 radishes, sliced (about 1 cup)
- 1/2 cup chopped scallions
- 3 1/2 cups shredded skinless cooked chicken, (about 1 1/2 pounds boneless, skinless chicken breast) (see Tip)

PREPARATION
1. To prepare dressing: Combine soy sauce, vinegar, brown sugar, sesame oil and chile-garlic sauce in a glass measuring cup; stir to blend. Heat canola oil in a small saucepan over medium-high heat. Add ginger and garlic; cook, stirring, until fragrant, 1 to 2 minutes.

Add the soy sauce mixture to the pan; bring to a simmer. Whisk in tahini and broth (or poaching liquid); cook until reduced slightly, 3 to 4 minutes. Let cool.
2. To prepare salad: Heat a small dry skillet over medium-low heat. Add sesame seeds and cook, stirring, until lightly browned and fragrant, 1 to 2 minutes. Transfer to a small plate to cool.
3. Combine cabbage, carrots, radishes, scallions and chicken in a large shallow bowl. Stir dressing to recombine and drizzle over the salad; toss to coat. Sprinkle the sesame seeds on top.

TIPS & NOTES

- **Make Ahead Tip**: Cover and refrigerate the dressing (Step 1) for up to 2 days.
- **Ingredient Notes:** Chile-garlic sauce is a spicy blend of chiles, garlic and other seasonings; it is found in the Asian section of the market.
- Napa cabbage has an elongated head and is pale green in color with tender, tapered white ribs. Its tightly packed, crinkled leaves have a crisp texture. Discard the cone-shaped core. One small head yields about 8 cups shredded.
- **Tip:** To poach chicken: Combine two 14-ounce cans reduced-sodium chicken broth, 2 chopped scallions, 2 slivers fresh ginger and 2 cloves garlic in a large skillet; bring to a simmer. Add 1 1/2 pounds boneless, skinless chicken breast and cook over medium heat until no longer pink inside, 10 to 15 minutes. The flavorful poaching liquid will keep, tightly covered, in the refrigerator for up to 2 days or in the freezer for up to 6 months.

NUTRITION

Per serving: 289 calories; 14 g fat (2 g sat, 7 g mono); 64 mg cholesterol; 14 g carbohydrates; 3 g added sugars; 28 g protein; 3 g fiber; 518 mg sodium; 355 mg potassium.
Nutrition Bonus: Vitamin A (100% daily value), Vitamin C (60% dv).
Carbohydrate Servings: 1
Exchanges: 1 1/2 vegetable, 3 lean meat, 2 fat

Roasted Tomato Soup

INGREDIENTS
- 1 1/2 pounds large tomatoes, such as beefsteak, cut in half crosswise
- 1 medium sweet onion, such as Vidalia, peeled and cut in half crosswise
- 3 large cloves garlic, unpeeled
- 1 tablespoon plus 1 teaspoon extra-virgin olive oil, divided
- 1/4 teaspoon salt, or to taste
- Freshly ground pepper, to taste
- 2 cups reduced-sodium chicken broth, or vegetable broth, divided

- 1/4 cup tomato juice
- 1 teaspoon tomato paste
- 1/4 teaspoon Worcestershire sauce
- 1 tablespoon fresh basil, chopped and brown sugar to taste
- 1/2 cup corn kernels, or frozen, thawed

PREPARATION
1. Preheat oven to 400°F. Coat a baking sheet with cooking spray.
2. Toss tomatoes, onion and garlic in a mixing bowl with 1 tablespoon oil. Season with salt and pepper. Spread on the prepared baking sheet and roast until the vegetables are soft and caramelized, about 30 minutes. Let cool.
3. Peel and seed the tomatoes. Trim off the onion ends. Peel the garlic. Place the vegetables in a food processor or blender with 1 cup broth and the remaining 1 teaspoon oil. Pulse to desired thickness and texture.
4. Transfer the vegetable puree to a large heavy pot or Dutch oven. Add the remaining 1 cup broth, tomato juice, tomato pate, Worcestershire sauce, basil and brown sugar (if using). Bring to a simmer over medium heat, stirring often. Ladle into 6 soup bowls, garnish with corn and serve.

TIPS & NOTES
- **Make Ahead Tip**: Cover and refrigerate for up to 2 days or freeze for up to 2 months.
- **Tip:** Removing Corn from the Cob: Stand an uncooked ear of corn on its stem end in a shallow bowl and slice the kernels off with a sharp, thin-bladed knife. This technique produces whole kernels that are good for adding to salads and salsas. If you want to use the corn kernels for soups, fritters or puddings, you can add another step to the process. After cutting the kernels off, reverse the knife and, using the dull side, press it down the length of the ear to push out the rest of the corn and its milk.

NUTRITION
Per serving: 95 calories; 4 g fat (1 g sat, 2 g mono); 1 mg cholesterol; 15 g carbohydrates; 0 g added sugars; 3 g protein; 3 g fiber; 340 mg sodium; 406 mg potassium.
Nutrition Bonus: Vitamin C (35% daily value), Vitamin A (20% dv).
Carbohydrate Servings: 1
Exchanges: 2 vegetable, 1 fat

Watermelon Gazpacho

INGREDIENTS

- 8 cups finely diced seedless watermelon, (about 6 pounds with the rind) (see Tip)
- 1 medium cucumber, peeled, seeded and finely diced
- 1/2 red bell pepper, finely diced
- 1/4 cup chopped fresh basil
- 1/4 cup chopped flat-leaf parsley
- 3 tablespoons red-wine vinegar
- 2 tablespoons minced shallot
- 2 tablespoons extra-virgin olive oil
- 3/4 teaspoon salt

PREPARATION

1. Mix watermelon, cucumber, bell pepper, basil, parsley, vinegar, shallot, oil and salt in a large bowl. Puree 3 cups of the mixture in a blender or food processor to the desired smoothness; transfer to another large bowl. Puree another 3 cups and add to the bowl. Stir in the remaining diced mixture. Serve chilled.

TIPS & NOTES

- **Make Ahead Tip**: Cover and refrigerate for up to 1 day.
- **Tip:** Melon selection & storage: Look for symmetrical unblemished melons, without flat sides, that have a creamy yellow spot on the bottom indicating ripeness. At 92% water, this fruit should feel heavy when you heft it. Precut melon flesh should be dense, firm and appear moist. Store in the refrigerator for up to a week or keep in a cool, dark spot. Cover the cut surface of melon with plastic wrap and refrigerate.

NUTRITION
Per serving: 116 calories; 5 g fat (1 g sat, 4 g mono); 0 mg cholesterol; 18 g carbohydrates; 0 g added sugars; 2 g protein; 2 g fiber; 296 mg sodium; 345 mg potassium.
Nutrition Bonus: Vitamin C (110% daily value), Vitamin A (45% dv).
Carbohydrate Servings: 1
Exchanges: 1 fruit, 1 fat

Grilled Lamb with Fresh Mint Chutney

INGREDIENTS
- Fresh Mint Chutney, (recipe follows)
- 8 rib lamb chops, (about 3 ounces each), trimmed
- 1 clove garlic, cut in half
- 1 teaspoon extra-virgin olive oil, or canola oil
- 1/4 teaspoon kosher salt
- Freshly ground pepper, to taste

PREPARATION
1. Prepare Fresh Mint Chutney.
2. Heat gas grill. Rub lamb chops with garlic, then brush with oil and season with salt and pepper. Grill the chops until cooked to desired doneness, 4 to 5 minutes per side for medium-rare. Serve with Fresh Mint Chutney.

NUTRITION

Per serving: 296 calories; 13 g fat (4 g sat, 6 g mono); 112 mg cholesterol; 6 g carbohydrates; 36 g protein;1 g fiber; 653 mg sodium; 486 mg potassium.
Nutrition Bonus: Selenium (57% daily value), Vitamin C (50% dv), Zinc (36% dv).
Carbohydrate Servings: 1/2
Exchanges: 1 vegetable, 5 lean meat

Pork Roast with Walnut-Pomegranate Filling

INGREDIENTS
PORK & FILLING
- 1/2 cup shelled walnuts
- 4 tablespoons pomegranate molasses, (see Note), divided
- 3 tablespoons extra-virgin olive oil
- 2 cloves garlic, minced
- 1/4 teaspoon salt, divided
- Freshly ground pepper, to taste
- 1 2-pound boneless center-cut pork loin roast, trimmed

SAUCE
- 1 1/2 cups pomegranate juice
- 1 1/2 cups reduced-sodium chicken broth
- 2 tablespoons honey
- 1/4 teaspoon salt
- 1 1/2 teaspoons cornstarch
- 1 tablespoon water

- 1 cup pomegranate seeds, (1 large fruit; see Tip) for garnish

PREPARATION
1. Preheat oven to 350°F. Line a roasting pan with foil. Coat a rack with cooking spray.
2. To prepare pork & filling: Toast walnuts in a small dry skillet over medium-low heat, stirring constantly, until fragrant, 2 to 3 minutes. Transfer to a small bowl and let cool. Place the walnuts in a sealable plastic bag and crush with a rolling pin. Transfer to a medium bowl
and mix in 2 tablespoons pomegranate molasses, oil, garlic, 1/8 teaspoon salt and pepper.
3. Using a sharp knife, make a vertical cut two-thirds of the way to the bottom of the pork. From there, slice outward horizontally to about 3/4 inch from the sides. Unfold the pork.
4. Place the pork between 2 sheets of plastic wrap. Using a meat mallet or heavy skillet, pound the pork to an even 1/2-inch thickness. Remove the plastic wrap. Using a spatula, spread the filling over the surface, leaving a 1-inch border. Starting at the short edge, roll the roast up fairly tightly, completely enclosing the filling. Tie the roast at 1 1/2-inch intervals with kitchen string.
5. Season the roast with the remaining 1/8 teaspoon salt and pepper and coat with the remaining 2 tablespoons pomegranate molasses. Set the roast seam-side down on the prepared rack. Roast until an instant-read thermometer inserted in the center registers 155°F (it will increase to 160°F as it rests), about 1 hour 10 minutes. Transfer the pork to a clean cutting board; tent with foil and let rest for 10 minutes.
6. Meanwhile, prepare sauce: Combine pomegranate juice, broth, honey and 1/4 teaspoon salt in a medium saucepan; bring to a boil over medium-high heat. Boil until the sauce has reduced to 1 cup, 15 to 25 minutes. Mix cornstarch and water in a small bowl; add to the sauce and cook, whisking, until slightly thickened, about 1 minute.
7. Remove the string and carve the roast into 3/4-inch-thick slices. Serve with the sauce and garnish each serving with pomegranate seeds.

TIPS & NOTES
- **Make Ahead Tip**: Prepare through Step 4. Wrap in plastic wrap and refrigerate for up to 8 hours. The sauce (Step 6) can be made ahead: cover and refrigerate for up to 2 days; reheat before serving. Equipment: Kitchen string
- **Note:** Pomegranate molasses has a bright, tangy flavor. (Don't confuse it with sweet grenadine syrup, which contains little or no pomegranate juice.) Find it in Middle Eastern markets and some large supermarkets near the vinegar or molasses.

To make your own: Simmer 4 cups pomegranate juice, uncovered, in a medium nonreactive saucepan over medium heat until thick enough to coat the back of a spoon, 45 to 50 minutes. (Do not let the syrup reduce too much or it will darken and become very sticky.) Makes about 1/2 cup (25 calories per tablespoon). Refrigerate the molasses in an airtight container for up to 3 months.

- **Tip:** To seed a pomegranate and avoid the enduring stains of pomegranate juice, work under water. Fill a large bowl with water. Hold the pomegranate in the water and slice off the crown. Lightly score the fruit into quarters, from crown to stem end. Keeping the fruit under water, break it apart, gently separating the plump seeds from the outer skin and white pith. The seeds will drop to the bottom of the bowl and the pith will float to the surface. Discard the pith. Pour the seeds into a colander. Rinse and pat dry.

NUTRITION
Per serving: 298 calories; 14 g fat (3 g sat, 7 g mono); 72 mg cholesterol; 16 g carbohydrates; 26 g protein;0 g fiber; 238 mg sodium; 534 mg potassium.

Green Beans with Poppy Seed Dressing

INGREDIENTS
- 1 teaspoon poppy seeds
- 2 tablespoons extra-virgin olive oil
- 1 tablespoon white-wine vinegar, or rice-wine vinegar
- 1 teaspoon Dijon mustard
- 1/2 teaspoon honey
- 1 tablespoon minced shallot
- 1/8 teaspoon salt, or to taste
- Freshly ground pepper, to taste
- 1 pound green beans, stem ends trimmed

PREPARATION
1. To prepare dressing: Heat a small dry skillet over medium-low heat. Add poppy seeds and toast, stirring, until fragrant, about 1 minute. Transfer to a small bowl (or jar) and let cool. Add oil, vinegar,
mustard, honey, shallot, salt and pepper; whisk (or shake) until blended.

2. To prepare beans: Cook beans in a large pot of boiling water until just tender, 5 to 7 minutes. Drain. Warm the dressing in a large skillet over medium heat. Add beans and toss to coat.

TIPS & NOTES
- **Make Ahead Tip**: Cover and refrigerate the dressing (step 1) for up to 2 days.

NUTRITION
Per serving: 113 calories; 8 g fat (1 g sat, 5 g mono); 0 mg cholesterol; 11 g carbohydrates; 1 g added sugars; 3 g protein; 4 g fiber; 104 mg sodium; 185 mg potassium.
Nutrition Bonus: Vitamin C (20% daily value), Fiber (15% dv), Vitamin A (15% dv).
Carbohydrate Servings: 1
Exchanges: 1 1/2 vegetable, 1 1/2 fat (mono)

Orange Slices with Warm Raspberries

INGREDIENTS
- 4 seedless oranges, such as navel oranges
- 2 tablespoons sugar, or Splenda Granular
- 1 tablespoon lemon juice
- 1/4 teaspoon ground cinnamon
- 2 cups frozen unsweetened raspberries, (not thawed)

PREPARATION
1. With a sharp knife, remove and discard the skin and white pith from oranges; slice the oranges crosswise and arrange on 4 dessert plates.
2. Combine sugar (or Splenda), lemon juice and cinnamon in a small saucepan; stir over low heat until bubbling. Add raspberries and stir gently until the berries are just thawed. Spoon over the orange slices and serve immediately.

NUTRITION

Per serving: 122 calories; 0 g fat (0 g sat, 0 g mono); 0 mg cholesterol; 30 g carbohydrates; 2 g protein; 5 gfiber; 2 mg sodium; 237 mg potassium.
Nutrition Bonus: Vitamin C (157% daily value), Fiber (20% dv).
Carbohydrate Servings: 1 1/2
Exchanges: 2 fruit
Nutrition Note: Per serving with Splenda: 1 Carbohydrate Serving; 100 calories; 25 g carbohydrate.

DAY 11
BREAKFAST
Spiced Apple Butter Bran Muffins
Skim milk (1 cup)
Grapefruit (1/2)
LUNCH

Honey-Mustard Turkey Burgers or Chicken & Blueberry Pasta Salad
Broccoli Slaw
Fat-free cheese (1 slice)
Oatmeal Chocolate Chip Cookies

SNACK

Frosted Grapes

DINNER

Herbed Scallop Kebabs
Whole-Wheat Couscous with Parmesan & Peas or Butternut & Barley Pilaf
Steamed cauliflower (1 cup) Stuffed Nectarines

DAY 11 RECIPES

Spiced Apple Butter Bran Muffins

INGREDIENTS
- 1/2 cup raisins
- 3/4 cup whole-wheat flour
- 3/4 cup all-purpose flour
- 2 1/2 teaspoons baking powder
- 1/4 teaspoon salt
- 1/2 teaspoon ground cinnamon
- 3/4 cup unprocessed wheat bran, or oat bran
- 1 large egg, lightly beaten
- 1/2 cup low-fat milk
- 1/2 cup spiced apple butter
- 1/2 cup packed light brown sugar, or 1/4 cup Splenda Sugar Blend for Baking
- 1/4 cup canola oil
- 3 tablespoons molasses
- 1 cup finely diced peeled apple

PREPARATION
1. Preheat oven to 375°F. Coat 12 standard 2 1/2-inch muffin cups with cooking spray. Place raisins in a small bowl and cover with hot water. Set aside.
2. Whisk whole-wheat flour, all-purpose flour, baking powder, salt and cinnamon in a large bowl. Stir in bran.
3. Whisk egg, milk, apple butter, brown sugar (or Splenda), oil and molasses in a large bowl until blended. Make a well in the dry ingredients and pour in the wet ingredients. Drain the raisins; add them and the diced apple to the bowl. Stir until just combined. Scoop the batter into the prepared pan (the cups will be very full).

4. Bake the muffins until the tops spring back when touched lightly, 18 to 22 minutes. Let cool in the pan for 5 minutes. Loosen the edges and turn the muffins out onto a wire rack to cool slightly before serving.

TIPS & NOTES
- Wrap leftover muffins individually in plastic wrap, place in a plastic storage container or ziplock bag and freeze for up to 1 month. To thaw, remove plastic wrap, wrap in a paper towel and microwave on Defrost for about 2 minutes.

NUTRITION
Per muffin: 197 calories; 6 g fat (1 g sat, 3 g mono); 18 mg cholesterol; 38 g carbohydrates; 4 g protein; 4 gfiber; 148 mg sodium; 221 mg potassium.
Nutrition Bonus: Fiber (16% daily value).
Carbohydrate Servings: 2
Exchanges: 2 starch, 1 fat
Nutrition Note: Per muffin with Splenda: 2 Carbohydrate Servings; 187 calories, 31 g carbohydrate

Honey-Mustard Turkey Burgers

INGREDIENTS
- 1/4 cup coarse-grained mustard
- 2 tablespoons honey
- 1 pound ground turkey breast
- 1/4 teaspoon salt
- 1/4 teaspoon freshly ground pepper
- 2 teaspoons canola oil
- 4 whole-wheat hamburger rolls, split and toasted
- Lettuce, tomato slices and red onion slices, for garnish

PREPARATION
1. Prepare a grill.
2. Whisk mustard and honey in a small bowl until smooth.
3. Combine turkey, 3 tablespoons of the mustard mixture, salt and pepper in a bowl; mix well. Form into four 1-inch-thick burgers.
4. Lightly brush the burgers on both sides with oil. Grill until no pink remains in center, 5 to 7 minutes per side. Brush the burgers with the remaining mustard mixture. Serve on rolls with lettuce, tomato and onion slices.

NUTRITION
Per serving: 317 calories; 11 g fat (3 g sat, 2 g mono); 65 mg cholesterol; 31 g carbohydrates; 26 g protein;3 g fiber; 593 mg sodium; 387 mg potassium.

Nutrition Bonus: Folate (20% daily value), Iron (20% dv), Calcium (15% dv).
Carbohydrate Servings: 2
Exchanges: 2 starch, 4 lean meat

Chicken & Blueberry Pasta Salad

INGREDIENTS
- 1 pound boneless, skinless chicken breast, trimmed of fat
- 8 ounces whole-wheat fusilli or radiatore
- 3 tablespoons extra-virgin olive oil
- 1 large shallot, thinly sliced
- 1/3 cup reduced-sodium chicken broth
- 1/3 cup crumbled feta cheese
- 3 tablespoons lime juice
- 1 cup fresh blueberries
- 1 tablespoon chopped fresh thyme
- 1 teaspoon freshly grated lime zest
- 1/4 teaspoon salt

PREPARATION
1. Place chicken in a skillet or saucepan and add enough water to cover; bring to a boil. Cover, reduce heat to low and simmer gently until cooked through and no longer pink in the middle, 10 to 12 minutes. Transfer the chicken to a cutting board to cool. Shred into bite-size strips.
2. Bring a large pot of water to a boil. Cook pasta until just tender, about 9 minutes or according to package directions. Drain. Place in a large bowl.
3. Meanwhile, place oil and shallot in a small skillet and cook over medium-low heat, stirring occasionally, until softened and just beginning to brown, 2 to 5 minutes. Add broth, feta and lime juice and cook, stirring occasionally, until the feta begins to melt, 1 to 2 minutes.
4. Add the chicken to the bowl with the pasta. Add the dressing, blueberries, thyme, lime zest and salt and toss until combined.

TIPS & NOTES
- **Make Ahead Tip**: Add everything except the blueberries and dressing to the pasta salad. Cover and refrigerate pasta salad, blueberries and dressing separately for up to 1 day. Toss together just before serving.

NUTRITION

Per serving: 315 calories; 11 g fat (3 g sat, 6 g mono); 49 mg cholesterol; 33 g carbohydrates; 0 g added sugars; 23 g protein; 5 g fiber; 238 mg sodium; 207 mg potassium.

Nutrition Bonus: Selenium (60% daily value), Fiber (20% dv).
Carbohydrate Servings: 2
Exchanges: 2 starch, 2 very lean meat, 2 fat

Broccoli Slaw

INGREDIENTS
- 4 slices turkey bacon
- 1 12- to 16-ounce bag shredded broccoli slaw, or 1 large bunch broccoli (about 1 1/2 pounds)
- 1/4 cup low-fat or nonfat plain yogurt
- 1/4 cup reduced-fat mayonnaise
- 3 tablespoons cider vinegar
- 2 teaspoons sugar
- 1/2 teaspoon salt, or to taste
- Freshly ground pepper, to taste
- 1 8-ounce can low-sodium sliced water chestnuts, rinsed and coarsely chopped
- 1/2 cup finely diced red onion, (1/2 medium)

PREPARATION
1. Cook bacon in a large skillet over medium heat, turning frequently, until crisp, 5 to 8 minutes. (Alternatively, microwave on High for 2 1/2 to 3 minutes.) Drain bacon on paper towels. Chop coarsely.
2. If using whole broccoli, trim about 3 inches off the stems. Chop the rest into 1/4-inch pieces.
3. Whisk yogurt, mayonnaise, vinegar, sugar, salt and pepper in a large bowl. Add water chestnuts, onion, bacon and broccoli; toss to coat. Chill until serving time.

TIPS & NOTES
- **Make Ahead Tip:** Cover and chill for up to 2 days.

NUTRITION

Per serving: 80 calories; 3 g fat (1 g sat, 1 g mono); 5 mg cholesterol; 9 g carbohydrates; 1 g added sugars; 3 g protein; 3 g fiber; 271 mg sodium; 181 mg potassium.
Nutrition Bonus: Vitamin C (70% daily value).
Carbohydrate Servings: 1/2
Exchanges: 2 vegetable, 1 fat

Oatmeal Chocolate Chip Cookies

INGREDIENTS
- 2 cups rolled oats, (not quick-cooking)
- 1/2 cup whole-wheat pastry flour, (see Ingredient Note)
- 1/2 cup all-purpose flour
- 1 teaspoon ground cinnamon
- 1/2 teaspoon baking soda
- 1/2 teaspoon salt
- 1/2 cup tahini, (see Ingredient Note)
- 4 tablespoons cold unsalted butter, cut into pieces
- 2/3 cup granulated sugar
- 2/3 cup packed light brown sugar
- 1 large egg
- 1 large egg white
- 1 tablespoon vanilla extract
- 1 cup semisweet or bittersweet chocolate chips
- 1/2 cup chopped walnuts

PREPARATION
1. Position racks in upper and lower thirds of oven; preheat to 350°F. Line 2 baking sheets with parchment paper.
2. Whisk oats, whole-wheat flour, all-purpose flour, cinnamon, baking soda and salt in a medium bowl. Beat tahini and butter in a large bowl with an electric mixer until blended into a paste. Add granulated sugar and brown sugar; continue beating until well combined, the mixture will still be a little grainy. Beat in egg, then egg white, then vanilla. Stir in the oat mixture with a wooden spoon until just moistened. Stir in chocolate chips and walnuts.
3. With damp hands, roll 1 tablespoon of the batter into a ball, place it on a prepared baking sheet and flatten it until squat, but don't let the sides crack. Continue with the remaining batter, spacing the flattened balls 2 inches apart.
4. Bake the cookies until golden brown, about 16 minutes, switching the pans back to front and top to bottom halfway through. Cool on the pans for 2 minutes, then transfer the cookies to a wire rack to cool completely. Let the pans cool for a few minutes before baking another batch.

TIPS & NOTES

- **Make Ahead Tip**: Store in an airtight container for up to 2 days or freeze for longer storage.
- **Ingredient notes:** Whole-wheat pastry flour, lower in protein than regular whole-wheat flour, has less gluten-forming potential, making it a better choice

for tender baked goods. You can find it in the natural-foods section of large super markets and natural-foods stores. Store in the freezer.
- Tahini is a paste made from ground sesame seeds. Look for it in natural-foods stores and some supermarkets.

NUTRITION
Per cookie: 102 calories; 5 g fat (2 g sat, 1 g mono); 7 mg cholesterol; 14 g carbohydrates; 2 g protein; 1 gfiber; 45 mg sodium; 53 mg potassium.
Carbohydrate Servings: 1
Exchanges: 1 other carbohydrate, 1 fat

Frosted Grapes

INGREDIENTS
- 2 cups seedless grapes

PREPARATION
1. Wash and pat dry grapes. Freeze 45 minutes. Let stand for 2 minutes at room temperature before serving.

NUTRITION
Per serving: 55 calories; 0 g fat (0 g sat, 0 g mono); 0 mg cholesterol; 14 g carbohydrates; 1 g protein; 1 gfiber; 2 mg sodium; 153 mg potassium.
Carbohydrate Servings: 1
Exchanges: 1 fruit

Herbed Scallop Kebabs

INGREDIENTS
- 3 tablespoons lemon juice
- 1 1/2 tablespoons chopped fresh thyme
- 2 teaspoons extra-virgin olive oil
- 2 teaspoons freshly grated lemon zest
- 1 teaspoon freshly ground pepper
- 1/4 teaspoon salt, or to taste
- 1 1/4 pounds sea scallops, trimmed
- 1 lemon, cut into 8 wedges

PREPARATION
1. Preheat grill to medium-high. Place a fine-mesh nonstick grill topper on grill to heat.
2. Whisk lemon juice, thyme, oil, lemon zest, pepper and salt in a small bowl.

3. Toss scallops with 2 tablespoons of the lemon mixture; reserve the remaining mixture for basting the kebabs. Thread the scallops and the lemon wedges onto four 10-inch-long skewers (see Tip), placing 6 to 7 scallops and 2 lemon wedges on each skewer.
4. Lightly oil the grill rack (see Tip). Cook the kebabs, turning from time to time and basting with the reserved lemon mixture, until the scallops are opaque in the center, 8 to 12 minutes. Serve immediately.

TIPS & NOTES

- If using wooden skewers, soak them in water for 20 to 30 minutes first to prevent them from scorching.
- **To oil a grill rack:** Oil a folded paper towel, hold it with tongs and rub it over the rack. Do not use cooking spray on a hot grill.

NUTRITION
Per serving: 152 calories; 3 g fat (0 g sat, 2 g mono); 47 mg cholesterol; 5 g carbohydrates; 0 g added sugars; 24 g protein; 0 g fiber; 374 mg sodium; 478 mg potassium.
Nutrition Bonus: Selenium (44% daily value), Vitamin C (20% dv).
Exchanges: 3 1/2 very lean meat

Whole-Wheat Couscous with Parmesan & Peas

INGREDIENTS
- 1 14-ounce can reduced-sodium chicken broth, or vegetable broth
- 1/4 cup water
- 2 teaspoons extra-virgin olive oil
- 1 cup whole-wheat couscous
- 1 1/2 cups frozen peas
- 2 tablespoons chopped fresh dill
- 1 teaspoon freshly grated lemon zest
- Salt & freshly ground pepper, to taste
- 1/2 cup freshly grated Parmesan cheese

PREPARATION
Combine broth, water and oil in a large saucepan; bring to a boil. Stir in couscous and remove from heat. Cover and let plump for 5 minutes.
Meanwhile, cook peas on the stovetop or in the microwave according to package directions.
Add the peas, dill, lemon zest, salt and pepper to the couscous; mix gently and fluff with a fork. Serve hot, sprinkled with cheese.

NUTRITION

Per serving: 208 calories; 4 g fat (1 g sat, 2 g mono); 6 mg cholesterol; 35 g carbohydrates; 0 g added sugars; 10 g protein; 7 g fiber; 186 mg sodium; 45 mg potassium.
Carbohydrate Servings: 2
Exchanges: 2 starch

Butternut & Barley Pilaf

INGREDIENTS
- 2 teaspoons extra-virgin olive oil
- 1 medium onion, chopped
- 1 14-ounce can reduced-sodium chicken broth, or vegetable broth
- 1 3/4 cups water
- 1 cup pearl barley
- 2 cups cubed peeled butternut squash, (3/4-inch cubes) (see Tip)
- 1/3 cup chopped flat-leaf parsley
- 1 teaspoon freshly grated lemon zest
- 1 tablespoon lemon juice
- 1 clove garlic, minced
- 1/4 teaspoon salt, or to taste
- Freshly ground pepper, to taste

PREPARATION
1. Heat oil in a large saucepan over medium heat. Add onion and cook, stirring often, until softened, 2 to 3 minutes. Add broth, water, barley and squash; bring to a simmer, reduce heat to medium-low and simmer until the barley and squash are tender and most of the liquid has been absorbed, about 45 minutes. Add parsley, lemon zest, lemon juice, garlic, salt and pepper; mix gently.

TIPS & NOTES
- **Tip:** To save time, use conveniently peeled and cubed butternut squash, available in many supermarkets in the fall and winter.

NUTRITION
Per serving: 194 calories; 2 g fat (0 g sat, 1 g mono); 1 mg cholesterol; 40 g carbohydrates; 0 g added sugars; 6 g protein; 8 g fiber; 149 mg sodium; 457 mg potassium.
Nutrition Bonus: Vitamin A (180% daily value), Vitamin C (45% dv), Fiber (30% dv).
Carbohydrate Servings: 2
Exchanges: 2 starch,1 vegetable

Stuffed Nectarines

INGREDIENTS
- 1 nectarine, halved and pitted
- 4 gingersnaps, crushed
- 2 teaspoons melted butter
- 1 teaspoon brown sugar
- 1/2 teaspoon lemon juice
- 1/2 cup orange juice
- 1/4 cup low-fat vanilla yogurt

PREPARATION

1. Preheat oven to 350°F. Place nectarine halves cut-side up in a small baking dish. Combine gingersnaps, butter, sugar and lemon juice; divide between the nectarine halves. Pour orange juice around them. Cover with foil. Bake until tender, about 25 minutes. Serve with low-fat vanilla yogurt.

NUTRITION
Per serving: 176 calories; 5 g fat (3 g sat, 1 g mono); 11 mg cholesterol; 30 g carbohydrates; 2 g protein; 1 g fiber; 103 mg sodium; 361 mg potassium.
Carbohydrate Servings: 2
Exchanges: 1 fruit, 1 carbohydrate, 1 fat

DAY 12
BREAKFAST

Oatbran Bagel or Date-Oat Muffins
Skim milk (1 cup)
Vegetable Cream Cheese

LUNCH

Pasta, Tuna & Roasted Pepper Salad
Whole-wheat pita bread (1 medium pita)
Skim milk (1 cup)

SNACK

Strawberries (1 cup)

DINNER

Pampered Chicken or Southwestern Stuffed Acorn Squash
Carrot Saute with Ginger & Orange
Baked potato (1 medium)
Cranberry & Ruby Grapefruit Compote

DAY 12 RECIPES

Date-Oat Muffins

INGREDIENTS
- 1 cup plus 2 tablespoons old-fashioned oats
- 1/3 cup chopped walnuts, (optional)
- 1 cup whole-wheat flour
- 3/4 cup all-purpose flour
- 1/3 cup whole flaxseeds, ground (see Ingredient notes)
- 2 teaspoons baking powder
- 1/2 teaspoon baking soda
- 1/4 teaspoon salt
- 2 large eggs
- 2/3 cup packed light brown sugar
- 3/4 cup buttermilk, (see Tip)
- 1/2 cup orange juice
- 1/4 cup canola oil
- 2 tablespoons freshly grated orange zest
- 1 teaspoon vanilla extract
- 3/4 cup chopped pitted dates, (see Ingredient notes)

PREPARATION
1. Preheat oven to 400°F. Coat 12 muffin cups with cooking spray.
2. Spread 1 cup oats and the walnuts, if using, in 2 separate small baking pans. Bake, stirring once or twice, until light golden and fragrant, 4 to 6 minutes for the nuts and 8 to 10 minutes for the oats. Transfer to a plate to cool.
3. Meanwhile, whisk whole-wheat flour, all-purpose flour, flaxseeds, baking powder, baking soda and salt in a medium bowl.
4. Whisk eggs and brown sugar in a medium bowl until smooth. Whisk in buttermilk, orange juice, oil, orange zest and vanilla. Add to the dry ingredients and mix with a rubber spatula just until moistened. Fold in dates, the toasted oats and nuts, if using. Scoop batter into the prepared muffin cups (they'll be quite full). Sprinkle the tops with the remaining 2 tablespoons oats.
5. Bake the muffins until the tops are golden brown and spring back when touched lightly, 15 to 25 minutes. Let cool in the pan for 5 minutes. Loosen edges and turn muffins out onto a wire rack to cool slightly before serving.

TIPS & NOTES
- **Ingredient Notes:**
- Flaxseeds are one of the best plant sources of omega-3 fatty acids. They provide both soluble fiber, linked to reduced risk of heart disease, and insoluble fiber,

which provides valuable roughage. Flaxseeds are perishable, so purchase whole seeds (instead of ground flaxmeal), store in the refrigerator and grind in a clean coffee grinder or dry blender just before using.
- Look for packages of chopped pitted dates in the dried fruit section of your supermarket. Whole dates are sticky and cumbersome to chop.
- **Tip:** You can use buttermilk powder in place of fresh buttermilk. Or make "sour milk": mix 1 tablespoon lemon juice or vinegar to 1 cup milk.

NUTRITION

Per muffin: 252 calories; 9 g fat (1 g sat, 4 g mono); 36 mg cholesterol; 41 g carbohydrates; 6 g protein; 5 gfiber; 195 mg sodium; 194 mg potassium.
Carbohydrate Servings: 2
Exchanges: 2 1/2 starch, 1 1/2 fat

Vegetable Cream Cheese

INGREDIENTS
- 8 ounces light cream cheese
- 1/4 cup chopped scallions
- 1/4 cup finely chopped carrots
- 1/4 cup finely chopped daikon radish
- 2 tablespoons chopped fresh dill
- 1/4 teaspoon freshly ground pepper

PREPARATION
1. Blend all ingredients in a small bowl.

NUTRITION

Per tablespoon: 30 calories; 2 g fat (1 g sat, 1 g mono); 7 mg cholesterol; 2 g carbohydrates; 1 g protein; 1 g fiber; 56 mg sodium; 10 mg potassium.
Exchanges: 1/2 fat

Pasta, Tuna & Roasted Pepper Salad

INGREDIENTS
- 1 6-ounce can chunk light tuna in water, drained (see Note)
- 1 7-ounce jar roasted red peppers, rinsed and sliced (2/3 cup), divided
- 1/2 cup finely chopped red onion or scallions
- 2 tablespoons capers, rinsed, coarsely chopped if large
- 2 tablespoons nonfat plain yogurt
- 2 tablespoons chopped fresh basil

- 1 tablespoon extra-virgin olive oil
- 1 1/2 teaspoons lemon juice
- 1 small clove garlic, crushed and peeled
- 1/8 teaspoon salt, or to taste
- Freshly ground pepper, to taste
- 6 ounces whole-wheat penne or rigatoni, (1 3/4 cups)

PREPARATION
1. Put a large pot of lightly salted water on to boil.
2. Combine tuna, 1/3 cup red peppers, onion (or scallions) and capers in a large bowl.
3. Combine yogurt, basil, oil, lemon juice, garlic, salt, pepper and the remaining 1/3 cup red peppers in a blender or food processor. Puree until smooth.
4. Cook pasta until just tender, 10 to 14 minutes or according to package directions. Drain and rinse under cold water. Add to the tuna mixture along with the red pepper sauce; toss to coat.

TIPS & NOTES
- **Note:** Chunk light tuna, which comes from the smaller skipjack or yellowfin, has less mercury than canned white albacore tuna. The FDA/EPA advises that women who are or might become pregnant, nursing mothers and young children consume no more than 6 ounces of albacore a week; up to 12 ounces of canned light tuna is considered safe.

NUTRITION
Per serving: 270 calories; 5 g fat (1 g sat, 3 g mono); 13 mg cholesterol; 39 g carbohydrates; 0 g added sugars; 18 g protein; 6 g fiber; 539 mg sodium; 234 mg potassium.
Nutrition Bonus: Vitamin C (30% daily value), Fiber (23% dv), Magnesium (19% dv).
Carbohydrate Servings: 2
Exchanges: 2 starch, 2 very lean meat

Pampered Chicken

INGREDIENTS
- 4 boneless, skinless chicken breast halves, (about 1 pound), trimmed of fat
- 4 slices Monterey Jack cheese, (2 ounces)
- 2 egg whites
- 1/3 cup seasoned (Italian-style) breadcrumbs
- 2 tablespoons freshly grated Parmesan cheese
- 2 tablespoons chopped fresh parsley
- 1/4 teaspoon salt, or to taste

- 1/2 teaspoon freshly ground pepper
- 2 teaspoons extra-virgin olive oil
- Lemon wedges, for garnish

PREPARATION
1. Preheat oven to 400°F. Place a chicken breast, skinned-side down, on a cutting board. Keeping the blade of a sharp knife parallel to the board, make a horizontal slit along the thinner, long edge of the breast, cutting nearly through to the opposite side. Open the breast so it forms two flaps, hinged at the center. Place a slice of cheese on one flap, leaving a 1/2-inch border at the edge. Press remaining flap down firmly over the cheese and set aside. Repeat with the remaining breasts.
2. Lightly beat egg whites with a fork in a medium bowl. Mix breadcrumbs, Parmesan, parsley, salt and pepper in a shallow dish. Holding a stuffed breast together firmly, dip it in the egg whites and then roll in the breadcrumbs. Repeat with the remaining breasts.
3. Heat oil in a large ovenproof skillet over medium-high heat. Add the stuffed breasts and cook until browned on one side, about 2 minutes. Turn the breasts over and place the skillet in the oven.
4. Bake the chicken until no longer pink in the center, about 20 minutes. Serve with lemon wedges.

NUTRITION
Per serving: 255 calories; 11 g fat (4 g sat, 4 g mono); 78 mg cholesterol; 7 g carbohydrates; 31 g protein; 1 g fiber; 518 mg sodium; 268 mg potassium.
Nutrition Bonus: Selenium (40% daily value), Calcium (15% dv).
Carbohydrate Servings: 1/2
Exchanges: 1/2 starch, 4 very lean meat, 1 medium-fat meat

Southwestern Stuffed Acorn Squash

INGREDIENTS
- 3 acorn squash, (3/4-1 pound each)
- 5 ounces bulk turkey sausage
- 1 small onion, chopped
- 1/2 medium red bell pepper, chopped
- 1 clove garlic, minced
- 1 tablespoon chili powder
- 1 teaspoon ground cumin
- 2 cups chopped cherry tomatoes
- 1 15-ounce can black beans, rinsed (see Tip)
- 1/2 teaspoon salt

- Several dashes hot red pepper sauce, to taste
- 1 cup shredded Swiss cheese

PREPARATION
1. Preheat oven to 375°F. Lightly coat a large baking sheet with cooking spray.
2. Cut squash in half horizontally. Scoop out and discard seeds. Place the squash cut-side down on the prepared baking sheet. Bake until tender, about 45 minutes.
3. Meanwhile, lightly coat a large skillet with cooking spray; heat over medium heat. Add sausage and cook, stirring and breaking up with a wooden spoon, until lightly browned, 3 to 5 minutes. Add onion and bell pepper; cook, stirring often, until softened, 3 to 5 minutes. Stir in garlic, chili powder and cumin; cook for 30 seconds. Stir in tomatoes, beans, salt and hot sauce, scraping up any browned bits. Cover, reduce heat, and simmer until the tomatoes are broken down, 10 to 12 minutes.
4. When the squash are tender, reduce oven temperature to 325°. Fill the squash halves with the turkey mixture. Top with cheese. Place on the baking sheet and bake until the filling is heated through and the cheese is melted, 8 to 10 minutes.

TIPS & NOTES
- **Tip:** While we love the convenience of canned beans, they tend to be high in sodium. Give them a good rinse before adding to a recipe to rid them of some of their sodium (up to 35 percent) or opt for low-sodium or no-salt-added varieties. (Our recipes are analyzed with rinsed, regular canned beans.) Or, if you have the time, cook your own beans from scratch.

NUTRITION
Per serving: 259 calories; 7 g fat (4 g sat, 1 g mono); 29 mg cholesterol; 38 g carbohydrates; 15 g protein; 7 g fiber; 482 mg sodium; 884 mg potassium.
Nutrition Bonus: Vitamin C (80% daily value), Vitamin A (45% dv), Calcium (20% dv), Iron (15% dv)
Carbohydrate Servings: 1
Exchanges: 2 starch, 1 vegetable

Carrot Saute with Ginger & Orange

INGREDIENTS
- 2 teaspoons canola oil
- 3 cups grated carrots, (6 medium-large)
- 2 teaspoons minced fresh ginger
- 1/2 cup orange juice
- 1/4 teaspoon salt, or to taste
- Freshly ground pepper, to taste

PREPARATION

1. Heat oil in a large nonstick skillet over medium-high heat. Add carrots and ginger; cook, stirring often, until wilted, about 2 minutes. Stir in orange juice and salt; simmer, uncovered, until the carrots are tender and most of the liquid has evaporated, 1 to 2 minutes. Season with pepper and serve.

NUTRITION

Per serving: 69 calories; 3 g fat (0 g sat, 1 g mono); 0 mg cholesterol; 6 g carbohydrates; 0 g added sugars;1 g protein; 2 g fiber; 20 mg sodium; 330 mg potassium.
Nutrition Bonus: Vitamin A (200% daily value), Vitamin C (35% dv).
Carbohydrate Servings: 1
Exchanges: 2 vegetable, 1/2 fat (mono)

Cranberry & Ruby Grapefruit Compote

INGREDIENTS
- 1 3/4 cups fresh or frozen cranberries
- 1 1/4 cups water
- 2 3/4-by-2 1/2-inch strips orange zest
- 1/2 cup orange juice
- 1/2 cup sugar
- 1 cinnamon stick, (optional)
- 3 large red grapefruit
- Fresh mint sprigs, for garnish

PREPARATION

1. Combine cranberries, water, orange zest, orange juice, sugar and cinnamon stick (if using) in a medium saucepan. Bring to a boil over medium-high heat. Cook, stirring often, until the cranberries are tender and begin to pop, 3 to 5 minutes. Transfer to a large bowl. Cover loosely and refrigerate until thoroughly chilled, about 2 hours.
2. An hour or two before serving, prepare grapefruit: With a sharp knife, remove the skin and all the white pith from the fruit. Working over a bowl, cut the segments from their surrounding membranes. Squeeze juice from the membranes into the bowl before discarding. Add the segments and juice to the cranberry mixture. To serve, divide the compote among 6 dessert bowls and garnish with mint. Cranberry & Pear Variation: Instead of grapefruit, peel and core 3 to 4 Bartlett or Anjou pears; cut into 1/2-inch wedges. In Step 1, after

the mixture comes to a boil, add pears and reduce heat to medium-low. Simmer gently until the cranberries and pears are tender, 5 to 10 minutes. Cover loosely and refrigerate until thoroughly chilled, about 2 hours. Omit Step 2.

TIPS & NOTES
- **Make Ahead Tip**: Cover and refrigerate for up to 2 days.

NUTRITION
Per serving: 140 calories; 0 g fat (0 g sat, 0 g mono); 0 mg cholesterol; 36 g carbohydrates; 1 g protein; 3 gfiber; 2 mg sodium; 236 mg potassium.
Nutrition Bonus: Vitamin C (35% daily value), Fiber (16% dv).
Carbohydrate Servings: 2 1/2
Exchanges: 1 1/2 fruit, 1/2 other carbohydrate

DAY 13
BREAKFAST
Healthy Pancakes
Strawberries (1 cup)
Low-fat vanilla yogurt (8 oz.)
LUNCH
Chicken & White Bean Soup
Whole-wheat toast (1 slice)
Fat-free cheese (1 slice)
Orange (1 large)
SNACK
Nectarine (1 small)
DINNER
Oven-Fried Fish Fillets or Honey-Soy Broiled Salmon
Tarragon Tartar Sauce
Roasted Asparagus with Pine Nuts or Kale with Apples & Mustard
Brown rice (1/2 cup, cooked)
Salad of Boston Lettuce with Creamy Orange-Shallot Dressing

DAY 13 RECIPES

Healthy Pancakes
INGREDIENTS
- 2 1/2 cups whole-wheat flour
- 1 cup buttermilk powder, (see Note)
- 5 tablespoons dried egg whites, such as Just Whites (see Note)

- 1/4 cup sugar
- 1 1/2 tablespoons baking powder
- 2 teaspoons baking soda
- 1 teaspoon salt
- 1 cup flaxseed meal, (see Note)
- 1 cup nonfat dry milk and 1 1/2 cups nonfat milk
- 1/2 cup wheat bran, or oat bran
- 1/4 cup canola oil
- 1 teaspoon vanilla extract

PREPARATION

1. Whisk flour, buttermilk powder, dried egg whites, sugar, baking powder, baking soda and salt in a large bowl. Stir in flaxseed meal, dry milk and bran. (Makes 6 cups dry mix.)
2. Combine milk, oil and vanilla in a glass measuring cup.
3. Place 2 cups pancake mix in a large bowl. (Refrigerate the remaining pancake mix in an airtight container for up to 1 month or freeze for up to 3 months.) Make a well in the center of the pancake mix. Whisk in the milk mixture until just blended; do not overmix. (The batter will seem quite thin, but will thicken up as it stands.) Let stand for 5 minutes.
4. Coat a nonstick skillet or griddle with cooking spray and place over medium heat. Whisk the batter. Using 1/4 cup batter for each pancake, cook pancakes until the edges are dry and bubbles begin to form, about 2 minutes. Turn over and cook until golden brown, about 2 minutes longer. Adjust heat as necessary for even browning.

TIPS & NOTES

- **Notes:** Buttermilk powder, such as Saco Buttermilk Blend, is a useful substitute for fresh buttermilk. Look in the baking section or with the powdered milk in most markets.
- **Dried egg whites:** Dried egg whites are convenient in recipes calling for egg whites because there is no waste. Look for brands like Just Whites in the baking or natural-foods section of most supermarkets or online at bakerscatalogue.com.
- **Flaxseed meal:** You can find flaxseed meal in the natural-foods section of large supermarkets. You can also start with whole flaxseeds: Grind 2/3 cup whole flaxseeds to yield 1 cup.
- **Variations:** Chocolate-Chocolate Chip Pancakes: Fold 1/2 cup cocoa powder and 3 ounces chocolate chips into the batter. Blueberry: Fold 1 cup frozen

blueberries into the batter. Banana-Nut: Fold 1 cup thinly sliced bananas and 4 tablespoons finely chopped toasted pecans into the batter.

NUTRITION

Per serving: 272 calories; 13 g fat (2 g sat, 6 g mono); 8 mg cholesterol; 27 g carbohydrates; 12 g protein; 5 g fiber; 471 mg sodium; 336 mg potassium.
Nutrition Bonus: Calcium (24% daily value), Fiber (20% dv)
Carbohydrate Servings: 1/2
Exchanges: 2 starch, 1 very lean meat, 2 fat (mono)

Chicken & White Bean Soup

INGREDIENTS
- 2 teaspoons extra-virgin olive oil
- 2 leeks, white and light green parts only, cut into 1/4-inch rounds
- 1 tablespoon chopped fresh sage, or 1/4 teaspoon dried
- 2 14-ounce cans reduced-sodium chicken broth
- 2 cups water
- 1 15-ounce can cannellini beans, rinsed
- 1 2-pound roasted chicken, skin discarded, meat removed from bones and shredded (4 cups)

PREPARATION

1. Heat oil in a Dutch oven over medium-high heat. Add leeks and cook, stirring often, until soft, about 3 minutes. Stir in sage and continue cooking until aromatic, about 30 seconds. Stir in broth and water, increase heat to high, cover and bring to a boil. Add beans and chicken and cook, uncovered, stirring occasionally, until heated through, about 3 minutes. Serve hot.

TIPS & NOTES
- **Make Ahead Tip:** Cover and refrigerate for up to 2 days.

NUTRITION
Per serving: 172 calories; 4 g fat (1 g sat, 2 g mono); 54 mg cholesterol; 10 g carbohydrates; 0 g added sugars; 24 g protein; 3 g fiber; 350 mg sodium; 389 mg potassium.
Carbohydrate Servings: 1/2
Exchanges: 1 starch, 3 lean meat

Oven-Fried Fish Fillets

INGREDIENTS
- 1/3 cup fine, dry, unseasoned breadcrumbs
- 1/4 teaspoon salt
- Freshly ground pepper, to taste
- 1 pound Pacific sole fillets
- 1 tablespoon extra-virgin olive oil
- 1/2 cup Tarragon Tartar Sauce, (recipe follows)
- Lemon wedges

PREPARATION

1. Preheat oven to 450°F. Coat a baking sheet with cooking spray.
2. Place breadcrumbs, salt and pepper in a small dry skillet over medium heat. Cook, stirring, until toasted, about 5 minutes. Remove from heat. Brush both sides of each fish fillet with oil and dredge in the breadcrumb mixture. Place on the prepared baking sheet.
3. Bake the fish until opaque in the center, 5 to 6 minutes.
4. Meanwhile, make Tarragon Tartar Sauce.
5. To serve, carefully transfer the fish to plates using a spatula. Garnish with a dollop of the sauce and serve with lemon wedges.

NUTRITION
Per serving: 229 calories; 10 g fat (2 g sat, 4 g mono); 59 mg cholesterol; 11 g carbohydrates; 23 g protein;1 g fiber; 444 mg sodium; 472 mg potassium.
Nutrition Bonus: Selenium (57% daily value).
Carbohydrate Servings: 1
Exchanges: 1/2 starch, 3 lean meat

Honey-Soy Broiled Salmon

INGREDIENTS
- 1 scallion, minced
- 2 tablespoons reduced-sodium soy sauce
- 1 tablespoon rice vinegar
- 1 tablespoon honey
- 1 teaspoon minced fresh ginger
- 1 pound center-cut salmon fillet, skinned (see Tip) and cut into 4 portions
- 1 teaspoon toasted sesame seeds, (see Tip)

PREPARATION

1. Whisk scallion, soy sauce, vinegar, honey and ginger in a medium bowl until the honey is dissolved. Place salmon in a sealable plastic bag, add 3 tablespoons of the sauce and refrigerate; let marinate for 15 minutes. Reserve the remaining sauce.
2. Preheat broiler. Line a small baking pan with foil and coat with cooking spray.
3. Transfer the salmon to the pan, skinned-side down. (Discard the marinade.) Broil the salmon 4 to 6 inches from the heat source until cooked through, 6 to 10 minutes. Drizzle with the reserved sauce and garnish with sesame seeds.

TIPS & NOTES

- **Tips:** How to skin a salmon fillet: Place skin-side down. Starting at the tail end, slip a long knife between the fish flesh and the skin, holding down firmly with your other hand. Gently push the blade along at a 30° angle, separating the fillet from the skin without cutting through either.
- To toast sesame seeds, heat a small dry skillet over low heat. Add seeds and stir constantly, until golden and fragrant, about 2 minutes. Transfer to a small bowl and let cool.

NUTRITION

Per serving: 234 calories; 13 g fat (3 g sat, 5 g mono); 67 mg cholesterol; 6 g carbohydrates; 4 g added sugars; 23 g protein; 0 g fiber; 335 mg sodium; 444 mg potassium.
Nutrition Bonus: Selenium (60% daily value), excellent source of omega-3s.
Carbohydrate Servings: 1/2
Exchanges: 3 lean meat, 1/2 other carbohydrate

Tarragon Tartar Sauce

INGREDIENTS

- 1/2 cup nonfat or low-fat plain yogurt
- 1/2 cup reduced-fat mayonnaise
- 1 teaspoon sugar
- 1/2 teaspoon Dijon mustard
- 1/2 teaspoon lemon juice
- 1/4 cup finely chopped dill pickle
- 1 tablespoon drained capers, minced
- 2 tablespoons chopped fresh parsley
- 2 teaspoons chopped fresh tarragon, or 1/2 teaspoon dried
- 1 clove garlic, minced

PREPARATION

1. Whisk yogurt, mayonnaise, sugar, mustard and lemon juice in a small bowl. Stir in pickle, capers, parsley, tarragon and garlic.

TIPS & NOTES
- **Make Ahead Tip**: The sauce will keep, covered, in the refrigerator for up to 4 days.

NUTRITION

Per tablespoon: 22 calories; 2 g fat (0 g sat, 0 g mono); 2 mg cholesterol; 2 g carbohydrates; 0 g protein; 0 g fiber; 71 mg sodium; 6 mg potassium.
Exchanges: Per tablespoon: free food

Roasted Asparagus with Pine Nuts

INGREDIENTS
- 2 tablespoons pine nuts
- 1 1/2 pounds asparagus
- 1 large shallot, thinly sliced
- 2 teaspoons extra-virgin olive oil
- 1/4 teaspoon salt, divided
- Freshly ground pepper, to taste
- 1/4 cup balsamic vinegar

PREPARATION

1. Preheat oven to 350° F. Spread pine nuts in a small baking pan and toast in the oven until golden and fragrant, 7 to 10 minutes. Transfer to a small bowl to cool.
2. Increase oven temperature to 450° F. Snap off the tough ends of asparagus. Toss the asparagus with shallot, oil, 1/8 teaspoon salt and pepper. Spread in a single layer on a large baking sheet with sides. Roast, turning twice, until the asparagus is tender and browned, 10 to 15 minutes.
3. Meanwhile, bring vinegar and the remaining 1/8 teaspoon salt to a simmer in a small skillet over medium-high heat. Reduce heat to medium-low and simmer, swirling the pan occasionally, until slightly syrupy and reduced to 1 tablespoon, about 5 minutes. To serve, toss the asparagus with the reduced vinegar and sprinkle with the pine nuts.

NUTRITION
Per serving: 112 calories; 5 g fat (1 g sat, 3 g mono); 0 mg cholesterol; 12 g carbohydrates; 0 g added sugars; 5 g protein; 4 g fiber; 150 mg sodium; 491 mg potassium.

Nutrition Bonus: Vitamin C (30% daily value), Vitamin A (20% dv).
Carbohydrate Servings: 1
Exchanges: 2 vegetable, 1 fat (mono)

Kale with Apples & Mustard

INGREDIENTS
- 1 tablespoon extra-virgin olive oil
- 1-1 1/2 pounds pounds kale, ribs removed, coarsely chopped
- 2/3 cup water
- 2 Granny Smith apples, sliced
- 2 tablespoons cider vinegar
- 4 teaspoons whole-grain mustard
- 2 teaspoons brown sugar
- Pinch of salt

PREPARATION
1. Heat oil in a Dutch oven over medium heat. Add kale and cook, tossing with two large spoons, until bright green, about 1 minute. Add water, cover and cook, stirring occasionally, for 3 minutes. Stir in apples; cover and cook, stirring occasionally, until the kale is tender, 8 to 10 minutes more.
2. Meanwhile, whisk vinegar, mustard, brown sugar and salt in a small bowl. Add the mixture to the kale, increase heat to high and boil, uncovered, until most of the liquid evaporates, 3 to 4 minutes.

TIPS & NOTES
- **Tip:** A 1- to 1 1/2-pound bunch of kale yields 16 to 24 cups of chopped leaves. When preparing kale for this recipe, remove the tough ribs, chop or tear the kale as directed, then wash it—allowing some water to cling to the leaves. The moisture helps steam the kale during the first stages of cooking.

NUTRITION

Per serving: 107 calories; 4 g fat (1 g sat, 3 g mono); 0 mg cholesterol; 18 g carbohydrates; 2 g added sugars; 2 g protein; 3 g fiber; 134 mg sodium; 399 mg potassium.
Nutrition Bonus: Vitamin A (170% daily value), Vitamin C (100% dv).
Carbohydrate Servings: 1
Exchanges: 1/2 fruit, 1 1/2 vegetable, 1 fat (mono)

Salad of Boston Lettuce with Creamy Orange-Shallot Dressing

INGREDIENTS

DRESSING
- 1/4 cup reduced-fat mayonnaise
- 1/2 teaspoon Dijon mustard
- 1/4 cup orange juice
- 2 teaspoons finely chopped shallot
- Freshly ground pepper, to taste

SALAD
- 1 large head Boston lettuce, torn into bite-size pieces (5 cups)
- 1 cup julienned or grated carrot, (1 carrot)
- 1 cup cherry or grape tomatoes, rinsed and cut in half
- 2 tablespoons snipped fresh tarragon, or chives (optional)

PREPARATION
1. To prepare dressing: Whisk mayonnaise and mustard in a small bowl. Slowly whisk in orange juice until smooth. Stir in shallot. Season with pepper.
2. To prepare salad: Divide lettuce among 4 plates and scatter carrot and tomatoes on top. Drizzle the dressing over the salads and sprinkle with tarragon (or chives), if desired. Serve immediately.

NUTRITION
Per serving: 64 calories; 1 g fat (0 g sat, 0 g mono); 0 mg cholesterol; 12 g carbohydrates; 1 g added sugars; 2 g protein; 2 g fiber; 182 mg sodium; 386 mg potassium.
Nutrition Bonus: Vitamin A (120% daily value), Vitamin C (30% dv), Folate (16% dv).
Carbohydrate Servings: 1
Exchanges: 2 vegetable

DAY 14
BREAKFAST

Sunday Sausage Strata
Skim milk (1 cup)
Orange (1 large)
LUNCH

Barbecued Chicken Burritos or Tomato & Smoked Mozzarella Sandwiches
The Diet House Salad
Strawberries (1 cup)
SNACK

Melon (1 cup)

DINNER

Roasted Vegetable Pasta or Chicken & Sweet Potato Stew
Spinach Salad with Black Olive Vinaigrette
Low-fat Vanilla Yogurt (6 oz)

DAY 14 RECIPES

Sunday Sausage Strata

INGREDIENTS
- 1/2 pound turkey breakfast sausage, (four 2-ounce links), casing removed
- 2 medium onions, chopped (2 cups)
- 1 medium red bell pepper, seeded and diced (1 1/2 cups)
- 12 large eggs
- 4 cups 1% milk
- 1 teaspoon salt, or to taste
- Freshly ground pepper, to taste
- 6 cups cubed, whole-wheat country bread, (about 7 slices, crusts removed)
- 1 tablespoon Dijon mustard
- 1 1/2 cups grated Swiss cheese, (4 ounces)

PREPARATION
1. Coat a 9-by-13-inch baking dish (or similar shallow 3-quart baking dish) with cooking spray.
2. Cook sausage in a large nonstick skillet over medium heat, crumbling with a wooden spoon, until lightly browned, 3 to 4 minutes. Transfer to a plate lined with paper towels to drain. Add onions and bell pepper to the pan and cook, stirring often, until softened, 3 to 4 minutes.
3. Whisk eggs, milk, salt and pepper in a large bowl until blended.
4. Spread bread in the prepared baking dish. Scatter the sausage and the onion mixture evenly over the bread. Brush with mustard. Sprinkle with cheese. Pour in the egg mixture. Cover with plastic wrap and refrigerate for at least 2 hours or overnight.
5. Preheat oven to 350 degrees F. Bake the strata, uncovered, until puffed, lightly browned and set in the center, 55 to 65 minutes. Let cool for about 5 minutes before serving hot.

TIPS & NOTES
- **Make Ahead Tip**: Prepare through Step 4 the night before serving.

NUTRITION

Per serving: 255 calories; 13 g fat (45 g sat, 4 g mono); 229 mg cholesterol; 19 g carbohydrates; 17 gprotein; 2 g fiber; 513 mg sodium; 380 mg potassium.
Nutrition Bonus: Vitamin C (72% daily value), Calcium (23% dv).
Carbohydrate Servings: 1
Exchanges: 2/3 starch, 1/3 milk, 1/2 vegetable, 1 very lean protein, 1 1/3 medium-fat protein

Barbecued Chicken Burritos

INGREDIENTS

- 1 2-pound roasted chicken, skin discarded, meat removed from bones and shredded (4 cups)
- 1/2 cup prepared barbecue sauce
- 1 cup canned black beans, rinsed
- 1/2 cup frozen corn, thawed, or canned corn, drained
- 1/4 cup reduced-fat sour cream
- 4 leaves romaine lettuce
- 4 10-inch whole-wheat tortillas
- 2 limes, cut in wedges

PREPARATION

1. Place a large nonstick skillet over medium-high heat. Add chicken, barbecue sauce, beans, corn and sour cream; stir to combine. Cook until hot, 4 to 5 minutes.
2. Assemble the wraps by placing a lettuce leaf in the center of each tortilla and topping with one-fourth of the chicken mixture; roll as you would a burrito. Slice in half diagonally and serve warm, with lime wedges.

TIPS & NOTES

- Eat neat: Keeping the filling inside a wrap or burrito can be a challenge, especially if you're on the go. That's why we recommend wrapping your burrito in foil so you can pick it up and eat it without losing the filling, peeling back the foil as you go.

NUTRITION

Per serving: 404 calories; 8 g fat (2 g sat, 1 g mono); 80 mg cholesterol; 48 g carbohydrates; 32 g protein; 6 g fiber; 600 mg sodium; 531 mg potassium.
Nutrition Bonus: Fiber (24% daily value), Iron (20% dv).
Carbohydrate Servings: 2 1/2
Exchanges: 2 1/2 starch, 1 vegetable, 4 very lean meat

Tomato & Smoked Mozzarella Sandwiches

INGREDIENTS

- 1/3 cup sun-dried tomatoes, (not oil-packed)
- 1 clove garlic, crushed and peeled
- 1/4 teaspoon salt, plus more to taste
- 2 tablespoons extra-virgin olive oil
- 1 tablespoon lemon juice
- 1/8 teaspoon crushed red pepper
- 1/4 cup chopped California Ripe Olives
- 8 slices sourdough bread, preferably whole-grain
- 4 ounces fresh mozzarella, preferably smoked, cut into 1/4-inch-thick slices
- Freshly ground pepper, to taste
- 3 vine-ripened tomatoes, sliced
- 2 teaspoons balsamic vinegar
- 1 cup fresh basil leaves

PREPARATION

1. Place the sun-dried tomatoes in a bowl and cover with boiling water. Let plump for 10 minutes.
2. On a cutting board, mash the garlic and 1/4 teaspoon salt with the side of a knife until it's a smooth paste. Transfer to a bowl and whisk in 1 tablespoon oil, the lemon juice and crushed red pepper.
3. Drain the tomatoes and finely chop. Add to the bowl with the dressing, along with the olives; mix well.
4. Spread the tomato mixture on half the bread. Layer on cheese slices, some pepper, then the tomato slices; season with salt and vinegar. Top with several basil leaves. Brush the remaining 1 tablespoon oil over the remaining bread slices and set them on the sandwiches.

TIPS & NOTES

- **Make Ahead Tip**: Prepare the tomato spread (Steps 1-3); cover and refrigerate for up to 4 days.

NUTRITION

Per serving: 351 calories; 11 g fat (1 g sat, 5 g mono); 5 mg cholesterol; 40 g carbohydrates; 18 g protein; 7 g fiber; 740 mg sodium; 279 mg potassium.
Nutrition Bonus: Vitamin A (36% daily value), Calcium (32% dv), Vitamin C (27% dv), Iron (18% dv)
Carbohydrate Servings: 2
Exchanges: 1 very-lean meat, 2 fat, 1 vegetable, 2 starch

The Diet House Salad

INGREDIENTS
- 4 cups torn green leaf lettuce
- 1 cup sprouts
- 1 cup tomato wedges
- 1 cup peeled, sliced cucumber
- 1 cup shredded carrots
- 1/2 cup chopped radishes
- 1/2 cup Sesame Tamari Vinaigrette (recipe follows), or other dressing

PREPARATION

1. Toss lettuce, sprouts, tomato, cucumber, carrots and radishes in a large bowl with the dressing until the vegetables are coated.

NUTRITION
Per serving: 71 calories; 3 g fat (0 g sat, 1 g mono); 0 mg cholesterol; 11 g carbohydrates; 2 g protein; 3 gfiber; 334 mg sodium; 428 mg potassium.
Nutrition Bonus: Vitamin A (140% daily value), Vitamin C (30% dv), Folate (16% dv).
Carbohydrate Servings: 1
Exchanges: 2 vegetable, 1/2 fat

Roasted Vegetable Pasta

INGREDIENTS
- 1 medium zucchini, diced
- 1 red or yellow bell pepper, seeded and diced
- 1 large onion, thinly sliced
- 2 tablespoons extra-virgin olive oil, divided
- Salt & freshly ground pepper, to taste
- 2 large tomatoes, chopped
- 1/4 cup chopped fresh basil
- 2 cloves garlic, minced
- 12 ounces whole-wheat pasta
- 1/2 cup crumbled feta cheese

PREPARATION

1. Preheat oven to 450°F. Put a large pot of lightly salted water on to boil.
2. Toss zucchini, bell pepper and onion with 1 tablespoon oil in a large roasting pan or a large baking sheet with sides. Season with salt and pepper. Roast the vegetables, stirring every 5 minutes, until tender and browned, 10 to 20 minutes.

3. Meanwhile, combine tomatoes, basil, garlic and the remaining 1 tablespoon oil in a large bowl. Season with salt and pepper.
4. Cook pasta until just tender, 8 to 10 minutes. Drain and transfer to the bowl with the tomatoes. Add the roasted vegetables and toss well. Adjust seasoning with salt and pepper. Serve, passing feta cheese separately.

NUTRITION

Per serving: 288 calories; 12 g fat (4 g sat, 6 g mono); 17 mg cholesterol; 75 g carbohydrates; 17 g protein;6 g fiber; 226 mg sodium; 619 mg potassium.
Nutrition Bonus: Vitamin C (90% daily value), Fiber (34% dv), Vitamin A (25% dv).
Carbohydrate Servings: 2 1/2
Exchanges: 3 starch, 1 vegetable, 1 fat

Chicken & Sweet Potato Stew

INGREDIENTS
- 6 bone-in chicken thighs, skin removed, trimmed of fat
- 2 pounds sweet potatoes, peeled and cut into spears
- 1/2 pound white button mushrooms, thinly sliced
- 6 large shallots, peeled and halved
- 4 cloves garlic, peeled
- 1 cup dry white wine
- 2 teaspoons chopped fresh rosemary, or 1/2 teaspoon dried rosemary, crushed
- 1 teaspoon salt
- 1/2 teaspoon freshly ground pepper
- 1 1/2 tablespoons white-wine vinegar

PREPARATION

1. Place chicken, sweet potatoes, mushrooms, shallots, garlic, wine, rosemary, salt and pepper in a 6-quart slow cooker; stir to combine. Put the lid on and cook on low until the potatoes are tender, about 5 hours. Before serving, remove bones from the chicken, if desired, and stir in vinegar.

TIPS & NOTES
- **Make Ahead Tip:** Cover and refrigerate for up to 3 days or freeze for up to 1 month.
- For easy cleanup, try a slow-cooker liner. These heat-resistant, disposable liners fit neatly inside the insert and help prevent food from sticking to the bottom and sides of your slow cooker.

NUTRITION

Per serving: 285 calories; 6 g fat (2 g sat, 2 g mono); 50 mg cholesterol; 35 g carbohydrates; 0 g added sugars; 17 g protein; 5 g fiber; 519 mg sodium; 866 mg potassium.
Nutrition Bonus: Vitamin A (430% daily value), Potassium (25% dv), Fiber (20% dv).
Carbohydrate Servings: 2
Exchanges: 2 starch, 2 lean meat

Spinach Salad with Black Olive Vinaigrette

INGREDIENTS
- 3 tablespoons extra-virgin olive oil
- 1 1/2 tablespoons red-wine vinegar, or lemon juice
- 6 pitted Kalamata olives, finely chopped
- 1/4 teaspoon salt
- Freshly ground pepper, to taste
- 6 cups torn spinach leaves
- 1/2 cucumber, seeded and sliced
- 1/2 red onion, thinly sliced

PREPARATION
1. Whisk oil, vinegar (or lemon juice) and olives in a salad bowl. Season with salt and pepper. Add spinach, cucumbers and onions; toss well. Serve immediately.

NUTRITION

Per serving: 128 calories; 12 g fat (2 g sat, 9 g mono); 0 mg cholesterol; 3 g carbohydrates; 2 g protein; 1 gfiber; 271 mg sodium; 284 mg potassium.
Nutrition Bonus: Vitamin A (80% daily value), Folate (22% dv), Vitamin C (20% dv).
Exchanges: 1 vegetable, 2 fat

DAY 15
BREAKFAST

Morning Smoothie
Whole-wheat toast (1 slice)
Pear Butter
LUNCH

Romaine Salad with Chicken, Apricots & Mint
Whole-wheat pita bread (1 medium pita)
Raspberries (1 cup)
Skim milk (1 cup)
SNACK

Fat-free cheese (1 slice)
DINNER
Pacific Sole with Oranges & Pecans or Turkey Mushroom Loaves
Steamed Vegetable Ribbons
Rice Pilaf with Lime & Cashews or Mashed Roots with Buttermilk & Chives
Melon (1 cup)

DAY 15 RECIPES

Morning Smoothie

INGREDIENTS
- 1 1/4 cups orange juice, preferably calcium-fortified
- 1 banana
- 1 1/4 cups frozen berries, such as raspberries, blackberries, blueberries and/or strawberries
- 1/2 cup low-fat silken tofu, or low-fat plain yogurt
- 1 tablespoon sugar, or Splenda Granular (optional)

PREPARATION
1. Combine orange juice, banana, berries, tofu (or yogurt) and sugar (or Splenda), if using, in a blender; cover and blend until creamy. Serve immediately.

NUTRITION
Per serving: 139 calories; 2 g fat (0 g sat, 0 g mono); 0 mg cholesterol; 33 g carbohydrates; 0 g added sugars; 4 g protein; 4 g fiber; 19 mg sodium; 421 mg potassium.
Nutrition Bonus: Vitamin C (110% daily value), Fiber (16% dv).
Carbohydrate Servings: 2
Exchanges: 2 fruit, 1/2 low-fat milk

Pear Butter

INGREDIENTS
- 4 ripe but firm Bartlett pears, (1-1 1/4 pounds), peeled, cored and cut into 1-inch chunks
- 3/4 cup pear nectar

PREPARATION
1. Place pears and pear nectar in a heavy medium saucepan; bring to a simmer. Cover and simmer over medium-low heat, stirring occasionally, until the pears are very tender, 30 to 35 minutes. Cooking time will vary depending on the ripeness of the pears.

2. Mash the pears with a potato masher. Cook, uncovered, over medium-low heat, stirring often, until the puree has cooked down to a thick mass (somewhat thicker than applesauce), 20 to 30 minutes. Stir almost constantly toward the end of cooking. Scrape the pear butter into a bowl or storage container and let cool.

TIPS & NOTES
- **Make Ahead Tip**: Store in an airtight container in the refrigerator for up to 2 weeks or freeze for up to 6 months.

NUTRITION
Per tablespoon: 22 calories; 0 g fat (0 g sat, 0 g mono); 0 mg cholesterol; 6 g carbohydrates; 0 g protein; 1 g fiber; 1 mg sodium; 33 mg potassium.
Carbohydrate Servings: 1/2
Exchanges: 1/2 fruit

Romaine Salad with Chicken, Apricots & Mint

INGREDIENTS
MARINADE & DRESSING
- 1/2 cup dried apricots
- 1 cup hot water
- 2 cups loosely packed mint leaves, (about 1 bunch)
- 1 teaspoon freshly grated orange zest
- 1/2 cup orange juice
- 2 tablespoons honey
- 4 teaspoons Dijon mustard
- 4 teaspoons red-wine vinegar
- 1/2 teaspoon salt, or to taste
- Freshly ground pepper, to taste
- 1/4 cup extra-virgin olive oil

SALAD
- 1 pound boneless, skinless chicken breast, trimmed of fat
- 1 large head romaine lettuce, torn into bite-size pieces (10 cups)
- 6 fresh apricots, or plums, pitted and cut into wedges
- 1 cup loosely packed mint leaves, (about 1/2 bunch), roughly chopped
- 1/2 cup sliced almonds, toasted (see Tip)

PREPARATION
1. Preheat grill.
2. To prepare marinade & dressing: Soak dried apricots in hot water for 10 minutes. Drain and transfer apricots to a food processor. Add 2 cups mint, orange zest, orange juice, honey, mustard, vinegar, salt and pepper. Process

until smooth. With the motor running, gradually drizzle in oil. Reserve 1 cup for the dressing.
3. To prepare salad: Transfer the remaining marinade to a large sealable plastic bag. Add chicken, seal and turn to coat. Marinate in the refrigerator for 20 minutes.
4. Lightly oil the grill rack (hold a piece of oil-soaked paper towel with tongs and rub it over the grate). Grill the chicken over medium-high heat until no longer pink in the center, 6 to 8 minutes per side. (Discard the marinade.)
5. Meanwhile, combine lettuce, apricot (or plum) wedges and chopped mint in a large bowl. Add the reserved dressing and toss to coat. Divide the salad among 4 plates. Slice the chicken and arrange over the salads. Sprinkle with almonds and serve.

TIPS & NOTES
- **Make Ahead Tip**: The dressing will keep, covered, in the refrigerator for up to 2 days.
- **Tip**: To toast almonds: Spread on a baking sheet and bake at 350°F until golden brown and fragrant, 5 to 7 minutes. Toasted almonds will keep, tightly covered, at room temperature for up to 1 week.

NUTRITION
Per serving: 456 calories; 20 g fat (3 g sat, 13 g mono); 66 mg cholesterol; 33 g carbohydrates; 34 gprotein; 10 g fiber; 433 mg sodium; 1281 mg potassium.
Nutrition Bonus: Vitamin A (230% daily value), Vitamin C (110% dv), Fiber (41% dv).
Carbohydrate Servings: 2
Exchanges: 1 fruit, 3 vegetable, 4 lean meat, 1fat (mono)

Pacific Sole with Oranges & Pecans

INGREDIENTS
- 1 orange
- 10 ounces Pacific sole, (see Note) or tilapia fillets
- 1/4 teaspoon salt
- 1/4 teaspoon freshly ground pepper
- 2 teaspoons unsalted butter
- 1 medium shallot, minced
- 2 tablespoons white-wine vinegar
- 2 tablespoons chopped pecans, toasted (see Cooking Tip)
- 2 tablespoons chopped fresh dill

PREPARATION
1. Using a sharp paring knife, remove the skin and white pith from orange. Hold the fruit over a medium bowl and cut between the membranes to release individual orange sections into the bowl, collecting any juice as well. Discard membranes, pith and skin.
3. Sprinkle both sides of fillets with salt and pepper. Coat a large nonstick skillet with cooking spray and place over medium heat. Add the fillets and cook 1 minute for sole or 3 minutes for tilapia. Gently flip and cook until the fish is opaque in the center and just cooked through, 1 to 2 minutes for sole or 3 to 5 minutes for tilapia. Divide between 2 serving plates; tent with foil to keep warm.
4. Add butter to the pan and melt over medium heat. Add shallot and cook, stirring, until soft, about 30 seconds. Add vinegar and the orange sections and juice; loosen any browned bits on the bottom of the pan and cook for 30 seconds. Spoon the sauce over the fish and sprinkle each portion with pecans and dill. Serve immediately. Makes 2 servings.

TIPS & NOTES
- **Ingredient Note:** The term "sole" is widely used for many types of flatfish from both the Atlantic and Pacific. Flounder and Atlantic halibut are included in the group that is often identified as sole or grey sole. The best choices are Pacific, Dover or English sole. Other sole and flounder are overfished.
- **Cooking Tip:** To toast chopped nuts or seeds: Cook in a small dry skillet over medium-low heat, stirring constantly, until fragrant and lightly browned, 2 to 4 minutes.

NUTRITION
Per serving: 234 calories; 9 g fat (3 g sat, 3 g mono); 70 mg cholesterol; 11 g carbohydrates; 0 g added sugars; 28 g protein; 2 g fiber; 401 mg sodium; 556 mg potassium.
Nutrition Bonus: Vitamin C (70% daily value); Calcium (20% dv).
Carbohydrate Servings: 1
Exchanges: 1 fruit, 4 very lean meat, 1 fat

Turkey Mushroom Loaves

INGREDIENTS
- 1 tablespoon extra-virgin olive oil
- 2/3 cup finely diced celery
- 1/3 cup finely diced onion
- 12 ounces cremini mushrooms, finely chopped
- 1 large egg, at room temperature, lightly beaten
- 1 1/2 pounds 93%-lean ground turkey

- 1/3 ounce dried porcini mushrooms (1/2 cup), ground to a powder in a spice grinder or a mini food processor
- 1/3 cup dry whole-wheat breadcrumbs, (see Tip)
- 2 tablespoons tomato paste
- 1 tablespoon Worcestershire sauce
- 2 teaspoons fresh thyme or 1 teaspoon dried
- 1/2 teaspoon salt
- 1/2 teaspoon freshly ground pepper

PREPARATION
1. Preheat oven to 375°F. Coat a large rimmed baking sheet or roasting pan with cooking spray.
2. Heat oil in a large skillet over medium heat. Add celery and onion. Cook, stirring often, until softened, 2 to 3 minutes. Add cremini mushrooms. Cook, stirring occasionally, until they give off their moisture and it mostly evaporates, about 5 minutes. Pour into a large bowl; cool for 10 minutes.
3. Stir in egg, turkey, ground porcini, breadcrumbs, tomato paste, Worcestershire sauce, thyme, salt and pepper until well combined, taking care not to overmix. Use a scant 3/4 cup to form an oval loaf about 4 inches long and 21/2 inches wide. Transfer to the prepared pan. Make 5 more loaves with the remaining mixture.
4. Bake the loaves until lightly browned and an instant-read thermometer inserted into the center of one registers 165°F, 35 to 40 minutes. Slice and serve.

TIPS & NOTES
- **Tip:** If you can't find whole-wheat breadcrumbs, you can make your own. Trim crusts from firm sandwich bread. Tear the bread into pieces and process in a food processor until fine crumbs form. One slice makes about 1/3 cup. Spread the breadcrumbs on a baking sheet and bake at 250°F until dry and crispy, about 15 minutes.

NUTRITION

Per serving: 231 calories; 10 g fat (3 g sat, 2 g mono); 100 mg cholesterol; 10 g carbohydrates; 0 g added sugars; 26 g protein; 2 g fiber; 376 mg sodium; 389 mg potassium.
Nutrition Bonus: Selenium (24% daily value), Iron (15% dv).
Carbohydrate Servings: 1/2
Exchanges: 1 vegetable, 3 lean meat

Steamed Vegetable Ribbons

INGREDIENTS
- 2 large carrots, peeled
- 3 small zucchini
- 2 teaspoons extra-virgin olive oil
- 2 teaspoons lemon juice, or to taste
- 1/4 teaspoon salt, or to taste
- Freshly ground pepper, to taste

PREPARATION

1. With a swivel vegetable peeler, shave carrots lengthwise into wide ribbons. Repeat with zucchini, shaving long, wide strips from all sides until you reach the seedy core. Discard the core.
2. Bring 2 inches of water to a boil in a large saucepan fitted with a steamer basket. Add the carrots; cover and steam for 2 minutes. Place the zucchini over the carrots; cover and steam until the vegetables are just tender, 2 to 3 minutes more. Transfer the vegetables to a large bowl. Toss with oil, lemon juice, salt and pepper. Serve immediately.

NUTRITION
Per serving: 51 calories; 3 g fat (0 g sat, 2 g mono); 0 mg cholesterol; 7 g carbohydrates; 0 g added sugars;1 g protein; 2 g fiber; 179 mg sodium; 350 mg potassium.
Nutrition Bonus: Vitamin A (90% daily value), Vitamin C (30% dv).
Carbohydrate Servings: 1/2
Exchanges: 11/2 vegetable, 1/2 fat (mono)

Rice Pilaf with Lime & Cashews

INGREDIENTS
- 1 cup basmati rice
- 1 1/2 cups cold water
- 1 tablespoon canola oil
- 1 teaspoon black or yellow mustard seeds
- 2 tablespoons coarsely chopped cashews
- 2-3 tablespoons lime juice
- 2 tablespoons finely chopped fresh cilantro, or 12 fresh kari leaves (see Ingredient Note), chopped
- 2-3 fresh Thai, cayenne or serrano chiles, or 1 jalapeno pepper, seeded and minced
- 1/4 teaspoon turmeric and 1/4 teaspoon salt

PREPARATION
1. Place rice in a medium saucepan with enough water to cover by about 1 inch. Gently swish grains in the pan with your fingertips until the water becomes cloudy; drain. Repeat 3 or 4 times, until the water remains almost clear. Cover with 1 1/2 cups cold water; let soak for 30 minutes.
2. Bring the rice and water to a boil over medium-high heat. Cook, uncovered, stirring occasionally, until most of the liquid evaporates from the surface, 4 to 6 minutes. Cover the pan and reduce the heat to the lowest setting; cook for 5 minutes. Remove from the heat and let sit undisturbed for 5 minutes.
3. Meanwhile, heat oil in a small skillet over medium-high heat; add mustard seeds. When the seeds begin to pop, cover the pan until the popping stops. Reduce heat to medium; add cashews and cook, stirring, until golden brown, 30 seconds to 1 minute. Remove from the heat; add lime juice, cilantro (or kari leaves), chiles (or jalapeno), turmeric and salt. Add the mixture to the cooked rice; mix well. Brown-Rice Variation: If using brown basmati rice, rinse as directed in Step 1 then soak in 2 cups water. In Step 2, bring rice and water to a boil over medium-high heat. Reduce the heat to low, cover and simmer until the water is absorbed and the rice is tender, 25 to 30 minutes. Remove from the heat and let sit for 5 minutes. Proceed with Step 3.

TIPS & NOTES
- **Ingredient Note:** Olive-green kari leaves (also called curry leaves), a distant cousin to the citrus family, have a delicate aroma and flavor and are available in the produce section of Indian grocery stores. They last up to 3 weeks in the refrigerator or in the freezer for up to a month. Do not use the dried (and highly insipid) version of these leaves—substitute cilantro instead.

NUTRITION
Per serving: 161 calories; 4 g fat (1 g sat, 2 g mono); 0 mg cholesterol; 29 g carbohydrates; 3 g protein; 0 gfiber; 101 mg sodium; 36 mg potassium.
Carbohydrate Servings: 2
Exchanges: 1 1/2 starch, 1/2 fat

Mashed Roots with Buttermilk & Chives

INGREDIENTS
- 2 pounds celery root, (celeriac), peeled (see Tip) and cut into 1-inch pieces
- 1 pound rutabaga, peeled (see Tip) and cut into 1-inch pieces
- 1 pound Yukon Gold potatoes, peeled and cut into 1-inch pieces
- 5 cloves garlic, peeled
- 4 tablespoons unsalted butter, divided
- 3/4 cup nonfat buttermilk, (see Tip)

- 1/2 teaspoon salt
- 1/4 teaspoon freshly ground pepper
- 1/4 teaspoon ground nutmeg
- 1/3 cup snipped fresh chives

PREPARATION
1. Bring 1 inch of water to a simmer in a large pan or Dutch oven. Place celery root, rutabaga and potatoes in a large steamer basket over the water, cover and steam over medium-low heat for 20 minutes. Add garlic and continue steaming; checking the water level and replenishing as necessary; until the vegetables are fall-apart tender, 20 minutes more.
2. Remove the vegetables, drain the cooking liquid and return the vegetables to the pan. Add 2 tablespoons butter and mash until chunky-smooth. Gradually stir in buttermilk, salt, pepper and nutmeg.
3. Just before serving, stir in the remaining 2 tablespoons butter and chives.

TIPS & NOTES
- **Make Ahead Tip**: Prepare through Step 2 and refrigerate for up to 2 days. Reheat in a double boiler and stir in the remaining butter and chives (Step 3) just before serving.
- **Tips:** To peel celery root and rutabaga, cut off one end to create a flat surface to keep it steady. Cut off the skin with your knife, following the contour of the root. Or use a vegetable peeler and peel around the root at least three times to ensure all the fibrous skin has been removed.
- **No buttermilk? You can use buttermilk powder prepared according to package directions. Or make "sour milk":** mix 1 tablespoon lemon juice or vinegar to 1 cup milk.

NUTRITION
Per serving: 174 calories; 6 g fat (4 g sat, 2 g mono); 16 mg cholesterol; 26 g carbohydrates; 5 g protein; 4 g fiber; 290 mg sodium; 835 mg potassium.
Nutrition Bonus: Vitamin C (35% daily value), Potassium (22% dv),
Carbohydrate Servings: 1 1/2
Exchanges: 1 starch, 1 vegetable, 1 fat

DAY 16
BREAKFAST

Cocoa-Date Oatmeal
Skim milk (1 cup)
Melon (1 cup, cubes)

LUNCH

Skim milk (1 cup)
Five-Spice Chicken & Orange Salad
Apricot (1 cup, halves)

SNACK

Fat-free cheese (1 slice)
Whole-wheat toast (1 slice)

DINNER

Pork Medallions with a Port-&-Cranberry Pan Sauce or Grilled Sea Scallops with Cilantro & Black Bean Sauce
Quick-cooking barley (1/2 cup)
Roasted Florets
The Diet House Salad
Blueberry Torte or Frozen Raspberry Pie

DAY 16 RECIPES

Cocoa-Date Oatmeal

INGREDIENTS
- 1/4 cup chopped pitted dates, (10-12 dates)
- 1 cup old-fashioned rolled oats
- 2 tablespoons cocoa
- Pinch of salt
- 2 cups water

PREPARATION

1. Combine dates, oats, cocoa and salt in a 1-quart microwavable container. Slowly stir in the water. Partially cover with plastic wrap. Microwave on Medium for 4 or 5 minutes, then stir. Microwave on Medium again for 3 or 4 minutes, then stir. Continue cooking and stirring until the cereal is creamy.

TIPS & NOTES
- **Note:** The cooking times will vary considerably depending on the power of your microwave. New microwaves tend to cook much faster than older models.

NUTRITION
Per serving: 142 calories; 4 g fat (1 g sat, 1 g mono); 0 mg cholesterol; 61 g carbohydrates; 0 g added sugars; 8 g protein; 9 g fiber; 81 mg sodium; 497 mg potassium.
Nutrition Bonus: Fiber (16% daily value).
Carbohydrate Servings: 2
Exchanges: 11/2 starch, 1/2 fruit
Nutrition Note: Chocolate contains compounds called flavonoids, which can function as antioxidants and also seem to keep blood from clotting. Cocoa is unusually rich in two kinds of flavonoids, flavonols and proanthocyanidins, which appear to be especially potent. To get

Five-Spice Chicken & Orange Salad

INGREDIENTS
- 6 teaspoons extra-virgin olive oil, divided
- 1 teaspoon five-spice powder, (see Note)
- 1 teaspoon kosher salt, divided
- 1/2 teaspoon freshly ground pepper, plus more to taste
- 1 pound boneless, skinless chicken breasts, trimmed
- 3 oranges
- 12 cups mixed Asian or salad greens
- 1 red bell pepper, cut into thin strips
- 1/2 cup slivered red onion
- 3 tablespoons cider vinegar
- 1 tablespoon Dijon mustard

PREPARATION

1. Preheat oven to 450°F. Combine 1 teaspoon oil, five-spice powder, 1/2 teaspoon salt and 1/2 teaspoon pepper in a small bowl. Rub the mixture into both sides of the chicken breasts.
2. Heat 1 teaspoon oil in a large ovenproof nonstick skillet over medium-high heat. Add chicken breasts; cook until browned on one side, 3 to 5 minutes. Turn them over and transfer the pan to the oven. Roast until the chicken is just cooked through (an instant-read thermometer inserted into the center should read 165°F), 6 to 8 minutes. Transfer the chicken to a cutting board; let rest for 5 minutes.

3. Meanwhile, peel and segment two of the oranges (see Tip), collecting segments and any juice in a large bowl. (Discard membranes, pith and skin.) Add the greens, bell pepper and onion to the bowl. Zest and juice the remaining orange. Place the zest and juice in a small bowl; whisk in vinegar, mustard, the remaining 4 teaspoons oil, remaining 1/2 teaspoon salt and freshly ground pepper to taste. Pour the dressing over the salad; toss to combine. Slice the chicken and serve on the salad.

TIPS & NOTES
- **Make Ahead Tip**: Prepare through Step 2. Store the chicken in an airtight container in the refrigerator for up to 2 days. Slice and serve chilled.
- **Note:** Often a blend of cinnamon, cloves, fennel seed, star anise and Szechuan peppercorns, five-spice powder was originally considered a cure-all miracle blend encompassing the five elements (sour, bitter, sweet, pungent, salty). Look for it in the supermarket spice section.
- **Tip:** To segment citrus: With a sharp knife, remove the skin and white pith from the fruit. Working over a bowl, cut the segments from their surrounding membranes. Squeeze juice into the bowl before discarding the membranes.

NUTRITION
Per serving: 278 calories; 10 g fat (2 g sat, 6 g mono); 63 mg cholesterol; 23 g carbohydrates; 0 g added sugars; 26 g protein; 7 g fiber; 491 mg sodium; 450 mg potassium.
Nutrition Bonus: Vitamin C (170% daily value), Vitamin A (140% dv), Selenium (30% dv), Iron (15% dv).
Carbohydrate Servings: 1
Exchanges: 1 fruit, 1 1/2 vegetable, 3 lean meat, 1 1/2 fat

Pork Medallions with a Port-&-Cranberry Pan Sauce

INGREDIENTS
- 1/4 cup dried cranberries
- 1/4 cup port
- 1 pound pork tenderloin, trimmed
- Salt & freshly ground pepper to taste
- 1 teaspoon extra-virgin olive oil
- 2 cloves cloves garlic, peeled and halved
- 1 teaspoon balsamic vinegar
- 2 sage leaves
- 1/2 cup reduced-sodium chicken broth

PREPARATION

1. Combine cranberries and port in a small bowl. Set aside. Slice tenderloin into medallions 1 1/2 inches thick. Place between 2 layers of plastic wrap, and pound the medallions with the bottom of a saucepan until they are 1/2 inch thick. Season both sides with salt and pepper.
2. Heat oil in a nonstick skillet over medium-high heat. Sear medallions on one side until golden brown, 2 to 3 minutes. Turn and sear on the other side for 4 to 5 minutes; turn medallions again and continue cooking until golden brown and no longer pink in the center, 2 to 3 minutes. Remove to a serving platter and cover loosely to keep warm.
3. Add garlic to the pan and return to medium-high heat. Cook, stirring, 1 minute. Add port with cranberries, vinegar and sage leaves; cook for 1 minute, scraping skillet for browned bits. Pour in broth, swirl the pan and bring to a boil again. Continue cooking until sauce thickens and is reduced by half, about 3 minutes. Remove the garlic and sage. Season the sauce to taste with salt and pepper. Spoon over the pork and serve.

NUTRITION

Per serving: 194 calories; 5 g fat (2 g sat, 2 g mono); 64 mg cholesterol; 9 g carbohydrates; 0 g added sugars; 23 g protein; 0 g fiber; 137 mg sodium; 370 mg potassium.
Nutrition Bonus: Selenium (55% daily value).
Carbohydrate Servings: 1/2
Exchanges: 1/2 fruit, 4 1/2 lean meat

Grilled Sea Scallops with Cilantro & Black Bean Sauce

INGREDIENTS

- 2 tablespoons fermented black beans (see Note) or 1 tablespoon black bean-garlic sauce (see Note)
- 2 tablespoons canola oil, divided
- 2 large cloves garlic, peeled and finely grated or minced
- 2 tablespoons finely grated fresh ginger
- 1/3 cup Shao Hsing rice wine (see Note) or Japanese sake
- 1/4 cup mirin, (see Note)
- 2 teaspoons toasted sesame oil
- 1/2 bunch fresh cilantro, stems trimmed, plus sprigs for garnish
- 3 tablespoons lemon juice
- 1 1/2 pounds (24-30) large dry sea scallops, (see Note)
- 1/4 teaspoon freshly ground pepper, or to taste

PREPARATION

1. If using fermented black beans, place them in a small bowl, cover with water and let stand for 10 minutes. Drain and rinse.
2. Heat 1 tablespoon oil in a large skillet or wok over high heat. Add garlic and ginger and cook, stirring, until light golden and fragrant, 30 to 45 seconds. Add the black beans (or black bean-garlic sauce) and cook, stirring, for 1 minute. Carefully pour in rice wine (or sake), mirin and sesame oil; lower the heat to medium-low and simmer, lightly crushing the black beans, until the liquid is reduced by about half, about 3 minutes. Remove from heat.
3. Preheat grill to high.
4. Put cilantro, lemon juice and the remaining 1 tablespoon oil in a blender; process until smooth. Transfer the marinade to a large bowl, add scallops and gently toss to coat with the marinade. Divide the scallops among 6 skewers, spacing about 1/2 inch apart. Season with pepper. (Discard marinade.) Oil the grill rack (see Tip). Grill the scallops until golden and crisp on the edges and cooked through, 2 to 4 minutes per side. Serve with the black bean sauce and garnish with cilantro sprigs.

TIPS & NOTES

- **Make Ahead Tip**: The sauce (Steps 1-2) will keep for up to 5 days in the refrigerator. | Equipment: Six 10-inch skewers
- **Notes:** Fermented black beans, oxidized soybeans that are salt-dried, have a savory, salty and slightly bitter flavor. They are frequently used in Chinese stir-fries, marinades and sauces. Before using, they should be soaked in water 10-30 minutes to get rid of excess salt. When purchasing fermented black beans, look for shinny and firm beans, rather than dull and dry with salt spots. Once open, store in plastic in the refrigerator for up to 1 year.
- Black bean-garlic sauce, made from pureed salted and fermented black soybeans, is a widely used condiment in Chinese cooking and can be found with the Asian food in most supermarkets.
- Shao hsing (or Shaoxing) is a seasoned rice wine available in many Asian specialty markets and some large supermarkets. Japanese sake or dry sherry are acceptable substitutes.
- Mirin is a low-alcohol rice wine essential to Japanese cooking. Look for it in your supermarket with the Asian or gourmet ingredients. An equal portion of sherry or white wine with a pinch of sugar may be substituted.
- We prefer "dry" sea scallops (not treated with sodium tripolyphosphate, or STP). Scallops treated with STP ("wet" scallops) are mushy, less flavorful and will not brown properly.
- **Tip:** How to oil a grill rack: Oil a folded paper towel, hold it with tongs and rub it over the rack. (Do not use cooking spray on a hot grill.)

NUTRITION

Per serving: 196 calories; 6 g fat (1 g sat, 1 g mono); 37 mg cholesterol; 8 g carbohydrates; 0 g added sugars; 20 g protein; 0 g fiber; 183 mg sodium; 383 mg potassium.
Nutrition Bonus: Selenium (37% daily value), Magnesium (17% dv).
Carbohydrate Servings: 1/2
Exchanges: 1/2 other carbohydrate, 3 very lean meat, 1 fat

Roasted Florets

INGREDIENTS
- 8 cups bite-size cauliflower florets, or broccoli florets (about 1 head), sliced
- 2 tablespoons extra-virgin olive oil
- 1/2 teaspoon salt, or to taste
- Freshly ground pepper, to taste
- Lemon wedges, (optional)

PREPARATION
1. Preheat oven to 450°F. Place florets in a large bowl with oil, salt and pepper and toss to coat. Spread out on a baking sheet. Roast the vegetables, stirring once, until tender-crisp and browned in spots, 15 to 25 minutes. Serve hot or warm with lemon wedges, if desired.

NUTRITION

Per serving (cauliflower): 113 calories; 7 g fat (1 g sat, 5 g mono); 0 mg cholesterol; 7 g carbohydrates; 4 gprotein; 4 g fiber; 327 mg sodium; 433 mg potassium.
Carbohydrate Servings: 1/2
Exchanges: 2 vegetable, 11/2 fat (mono)
Nutrition Note: Per serving (broccoli): 101 calories; 7 g fat (1 g sat, 5 g mono); 0 mg cholesterol; 7 g carbohydrate; 4 g protein; 4 g fiber; 327 mg sodium.

The Diet House Salad

INGREDIENTS
- 4 cups torn green leaf lettuce
- 1 cup sprouts
- 1 cup tomato wedges
- 1 cup peeled, sliced cucumber
- 1 cup shredded carrots
- 1/2 cup chopped radishes
- 1/2 cup Sesame Tamari Vinaigrette (recipe follows), or other dressing

PREPARATION
1. Toss lettuce, sprouts, tomato, cucumber, carrots and radishes in a large bowl with the dressing until the vegetables are coated.

NUTRITION
Per serving: 71 calories; 3 g fat (0 g sat, 1 g mono); 0 mg cholesterol; 11 g carbohydrates; 2 g protein; 3 gfiber; 334 mg sodium; 428 mg potassium.
Nutrition Bonus: Vitamin A (140% daily value), Vitamin C (30% dv), Folate (16% dv).
Carbohydrate Servings: 1
Exchanges: 2 vegetable, 1/2 fat

Blueberry Torte

INGREDIENTS
- 1 1/2 cups all-purpose flour
- 1/2 cup sugar
- 1/2 teaspoon ground cinnamon
- 1 1/2 teaspoons baking powder
- 1/4 teaspoon salt
- 1/4 cup canola oil
- 2 large egg whites, lightly beaten
- 1 tablespoon melted butter
- 2 teaspoons vanilla extract, divided
- 1 large egg
- 2/3 cup low-fat sweetened condensed milk
- 2 tablespoons cornstarch
- 1 1/2 cups cups nonfat plain yogurt
- Grated zest of 1 lemon
- 3 cups blueberries, preferably wild
- Confectioners' sugar for dusting

PREPARATION
1. Preheat oven to 300°F. Coat a 9-inch springform pan or 8-inch square cake pan with cooking spray.
2. Stir together flour, sugar, cinnamon, baking powder and salt in a mixing bowl with a fork. Add oil, egg whites, butter and 1 teaspoon vanilla; mix with a fork or your fingertips until well blended. Press into the bottom of the prepared pan.
3. Whisk together egg, condensed milk and cornstarch in a mixing bowl until smooth. Add yogurt and whisk until smooth. Blend in lemon zest and the remaining 1 teaspoon vanilla. Pour over the crust. Sprinkle blueberries evenly over the top. Bake the torte until the top is just set, 1 1/4 to 1 1/2 hours. (The center will quiver slightly when the pan is gently shaken.) Let cool in the pan on

a rack. Loosen edges and remove the pan's outer ring. Serve warm or chilled, dusted with confectioners' sugar.

NUTRITION
Per serving: 221 calories; 6 g fat (1 g sat, 1 g mono); 23 mg cholesterol; 37 g carbohydrates; 5 g protein; 1 g fiber; 149 mg sodium; 226 mg potassium.
Carbohydrate Servings: 2 1/2
Exchanges: 2 1/2 other carbohydrate, 1 fat

Frozen Raspberry Pie

INGREDIENTS
CRUST
- 32 chocolate wafers, (about 6 1/2 ounces; see Note), plus 1 for garnish
- 1/4 cup confectioners' sugar
- 2 tablespoons canola oil
- 2 tablespoons skim milk
- 1 tablespoon butter

FILLING
- 3 cups raspberries, fresh or frozen (thawed)
- 2 tablespoons lemon juice
- 1/4 teaspoon salt
- 2 large egg whites, at room temperature (see Tip)
- 1/2 cup granulated sugar
- 1/2 teaspoon cream of tartar

PREPARATION
1. Preheat oven to 350°F. Coat a 9-inch pie pan with cooking spray.
2. To prepare crust: Process 32 wafers, confectioners' sugar, oil, milk and butter in a food processor until finely ground. Press the mixture into the bottom and up the sides of the prepared pan, creating an even, dense crust. Bake for 12 minutes. Cool on a wire rack to room temperature, about 1 hour, pressing any puffed parts of the crust back into the pan.
3. To prepare filling: Meanwhile, puree raspberries, lemon juice and salt in a blender or food processor until smooth. Strain through a fine-mesh sieve into a medium bowl, pressing with a rubber spatula to extract the juice; discard seeds.
4. Bring 1 inch of water to a slow simmer in a large saucepan. Combine egg whites, granulated sugar and cream of tartar in a 3-quart stainless-steel bowl. Beat with an electric mixer on medium speed until foamy. Set the bowl over the simmering water and continue to beat on medium speed, moving the mixer around, until the mixture is glossy and thick, about 3 1/2 minutes. Increase the speed to high, and continue beating over the simmering water until very stiff and glossy, about

3 1/2 minutes more (the eggs will be at a safe temperature, 160°F, at this point). Remove from the heat (be careful of the escaping steam) and continue beating on medium speed until room temperature, 3 to 5 minutes.
5. Fold the raspberry puree into the meringue until combined. Pour the raspberry filling into the pie crust; crumble the remaining chocolate wafer over the top. Place the pie on a level surface in your freezer and freeze until solid, at least 6 hours. To serve, let the pie stand at room temperature until softened slightly, about 10 minutes, before slicing.

TIPS & NOTES
- **Make Ahead Tip**: Cover with plastic wrap and store in the freezer for up to 2 weeks.
- **Note:** Look for chocolate wafer cookies without any partially hydrogenated oils. Our two favorites were both from Newman's Own Organics: Tops & Bottoms and Chocolate Alphabet Cookies. Chocolate Snaps from Mi-Del will also work, but the chocolate flavor isn't as rich.
- **Tip:** To get the most volume from beaten eggs, it's best for them to be at room temperature. Either set the eggs out on the counter for 15 minutes or submerge them in their shells in a bowl of lukewarm (not hot) water for 5 minutes.
- Storage smarts: For long-term freezer storage, wrap your food in a layer of plastic wrap followed by a layer of foil. The plastic will help prevent freezer burn while the foil will help keep off-odors from seeping into the food.

NUTRITION
Per serving: 220 calories; 7 g fat (1 g sat, 2 g mono); 4 mg cholesterol; 37 g carbohydrates; 3 g protein; 4 gfiber; 165 mg sodium; 126 mg potassium.
Carbohydrate Servings: 2 1/2
Exchanges: 2 1/2 other carbohydrates, 1 1/2 fat

DAY 17
BREAKFAST
Greek Potato & Feta Omelet
Strawberries (1 cup)
LUNCH
Steak Salad-Stuffed Pockets or Burgers with Caramelized Onions
Skim milk (1 cup)
SNACK
Cucumbers & Cottage Cheese
Nectarine (1 small)
DINNER

Chicken Tabbouleh or Portobello "Philly Cheese Steak" Sandwich
Sliced Tomato Salad
Chocolate Velvet Pudding

DAY 17 RECIPES

Greek Potato & Feta Omelet

INGREDIENTS
- 2 teaspoons extra-virgin olive oil, divided
- 1 cup frozen hash brown potatoes, or cooked potatoes cut into 1/2-inch cubes
- 1/3 cup chopped scallions
- 4 large eggs
- 1/8 teaspoon salt
- Freshly ground pepper to taste
- 1/4 cup crumbled feta cheese

PREPARATION
1. Heat 1 teaspoon oil in a medium nonstick skillet over medium-high heat. Add potatoes and cook, shaking the pan and tossing the potatoes, until golden brown, 4 to 5 minutes. Add scallions and cook for 1 minute longer. Transfer to a plate. Wipe out the pan.
2. Blend eggs, salt and pepper in a medium bowl. Stir in feta and the potato mixture.
3. Preheat broiler. Brush the pan with the remaining 1 teaspoon oil; heat over medium heat. Add the egg mixture and tilt to distribute evenly. Reduce heat to medium-low and cook until the bottom is light golden, lifting the the edges to allow uncooked egg to flow underneath, 3 to 4 minutes. Place the pan under the broiler and cook until the top is set, 1 1/2 to 2 1/2 minutes. Slide the omelet onto a plate and cut into wedges.

NUTRITION
Per serving: 294 calories; 17 g fat (5 g sat, 7 g mono); 380 mg cholesterol; 18 g carbohydrates; 16 gprotein; 3 g fiber; 433 mg sodium; 442 mg potassium.
Nutrition Bonus: Vitamin A (15% daily value), Vitamin C (15% dv).
Carbohydrate Servings: 1
Exchanges: 1 starch; 2 medium-fat meat; 1 1/2 fat (mono)

Steak Salad-Stuffed Pockets

INGREDIENTS
- 1/4 cup lemon juice
- 3 tablespoons extra-virgin olive oil

- 2 teaspoons Dijon mustard
- 1/4 teaspoon salt, or to taste
- Freshly ground pepper, to taste
- 1 pound top round steak, 1 1/2 inches thick, trimmed
- 4 cups romaine lettuce, chopped
- 1 medium cucumber, diced
- 1 large tomato, diced
- 8 4-inch whole-wheat pitas, or four 8-inch pitas, split open (see Tip)

PREPARATION

1. Position rack in upper third of oven; preheat broiler.

2. Whisk lemon juice, oil, mustard, salt and pepper in a large bowl. Place steak in a shallow dish and pour half the dressing over it. Let marinate at room temperature, turning once, for 10 minutes.

3. Meanwhile, prepare the salad by adding lettuce, cucumber and tomato to the remaining dressing in the bowl; toss to coat.

4. Transfer the meat to a broiling pan. Broil for 5 minutes on each side for medium-rare, or until it reaches desired doneness. Transfer to a cutting board, let rest for 3 minutes, then slice thinly against the grain. Mix the meat with the salad and fill each pita. Serve immediately.

TIPS & NOTES

- **Tip:** Warm pitas on the bottom rack of the oven while the steak is broiling.

NUTRITION

Per serving: 408 calories; 16 g fat (3 g sat, 8 g mono); 71 mg cholesterol; 36 g carbohydrates; 0 g added sugars; 32 g protein; 6 g fiber; 534 mg sodium; 774 mg potassium.

Nutrition Bonus: Vitamin A (70% daily value), Selenium (66% dv), Vitamin C (45% dv), Folate (29% dv), Iron (25% dv), Magnesium (20% dv).

Carbohydrate Servings: 2

Exchanges: 2 starch, 1 vegetable, 4 lean meat, 2 fat

Burgers with Caramelized Onions

INGREDIENTS

- 3 tablespoons bulgur
- 1/4 cup boiling water, plus 2 tablespoons water, divided
- 2 teaspoons extra-virgin olive oil
- 2 cups sliced onions
- 1 teaspoon sugar
- 1 teaspoon balsamic vinegar
- 1/4 teaspoon salt, divided
- 8 ounces 92%-lean ground beef
- 1 tablespoon tomato paste, (see Tips for Two)
- 2 tablespoons chopped fresh parsley
- 1/4 teaspoon freshly ground pepper
- 2 whole-wheat hamburger buns, split and toasted
- Lettuce, for garnish

PREPARATION

1. Combine bulgur and 1/4 cup boiling water in a small bowl; let stand until most of the water is absorbed, 20 to 30 minutes.

2. Meanwhile, heat oil in a nonstick skillet over medium-low heat. Add onions and sugar; cook, stirring occasionally, until the onions are very tender and golden, about 15 minutes. Stir in 2 tablespoons water, vinegar and 1/8 teaspoon salt. Keep warm over very low heat, stirring occasionally.

3. Preheat the grill or broiler to high. Combine the bulgur, beef, tomato paste, parsley, the remaining 1/8 teaspoon salt and pepper in a medium bowl; knead thoroughly to combine. Shape into two 3/4-inch-thick patties. Grill or broil on a lightly oiled rack until browned and cooked through, about 5 minutes per side. Place the patties on buns, top with the caramelized onions and garnish with lettuce.

TIPS & NOTES

- **Tips for Two:** Transfer leftover tomato paste to an airtight container and refrigerate for up to 1 week or freeze for up to 3 months. Add to soups, chilis and sauces; stir into rice with oregano and cilantro to serve alongside Mexican dishes.

NUTRITION

Per serving: 403 calories; 15 g fat (5 g sat, 8 g mono); 72 mg cholesterol; 38 g carbohydrates; 30 g protein; 7 g fiber; 644 mg sodium; 714 mg potassium.

Nutrition Bonus: Zinc (47% daily value), Iron (25% dv), Magnesium (23% dv), Potassium (20% dv), Vitamin A & Vitamin C (15% dv).

Carbohydrate Servings: 2

Exchanges: 2 starch, 1 vegetable, 3 lean meat, 1 fat

Cucumbers & Cottage Cheese

INGREDIENTS

- 1/2 cup low-fat cottage cheese
- 1/4 teaspoon spice blend, such as Jane's Krazy Mixed-Up Salt
- 1/2 cucumber, cut into spears

PREPARATION

Sprinkle cottage cheese with spice blend. Dip cucumbers into the cottage cheese.

NUTRITION

Per serving: 104 calories; 1 g fat (1 g sat, 0 g mono); 5 mg cholesterol; 9 g carbohydrates; 15 g protein; 1 g fiber; 599 mg sodium; 318 mg potassium.

Carbohydrate Servings: 1/2

Exchanges: 1 vegetable, 2 very lean meat

Chicken Tabbouleh

INGREDIENTS

- 3 cups water
- 1 cup bulgur
- 3 cups cubed skinless cooked chicken, (1-inch cubes)
- 1 cup chopped fresh parsley
- 1 cup chopped scallions
- 1/3 cup currants
- 1/4 cup frozen orange juice concentrate
- 2 tablespoons lemon juice
- 1 tablespoon extra-virgin olive oil
- 1 teaspoon ground cumin
- 1/4 teaspoon cayenne pepper, or to taste
- 1/4 teaspoon salt
- Freshly ground pepper, to taste

PREPARATION

1. Bring water to a boil in a large saucepan. Add bulgur and remove from the heat. Let stand until most of the water is absorbed, 20 to 30 minutes.

2. Drain bulgur well, squeezing out excess moisture. Transfer to a large bowl. Add chicken, parsley, scallions and currants.

3. Whisk orange juice concentrate, lemon juice, oil, cumin and cayenne in a small bowl until blended. Toss with the bulgur mixture. Season with salt and pepper and serve.

TIPS & NOTES

- **To poach chicken breasts:** Place boneless, skinless chicken breasts in a medium skillet or saucepan and add lightly salted water to cover; bring to a boil. Cover, reduce heat to low and simmer gently until chicken is cooked through and no longer pink in the middle, 10 to 12 minutes.

- **Ingredient note:** Bulgur is made by parboiling, drying and coarsely grinding or cracking wheat berries. Don't confuse bulgur with cracked wheat, which is simply that, cracked wheat. Since the parboiling step is skipped, cracked wheat must be cooked for up to an hour whereas bulgur simply needs a quick soak in hot water for most uses. Look for it in the natural-foods section of large supermarkets, near other grains.

NUTRITION

Per serving: 260 calories; 5 g fat (1 g sat, 3 g mono); 60 mg cholesterol; 31 g carbohydrates; 0 g added sugars; 26 g protein; 6 g fiber; 166 mg sodium; 536 mg potassium.

Nutrition Bonus: Vitamin C (60% daily value), Fiber (24% dv), Potassium (15% dv).

Carbohydrate Servings: 1 1/2

Exchanges: 2 starch, 3 very lean meat

Portobello "Philly Cheese Steak" Sandwich

INGREDIENTS

- 2 teaspoons extra-virgin olive oil
- 1 medium onion, sliced
- 4 large portobello mushrooms, stems and gills removed (see Tip), sliced
- 1 large red bell pepper, thinly sliced
- 2 tablespoons minced fresh oregano, or 2 teaspoons dried
- 1/2 teaspoon freshly ground pepper
- 1 tablespoon all-purpose flour
- 1/4 cup vegetable broth, or reduced-sodium chicken broth

- 1 tablespoon reduced-sodium soy sauce
- 3 ounces thinly sliced reduced-fat provolone cheese
- 4 whole-wheat buns, split and toasted

PREPARATION

1. Heat oil in a large nonstick skillet over medium-high heat. Add onion and cook, stirring often, until soft and beginning to brown, 2 to 3 minutes. Add mushrooms, bell pepper, oregano and pepper and cook, stirring often, until the vegetables are wilted and soft, about 7 minutes.

2. Reduce heat to low; sprinkle the vegetables with flour and stir to coat. Stir in broth and soy sauce; bring to a simmer. Remove from the heat, lay cheese slices on top of the vegetables, cover and let stand until melted, 1 to 2 minutes.

3. Divide the mixture into 4 portions with a spatula, leaving the melted cheese layer on top. Scoop a portion onto each toasted bun and serve immediately.

TIPS & NOTES

- The dark gills found on the underside of a portobello are edible, but if you like you can scrape them off with a spoon.

NUTRITION

Per serving: 268 calories; 10 g fat (4 g sat, 4 g mono); 15 mg cholesterol; 35 g carbohydrates; 13 g protein; 7 g fiber; 561 mg sodium; 704 mg potassium.

Nutrition Bonus: Vitamin C (140% daily value), Selenium (49% dv), Vitamin A (30% dv), Calcium (25% dv), Potassium (20% dv), Magnesium (16% dv).

Carbohydrate Servings: 2

Exchanges: 2 starch, 1 vegetable, 1 high-fat meat

Sliced Tomato Salad

INGREDIENTS

- 4 tomatoes, sliced
- 1/4 cup thinly sliced red onion
- 8 anchovies
- 1/2 teaspoon dried oregano
- Salt & freshly ground pepper, to taste
- 2 tablespoons extra-virgin olive oil
- 1 tablespoon white-wine vinegar

PREPARATION

Arrange tomato slices on a platter. Top with onion, anchovies, oregano, salt and pepper. Drizzle with oil and vinegar.

NUTRITION

Per serving: 44 calories; 1 g fat (0 g sat, 0 g mono); 3 mg cholesterol; 8 g carbohydrates; 0 g added sugars; 3 g protein; 2 g fiber; 300 mg sodium; 403 mg potassium.

Nutrition Bonus: Vitamin C (35% daily value), Vitamin A (25% dv).

Carbohydrate Servings: 1/2

Exchanges: 1 vegetable, 1 1/2 fat

Chocolate Velvet Pudding

INGREDIENTS

- 1 large egg
- 1/3 cup nonfat sweetened condensed milk
- 1/4 cup unsweetened cocoa powder
- 2 tablespoons cornstarch
- 1/8 teaspoon salt

- 2 cups low-fat milk
- 1 ounce bittersweet or semisweet (not unsweetened) chocolate, chopped
- 2 teaspoons vanilla extract

PREPARATION

1. Whisk egg, condensed milk, cocoa, cornstarch and salt in a heavy saucepan until smooth. Gradually whisk in milk. Bring to a boil over medium-low heat, whisking constantly, until thickened, 7 to 9 minutes.

2. Remove from the heat; add chocolate and vanilla, whisking until the chocolate melts. Transfer to a bowl. Place plastic wrap directly on the surface to prevent a skin from forming. Serve warm or refrigerate until ready to serve.

NUTRITION

Per serving: 196 calories; 5 g fat (3 g sat, 1 g mono); 64 mg cholesterol; 30 g carbohydrates; 9 g protein; 2 g fiber; 183 mg sodium; 348 mg potassium.

Nutrition Bonus: Calcium (23% daily value).

Carbohydrate Servings: 2

Exchanges: 2 other carbohydrate

DAY 18
BREAKFAST
Overnight Oatmeal
Skim milk (1 cup)
Grapefruit (1/2)
LUNCH
Skim Milk
Grilled Chicken Caesar Salad
Whole-wheat pita bread (1 medium pita)
Nectarine (1 small)
SNACK
Blueberries (1 cup)
DINNER

Chicken-Sausage & Kale Stew or Puerto Rican Fish Stew (Bacalao)
Mexican Coleslaw
Brown rice (1 cup, cooked)
Strawberry Frozen Yogurt or Chocolate Bark with Pistachios & Dried Cherries

DAY 18 RECIPES

Overnight Oatmeal

INGREDIENTS
- 8 cups water
- 2 cups steel-cut oats, (see Ingredient note)
- 1/3 cup dried cranberries
- 1/3 cup dried apricots, chopped
- 1/4 teaspoon salt, or to taste

PREPARATION
1. Combine water, oats, dried cranberries, dried apricots and salt in a 5- or 6-quart slow cooker. Turn heat to low. Put the lid on and cook until the oats are tender and the porridge is creamy, 7 to 8 hours. Stovetop Variation Halve the above recipe to accommodate the size of most double boilers: Combine 4 cups water, 1 cup steel-cut oats, 3 tablespoons dried cranberries, 3 tablespoons dried apricots
and 1/8 teaspoon salt in the top of a double boiler. Cover and cook over boiling water for about 1 1/2 hours, checking the water level in the bottom of the double boiler from time to time.

TIPS & NOTES
- **Ingredient Note:** Steel-cut oats, sometimes labeled "Irish oatmeal," look like small pebbles. They are toasted oat groats—the oat kernel that has been removed from the husk that have been cut in 2 or 3 pieces. Do not substitute regular rolled oats, which have a shorter cooking time, in the slow-cooker oatmeal recipe.
- For easy cleanup, try a slow-cooker liner. These heat-resistant, disposable liners fit neatly inside the insert and help prevent food from sticking to the bottom and sides of your slow cooker.

NUTRITION
Per serving: 193 calories; 3 g fat (0 g sat, 1 g mono); 0 mg cholesterol; 34 g carbohydrates; 0 g added sugars; 6 g protein; 9 g fiber; 77 mg sodium; 195 mg potassium.
Nutrition Bonus: Fiber (36% daily value).

Carbohydrate Servings: 2
Exchanges: 2 starch, 1/2 fruit

Grilled Chicken Caesar Salad

INGREDIENTS
- 1 pound boneless, skinless chicken breasts, trimmed of fat
- 1 teaspoon canola oil
- 1/4 teaspoon salt, or to taste
- Freshly ground pepper, to taste
- 8 cups washed, dried and torn romaine lettuce
- 1 cup fat-free croutons
- 1/2 cup Caesar Salad Dressing, (recipe follows)
- 1/2 cup Parmesan curls, (see Tip)
- Lemon wedges

PREPARATION

1. Prepare a grill or preheat broiler.
2. Rub chicken with oil and season with salt and pepper. Grill or broil chicken until browned and no trace of pink remains in the center, 3 to 4 minutes per side.
3. Combine lettuce and croutons in a large bowl. Toss with Caesar Salad Dressing and divide among 4 plates. Cut chicken into 1/2-inch slices and fan over salad. Top with Parmesan curls. Serve immediately, with lemon wedges.

TIPS & NOTES
- **Tip:** To make parmesan curls, start with a piece of cheese that is at least 4 ounces. Use a swivel-bladed vegetable peeler to shave off curls.

NUTRITION
Per serving: 278 calories; 6 g fat (2 g sat, 2 g mono); 74 mg cholesterol; 14 g carbohydrates; 34 g protein; 1 g fiber; 662 mg sodium; 308 mg potassium.
Carbohydrate Servings: 1
Exchanges: 1/2 starch, 2 vegetable, 4 very lean meat, For Caesar Salad Dressing, free food

Chicken-Sausage & Kale Stew

INGREDIENTS
- 1 tablespoon extra-virgin olive oil
- 1 large onion, diced
- 4 cups kale, torn into bite-size pieces and rinsed
- 2 14-ounce cans reduced-sodium chicken broth
- 4 plum tomatoes, chopped

- 2 cups diced cooked potatoes, (see Note), preferably red-skinned
- 1 teaspoon chopped fresh rosemary
- 1/2 teaspoon freshly ground pepper
- 1 12-ounce package cooked chicken sausages, halved lengthwise and sliced
- 1 tablespoon cider vinegar

PREPARATION

1. Heat oil in a Dutch oven over medium-high heat. Add onion and kale and cook, stirring often, until the onion starts to soften, 5 to 7 minutes.
2. Stir in broth, tomatoes, potatoes, rosemary and pepper. Cover, increase heat to high and bring to a boil, stirring occasionally. Reduce heat and simmer, covered, until the vegetables are just tender, about 15 minutes. Stir in sausage and vinegar and continue to cook, stirring often, until heated through, about 2 minutes more.

TIPS & NOTES

- **Make Ahead Tip**: Cover and refrigerate for up to 2 days.
- **Note:** Convenient cooked and diced potatoes can be found in the refrigerated section of the produce and/or dairy department of the supermarket.

NUTRITION

Per serving: 214 calories; 7 g fat (1 g sat, 2 g mono); 40 mg cholesterol; 25 g carbohydrates; 0 g added sugars; 14 g protein; 3 g fiber; 346 mg sodium; 689 mg potassium.
Nutrition Bonus: Vitamin A (140% daily value), Vitamin C (120% dv), Potassium (20% dv).
Carbohydrate Servings: 2
Exchanges: 1 1/2 starch, 1 vegetable, 2 lean meat

Puerto Rican Fish Stew (Bacalao)

INGREDIENTS

- 2 tablespoons extra-virgin olive oil
- 1 medium onion, chopped
- 4 cloves garlic, minced
- 1 pound flaky white fish, such as haddock, tilapia or cod (see Tip), cut into 1 1/2-inch pieces
- 1 14-ounce can diced tomatoes
- 1 Anaheim or poblano chile pepper, chopped
- 1/4 cup packed chopped fresh cilantro
- 2 tablespoons sliced pimento-stuffed green olives
- 1 tablespoon capers, rinsed

- 1 teaspoon dried oregano
- 1/2 teaspoon salt
- 1/2 cup water, as needed
- 1 avocado, chopped (optional)

PREPARATION
1. Heat oil in a large high-sided skillet or Dutch oven over medium heat. Add onion and cook, stirring occasionally, until softened, about 2 minutes. Add garlic and cook, stirring, for 1 minute.
2. Add fish, tomatoes and their juices, chile pepper, cilantro, olives, capers, oregano and salt; stir to combine. Add up to 1/2 cup water if the mixture seems dry. Cover and simmer for 20 minutes. Remove from the heat. Serve warm or at room temperature, garnished with avocado (if using).

TIPS & NOTES
- **Tip:** Opt for firmer hook-and-line-caught haddock or U.S.-farmed tilapia. Cod also works, but will be more flaky. For more information about sustainable seafood visit Monterey Bay Aquarium Seafood Watch at seafoodwatch.org.

NUTRITION
Per serving: 215 calories; 8 g fat (1 g sat, 6 g mono); 65 mg cholesterol; 9 g carbohydrates; 23 g protein; 2 g fiber; 697 mg sodium; 475 mg potassium.
Nutrition Bonus: Vitamin C (70% daily value), Iron & Vitamin A (15% dv).
Carbohydrate Servings: 1/2
Exchanges: 1 vegetable, 3 lean meat

Mexican Coleslaw

INGREDIENTS
- 6 cups very thinly sliced green cabbage, (about 1/2 head) (see Tip)
- 1 1/2 cups peeled and grated carrots, (2-3 medium)
- 1/3 cup chopped cilantro
- 1/4 cup rice vinegar
- 2 tablespoons extra-virgin olive oil
- 1/4 teaspoon salt

PREPARATION

1. Place cabbage and carrots in a colander; rinse thoroughly with cold water to crisp. Let drain for 5 minutes.
2. Meanwhile, whisk cilantro, vinegar, oil and salt in a large bowl. Add cabbage and carrots; toss well to coat.

TIPS & NOTES

- **Make Ahead Tip**: Cover and refrigerate for up to 1 day. Toss again to refresh just before serving.
- **Tip:** To make this coleslaw even faster, use a coleslaw mix containing cabbage and carrots from the produce section of the supermarket.

NUTRITION

Per serving: 53 calories; 4 g fat (1 g sat, 3 g mono); 0 mg cholesterol; 5 g carbohydrates; 0 g added sugars;1 g protein; 2 g fiber; 97 mg sodium; 199 mg potassium.
Nutrition Bonus: Vitamin A (50% daily value), Vitamin C (30% dv), phytochemicals sulforaphane and indoles.
Exchanges: 1 vegetable, 1/2 fat (mono

Strawberry Frozen Yogurt

INGREDIENTS

- 4 cups strawberries, hulled
- 1/3 cup sugar
- 2 tablespoons orange juice
- 1/2 cup nonfat or low-fat plain yogurt

PREPARATION

1. Place berries in a food processor and process until smooth, scraping down the sides as necessary. Add sugar and orange juice; process for a few seconds. Add yogurt and pulse several times until
blended. Transfer to a bowl. Cover and refrigerate until chilled, about 1 hour or overnight.

2. Pour the strawberry mixture into an ice cream maker and freeze according to manufacturer's directions. Serve immediately or transfer to a storage container and let harden in the freezer for 1 to 1 1/2 hours. Serve in chilled dishes.

TIPS & NOTES

- **Make Ahead Tip**: Freeze for up to 1 week. Let soften in the refrigerator for 1/2 hour before serving. | Equipment: Ice cream maker

NUTRITION

Per serving: 82 calories; 0 g fat (0 g sat, 0 g mono); 0 mg cholesterol; 20 g carbohydrates; 1 g protein; 2 gfiber; 12 mg sodium; 170 mg potassium.
Nutrition Bonus: Vitamin C (100% daily value).

Carbohydrate Servings: 1
Exchanges: 1 fruit

Chocolate Bark with Pistachios & Dried Cherries

INGREDIENTS
- 3/4 cup roasted, shelled pistachios, (3 ounces), coarsely chopped
- 3/4 cup dried cherries, or dried cranberries
- 1 teaspoon freshly grated orange zest
- 24 ounces bittersweet chocolate, finely chopped, divided

PREPARATION
1. Line the bottom and sides of a jelly-roll pan or baking sheet with foil. (Take care to avoid wrinkles.) Toss pistachios with cherries (or cranberries) in a medium bowl. Divide the mixture in half; stir orange zest into 1 portion.
2. Melt 18 ounces chocolate in a double boiler over hot water. (Alternatively, microwave on low in 30-second bursts.) Stir often with a rubber spatula so it melts evenly.
3. Remove the top pan and wipe dry (or remove the bowl from the microwave). Stir in the remaining 6 ounces chocolate, in 2 additions, until thoroughly melted and smooth.
4. Add the pistachio mixture containing the orange zest to the chocolate; stir to mix well. Working quickly, scrape the chocolate onto the prepared pan, spreading it to an even 1/4-inch thickness with a rubber spatula. Sprinkle the remaining pistachio mixture on top; gently press it into the chocolate with your fingertips. Refrigerate, uncovered, just until set, about 20 minutes.
5. Invert the pan onto a large cutting board. Remove the pan and peel off the foil. Using the tip of a sharp knife, score the chocolate lengthwise with 6 parallel lines. Break bark along the score lines. Break the strips of bark into 2- to 3-inch chunks.

TIPS & NOTES
- **Make Ahead Tip**: Store in an airtight container in the refrigerator for up to 2 weeks.

NUTRITION
Per piece: 79 calories; 5 g fat (2 g sat, 0 g mono); 0 mg cholesterol; 11 g carbohydrates; 1 g protein; 2 gfiber; 0 mg sodium; 26 mg potassium.
Carbohydrate Servings: 1
Exchanges: 1/2 fruit, 1 fat

DAY 19
BREAKFAST

Tofu Scrambled Egg
Salsa Cornbread
Strawberries (1 cup)

LUNCH

Turkey & Balsamic Onion Quesadillas or Arugula & Chicken Sausage Bread Pudding
The Diet House Salad
Melon (1 cup, cubes)

SNACK

Low-fat vanilla yogurt (8 oz.)

DINNER

Salmon on a Bed of Lentils or Scallop Piccata on Angel Hair
Sesame Green Beans
Plum Fool

DAY 19 RECIPES

Tofu Scrambled Egg

INGREDIENTS
- 1 large egg and 1/2 teaspoon dried tarragon
- Dash of hot sauce, such as
- Pinch of salt
- Freshly ground pepper, to taste
- 1 teaspoon extra-virgin olive oil, or canola oil
- 2 tablespoons crumbled tofu, (silken or regular)

PREPARATION
1. Blend egg, tarragon, hot sauce, salt and pepper in a small bowl with a fork. Heat oil in a small nonstick skillet over medium-low heat. Add tofu and cook, stirring, until warmed through, 20 to 30 seconds. Add egg mixture and stir until the egg is set, but still creamy, 20 to 30 seconds. Serve immediately.

NUTRITION

Per serving: 140 calories; 11 g fat (2 g sat, 6 g mono); 212 mg cholesterol; 2 g carbohydrates; 0 g added sugars; 9 g protein; 1 g fiber; 230 mg sodium; 93 mg potassium.
Nutrition Bonus: Selenium (23% daily value).
Exchanges: 1 medium-fat meat. 1 fat (mono)

Salsa Cornbread

INGREDIENTS
- 1 cup all-purpose flour
- 1/2 cup whole-wheat flour
- 1/2 cup cornmeal
- 2 teaspoons baking powder
- 1/2 teaspoon salt
- Freshly ground pepper, to taste
- 3 large eggs, lightly beaten
- 1/2 cup buttermilk, or equivalent buttermilk powder
- 1 tablespoon butter, melted
- 1 tablespoon honey
- 1/2 cup drained canned corn kernels
- 1 small onion, diced
- 1/2 cup chopped tomato
- 1 clove garlic, minced
- 1 jalapeno pepper, seeded and minced
- 1/2 cup grated Cheddar cheese

PREPARATION
1. Preheat oven to 425° F. Place a 9-inch cast-iron skillet (or similar ovenproof skillet, see Tip) in the oven to heat.
2. Whisk all-purpose flour, whole-wheat flour, cornmeal, baking powder, salt and pepper in a large mixing bowl.
3. Whisk eggs, buttermilk, butter and honey in a medium bowl. Add the egg mixture to the dry ingredients; mix with a rubber spatula. Stir in corn, onion, tomato, garlic and jalapeno.
4. Remove the skillet from the oven and coat it with cooking spray. Pour in the batter, spreading evenly. Sprinkle cheese over the top.
Bake the cornbread until golden brown and a knife inserted into the center comes out clean, 20 to 25 minutes. Serve warm.

TIPS & NOTES
- **Tip:** If you do not have an ovenproof skillet of the correct size, use an 8-by-8-inch glass baking dish. Do not preheat the empty baking dish in the oven before filling it.

NUTRITION
Per serving: 138 calories; 4 g fat (2 g sat, 1 g mono); 70 mg cholesterol; 20 g carbohydrates; 6 g protein; 1 g fiber; 319 mg sodium; 91 mg potassium.
Carbohydrate Servings: 1
Exchanges: 1 starch, 1 fat

Turkey & Balsamic Onion Quesadillas

INGREDIENTS
- 1 small red onion, thinly sliced
- 1/4 cup balsamic vinegar
- 4 10-inch whole-wheat tortillas
- 1 cup shredded sharp Cheddar cheese
- 8 slices deli turkey, preferably smoked (8 ounces)

PREPARATION
1. Combine onion and vinegar in a bowl; let marinate for 5 minutes. Drain, reserving the vinegar for another use, such as salad dressing.
2. Warm 2 tortillas in a large nonstick skillet over medium-high heat for about 45 seconds, then flip. Pull the tortillas up the edges of the pan so they are no longer overlapping. Working on one half of each tortilla, sprinkle one-fourth of the cheese, cover with 2 slices of turkey and top with one-fourth of the onion. Fold the tortillas in half, flatten gently with a spatula and cook until the cheese starts to melt, about 2 minutes. Flip and cook until the second side is golden, 1 to 2 minutes more. Transfer to a plate and cover to keep warm. Make 2 more quesadillas with the remaining ingredients.

NUTRITION
Per serving: 328 calories; 12 g fat (6 g sat, 0 g mono); 56 mg cholesterol; 30 g carbohydrates; 24 g protein; 2 g fiber; 871 mg sodium; 33 mg potassium.
Nutrition Bonus: Calcium (30% daily value).
Carbohydrate Servings: 1 1/2
Exchanges: 1 1/2 starch, 3 lean meat

Arugula & Chicken Sausage Bread Pudding

INGREDIENTS
CUSTARD
- 4 large egg whites
- 4 large eggs
- 1 cup skim milk

SEASONINGS
- 2 tablespoons Dijon mustard
- 1/4 teaspoon salt
- 1/4 teaspoon freshly ground pepper
- 1/2 cup sliced fresh basil

BREAD & FILLING
- 4 cups whole-grain bread, crusts removed if desired, cut into 1-inch cubes (about 1/2 pound, 4-6 slices)

- 5 cups chopped arugula, wilted (see Tip)
- 3/4 cup chopped artichoke hearts, frozen (thawed) or canned
- 1 cup diced cooked chicken sausage, (5 ounces)

TOPPING
- 3/4 cup shredded fontina cheese

PREPARATION
1. Preheat oven to 375 degrees F. Coat an 11-by-7-inch glass baking dish or a 2-quart casserole with cooking spray.
2. To prepare custard: Whisk egg whites, eggs and milk in a medium bowl. Add mustard, salt, pepper and basil: whisk to combine.
3. Toss bread, arugula, artichokes and sausage in a large bowl. Add the custard and toss well to coat. Transfer to the prepared baking dish and push down to compact. Cover with foil.
4. Bake until the custard has set, 40 to 45 minutes. Uncover, sprinkle with cheese and continue baking until the pudding is puffed and golden on top, 15 to 20 minutes more. Transfer to a wire rack and cool for 15 to 20 minutes before serving.

TIPS & NOTES
- **Make Ahead Tip**: Prepare the pudding through Step 3; refrigerate overnight. Let stand at room temperature while the oven preheats. Bake as directed in Step 4.
- **Tip:** To wilt greens, rinse greens thoroughly in cool water. Transfer them to a large microwave-safe bowl. Cover with plastic wrap and punch several holes in the wrap. Microwave on high until wilted, 2 to 3 minutes. Squeeze out any excess moisture from the greens before adding them to the recipe.

NUTRITION
Per serving: 272 calories; 11 g fat (4 g sat, 3 g mono); 174 mg cholesterol; 24 g carbohydrates; 20 gprotein; 5 g fiber; 696 mg sodium; 435 mg potassium.
Nutrition Bonus: Folate (29% daily value), Calcium & Vitamin A (25% dv), Iron & Vitamin C (15% dv).
Carbohydrate Servings: 1
Exchanges: 1 starch, 1 vegetable, 2 medium-fat meat

The Diet House Salad

INGREDIENTS
- 4 cups torn green leaf lettuce
- 1 cup sprouts
- 1 cup tomato wedges
- 1 cup peeled, sliced cucumber
- 1 cup shredded carrots

- 1/2 cup chopped radishes
- 1/2 cup Sesame Tamari Vinaigrette (recipe follows), or other dressing

PREPARATION

1. Toss lettuce, sprouts, tomato, cucumber, carrots and radishes in a large bowl with the dressing until the vegetables are coated.

NUTRITION

Per serving: 71 calories; 3 g fat (0 g sat, 1 g mono); 0 mg cholesterol; 11 g carbohydrates; 2 g protein; 3 gfiber; 334 mg sodium; 428 mg potassium.
Nutrition Bonus: Vitamin A (140% daily value), Vitamin C (30% dv), Folate (16% dv).
Carbohydrate Servings: 1
Exchanges: 2 vegetable, 1/2 fat

Salmon on a Bed of Lentils

INGREDIENTS
- 2 teaspoons extra-virgin olive oil
- 1 tablespoon finely chopped shallots
- 2 teaspoons minced garlic
- 2 1/2 cups reduced-sodium chicken broth
- 1 cup green or brown lentils, rinsed
- 1 small onion, peeled and studded with a clove
- 1 1/2 teaspoons chopped fresh thyme, or 1/2 teaspoon dried
- 1/4 teaspoon salt
- Freshly ground pepper, to taste
- 2 carrots, peeled and finely chopped
- 2 small white turnips, peeled and finely chopped
- 1 pound salmon fillet, skin removed, cut into 4 portions
- 2 tablespoons chopped fresh parsley
- 1 lemon, quartered

PREPARATION
1. Heat oil in a Dutch oven or deep sauté pan over medium heat. Add shallots and garlic and cook, stirring, until softened, about 30 seconds. Add broth, lentils, onion, thyme, salt and pepper. Bring to a boil, reduce heat to low and simmer, covered, until the lentils are tender, 25 minutes.
2. Add carrots and turnips; simmer until the vegetables are tender, about 10 minutes more. Remove the onion. Add more broth if necessary; the mixture should be slightly soupy. Taste and adjust seasonings. Lay salmon fillets on top, cover the pan and cook until the salmon is opaque in the center, 8 to 10 minutes.
3. Serve in shallow bowls, garnished with parsley and lemon wedges.

NUTRITION
Per serving: 382 calories; 11 g fat (2 g sat, 4 g mono); 65 mg cholesterol; 35 g carbohydrates; 0 g added sugars; 36 g protein; 9 g fiber; 342 mg sodium; 1142 mg potassium.
Nutrition Bonus: Vitamin A (80% daily value), Potassium (56% dv), Fiber (36% dv), Vitamin C(20% dv), Iron (20% dv).
Carbohydrate Servings: 2
Exchanges: 1 1/2 starch, 1 vegetable, 4 lean meat

Scallop Piccata on Angel Hair

INGREDIENTS
- 1 pound dry sea scallops, tough muscle removed (see Ingredient note)
- 1/4 teaspoon kosher salt
- 1/4 teaspoon freshly ground pepper
- 1 tablespoon extra-virgin olive oil
- 8 ounces whole-wheat angel hair pasta
- 1/2 cup white wine
- 1/2 cup clam juice
- 2 teaspoons cornstarch
- 1/4 cup chopped garlic
- 3 tablespoons lemon juice
- 1 tablespoon capers, rinsed and chopped
- 2 teaspoons butter
- 2 tablespoons chopped fresh parsley

PREPARATION
1. Put a large pot of water on to boil.
2. Sprinkle scallops on both sides with salt and pepper. Heat oil in a large nonstick skillet over medium-high heat. Reduce heat to medium and add the scallops; cook, turning once, until browned on both sides, about 6 minutes total. Transfer to a plate.
3. Cook pasta in the boiling water until not quite tender, about 4 minutes. Drain and rinse.
4. Whisk wine, clam juice and cornstarch in a small bowl until smooth.
5. Cook garlic in the pan over medium-high heat, stirring often, until softened, 1 to 2 minutes. Add the wine mixture; bring to a boil and cook until thickened, about 2 minutes. Stir in lemon juice, capers and butter; cook until the butter melts, 1 to 2 minutes.
6. Return the scallops to the pan, add the pasta and cook, stirring gently, until heated through and coated with the sauce, about 1 minute. Stir in parsley and serve immediately.

TIPS & NOTES
- **Ingredient Note:** We prefer cooking with "dry" sea scallops (not treated with sodium tripolyphosphate, or STP). Scallops that have been treated with STP ("wet" scallops) have been subjected to a chemical bath and are not only mushy and less flavorful, but will not brown properly.

NUTRITION
Per serving: 387 calories; 7 g fat (2 g sat, 3 g mono); 42 mg cholesterol; 50 g carbohydrates; 0 g added sugars; 28 g protein; 7 g fiber; 465 mg sodium; 514 mg potassium.
Nutrition Bonus: Selenium (96% daily value), Magnesium (29% dv), Vitamin C (25% dv), Zinc (17% dv).
Carbohydrate Servings: 3
Exchanges: 3 starch, 3 very lean meat, 1 fat

Sesame Green Beans

INGREDIENTS
- 1 pound green beans, trimmed
- 2 teaspoons extra-virgin olive oil
- 2 teaspoons toasted sesame seeds, (see Tip)
- 1 teaspoon sesame oil
- Salt & freshly ground pepper, to taste

PREPARATION

1. Preheat oven to 500°F.
2. Toss green beans with olive oil. Spread in an even layer on a rimmed baking sheet. Roast, turning once halfway through cooking, until tender and beginning to brown, about 10 minutes. Toss with sesame seeds, sesame oil, salt and pepper.

TIPS & NOTES
- **Tip:** To toast sesame seeds: Place in a small dry skillet and cook over medium-low heat, stirring constantly, until fragrant and lightly browned, 2 to 4 minutes.

NUTRITION
Per serving: 67 calories; 4 g fat (1 g sat, 3 g mono); 0 mg cholesterol; 7 g carbohydrates; 0 g added sugars;2 g protein; 4 g fiber; 73 mg sodium; 280 mg potassium.
Nutrition Bonus: Vitamin C (15% daily value).
Carbohydrate Servings: 1/2
Exchanges: 1 vegetable

Plum Fool

INGREDIENTS
- 1 pound plums, pitted and sliced (about 2 1/2 cups)
- 1/4-1/2 cup sugar, or Splenda Granular
- 1/2 teaspoon grated fresh ginger
- 1/2 teaspoon ground cinnamon
- 1 1/2 cups low-fat vanilla yogurt
- 1/3 cup whipping cream

PREPARATION

1. Set aside a few plum slices for garnish. Combine the remaining plum slices, 1/4 cup sugar (or Splenda), ginger and cinnamon in a small heavy saucepan. Bring to a simmer, stirring, over medium heat. Cook until the mixture has softened into a chunky puree, 15
to 20 minutes. Taste and add more sugar (or Splenda), if desired. Transfer to a bowl and chill until cool, about 1 hour.
2. Meanwhile, set a fine-mesh stainless-steel sieve over a bowl. Spoon in yogurt and let drain in the refrigerator until reduced to 1 cup, about 1 hour.
3. Whip cream to soft peaks in a chilled bowl. Gently fold in the drained yogurt with a rubber spatula. Fold this mixture into the fruit puree, leaving distinct swirls. Spoon into 6 dessert dishes and cover with plastic wrap. Refrigerate for at least 1 hour or up to 2 days. Garnish with the reserved plum slices before serving.

NUTRITION
Per serving: 156 calories; 5 g fat (3 g sat, 2 g mono); 18 mg cholesterol; 25 g carbohydrates; 4 g protein; 1 g fiber; 45 mg sodium; 259 mg potassium.
Nutrition Bonus: Calcium (12% daily value), Vitamin C (12% dv).
Carbohydrate Servings: 1 1/2
Exchanges: 11/2 fruit, 1 fat
Nutrition Note: Per serving with Splenda: 1 Carbohydrate Serving, 128 calories, 18 g carbohydrate.

DAY 20
BREAKFAST

Cranberry Muesli
Skim milk (1 cup)
Grapefruit (1/2)

LUNCH

Skim milk (1 cup)
Penne with Braised Squash & Greens or Southwestern Beef & Bean Burger Wraps

SNACK

Banana (1/2 cup, sliced)

DINNER

Pampered Chicken or Seared Scallops with Grapefruit Sauce
Sliced Fennel Salad
Quick-cooking barley (1 cup)
Steamed cauliflower (1/2 cup)
One-Bowl Chocolate Cake

DAY 20 RECIPES

Cranberry Muesli

INGREDIENTS
- 1/2 cup low-fat plain yogurt
- 1/2 cup unsweetened or fruit-juice-sweetened cranberry juice
- 6 tablespoons old-fashioned rolled oats, (not quick-cooking or steel-cut)
- 2 tablespoons dried cranberries
- 1 tablespoon unsalted sunflower seeds
- 1 tablespoon wheat germ
- 2 teaspoons honey
- 1/4 teaspoon vanilla extract
- 1/8 teaspoon salt

PREPARATION
1. Combine yogurt, juice, oats, cranberries, sunflower seeds, wheat germ, honey, vanilla and salt in a medium bowl; cover and refrigerate for at least 8 hours and up to 1 day.

TIPS & NOTES
- **Make Ahead Tip**: Cover and refrigerate for up to 1 day.

NUTRITION
Per serving: 209 calories; 4 g fat (1 g sat, 1 g mono); 4 mg cholesterol; 37 g carbohydrates; 8 g protein; 3 gfiber; 190 mg sodium; 266 mg potassium.
Nutrition Bonus: Calcium (15% daily value)
Carbohydrate Servings: 2 1/2
Exchanges: 1 starch, 1 fruit, 1/2 other carbohydrate, 1/2 fat

Penne with Braised Squash & Greens

INGREDIENTS
- 2 teaspoons extra-virgin olive oil
- 4 ounces cubed smoked tofu
- 1 medium onion, chopped
- 3 cloves garlic, minced
- Pinch of crushed red pepper
- 1 1/2 cups vegetable broth
- 1 pound butternut squash, peeled and cut into 3/4-inch cubes (3 cups)
- 1 small bunch Swiss chard, stems removed, leaves cut into 1-inch pieces
- 8 ounces whole-wheat penne, rigatoni or fusilli
- 1/2 cup freshly grated Parmesan cheese
- 1/4 teaspoon salt, or to taste
- Freshly ground pepper, to taste

PREPARATION
1. Put a large pot of water on to boil for cooking pasta.
2. Heat oil in a large nonstick skillet over medium heat. Add tofu and cook, stirring, until lightly browned, 3 to 5 minutes. Transfer to a plate. Add onion to the pan; cook, stirring often, until softened and golden, 2 to 3 minutes. Add garlic and crushed red pepper; cook, stirring, for 30 seconds. Return the tofu to the pan and add broth and squash; bring to a simmer. Cover and cook for 10 minutes. Add chard and stir to immerse. Cover and cook until the squash and chard are tender, about 5 minutes.
3. Meanwhile, cook pasta until just tender, 8 to 10 minutes or according to package directions. Drain and return to the pot. Add the squash mixture, Parmesan, salt and pepper; toss to coat.

NUTRITION
Per serving: 386 calories; 5 g fat (2 g sat, 1 g mono); 18 mg cholesterol; 63 g carbohydrates; 16 g protein; 9 g fiber; 660 mg sodium; 755 mg potassium.
Nutrition Bonus: Vitamin A (340% daily value), Vitamin C (80% dv), Calcium (25% dv), Potassium (22% dv).
Carbohydrate Servings: 4
Exchanges: 4 starch, 1 vegetable, 1 medium-fat meat, 1/2 fat

Southwestern Beef & Bean Burger Wraps

INGREDIENTS
- 12 ounces 93%-lean ground beef
- 1 cup refried beans
- 1/2 cup chopped fresh cilantro
- 1 tablespoon chopped pickled jalapenos
- 1 avocado, peeled and pitted
- 1/2 cup prepared salsa
- 1/8 teaspoon garlic powder
- 4 whole-wheat tortillas, warmed (see Tip)
- 2 cups shredded romaine lettuce
- 1/2 cup shredded pepper Jack cheese
- 1 lime, cut into 4 wedges

PREPARATION
1. Position oven rack in upper third of oven; preheat broiler. Coat a broiler pan with cooking spray.
2. Gently combine ground beef, beans, cilantro and jalapenos in a medium bowl (do not overmix). Shape into four 5-by-2-inch oblong patties and place on the prepared pan.
3. Broil the patties until an instant-read thermometer inserted into the center reads 165°F, 12 to 14 minutes.
4. Meanwhile, mash together avocado, salsa and garlic powder in a small bowl.
5. Place tortillas on a clean work surface. Spread each with the guacamole, then sprinkle with lettuce and cheese. Top each with a burger and roll into a wrap. Serve immediately, with lime wedges.

TIPS & NOTES
- **Tip:** To warm tortillas: Wrap in foil; bake at 300°F until steaming, about 5 minutes. Or wrap in barely damp paper towels and microwave on High for 30 to 45 seconds.

NUTRITION
Per serving: 455 calories; 20 g fat (6 g sat, 7 g mono); 62 mg cholesterol; 42 g carbohydrates; 28 g protein; 9 g fiber; 716 mg sodium; 749 mg potassium.
Nutrition Bonus: Vitamin C (50% daily value), Vitamin A (45% dv), Fiber & Zinc (40% dv), Folate & Potassium (23% dv), Magnesium (20% dv)
Carbohydrate Servings: 2
Exchanges: 2 1/2 starch, 1 vegetable, 3 lean meat, 1 fat

Pampered Chicken

INGREDIENTS

- 4 boneless, skinless chicken breast halves, (about 1 pound), trimmed of fat
- 4 slices Monterey Jack cheese, (2 ounces)
- 2 egg whites
- 1/3 cup seasoned (Italian-style) breadcrumbs
- 2 tablespoons freshly grated Parmesan cheese
- 2 tablespoons chopped fresh parsley
- 1/4 teaspoon salt, or to taste
- 1/2 teaspoon freshly ground pepper
- 2 teaspoons extra-virgin olive oil
- Lemon wedges, for garnish

PREPARATION

1. Preheat oven to 400°F. Place a chicken breast, skinned-side down, on a cutting board. Keeping the blade of a sharp knife parallel to the board, make a horizontal slit along the thinner, long edge of the breast, cutting nearly through to the opposite side. Open the breast so it forms two flaps, hinged at the center. Place a slice of cheese on one flap, leaving a 1/2-inch border at the edge. Press remaining flap down firmly over the cheese and set aside. Repeat with the remaining breasts.
2. Lightly beat egg whites with a fork in a medium bowl. Mix breadcrumbs, Parmesan, parsley, salt and pepper in a shallow dish. Holding a stuffed breast together firmly, dip it in the egg whites and then roll in the breadcrumbs. Repeat with the remaining breasts.
3. Heat oil in a large ovenproof skillet over medium-high heat. Add the stuffed breasts and cook until browned on one side, about 2 minutes. Turn the breasts over and place the skillet in the oven.
4. Bake the chicken until no longer pink in the center, about 20 minutes. Serve with lemon wedges.

NUTRITION

Per serving: 255 calories; 11 g fat (4 g sat, 4 g mono); 78 mg cholesterol; 7 g carbohydrates; 31 g protein; 1 g fiber; 518 mg sodium; 268 mg potassium.
Nutrition Bonus: Selenium (40% daily value), Calcium (15% dv).
Carbohydrate Servings: 1/2
Exchanges: 1/2 starch, 4 very lean meat, 1 medium-fat meat

Seared Scallops with Grapefruit Sauce

INGREDIENTS
- 1 small pink grapefruit
- 8 ounces dry sea scallops, (see Note)
- 1/8 teaspoon kosher salt
- 1/8 teaspoon freshly ground pepper
- 3 teaspoons canola oil, divided
- 1 shallot, thinly sliced
- 2 tablespoons dry vermouth, or dry white wine
- 1 tablespoon honey
- 1 tablespoon chopped fresh mint

PREPARATION
1. Remove skin and white pith from grapefruit using a sharp knife and discard. Hold the fruit over a bowl and cut between the membrane to release individual sections into the bowl, collecting the juice as well. Squeeze any remaining juice from the membranes into the bowl. Discard the seeds and membranes. Drain the juice into a measuring cup and add water, if necessary, to make 1/4 cup.
2. Sprinkle both sides of scallops with salt and pepper. Heat 2 teaspoons oil in a medium nonstick skillet over medium-high heat. Add the scallops and cook until golden, 3 to 4 minutes per side. Transfer the scallops to a plate and cover with foil to keep warm.
3. Add the remaining 1 teaspoon oil to the pan. Add shallot and cook, stirring often, until softened, about 1 minute. Add the reserved grapefruit juice and vermouth (or wine) and bring to a boil. Boil until reduced by half, about 3 minutes. Reduce heat to low and add honey, the grapefruit sections and mint. Return the scallops to the pan and reheat gently, turning to coat with the sauce.

TIPS & NOTES
- **Note:** Be sure to buy "dry" sea scallops (scallops that have not been treated with sodium tripolyphosphate, or STP). Scallops that have been treated with STP ("wet" scallops) have been subjected to a chemical bath and are not only mushy and less flavorful, but will not brown properly.

NUTRITION
Per serving: 258 calories; 8 g fat (1 g sat, 4 g mono); 37 mg cholesterol; 23 g carbohydrates; 20 g protein; 1 g fiber; 257 mg sodium; 589 mg potassium.
Nutrition Bonus: Vitamin C (70% daily value), Vitamin A (25% dv), Magnesium (20% dv), Potassium (17% dv).
Carbohydrate Servings: 112
Exchanges: 1 fruit, 1/2 other carbohydrates, 3 very lean meat, 1 1/2 fat

Sliced Fennel Salad

INGREDIENTS

- 1 large fennel bulb
- 1 tablespoon extra-virgin olive oil
- 1 tablespoon lemon juice
- 1/8 teaspoon salt
- Freshly ground pepper, to taste

PREPARATION

1. Trim base from fennel bulb. Remove and discard the fennel stalks; reserve some of the feathery leaves for garnish. Pull off and discard any discolored parts from the bulb. Stand the bulb upright and cut vertically into very thin slices. Arrange the slices on 4 salad plates.
2. Whisk oil, lemon juice and salt in a small bowl. Drizzle the mixture over the fennel and garnish with a grinding of pepper and a few fennel leaves.

NUTRITION

Per serving: 51 calories; 4 g fat (0 g sat, 3 g mono); 0 mg cholesterol; 5 g carbohydrates; 0 g added sugars;1 g protein; 2 g fiber; 103 mg sodium; 247 mg potassium.
Nutrition Bonus: Vitamin C (15% daily value).
Exchanges: vegetable, 1 fat (mono)

One-Bowl Chocolate Cake

INGREDIENTS

- 3/4 cup plus 2 tablespoons whole-wheat pastry flour, (see Ingredient Note)
- 1/2 cup granulated sugar
- 1/3 cup unsweetened cocoa powder
- 1 teaspoon baking powder
- 1 teaspoon baking soda
- 1/4 teaspoon salt
- 1/2 cup nonfat buttermilk, (see Tip)
- 1/2 cup packed light brown sugar
- 1 large egg, lightly beaten
- 2 tablespoons canola oil
- 1 teaspoon vanilla extract
- 1/2 cup hot strong black coffee
- Confectioners' sugar, for dusting

PREPARATION
1. Preheat oven to 350°F. Coat a 9-inch round cake pan with cooking spray. Line the pan with a circle of wax paper.
2. Whisk flour, granulated sugar, cocoa, baking powder, baking soda and salt in a large bowl. Add buttermilk, brown sugar, egg, oil and vanilla. Beat with an electric mixer on medium speed for 2 minutes. Add hot coffee and beat to blend. (The batter will be quite thin.) Pour the batter into the prepared pan.
3. Bake the cake until a skewer inserted in the center comes out clean, 30 to 35 minutes. Cool in the pan on a wire rack for 10 minutes; remove from the pan, peel off the wax paper and let cool completely. Dust the top with confectioners' sugar before slicing.

TIPS & NOTES

- **Ingredient Note:** Whole-wheat pastry flour, lower in protein than regular whole-wheat flour, has less gluten-forming potential, making it a better choice for tender baked goods. You can find it in the natural-foods section of large super markets and natural-foods stores. Store in the freezer.
- **Tip:** No buttermilk? You can use buttermilk powder prepared according to package directions. Or make "sour milk": mix 1 tablespoon lemon juice or vinegar to 1 cup milk.

NUTRITION
Per serving: 139 calories; 3 g fat (1 g sat, 2 g mono); 18 mg cholesterol; 26 g carbohydrates; 2 g protein; 2 g fiber; 212 mg sodium; 60 mg potassium.
Carbohydrate Servings: 1 1/2
Exchanges: 1 1/2 other carbohydrate

DAY 21
BREAKFAST
Skim milk (1 cup)
Zucchini-Walnut Loaf
Banana (1 cup, sliced)
LUNCH
Curried Tofu Salad
Whole-wheat pita bread (1 medium pita)
Orange (1 large)
SNACK
Nonfat plain yogurt (8 oz.)
DINNER
Roast Salmon with Salsa or Pan-Roasted Chicken & Gravy

Brown rice (1 cup, cooked)
North African Spiced Carrots
Rainbow Chopped Salad
Frozen Raspberry Mousse or Raspberry-Chocolate Chip Frozen Yogurt

DAY 21 RECIPES

Zucchini-Walnut Loaf

INGREDIENTS

- 3/4 cup whole-wheat flour
- 3/4 cup all-purpose flour
- 1 teaspoon baking powder and 1/4 teaspoon baking soda
- 1/4 teaspoon salt
- 1 teaspoon ground cinnamon
- 1/4 teaspoon ground nutmeg
- 2 large egg whites, at room temperature (see Tip)
- 1 cup sugar, or 1/2 cup
- 1/2 cup unsweetened applesauce
- 2 tablespoons canola oil
- 1/4 teaspoon lemon extract, (optional)
- 1 cup grated zucchini, lightly packed (about 8 ounces)
- 2 tablespoons chopped walnuts

PREPARATION

1. Preheat oven to 350°F. Coat 2 mini 6-by-3-inch loaf pans with cooking spray.
2. Whisk whole-wheat flour, all-purpose flour, baking powder, baking soda, salt, cinnamon and nutmeg in a large bowl.
3. Whisk egg whites, sugar (or Splenda), applesauce, oil and lemon extract (if using) in a medium bowl. Stir in zucchini.
4. Make a well in the dry ingredients; slowly, mix in the zucchini mixture with a rubber spatula. Fold in walnuts. Do not overmix. Transfer the batter to the prepared pans.
5. Bake the loaves until a toothpick comes out almost clean, 40 to 45 minutes. Cool in the pan on a wire rack for about 5 minutes, then turn out onto the rack to cool completely.

TIPS & NOTES

- **Tip:** To bring cold eggs to room temperature quickly: Place in a mixing bowl and set it in a larger bowl of warm water for a few minutes; the eggs will beat to a greater volume.

NUTRITION

Per slice: 118 calories; 3 g fat (0 g sat, 1 g mono); 0 mg cholesterol; 22 g carbohydrates; 2 g protein; 1 gfiber; 88 mg sodium; 37 mg potassium.
Carbohydrate Servings: 1 1/2
Exchanges: 1 1/2 starch

Curried Tofu Salad

INGREDIENTS
- 3 tablespoons low-fat plain yogurt
- 2 tablespoons reduced-fat mayonnaise
- 2 tablespoons prepared mango chutney
- 2 teaspoons hot curry powder, preferably Madras
- 1/4 teaspoon salt
- Freshly ground pepper, to taste
- 1 14-ounce package extra-firm water-packed tofu, drained, rinsed and finely crumbled (see Ingredient note)
- 2 stalks celery, diced
- 1 cup red grapes, sliced in half
- 1/2 cup sliced scallions and 1/4 cup chopped walnuts

PREPARATION
1. Whisk yogurt, mayonnaise, chutney, curry powder, salt and pepper in a large bowl. Stir in tofu, celery, grapes, scallions and walnuts.

TIPS & NOTES
- **Make Ahead Tip:** Cover and refrigerate for up to 2 days.
- **Ingredient Note:** We prefer water-packed tofu from the refrigerated section of the supermarket. Crumbling it into uneven pieces creates more surface area, improving the texture and avoiding the blocky look that turns many people away.

NUTRITION
Per serving: 140 calories; 8 g fat (1 g sat, 2 g mono); 2 mg cholesterol; 13 g carbohydrates; 3 g added sugars; 7 g protein; 2 g fiber; 241 mg sodium; 271 mg potassium.
Nutrition Bonus: Calcium (15% daily value).
Carbohydrate Servings: 1
Exchanges: 1 other carb, 1 medium-fat meat

Roast Salmon with Salsa

INGREDIENTS

- 2 medium plum tomatoes, chopped
- 1 small onion, roughly chopped
- 1 clove garlic, peeled and quartered
- 1 fresh jalapeno pepper, seeded and chopped
- 2 teaspoons cider vinegar
- 1 teaspoon chili powder
- 1/2 teaspoon ground cumin
- 1/2 teaspoon salt
- 2-4 dashes hot sauce
- 1 1/2 pounds salmon fillet, skinned and cut into 6 portions

PREPARATION

1. Preheat oven to 400°F.
2. Place tomatoes, onion, garlic, jalapeno, vinegar, chili powder, cumin, salt and hot sauce to taste in a food processor; process until finely diced and uniform.
3. Place salmon in a large roasting pan; spoon the salsa on top. Roast until the salmon is flaky on the outside but still pink inside, about 15 minutes.

NUTRITION

Per serving: 227 calories; 13 g fat (3 g sat, 5 g mono); 65 mg cholesterol; 3 g carbohydrates; 0 g added sugars; 23 g protein; 1 g fiber; 269 mg sodium; 474 mg potassium.
Nutrition Bonus: Good source of omega-3s
Exchanges: 1/2 vegetable, 3.5 lean meat

Pan-Roasted Chicken & Gravy

INGREDIENTS

- 1 large clove garlic, minced
- 1/2 teaspoon kosher salt
- 1/4 teaspoon ground white pepper
- 1 1/2 teaspoons fresh thyme leaves
- 1 3 1/2-pound chicken, giblets removed
- 1 teaspoon peanut or canola oil
- 2 teaspoons butter, softened, divided
- 2 teaspoons all-purpose flour
- 1 1/2 cups reduced-sodium chicken broth
- 1 tablespoon minced fresh flat-leaf parsley, for garnish

PREPARATION
1. Preheat oven to 400°F.
2. Mash garlic and salt into a paste in a small bowl, using the back of a spoon. Stir in pepper and thyme.
3. With a sharp knife, remove any excess fat from chicken. Dry the inside with a paper towel. With your fingers, loosen the skin over the breasts and thighs to make pockets, being careful not to tear the skin. Rub the garlic mixture over the breast and thigh meat.
4. Heat oil and 1 teaspoon butter in a 12-inch cast-iron skillet over medium heat. Add the chicken and cook, turning often, until nicely browned on all sides, about 10 minutes.
5. Transfer the pan to the oven and roast the chicken until the internal temperature in the thickest part of the thigh reaches 165°F, 50 minutes to 1 hour. Transfer the chicken to a clean cutting board; tent with foil.
6. Meanwhile, mash the remaining 1 teaspoon butter and flour in a small bowl until a paste forms. Place the pan (use caution, the handle will be hot) over medium-high heat. Add broth and bring to a simmer, stirring to scrape up any browned bits. Gradually whisk in the butter-flour paste a few bits at a time, until the gravy thickens, about 8 minutes. Remove from the heat and let stand for 5 minutes, allowing any fat to rise to the top. Skim off the fat with a spoon. Carve the chicken and serve with the gravy. Garnish with parsley, if desired.

NUTRITION

Per serving: 223 calories; 10 g fat (3 g sat, 3 g mono); 95 mg cholesterol; 1 g carbohydrates; 0 g added sugars; 31 g protein; 0 g fiber; 216 mg sodium; 253 mg potassium.
Exchanges: 4 lean meats

North African Spiced Carrots

INGREDIENTS
- 1 tablespoon extra-virgin olive oil
- 4 cloves garlic, minced
- 2 teaspoons paprika
- 1 teaspoon ground cumin
- 1 teaspoon ground coriander
- 3 cups sliced carrots, (4 medium-large)
- 1 cup water
- 3 tablespoons lemon juice
- 1/8 teaspoon salt, or to taste
- 1/4 cup chopped fresh parsley

PREPARATION
1. Heat oil in a large nonstick skillet over medium heat. Add garlic, paprika, cumin and coriander; cook, stirring, until fragrant but not browned, about 20 seconds. Add carrots, water, lemon juice and salt; bring to a simmer. Reduce heat to low, cover and cook until almost tender, 5 to 7 minutes. Uncover and simmer, stirring often, until the carrots are just tender and the liquid is syrupy, 2 to 4 minutes. Stir in parsley. Serve hot or at room temperature.

NUTRITION
Per serving: 51 calories; 3 g fat (0 g sat, 2 g mono); 0 mg cholesterol; 7 g carbohydrates; 0 g added sugars;1 g protein; 2 g fiber; 86 mg sodium; 186 mg potassium.
Nutrition Bonus: Vitamin A (210% daily value), Vitamin C (15% dv).
Carbohydrate Servings: 1/2
Exchanges: 1 vegetable, 1/2 fat (mono)

Rainbow Chopped Salad

INGREDIENTS
ORANGE-OREGANO DRESSING
- 1/2 teaspoon orange zest
- 1/2 cup orange juice, preferably freshly squeezed
- 1/4 cup cider vinegar
- 1 tablespoon extra-virgin olive oil
- 2 teaspoons fresh oregano, chopped, or 3/4 teaspoon dried
- 1 teaspoon Dijon mustard
- 1/2 teaspoon salt
- 1/2 teaspoon freshly ground pepper

SALAD
- 1 1/2 cups bell peppers, chopped
- 1 1/2 cups broccoli florets, chopped
- 1 cup shredded carrots
- 1/2 cup radishes, diced
- 1 tablespoon red onion, minced
- 1/2 cup Orange-Oregano Dressing

PREPARATION
1. To prepare dressing: Place orange zest and juice, vinegar, oil, oregano, mustard, salt and pepper in a jar. Cover and shake to combine. (Makes about 1 cup.)
2. To prepare salad: Combine bell peppers, broccoli, carrots, radishes and onion in a medium bowl. Add 1/2 cup of the dressing and toss to coat. Refrigerate until ready to serve. (Refrigerate extra dressing for up to 1 week.)

TIPS & NOTES
- **Make Ahead Tip**: Cover and refrigerate dressing for up to 1 week.

NUTRITION
Per serving: 52 calories; 1 g fat (0 g sat, 1 g mono); 0 mg cholesterol; 9 g carbohydrates; 0 g added sugars;2 g protein; 3 g fiber; 111 mg sodium; 350 mg potassium.
Nutrition Bonus: Vitamin C (173% daily value), Vitamin A (143% dv)
Carbohydrate Servings: 1/2
Exchanges: 1 1/2 vegetable, 1/2 fat

Frozen Raspberry Mousse

INGREDIENTS
- 6 cups fresh raspberries, or two 12-ounce packages unsweetened frozen raspberries, thawed
- 1/4 cup confectioners' sugar, or
- 2 tablespoons orange juice
- 1 teaspoon unflavored gelatin
- 8 teaspoons dried egg whites, (see Ingredient notes), reconstituted in 1/2 cup warm water according to package directions (equivalent to 4 egg whites)
- 2/3 cup sugar
- 1/3 cup whipping cream
- 2 cups fresh raspberries, blueberries, blackberries and/or strawberries for garnish
- Mint sprigs, for garnish

PREPARATION
1. Place a small mixing bowl in the freezer to chill for Step 5.
2. Puree raspberries in a food processor until smooth. Pass through a fine sieve set over a large bowl; discard seeds. Measure out 1 cup raspberry puree, whisk in confectioners' sugar (or Splenda), cover and set aside in the refrigerator for sauce.
3. Place orange juice in a small saucepan. Sprinkle in gelatin. Let soften for 1 minute. Place over low heat and stir until the gelatin has completely dissolved. Let stand for 5 minutes.
4. Meanwhile, beat reconstituted egg whites in a large mixing bowl with an electric mixer until soft peaks form. Gradually add sugar, beating until the meringue is stiff and glossy.
5. Beat cream in the chilled bowl until soft peaks form.
6. Add the melted gelatin to the remaining raspberry puree and whisk until blended. Set the bowl over a bowl of ice water and stir just until the mixture

starts to thicken slightly, 5 to 10 minutes. Add one-fourth of the meringue to the raspberry puree and whisk until blended. Using a whisk, fold in the remaining meringue. With a rubber spatula, fold in the whipped cream. Scrape the mousse into a 6-cup metal bowl (or other decorative mold) or a 9-by-5-inch metal loaf pan. Cover with plastic wrap and foil and freeze until firm, at least 6 hours.

7. To serve, fill a bowl or basin (large enough to hold the mold comfortably) with very hot water. Run a knife around the edges of the mold. Quickly dip the mold in hot water, then invert a serving platter over the top. Grasping the mold and platter, jerk downward several times. If the mousse does not release, dip in hot water again and repeat. Cut the mousse into wedges or slices. Serve with the reserved raspberry sauce and garnish each serving with a scattering of berries and a mint sprig.

TIPS & NOTES
- **Make Ahead Tip**: Cover and freeze for up to 4 days.
- **Substituting with Splenda:** In the test Kitchen, sucralose is the only alternative sweetener we test with when we feel it is appropriate. For nonbaking recipes, we use Splenda Granular (boxed, not in a packet). For baking, we use Splenda Sugar Blend for Baking, a mix of sugar and sucralose. It can be substituted in recipes (1/2 cup of the blend for each 1 cup of sugar) to reduce sugar calories by half while maintaining some of the baking properties of sugar. If you make a similar blend with half sugar and half Splenda Granular, substitute this homemade mixture cup for cup.
- When choosing any low- or no-calorie sweetener, be sure to check the label to make sure it is suitable for your intended use.
- Dried egg whites are pasteurized so this product is a wise choice in dishes that call for an uncooked meringue. They are also convenient in recipes calling for egg whites because there is no waste. Look for brands like Just Whites in the baking or natural-foods section of most supermarkets.
- A stand-up mixer makes beating egg whites easier, but a hand-held electric mixer will work fine.

NUTRITION
Per serving: 168 calories; 4 g fat (2 g sat, 1 g mono); 11 mg cholesterol; 29 g carbohydrates; 3 g protein; 6 g fiber; 33 mg sodium; 184 mg potassium.
Nutrition Bonus: Vitamin C (45% daily value), Fiber (24% dv).
Carbohydrate Servings: 2
Exchanges: 2 fruit, 1 fat

Raspberry-Chocolate Chip Frozen Yogurt

INGREDIENTS

- 3 cups fresh or frozen (not thawed) raspberries
- 2 cups low-fat plain yogurt
- 1/3 cup sugar
- 1 1/2 teaspoons vanilla extract
- 1/2 cup chocolate chips, preferably mini

PREPARATION

1. Place raspberries, yogurt, sugar and vanilla in a food processor and process until smooth.
2. Transfer the mixture to an ice cream maker (or see "No Ice Cream Maker?" below). Freeze according to manufacturer's directions, or until desired consistency. Add chocolate chips during the last 5 minutes of freezing. Transfer to an airtight container and freeze until ready to serve. No Ice Cream Maker? Pour the mixture into a 9-by-13-inch pan and place in the freezer. Stir every few hours, until the mixture is firm along the edges and semi-firm in the center, 2 to 6 hours (using frozen berries will shorten the freezing time). Transfer to a food processor and process until smooth. Transfer to an airtight container, stir in chocolate chips, cover and freeze until ready to serve.

TIPS & NOTES

- **Make Ahead Tip**: Store in an airtight container in the freezer for up to 1 week. Let stand at room temperature for about 30 minutes before serving.

NUTRITION
Per serving: 147 calories; 4 g fat (2 g sat, 1 g mono); 4 mg cholesterol; 25 g carbohydrates; 4 g protein; 4 gfiber; 45 mg sodium; 253 mg potassium.
Nutrition Bonus: Vitamin C (20% daily value), Calcium (15% dv).
Carbohydrate Servings: 1 1/2
Exchanges: 1/2 reduced fat milk, 1 other carbohydrate

DAY 22
BREAKFAST
Oatbran Bagel or Banana-Nut-Chocolate Chip Quick Bread
Skim milk (1 cup)
Vegetable Cream Cheese
LUNCH
Skim milk (1 cup)
Bistro Beef Salad

Toasted Pita Crisps
Apricot (1 cup, halves)

SNACK

Carrot sticks (1 cup)
Fat-free cheese (1 slice)

DINNER

Chicken, Broccoli Rabe & Feta on Toast or Gorgonzola & Prune Stuffed Chicken
Spiced Corn & Rice Pilaf
Apple (1 cup Quartered)

DAY 22 RECIPES

Banana-Nut-Chocolate Chip Quick Bread

INGREDIENTS
- 1 1/2 cups whole-wheat pastry flour, (see Ingredient Note) or whole-wheat flour
- 1 cup all-purpose flour
- 1 1/2 teaspoons baking powder
- 1 teaspoon ground cinnamon
- 1/2 teaspoon baking soda
- 1/4 teaspoon ground nutmeg
- 1/4 teaspoon salt
- 2 large eggs
- 1 cup nonfat buttermilk, (see Tip)
- 2/3 cup brown sugar
- 2 tablespoons butter, melted
- 2 tablespoons canola oil
- 1 teaspoon vanilla extract
- 2 cups diced bananas
- 1/2 cup chopped toasted walnuts, (see Tip), plus more for topping if desired
- 1/2 cup mini chocolate chips

PREPARATION
1. Preheat oven to 400°F for muffins, mini loaves and mini Bundts or 375°F for a large loaf. (See pan options, below.) Coat pan(s) with cooking spray.
2. Whisk whole-wheat flour, all-purpose flour, baking powder, cinnamon, baking soda, nutmeg and salt in a large bowl. Whisk eggs, buttermilk, brown sugar, butter, oil and vanilla in another large bowl until well combined.
3. Make a well in the dry ingredients and stir in the wet ingredients until just combined. Add bananas, walnuts and chocolate chips. Stir just to combine; do not overmix. Transfer the batter to the prepared pan(s). Top with additional walnuts, if desired.

4. Bake until golden brown and a skewer inserted in the center comes out clean, 22 to 25 minutes for muffins or mini Bundts, 35 minutes for mini loaves, 1 hour 10 minutes for a large loaf. Let cool in the pan(s) for 10 minutes, then turn out onto a wire rack. Let muffins and mini Bundts cool for 5 minutes more, mini loaves for 30 minutes, large loaves for 40 minutes. Pan options: 1 large loaf (9-by-5-inch pan) 3 mini loaves (6-by-3-inch pan, 2-cup capacity) 6 mini Bundt cakes (6-cup mini Bundt pan, scant 1-cup capacity per cake) 12 muffins (standard 12-cup, 2 1/2-inch muffin pan)

TIPS & NOTES
- **Make Ahead Tip**: Store, individually wrapped, at room temperature for up to 2 days or in the freezer for up to 1 month.
- **Ingredient note:** Whole-wheat pastry flour, lower in protein than regular whole-wheat flour, has less gluten-forming potential, making it a better choice for tender baked goods. You can find it in the natural-foods section of large super markets and natural-foods stores. Store in the freezer.
- **Tips:** No buttermilk? You can use buttermilk powder prepared according to package directions. Or make "sour milk": mix 1 tablespoon lemon juice or vinegar to 1 cup milk.

- To toast chopped walnuts, place in a small dry skillet and cook over medium-low heat, stirring constantly, until fragrant and lightly browned, 2 to 4 minutes.

NUTRITION
Per serving: 273 calories; 11 g fat (3 g sat, 3 g mono); 41 mg cholesterol; 40 g carbohydrates; 7 g protein; 3 g fiber; 184 mg sodium; 178 mg potassium.
Carbohydrate Servings: 2 1/2
Exchanges: 1 starch, 1 1/2 other carbohydrate, 2 fat

Vegetable Cream Cheese

INGREDIENTS
- 8 ounces light cream cheese
- 1/4 cup chopped scallions
- 1/4 cup finely chopped carrots
- 1/4 cup finely chopped daikon radish
- 2 tablespoons chopped fresh dill
- 1/4 teaspoon freshly ground pepper

PREPARATION
1. Blend all ingredients in a small bowl.

NUTRITION
Per tablespoon: 30 calories; 2 g fat (1 g sat, 1 g mono); 7 mg cholesterol; 2 g carbohydrates; 1 g protein; 1 g fiber; 56 mg sodium; 10 mg potassium.
Exchanges: 1/2 fat

Bistro Beef Salad

INGREDIENTS
- 4 red potatoes, scrubbed and cut into quarters (1 pound)
- Salt, to taste
- 2 tablespoons chopped shallots
- 2 tablespoons white-wine vinegar
- 1 tablespoon Dijon mustard
- 1 tablespoon chopped fresh parsley
- 1 tablespoon chopped fresh tarragon, or 1 teaspoon dried
- 2 tablespoons cold water
- 1 tablespoon extra-virgin olive oil
- Freshly ground black pepper, to taste
- 1 large head red leaf lettuce, torn (8 cups)
- 2 cups red or yellow cherry tomatoes, cut in half
- 12 ounces cooked roast beef, or steak, thinly sliced

PREPARATION
1. Place potatoes in a medium saucepan and cover with lightly salted water by 1 inch. Bring to a boil over medium heat and cook until tender, about 15 minutes.
2. Meanwhile, whisk shallots, vinegar, mustard, parsley, tarragon and water in a small bowl. Slowly whisk in oil. Season with salt and pepper.
3. Drain the potatoes and rinse with cold water. Divide lettuce among 4 plates; arrange the potatoes, tomatoes and beef on top. Drizzle with the dressing and serve.

NUTRITION
Per serving: 355 calories; 15 g fat (5 g sat, 7 g mono); 69 mg cholesterol; 25 g carbohydrates; 28 g protein;3 g fiber; 283 mg sodium; 615 mg potassium.
Nutrition Bonus: Vitamin A (100% daily value), Vitamin C (70% dv), Zinc (44% dv), Selenium (29% dv), Iron (25% dv).
Carbohydrate Servings: 2
Exchanges: 2 starch, 2 vegetable, 3 lean meat, 1 fat

Toasted Pita Crisps

INGREDIENTS
- 4 whole-wheat pita breads
- Olive oil cooking spray, or extra-virgin olive oil

PREPARATION

1. Preheat oven to 425°F.
2. Cut pitas into 4 triangles each. Separate each triangle into 2 halves at the fold. Arrange, rough side up, on a baking sheet. Spritz lightly with cooking spray or brush lightly with oil. Bake until crisp, 8 to 10 minutes.

TIPS & NOTES
- **Make Ahead Tip**: Store in an airtight container at room temperature for up to 1 week or in the freezer for up to 2 months.

NUTRITION
Per crisp: 23 calories; 0 g fat (0 g sat, 0 g mono); 0 mg cholesterol; 4 g carbohydrates; 0 g added sugars; 1 g protein; 1 g fiber; 43 mg sodium; 14 mg potassium.
Exchanges: 1/3 starch

Chicken, Broccoli Rabe & Feta on Toast

INGREDIENTS
- 4 thick slices whole-wheat country bread
- 1 clove garlic, peeled (optional), plus 1/4 cup chopped garlic
- 4 teaspoons extra-virgin olive oil, divided
- 1 pound chicken tenders, cut crosswise into 1/2-inch pieces
- 1 bunch broccoli rabe, stems trimmed, cut into 1-inch pieces, or 2 bunches broccolini, chopped (see Ingredient note)
- 2 cups cherry tomatoes, halved
- 1 tablespoon red-wine vinegar
- 1/8 teaspoon salt
- Freshly ground pepper, to taste
- 3/4 cup crumbled feta cheese

PREPARATION

1. Grill or toast bread. Lightly rub with peeled garlic clove, if desired. Discard the garlic.
2. Heat 2 teaspoons oil in a large nonstick skillet over high heat until shimmering but not smoking. Add chicken; cook, stirring occasionally, until just cooked through and no longer pink in the

middle, 4 to 5 minutes. Transfer the chicken and any juices to a plate; cover to keep warm.
3. Add the remaining 2 teaspoons oil to the pan. Add chopped garlic and cook, stirring constantly, until fragrant but not brown, about 30 seconds. Add broccoli rabe (or broccolini) and cook, stirring often, until bright green and just wilted, 2 to 4 minutes. Stir in tomatoes, vinegar, salt and pepper; cook, stirring occasionally, until the tomatoes are beginning to break down, 2 to 4 minutes. Return the chicken and juices to the pan, add feta cheese and stir to combine. Cook until heated through, 1 to 2 minutes. Serve warm over garlic toasts.

TIPS & NOTES
- **Ingredient Note:** Pleasantly pungent and mildly bitter, broccoli rabe, or rapini, is a member of the cabbage family and commonly used in Mediterranean cooking. Broccolini (a cross between broccoli and Chinese kale) is sweet and tender - the florets and stalks are edible.

NUTRITION
Per serving: 313 calories; 11 g fat (5 g sat, 5 g mono); 85 mg cholesterol; 26 g carbohydrates; 35 g protein; 4 g fiber; 653 mg sodium; 423 mg potassium.
Nutrition Bonus: Vitamin C (160% daily value), Vitamin A (140% dv), Selenium (28% dv), Calcium (20% dv).
Carbohydrate Servings: 2
Exchanges: 1 starch, 2 vegetable, 4 lean meat

Gorgonzola & Prune Stuffed Chicken

INGREDIENTS
- 1/2 cup chopped prunes, divided
- 1/3 cup crumbled Gorgonzola cheese
- 1/4 cup coarse dry whole-wheat breadcrumbs, (see Note)
- 1 teaspoon minced fresh thyme, divided
- 4 boneless, skinless chicken breasts, (1-1 1/4 pounds), trimmed (see Tip)
- 1/2 teaspoon salt
- 1/2 teaspoon freshly ground pepper
- 1 tablespoon plus 1 teaspoon extra-virgin olive oil, divided
- 1 shallot, minced
- 1/2 cup red wine
- 1 cup reduced-sodium chicken broth
- 4 teaspoons all-purpose flour

PREPARATION

1. Combine 1/4 cup prunes, Gorgonzola, breadcrumbs and 1/2 teaspoon thyme in a small bowl. Cut a horizontal slit along the thin edge of each chicken breast, nearly through to the opposite side. Stuff each breast with about 2 1/2 tablespoons filling. Use a couple of toothpicks to seal the opening. Season with salt and pepper.
2. Heat 1 tablespoon oil in a large nonstick skillet over medium-high heat. Add the chicken and cook until golden, about 4 minutes per side. Transfer to a plate.
3. Add the remaining 1 teaspoon oil, shallot and the remaining 1/2 teaspoon thyme to the pan; cook, stirring, until fragrant, about 1 minute. Add wine and the remaining 1/4 cup prunes. Reduce heat to medium; cook, scraping up any browned bits, until most of the wine evaporates, about 2 minutes. Whisk broth and flour in a small bowl until smooth; add to the pan and cook, stirring, until thickened, about 2 minutes.
4. Reduce heat to low, return the chicken and any juices to the pan and turn to coat with sauce. Cover and cook until the chicken is cooked through, 3 to 5 minutes more. Remove toothpicks, slice the chicken and top with the sauce.

TIPS & NOTES

- **Note:** We like Ian's brand of coarse dry whole-wheat breadcrumbs, labeled "Panko breadcrumbs." Find them in the natural-foods section of large supermarkets. Or, make your own breadcrumbs: Trim crusts from firm sandwich bread. Tear the bread into pieces and process in a food processor until coarse crumbs form. One slice makes about 1/3 cup. Spread the breadcrumbs on a baking sheet and bake at 250°F until dry and crisp, about 15 minutes.
- **Tip:** To select chicken breasts: Our recommended serving size is 4-ounces (uncooked), so look for small breasts. If yours are closer to 5 ounces each, remove the tender (about 1 ounce) from the underside to get the correct portion size. Wrap and freeze the leftover tenders; when you have gathered enough, use them in a stir-fry, for chicken fingers or in soups.

NUTRITION

Per serving: 318 calories; 9 g fat (3 g sat, 4 g mono); 75 mg cholesterol; 21 g carbohydrates; 0 g added sugars; 31 g protein; 2 g fiber; 541 mg sodium; 492 mg potassium.
Nutrition Bonus: Selenium (30% daily value).
Carbohydrate Servings: 1 1/2
Exchanges: 1/2 starch, 1 fruit, 4 lean meat

Spiced Corn & Rice Pilaf

INGREDIENTS

- 2 teaspoons extra-virgin olive oil
- 1/4 cup finely chopped onion
- 1 3-inch cinnamon stick
- 3/4 teaspoon cumin seeds
- 1/4 teaspoon ground cardamom
- 1/4 teaspoon salt
- 1 cup brown basmati or long-grain brown rice
- 2 3/4 cups reduced-sodium chicken broth, or vegetable broth
- 2 tablespoons hulled pumpkin seeds
- 1 cup fresh corn kernels, (from 2 ears) or frozen

PREPARATION

1. Heat oil in a large saucepan over medium-high heat. Add onion and cook, stirring often, until lightly browned, about 3 minutes. Add cinnamon stick, cumin seeds, cardamom, salt and rice; cook, stirring often, until spices are fragrant, about 1 minute.
2. Stir in broth and bring to a boil. Reduce heat to low; cover and simmer until the liquid is absorbed and the rice is tender, 35 to 40 minutes.
3. Meanwhile, toast pumpkin seeds in a small dry skillet over medium-low heat, stirring constantly, until fragrant, 1 to 2 minutes. Transfer to a bowl to cool.
4. When the rice is ready, stir in corn, cover and cook until heated through, about 5 minutes. Remove the cinnamon stick. Fluff the pilaf with a fork and fold in the toasted pumpkin seeds.

NUTRITION

Per serving: 129 calories; 3 g fat (1 g sat, 2 g mono); 2 mg cholesterol; 22 g carbohydrates; 0 g added sugars; 4 g protein; 2 g fiber; 126 mg sodium; 80 mg potassium.
Carbohydrate Servings: 1 1/2
Exchanges: 11/2 starch, 1/2 fat (mono)

DAY 23
BREAKFAST

Skim milk (1 cup)
Cereal (dry, 1 cup) and Banana (1 cup, sliced)

LUNCH

Bacony Barley Salad with Marinated Shrimp or Kusa Mihshi
Whole-wheat pita bread (1/2 medium pita)
Apricot (1/2 cup, halves)

SNACK

Low-fat Vanilla Yogurt (6 oz)
Carrot sticks (1/2 Cup)

DINNER

Rosemary & Garlic Crusted Pork Loin with Butternut Squash & Potatoes or Shrimp & Pesto Pasta
Steamed cauliflower (1 cup)
Blueberries with Lemon Cream

DAY 23 RECIPES

Bacony Barley Salad with Marinated Shrimp

INGREDIENTS
- 3 strips bacon, chopped
- 1 1/3 cups water
- 1/2 teaspoon salt
- 2/3 cup quick-cooking barley
- 1 pound peeled cooked shrimp, (21-25 per pound; thawed if frozen), tails removed, coarsely chopped
- 1/3 cup lime juice
- 2 cups cherry tomatoes, halved
- 1/2 cup finely diced red onion
- 1/2 cup chopped fresh cilantro
- 2 tablespoons extra-virgin olive oil
- Freshly ground pepper, to taste
- 1 avocado, peeled and diced

PREPARATION

1. Cook bacon in a small saucepan over medium heat, stirring often, until crispy, about 4 minutes. Drain on paper towel; discard fat.

2. Add water and salt to the pan and bring to a boil. Add barley and return to a simmer. Reduce heat to low, cover and simmer until all the liquid is absorbed, 10 to 12 minutes.
3. Combine shrimp and lime juice in a large bowl. Add the cooked barley; toss to coat. Let stand for 10 minutes, stirring occasionally, to allow the barley to absorb some of the lime juice. Add tomatoes, onion, cilantro and the bacon; toss to coat. Add oil and pepper and toss again. Stir in avocado and serve.

TIPS & NOTES
- **Make Ahead Tip**: Prepare without avocado, cover and refrigerate for up to 2 days. Stir in the avocado just before serving.

NUTRITION
Per serving: 393 calories; 19 g fat (3 g sat, 11 g mono); 235 mg cholesterol; 3 g carbohydrates; 35 gprotein; 7 g fiber; 752 mg sodium; 859 mg potassium.
Nutrition Bonus: Vitamin C (50% daily value), Fiber (29% dv), Iron (25% dv), Folate (15% dv).
Carbohydrate Servings: 1 1/2
Exchanges: 1 starch, 1 vegetable, 4 very lean meat, 3 fat (mono)

Warm Salad with Chicken Paillards & Chèvre

INGREDIENTS
- 12 cups arugula, tough stems removed (about 8 ounces)
- 8 green olives, pitted and quartered
- 8 large dates, pitted and quartered
- 2 oranges, peeled, sectioned and sliced into chunks
- 1 pound boneless, skinless chicken breasts, trimmed of fat
- 1/3 cup seasoned Italian breadcrumbs
- 4 teaspoons extra-virgin olive oil, divided
- 1/4 cup frozen orange juice concentrate, thawed
- 2 tablespoons water
- 2 tablespoons cider vinegar
- 2 tablespoons Dijon mustard
- 1/8 teaspoon salt
- Freshly ground pepper, to taste
- 3 ounces aged or fresh goat cheese, crumbled (see Note)

PREPARATION
1. Place arugula, olives, dates and orange chunks in a large salad bowl.

2. Lay each chicken breast between 2 large pieces of plastic wrap. Gently pound with the smooth side of a meat mallet or a heavy saucepan until 1/4 inch thick. Place breadcrumbs on a large plate and dredge the chicken in them.
3. Heat 2 teaspoons oil in a large nonstick skillet over medium-high heat. Add 2 chicken breasts and cook until golden and just cooked through, about 2 minutes per side. Transfer to a platter, cover and keep warm. Reduce heat to medium, add the remaining 2 teaspoons oil to the pan and repeat with the remaining chicken. Transfer to the platter and cover.
4. Add orange juice concentrate, water and vinegar to the pan. Stir in mustard and let the dressing boil for 30 seconds. Season with salt and pepper. Add half the warm dressing to the salad; gently toss to mix.
5. To serve, cut chicken into thin slices. Top salad with chicken, goat cheese and the remaining dressing.

TIPS & NOTES
- **Note:** Goat cheese, also known as chèvre (French for goat), is earthy-tasting and slightly tart. Fresh goat cheese is creamy and commonly available. Aged goat cheese has a nutty, sharp flavor and is drier and firmer. Look for aged goat cheese in a well-stocked cheese section at larger supermarkets and specialty cheese shops.

NUTRITION
Per serving: 427 calories; 18 g fat (7 g sat, 8 g mono); 85 mg cholesterol; 35 g carbohydrates; 33 g protein;5 g fiber; 657 mg sodium; 792 mg potassium.
Nutrition Bonus: Vitamin C (110% daily value), Vitamin A (40% dv), Calcium (35% dv), Folate (28% dv), Potassium (23% dv).
Carbohydrate Servings: 2
Exchanges: 1.5 fruit, 2 vegetable, 4 very lean meat, 3.5 fat

Rosemary & Garlic Crusted Pork Loin with Butternut Squash & Potatoes
INGREDIENTS
- 3 tablespoons chopped fresh rosemary, or 1 tablespoon dried
- 4 cloves garlic, minced
- 1 teaspoon kosher salt, divided
- 1/2 teaspoon freshly ground pepper, plus more to taste
- 1 2-pound boneless center-cut pork loin roast, trimmed
- 1 1/2 pounds small Yukon Gold potatoes, scrubbed and cut into 1-inch cubes
- 4 teaspoons extra-virgin olive oil, divided
- 1 pound butternut squash, peeled, seeded and cut into 1-inch cubes
- 1/2 cup port, or prune juice
- 1/2 cup reduced-sodium chicken broth

PREPARATION
1. Preheat oven to 400°F.
2. Combine rosemary, garlic, 1/2 teaspoon salt and 1/2 teaspoon pepper in a mortar and crush with the pestle to form a paste. (Alternatively, finely chop the ingredients together on a cutting board.)
3. Coat a large roasting pan with cooking spray. Place pork in the pan and rub the rosemary mixture all over it. Toss potatoes with 2 teaspoons oil and 1/4 teaspoon salt in a medium bowl; scatter along one side of the pork.
4. Roast the pork and potatoes for 30 minutes. Meanwhile, toss squash with the remaining 2 teaspoons oil, 1/4 teaspoon salt and pepper in a medium bowl.
5. Remove the roasting pan from the oven. Carefully turn the pork over. Scatter the squash along the other side of the pork.
6. Roast the pork until an instant-read thermometer inserted in the center registers 155°F, 30 to 40 minutes more. Transfer the pork to a carving board; tent with foil and let stand for 10 to 15 minutes. If the vegetables are tender, transfer them to a bowl, cover and keep them warm. If not, continue roasting until they are browned and tender, 10 to 15 minutes more.
7. After removing the vegetables, place the roasting pan over medium heat and add port (or prune juice); bring to a boil, stirring to scrape up any browned bits. Simmer for 2 minutes. Add broth and bring to a simmer. Simmer for a few minutes to intensify the flavor. Add any juices that have accumulated on the carving board.
8. To serve, cut the strings from the pork and carve. Serve with the roasted vegetables and pan sauce.

TIPS & NOTES
- By placing the potatoes along one side of the roast and the squash along the other, you have the flexibility of removing one of the vegetables if it is done before the other.

NUTRITION
Per serving: 299 calories; 10 g fat (3 g sat, 5 g mono); 63 mg cholesterol; 23 g carbohydrates; 1 g added sugars; 25 g protein; 3 g fiber; 365 mg sodium; 451 mg potassium.
Nutrition Bonus: Vitamin A (110% daily value), Vitamin C (45% dv).
Carbohydrate Servings: 1 1/2
Exchanges: 11/2 starch, 3 lean meat

Chicken Tacos with Charred Tomatoes

INGREDIENTS
- 2 plum tomatoes, cored
- 8 ounces boneless, skinless chicken breast, trimmed of fat

- 1/4 teaspoon salt
- 1/8 teaspoon freshly ground pepper
- 2 teaspoons canola oil, divided
- 1/2 cup finely chopped white onion
- 1 clove garlic, minced
- 1 small jalapeño pepper, seeded and minced
- 2 teaspoons lime juice, plus lime wedges for garnish
- 2 teaspoons chopped fresh cilantro
- 2 scallions, chopped
- 6 small corn tortillas, heated (see Tip)

PREPARATION
1. Heat a medium skillet over high heat until very hot. Add tomatoes and cook, turning occasionally with tongs, until charred on all sides, 8 to 10 minutes. Transfer to a plate to cool slightly. Cut the tomatoes in half crosswise; squeeze to discard seeds. Remove cores and chop the remaining pulp and skin.
2. Cut chicken into 1-inch chunks; sprinkle with salt and pepper. Add 1 teaspoon oil to the pan and heat over high heat until very hot. Add the chicken and cook, stirring occasionally, until it is browned and no longer pink in the middle, 3 to 5 minutes. Transfer to a plate.
3. Reduce the heat to medium and add the remaining 1 teaspoon oil. Add onion and cook, stirring, until softened, about 2 minutes. Add garlic and jalapeño and cook, stirring, until fragrant, about 30 seconds. Add lime juice, the chicken and tomatoes. Cook, stirring, until heated through, 1 to 2 minutes. Stir in cilantro and scallions. Divide the chicken mixture among tortillas. Serve with lime wedges.

TIPS & NOTES
- **Tip:** Wrap tortillas in barely damp paper towels and microwave on High for 30 to 45 seconds.

NUTRITION
Per serving: 297 calories; 9 g fat (1 g sat, 4 g mono); 63 mg cholesterol; 27 g carbohydrates; 0 g added sugars; 27 g protein; 2 g fiber; 415 mg sodium; 463 mg potassium.
Nutrition Bonus: Selenium & Vitamin C (30% daily value), Vitamin A (20% dv).
Carbohydrate Servings: 2
Exchanges: 2 starch, 3 very lean meat, 1 fat

DAY 24
BREAKFAST

Healthy Pancakes
Strawberries (1 cup)
Low-fat vanilla yogurt (8 oz.)

LUNCH

Shrimp & Plum Kebabs or Beef Tataki
Roasted Tomato Soup
Whole-wheat toast (1 slice)
Ginger-Orange Biscotti

SNACK

Banana (1 cup, sliced)

DINNER

Sausage, Mushroom & Spinach Lasagna or Penne with Vodka Sauce & Capicola
Sliced Tomato Salad
Steamed asparagus (1/2 cup)
Apricot (1/2 cup, halves)
Whole-wheat toast (1 slice)

DAY 24 RECIPES

Healthy Pancakes

INGREDIENTS

- 2 1/2 cups whole-wheat flour
- 1 cup buttermilk powder, (see Note)
- 5 tablespoons dried egg whites, such as Just Whites (see Note)
- 1/4 cup sugar
- 1 1/2 tablespoons baking powder
- 2 teaspoons baking soda and 1 teaspoon salt
- 1 cup flaxseed meal, (see Note)
- 1 cup nonfat dry milk
- 1/2 cup wheat bran, or oat bran
- 1 1/2 cups nonfat milk
- 1/4 cup canola oil
- 1 teaspoon vanilla extract

PREPARATION

1. Whisk flour, buttermilk powder, dried egg whites, sugar, baking powder, baking soda and salt in a large bowl. Stir in flaxseed meal, dry milk and bran. (Makes 6 cups dry mix.)

2. Combine milk, oil and vanilla in a glass measuring cup.
3. Place 2 cups pancake mix in a large bowl. (Refrigerate the remaining pancake mix in an airtight container for up to 1 month or freeze for up to 3 months.) Make a well in the center of the pancake mix. Whisk in the milk mixture until just blended; do not overmix. (The batter will seem quite thin, but will thicken up as it stands.) Let stand for 5 minutes.
4. Coat a nonstick skillet or griddle with cooking spray and place over medium heat. Whisk the batter. Using 1/4 cup batter for each pancake, cook pancakes until the edges are dry and bubbles begin to form, about 2 minutes. Turn over and cook until golden brown, about 2 minutes longer. Adjust heat as necessary for even browning.

TIPS & NOTES
- **Notes:** Buttermilk powder, such as Saco Buttermilk Blend, is a useful substitute for fresh buttermilk. Look in the baking section or with the powdered milk in most markets.
- **Dried egg whites:** Dried egg whites are convenient in recipes calling for egg whites because there is no waste. Look for brands like Just Whites in the baking or natural-foods section of most supermarkets or online at bakerscatalogue.com.
- **Flaxseed meal:** You can find flaxseed meal in the natural-foods section of large supermarkets. You can also start with whole flaxseeds: Grind 2/3 cup whole flaxseeds to yield 1 cup.
- **Variations:** Chocolate-Chocolate Chip Pancakes: Fold 1/2 cup cocoa powder and 3 ounces chocolate chips into the batter. Blueberry: Fold 1 cup frozen blueberries into the batter. Banana-Nut: Fold 1 cup thinly sliced bananas and 4 tablespoons finely chopped toasted pecans into the batter.

NUTRITION
Per serving: 272 calories; 13 g fat (2 g sat, 6 g mono); 8 mg cholesterol; 27 g carbohydrates; 12 g protein; 5 g fiber; 471 mg sodium; 336 mg potassium.
Nutrition Bonus: Calcium (24% daily value), Fiber (20% dv)
Carbohydrate Servings: 1/2
Exchanges: 2 starch, 1 very lean meat, 2 fat (mono)

Shrimp & Plum Kebabs

INGREDIENTS
- 3 tablespoons canola oil, or toasted sesame oil
- 2 tablespoons chopped fresh cilantro
- 1 teaspoon freshly grated lime zest
- 3 tablespoons lime juice
- 1/2 teaspoon salt

- 12 raw shrimp, (8-12 per pound), peeled and deveined
- 3 jalapeño peppers, stemmed, seeded and quartered lengthwise
- 2 plums, pitted and cut into sixths

PREPARATION
1. Whisk oil, cilantro, lime zest, lime juice and salt in a large bowl. Set aside 3 tablespoons of the mixture in a small bowl to use as dressing. Add shrimp, jalapeños and plums to the remaining marinade; toss to coat.
2. Preheat grill to medium-high.
3. Make 4 kebabs, alternating shrimp, jalapeños and plums evenly among four 10-inch skewers. (Discard the marinade.) Grill the kebabs, turning once, until the shrimp are cooked through, about 8 minutes total. Drizzle with the reserved dressing.

TIPS & NOTES
- **Make Ahead Tip**: Equipment: Four 10-inch skewers

NUTRITION
Per serving: 194 calories; 8 g fat (1 g sat, 4 g mono); 221 mg cholesterol; 5 g carbohydrates; 0 g added sugars; 24 g protein; 1 g fiber; 446 mg sodium; 292 mg potassium.
Nutrition Bonus: Selenium (64% daily value), Iron & Vitamin C (20% dv).
Exchanges: 1 vegetable, 3 very lean meat, 1 fat

Beef Tataki

INGREDIENTS
- 1 cup matchstick-cut red radishes, or peeled daikon radish (see Note)
- 1 cup matchstick-cut carrots
- 1/2 cup thinly sliced onion
- 1/4 cup reduced-sodium soy sauce
- 2 tablespoons plus 2 teaspoons lemon juice
- 2 tablespoons finely chopped scallions
- 2 teaspoons finely grated fresh ginger
- 1 pound boneless sirloin steak, 3/4-1 inch thick, trimmed
- 1/4 teaspoon salt
- 1/4 teaspoon freshly ground pepper
- 2 teaspoons canola oil

PREPARATION
1. Place radishes (or daikon), carrot and onion in a medium bowl. Cover with cold water and let soak for 5 minutes. Drain.

2. Combine soy sauce, lemon juice, scallions and ginger in a small bowl. Add 2 tablespoons of the mixture to the drained vegetables and toss. Set aside the remaining sauce.
3. Season steak on both sides with salt and pepper. Heat oil in a large nonstick skillet over medium-high heat. Cook the steak 3 to 4 minutes per side for medium-rare. Let rest on a cutting board for 5 minutes, then thinly slice and serve with the vegetables, drizzled with the reserved sauce.

TIPS & NOTES
- **Note:** Daikon is a long, white radish; it can be found in Asian groceries and most natural-foods stores.

NUTRITION

Per serving: 196 calories; 7 g fat (2 g sat, 3 g mono); 42 mg cholesterol; 8 g carbohydrates; 24 g protein; 2 g fiber; 617 mg sodium; 551 mg potassium.
Nutrition Bonus: Vitamin A (110% daily value), Zinc (27% dv), Vitamin C (20% dv)
Carbohydrate Servings: 1/2
Exchanges: 1 vegetable, 3 lean meat

Roasted Tomato Soup

INGREDIENTS
- 1 1/2 pounds large tomatoes, such as beefsteak, cut in half crosswise
- 1 medium sweet onion, such as Vidalia, peeled and cut in half crosswise
- 3 large cloves garlic, unpeeled
- 1 tablespoon plus 1 teaspoon extra-virgin olive oil, divided
- 1/4 teaspoon salt, or to taste
- Freshly ground pepper, to taste
- 2 cups reduced-sodium chicken broth, or vegetable broth, divided
- 1/4 cup tomato juice
- 1 teaspoon tomato paste
- 1/4 teaspoon Worcestershire sauce
- 1 tablespoon fresh basil, chopped
- Brown sugar, to taste (optional)
- 1/2 cup corn kernels, (fresh, from 1 ear, see Tip) or frozen, thawed

PREPARATION
1. Preheat oven to 400°F. Coat a baking sheet with cooking spray.
2. Toss tomatoes, onion and garlic in a mixing bowl with 1 tablespoon oil. Season with salt and pepper. Spread on the prepared baking sheet and roast until the vegetables are soft and caramelized, about 30 minutes. Let cool.

3. Peel and seed the tomatoes. Trim off the onion ends. Peel the garlic. Place the vegetables in a food processor or blender with 1 cup broth and the remaining 1 teaspoon oil. Pulse to desired thickness and texture.
4. Transfer the vegetable puree to a large heavy pot or Dutch oven. Add the remaining 1 cup broth, tomato juice, tomato pate, Worcestershire sauce, basil and brown sugar (if using). Bring to a simmer over medium heat, stirring often. Ladle into 6 soup bowls, garnish with corn and serve.

TIPS & NOTES
- **Make Ahead Tip**: Cover and refrigerate for up to 2 days or freeze for up to 2 months.
- **Tip:** Removing Corn from the Cob: Stand an uncooked ear of corn on its stem end in a shallow bowl and slice the kernels off with a sharp, thin-bladed knife. This technique produces whole kernels that are good for adding to salads and salsas. If you want to use the corn kernels for soups, fritters or puddings, you can add another step to the process. After cutting the kernels off, reverse the knife and, using the dull side, press it down the length of the ear to push out the rest of the corn and its milk.

NUTRITION
Per serving: 95 calories; 4 g fat (1 g sat, 2 g mono); 1 mg cholesterol; 15 g carbohydrates; 0 g added sugars; 3 g protein; 3 g fiber; 340 mg sodium; 406 mg potassium.
Nutrition Bonus: Vitamin C (35% daily value), Vitamin A (20% dv).
Carbohydrate Servings: 1
Exchanges: 2 vegetable, 1 fat

Ginger-Orange Biscotti

INGREDIENTS
- 3/4 cup whole-wheat pastry flour
- 3/4 cup all-purpose flour
- 1 cup sugar, or 1/2 cup Splenda Sugar Blend for Baking
- 1/2 cup cornmeal
- 2 teaspoons ground ginger
- 1 teaspoon baking powder
- 1/2 teaspoon baking soda
- 1/4 teaspoon salt
- 2 large eggs and 2 large egg whites
- 2 teaspoons freshly grated orange zest
- 1 tablespoon orange juice

PREPARATION
1. Preheat oven to 325°F. Line a baking sheet with parchment paper or a silicone baking mat.
2. Whisk whole-wheat flour, all-purpose flour, sugar (or Splenda), cornmeal, ginger, baking powder, baking soda and salt in a medium bowl. Whisk eggs, egg whites, orange zest and orange juice in a large bowl until blended. Stir in the dry ingredients with a wooden spoon until just combined.
3. Divide the dough in half. With dampened hands, form each piece into a 14-by-1 1/2-inch log. Place the logs side by side on the prepared baking sheet
4. Bake until firm, 20 to 25 minutes. Cool on the pan on a wire rack. Reduce oven temperature to 300°.
5. Slice the logs on the diagonal into cookies 1/2 inch thick. Arrange, cut-side down, on 2 ungreased baking sheets. Bake until golden brown and crisp, 15 to 20 minutes. (Rotate the baking sheets if necessary to ensure even browning.) Transfer the biscotti to a wire rack to cool.

TIPS & NOTES
- **Make Ahead Tip**: Store in an airtight container for up to 2 weeks.

NUTRITION
Per biscotti: 34 calories; 0 g fat (0 g sat, 0 g mono); 8 mg cholesterol; 8 g carbohydrates; 1 g protein; 0 gfiber; 34 mg sodium; 9 mg potassium.
Carbohydrate Servings: 1/2
Exchanges: 1/2 other carbohydrate
Nutrition Note: Per biscotti with Splenda: 0 Carbohydrate Servings; 28 calories; 5 g carbohydrate.

Sausage, Mushroom & Spinach Lasagna

INGREDIENTS
- 8 ounces whole-wheat lasagna noodles
- 1 pound lean spicy Italian turkey sausage, casings removed, or vegetarian sausage-style soy product
- 4 cups sliced mushrooms, (10 ounces)
- 1/4 cup water
- 1 pound frozen spinach, thawed
- 1 28-ounce can crushed tomatoes, preferably chunky
- 1/4 cup chopped fresh basil
- 1/4 teaspoon salt
- Freshly ground pepper, to taste
- 1 pound part-skim ricotta cheese, (2 cups)
- 8 ounces part-skim mozzarella cheese, shredded (about 2 cups), divided

PREPARATION
1. Preheat oven to 350°F. Coat a 9-by-13-inch baking dish with cooking spray.
2. Bring a large pot of water to a boil. Add noodles and cook until not quite tender, about 2 minutes less than the package directions. Drain; return the noodles to the pot, cover with cool water and set aside.
3. Coat a large nonstick skillet with cooking spray and heat over medium-high heat. Add sausage; cook, crumbling with a wooden spoon, until browned, about 4 minutes. Add mushrooms and water; cook, stirring occasionally and crumbling the sausage more, until it is cooked through, the water has evaporated and the mushrooms are tender, 8 to 10 minutes. Squeeze spinach to remove excess water, then stir into the pan; remove from heat.
4. Mix tomatoes with basil, salt and pepper in a medium bowl.
5. To assemble lasagna: Spread 1/2 cup of the tomatoes in the prepared baking dish. Arrange a layer of noodles on top, trimming to fit if necessary. Evenly dollop half the ricotta over the noodles. Top with half the sausage mixture, one-third of the remaining tomatoes and one-third of the mozzarella. Continue with another layer of noodles, the remaining ricotta, the remaining sausage, half the remaining tomatoes and half the remaining mozzarella. Top with a third layer of noodles and the remaining tomatoes.
6. Cover the lasagna with foil and bake until bubbling and heated through, 1 hour to 1 hour 10 minutes. Remove the foil; sprinkle the remaining mozzarella on top. Return to the oven and bake until the cheese is just melted but not browned, 8 to 10 minutes. Let rest for 10 minutes before serving. Vegetarian Variation: Use a sausage-style soy product, such as Gimme Lean, or simply omit the sausage altogether.

TIPS & NOTES
- **Make Ahead Tip**: Prepare through Step 5 up to 1 day ahead.
- **Ingredient Note:** Whole-wheat lasagna noodles are higher in fiber than white noodles. They can be found in health-food stores and some large supermarkets.
- **Vegetarian Variation:** Use a sausage-style soy product, such as Gimme Lean, or simply omit the sausage altogether.

NUTRITION
Per serving: 333 calories; 14 g fat (5 g sat, 3 g mono); 41 mg cholesterol; 28 g carbohydrates; 26 g protein;7 g fiber; 655 mg sodium; 607 mg potassium.
Nutrition Bonus: Vitamin A (128% daily value), Calcium (23% dv), Iron (21% dv), Folate (19% dv), Potassium (17% dv).
Carbohydrate Servings: 1 1/2
Exchanges: 1 starch, 1 1/2 vegetable, 1 lean meat, 2 medium-fat meat

Penne with Vodka Sauce & Capicola

INGREDIENTS
- 12 ounces whole-wheat penne
- 1 2-ounce piece capicola, or pancetta, finely diced (see Tip)
- 1 small onion, chopped
- 3 cloves garlic, chopped
- 1/2 cup vodka
- 1 28-ounce can crushed tomatoes
- 1/4 cup half-and-half
- 2 teaspoons Worcestershire sauce
- 1/4-1/2 teaspoon crushed red pepper
- 1/4 cup chopped fresh basil
- Freshly ground pepper, to taste

PREPARATION
1. Bring a large pot of water to a boil. Cook penne until just tender, 12 minutes or according to package directions.
2. Meanwhile, cook capicola (or pancetta) in a large saucepan over medium heat until crisp, about 4 minutes. Drain on a paper towel.
3. Return the saucepan to medium-low heat; add onion and garlic and cook until the onion is translucent, about 1 minute. Increase heat to high; add vodka and bring to a boil. Boil until reduced by about half, about 2 minutes. Stir in tomatoes, half-and-half, Worcestershire sauce and crushed red pepper to taste; reduce to a simmer and cook until thickened, about 10 minutes.
4. Drain the pasta; serve topped with the sauce and sprinkled with the capicola (or pancetta), basil and pepper.

NUTRITION
Per serving: 311 calories; 3 g fat (1 g sat, 1 g mono); 9 mg cholesterol; 47 g carbohydrates; 0 g added sugars; 11 g protein; 5 g fiber; 264 mg sodium; 517 mg potassium.
Nutrition Bonus: Vitamin C (25% daily value), Iron, Magnesium & Vitamin A (20% dv).
Carbohydrate Servings: 3
Exchanges: 3 starch, 1 vegetable

Sliced Tomato Salad

INGREDIENTS
- 4 tomatoes, sliced
- 1/4 cup thinly sliced red onion
- 8 anchovies
- 1/2 teaspoon dried oregano

- Salt & freshly ground pepper, to taste
- 2 tablespoons extra-virgin olive oil
- 1 tablespoon white-wine vinegar

PREPARATION

1. Arrange tomato slices on a platter. Top with onion, anchovies, oregano, salt and pepper. Drizzle with oil and vinegar.

NUTRITION
Per serving: 44 calories; 1 g fat (0 g sat, 0 g mono); 3 mg cholesterol; 8 g carbohydrates; 0 g added sugars; 3 g protein; 2 g fiber; 300 mg sodium; 403 mg potassium.
Nutrition Bonus: Vitamin C (35% daily value), Vitamin A (25% dv).
Carbohydrate Servings: 1/2
Exchanges: 1 vegetable, 1 1/2 fat

DAY 25
BREAKFAST
Spiced Apple Cider Muffins
Skim milk (1 cup)
Grapefruit (1/2)
LUNCH
Skim milk (1 cup)
Nouveau Niçoise or Blackened Salmon Sandwich
Wasa crispbread (1 cracker)
SNACK
Low-fat cottage cheese (1/2 cup)
Carrot sticks (1/2 cup)
DINNER
Turkey Cutlets with Peas & Spring Onions or Miso Chicken Stir-Fry
Quick-cooking barley (3/4 cup) and Strawberries (1 cup)

DAY 25 RECIPES

Spiced Apple Cider Muffins

INGREDIENTS
STREUSEL
- 2 tablespoons packed light brown sugar
- 4 teaspoons whole-wheat flour

- 1/2 teaspoon ground cinnamon
- 1 tablespoon butter, cut into small pieces
- 2 tablespoons finely chopped walnuts, (optional)

MUFFINS
- 1 cup whole-wheat flour
- 1 cup all-purpose flour
- 1 1/2 teaspoons baking powder
- 1/2 teaspoon baking soda
- 1/4 teaspoon salt
- 1 tablespoon ground cinnamon
- 1/2 teaspoon ground nutmeg
- 1 large egg
- 1/3 cup packed light brown sugar
- 1/2 cup apple butter, such as Smucker's
- 1/3 cup maple syrup
- 1/3 cup apple cider
- 1/3 cup low-fat plain yogurt
- 1/4 cup canola oil

PREPARATION
1. Preheat oven to 400°F. Coat 12 muffin cups with cooking spray.
2. To prepare streusel: Mix brown sugar, whole-wheat flour and cinnamon in a small bowl. Cut in butter with a pastry blender or your fingers until the mixture resembles coarse crumbs. Stir in walnuts, if using.
3. To prepare muffins: Whisk whole-wheat flour, all-purpose flour, baking powder, baking soda, salt, cinnamon and nutmeg in a large bowl.
4. Whisk egg and brown sugar in a medium bowl until smooth. Whisk in apple butter, syrup, cider, yogurt and oil. Make a well in the dry ingredients; add the wet ingredients and stir with a rubber spatula until just combined. Scoop the batter into the prepared muffin cups (they'll be quite full). Sprinkle with the streusel.
5. Bake the muffins until the tops are golden brown and spring back when touched lightly, 15 to 25 minutes. Let cool in the pan for 5 minutes. Loosen edges and turn muffins out onto a wire rack to cool slightly before serving.

NUTRITION
Per muffin: 209 calories; 7 g fat (1 g sat, 3 g mono); 21 mg cholesterol; 34 g carbohydrates; 4 g protein; 2 gfiber; 162 mg sodium; 40 mg potassium.
Carbohydrate Servings: 2 1/2
Exchanges: 2 starch, 1 fat

Nouveau Niçoise

INGREDIENTS
- 8 cups water
- 8 ounces green beans, trimmed and halved
- 8 small red potatoes
- 2 eggs
- 1/4 cup minced shallots
- 1/4 cup red-wine vinegar
- 2 tablespoons Dijon mustard
- 1/4 teaspoon salt
- 1/4 teaspoon freshly ground pepper
- 3 tablespoons extra-virgin olive oil
- 6 cups mixed salad greens
- 2 6-ounce cans chunk light tuna, drained (see Note)
- 12 Nicoise or Kalamata olives

PREPARATION
1. Bring water to a boil in a 3- to 4-quart saucepan. Add green beans and cook until just tender and bright green, 1 to 2 minutes. Using a slotted spoon, transfer the beans to a colander, rinse under cold water and set aside in a large bowl. Carefully place potatoes and eggs into the boiling water. Cook the eggs until hard, 12 minutes. Using a slotted spoon, transfer the eggs to the colander, rinse under cold water until cool and set aside. Continue cooking the potatoes until fork-tender, 3 minutes more. Drain the potatoes; rinse under cold water until cool enough to handle.
2. Meanwhile, combine shallots, vinegar, mustard, salt and pepper in a small bowl. Slowly whisk in oil.
3. Cut the potatoes into quarters or eighths, depending on their size. Add to the bowl with the beans. Add greens, tuna and the dressing. Toss well. Peel the eggs and cut into wedges. Divide the salad among 4 plates. Top with egg wedges and olives. Serve immediately.

TIPS & NOTES
- **Make Ahead Tip**: Cook green beans, potatoes and eggs; dry, cover and refrigerate for up to 1 day.
- **Note:** Chunk light tuna, which comes from the smaller skipjack or yellowfin, has less mercury than canned white albacore tuna. The FDA/EPA advises that women who are or might become pregnant, nursing mothers and young children consume no more than 6 ounces of albacore a week; up to 12 ounces of canned light tuna is considered safe.

NUTRITION

Per serving: 436 calories; 16 g fat (3 g sat, 11 g mono); 159 mg cholesterol; 38 g carbohydrates; 0 g added sugars; 33 g protein; 6 g fiber; 547 mg sodium; 1140 mg potassium.
Nutrition Bonus: Vitamin C (90% daily value), Potassium (33% dv), Vitamin A (30% dv), Folate (26% dv), Iron (15% dv).
Carbohydrate Servings: 2
Exchanges: 2 starch, 2 vegetable, 3 very lean meat, 3 fat

Blackened Salmon Sandwich

INGREDIENTS
- 1 pound wild salmon fillet, (see Ingredient Note), skinned (see Tip) and cut into 4 portions
- 2 teaspoons blackening or Cajun seasoning
- 1 small avocado, pitted
- 2 tablespoons low-fat mayonnaise
- 4 crusty whole-wheat rolls, split and toasted
- 1 cup arugula
- 2 plum tomatoes, thinly sliced and 1/2 cup thinly sliced red onion

PREPARATION
1. Oil grill rack (see Tip); preheat grill to high.
2. Rub salmon on both sides with blackening (or Cajun) seasoning. Grill until cooked through, 3 to 4 minutes per side.
3. Mash avocado and mayonnaise in a small bowl.
4. To assemble sandwiches, spread some of the avocado mixture on each roll and top with salmon, arugula, tomato and onion.

TIPS & NOTES
- **Ingredient note:** Wild-caught salmon from the Pacific (Alaska, California, Washington and Oregon) is considered the best choice for the environment. For more information, visit Monterey Bay Aquarium Seafood Watch (mbayaq.org/cr/seafoodwatch.asp).
- **Tips:** To skin a salmon fillet, place salmon on a clean cutting board, skin side down. Starting at the tail end, slip the blade of a long, sharp knife between the fish flesh and the skin, holding the skin down firmly with your other hand. Gently push the blade along at a 30° angle, separating the fillet from the skin without cutting through either.
- To oil a grill rack, oil a folded paper towel, hold it with tongs and rub it over the rack. (Do not use cooking spray on a hot grill.) When grilling delicate foods like tofu and fish, it is helpful to spray the food with cooking spray.

NUTRITION
Per serving: 404 calories; 14 g fat (3 g sat, 6 g mono); 53 mg cholesterol; 43 g carbohydrates; 31 g protein;6 g fiber; 748 mg sodium; 775 mg potassium.
Nutrition Bonus: Fiber (24% daily value), Potassium (22% dv), Vitamin C (18% dv), Folate (15% dv), good source of omega-3s.
Carbohydrate Servings: 2 1/2
Exchanges: 2 starch, 1 1/2 vegetable, 4 lean meat, 1 fat (mono)

Turkey Cutlets with Peas & Spring Onions

INGREDIENTS
- 1/2 cup all-purpose flour
- 1/2 teaspoon salt, divided
- 1/4 teaspoon freshly ground pepper
- 1 pound 1/4-inch-thick turkey breast cutlets, or steaks
- 2 tablespoons extra-virgin olive oil, divided
- 4 ounces shiitake mushrooms, stemmed and sliced (about 1 1/2 cups)
- 1 bunch spring onions, or scallions, sliced, whites and greens separated
- 1 cup reduced-sodium chicken broth
- 1/2 cup dry white wine
- 1 cup peas, fresh or frozen, thawed
- 1 teaspoon freshly grated lemon zest

PREPARATION
1. Whisk flour, 1/4 teaspoon salt and pepper in a shallow dish. Dredge each turkey cutlet (or steak) in the flour mixture. Heat 1 tablespoon oil in a large nonstick skillet over medium-high heat. Add the turkey and cook until lightly golden, 2 to 3 minutes per side. Transfer to a plate; cover with foil to keep warm.
2. Add the remaining 1 tablespoon oil to the pan and heat over medium-high heat. Add mushrooms and onion (or scallion) whites and cook, stirring often, until the mushrooms are browned and the whites are slightly softened, 2 to 3 minutes. Add broth, wine and the remaining 1/4 teaspoon salt; cook, stirring occasionally, until the sauce is slightly reduced, 2 to 3 minutes. Stir in peas and onion (or scallion) greens and cook, stirring, until heated through, about 1 minute. Stir in lemon zest. Nestle the turkey into the vegetables along with any accumulated juices from the plate. Cook, turning the cutlets once, until heated through, 1 to 2 minutes.

NUTRITION
Per serving: 313 calories; 8 g fat (1 g sat, 5 g mono); 45 mg cholesterol; 23 g carbohydrates; 34 g protein; 3 g fiber; 571 mg sodium; 223 mg potassium.
Nutrition Bonus: Iron (15% daily value), Vitamin A & C (20% dv).
Carbohydrate Servings: 1

Exchanges: 1 starch, 1 vegetable, 4 lean meat, 1 fat

Miso Chicken Stir-Fry

INGREDIENTS
- 1/4 cup reduced-sodium chicken broth, (see Tips for Two)
- 3 tablespoons miso, preferably white (see Note)
- 2 tablespoons rice vinegar
- 1 tablespoon mirin, (see Note)
- 2 teaspoons minced fresh ginger
- 1 teaspoon canola oil
- 8 ounces boneless, skinless chicken breast, trimmed of fat and thinly sliced
- 1 cup thinly sliced carrots
- 1/4 cup water
- 1 medium red bell pepper, thinly sliced
- 1 cup frozen peas, thawed

PREPARATION
1. Combine broth, miso, vinegar, mirin and ginger in a small bowl.
2. Heat oil in a large nonstick skillet over medium-high heat. Add chicken and cook, stirring occasionally, until browned and cooked through, about 3 minutes. Transfer to a plate.
3. Add carrots and water to the pan; cover and cook, stirring occasionally, until tender-crisp, about 2 minutes. Stir in the miso mixture, bell pepper, peas and the chicken. Cook, stirring occasionally, until the peas are heated through and the sauce is slightly thickened, 1 to 2 minutes.

TIPS & NOTES
- **Tips for Two:** Leftover canned broth keeps for up to 5 days in the refrigerator or up to 3 months in your freezer. Leftover broths in aseptic packages keep for up to 1 week in the refrigerator. Add to soups, sauces and stews; use for cooking rice and grains; add a little when reheating leftovers to prevent them drying out.
- **Notes:** Miso is fermented soybean paste made by inoculating a mixture of soybeans, salt and grains (usually barley or rice) with koji, a beneficial mold. Aged for up to 3 years, miso is undeniably salty, but a little goes a long way. Akamiso (red miso), made from barley or rice and soybeans, is salty and tangy, and the most commonly used miso in Japan. Use in marinades for meat and oily fish, and in long-simmered dishes. Shiromiso (sweet or white miso), made with soy and rice, is yellow and milder in flavor; use for soup, salad dressings and sauces for fish or chicken.

- Mirin is a low-alcohol rice wine essential to Japanese cooking. Look for it in the Asian or gourmet-ingredients section of your supermarket. An equal portion of sherry or white wine with a pinch of sugar may be substituted for mirin.

NUTRITION
Per serving: 302 calories; 6 g fat (1 g sat, 2 g mono); 63 mg cholesterol; 29 g carbohydrates; 28 g protein; 7 g fiber; 776 mg sodium; 601 mg potassium.
Nutrition Bonus: Vitamin A (280% daily value), Vitamin C (210% dv), Selenium (30% dv), Potassium (17% dv).
Carbohydrate Servings: 112
Exchanges: 1 starch, 2 vegetable, 3 very lean meat

DAY 26
BREAKFAST

Skim milk (1 cup)
Overnight Oatmeal
Grapefruit (1/2)

LUNCH

Stir-Fry of Pork with Vietnamese Flavors or Shrimp Banh Mi
Quick Kimchi
Whole-wheat toast (1 slice)

SNACK

Almonds (1 oz.)
Skim milk (1 cup)

DINNER

Corn & Broccoli Calzones or Peanut Noodles with Shredded Chicken & Vegetables
Arugula-Mushroom Salad
Sliced Tomato Salad
Mango Sorbet

DAY 26 RECIPES

Overnight Oatmeal

INGREDIENTS
- 8 cups water
- 2 cups steel-cut oats, (see Ingredient note)
- 1/3 cup dried cranberries
- 1/3 cup dried apricots, chopped
- 1/4 teaspoon salt, or to taste

PREPARATION

1. Combine water, oats, dried cranberries, dried apricots and salt in a 5- or 6-quart slow cooker. Turn heat to low. Put the lid on and cook until the oats are tender and the porridge is creamy, 7 to 8 hours. Stovetop Variation Halve the above recipe to accommodate the size of most double boilers: Combine 4 cups water, 1 cup steel-cut oats, 3 tablespoons dried cranberries, 3 tablespoons dried apricots and 1/8 teaspoon salt in the top of a double boiler. Cover and cook over boiling water for about 1 1/2 hours, checking the water level in the bottom of the double boiler from time to time.

TIPS & NOTES

- **Ingredient Note:** Steel-cut oats, sometimes labeled "Irish oatmeal," look like small pebbles. They are toasted oat groats—the oat kernel that has been removed from the husk that have been cut in 2 or 3 pieces. Do not substitute regular rolled oats, which have a shorter cooking time, in the oatmeal recipe.
- For easy cleanup, try a slow-cooker liner. These heat-resistant, disposable liners fit neatly inside the insert and help prevent food from sticking to the bottom and sides of your slow cooker.

NUTRITION

Per serving: 193 calories; 3 g fat (0 g sat, 1 g mono); 0 mg cholesterol; 34 g carbohydrates; 0 g added sugars; 6 g protein; 9 g fiber; 77 mg sodium; 195 mg potassium.
Nutrition Bonus: Fiber (36% daily value).
Carbohydrate Servings: 2
Exchanges: 2 starch, 1/2 fruit

Stir-Fry of Pork with Vietnamese Flavors

INGREDIENTS

- 2 tablespoons finely chopped fresh ginger
- 2 serrano or jalapeño peppers, seeded and finely chopped
- 4 cloves garlic, finely chopped
- 3 tablespoons fish sauce, divided
- 2 tablespoons orange juice, divided
- 1 teaspoon cornstarch
- 1/2 teaspoon freshly ground pepper
- 1 pound pork tenderloin, trimmed and cut across the grain into 1/4-inch-thick slices
- 1 tablespoon sugar
- 3 teaspoons canola oil, divided
- 2 cups finely sliced onions, (2-4 onions)
- 1/4 cup sliced fresh cilantro leaves

PREPARATION

1. Combine ginger, peppers, garlic, 1 tablespoon of the fish sauce, 1 tablespoon of the orange juice, cornstarch and black pepper in a shallow dish. Add pork and toss to coat it with marinade. Set aside to marinate for 10 to 20 minutes.
2. Mix sugar, the remaining 2 tablespoons fish sauce and 1 tablespoon orange juice in a small bowl.
3. Heat a wok over high heat. Swirl in 1 teaspoon of the oil. Add onions and cook, stirring, until limp and caramelized, about 5 minutes. Transfer the onions to a plate. Wipe out the pan. Add the remaining 2 teaspoons oil to the pan and increase heat to high. Slowly drop in pork and stir-fry until browned and just cooked through, 2 to 3 minutes. Add the reserved fish sauce/orange juice mixture and the reserved onions; toss until the pork is coated with sauce. Sprinkle with cilantro and serve over rice.

NUTRITION
Per serving: 243 calories; 7 g fat (1 g sat, 4 g mono); 68 mg cholesterol; 19 g carbohydrates; 3 g added sugars; 25 g protein; 3 g fiber; 575 mg sodium; 615 mg potassium.
Nutrition Bonus: Selenium (44% daily value), Vitamin C (28% dv), Potassium (18% dv).
Carbohydrate Servings: 1
Exchanges: 1 1/2 vegetable, 3 lean meat

Shrimp Banh Mi

INGREDIENTS
- 1 large carrot, peeled and shredded
- 2 tablespoons rice vinegar
- 1/3 cup chopped fresh cilantro
- 2 1/2 tablespoons reduced-fat mayonnaise
- 2 1/2 tablespoons low-fat plain yogurt
- 3/4 teaspoon fish sauce, (see Ingredient note)
- 1 tablespoon lime juice
- 1/4 teaspoon cayenne pepper
- 3 12-inch baguettes, halved lengthwise
- 1 pound peeled cooked shrimp, (21-25 per pound; thawed if frozen), tails removed (see Tip)
- 18 thin slices cucumber
- 3 scallions, thinly sliced lengthwise and cut into 2-inch pieces

PREPARATION
1. Place carrot and vinegar in a small bowl; stir to combine. Let marinate while preparing the rest of the ingredients.
2. Place cilantro, mayonnaise, yogurt, fish sauce, lime juice and cayenne in a medium bowl; stir to combine. Spread 2 teaspoons of this sauce on the bottom half of each baguette. Add shrimp to the remaining sauce; toss to coat. Using a slotted spoon, divide carrot among the baguettes (discard vinegar). Top with shrimp, cucumber and scallions. Cut each baguette into two 6-inch sandwiches.

TIPS & NOTES
- **Ingredient Note:** Fish sauce: A pungent Southeast Asian sauce made from salted, fermented fish. Found in the Asian section of large supermarkets and in Asian specialty markets.
- **Tip:** To defrost frozen shrimp, place in a colander under cold running water until thawed.

NUTRITION
Per serving: 247 calories; 4 g fat (1 g sat, 1 g mono); 153 mg cholesterol; 30 g carbohydrates; 24 g protein;5 g fiber; 504 mg sodium; 993 mg potassium.
Nutrition Bonus: Vitamin A (50% daily value), Vitamin C (25% dv), Folate (20% dv), Magnesium (17% dv).
Carbohydrate Servings: 1 1/2
Exchanges: 2 starch, 2 very lean meat

Quick Kimchi

INGREDIENTS
- 1 small head napa (Chinese) cabbage, cored and cut into 1-inch squares (about 8 cups)
- 2 cloves garlic, minced
- 1/4 cup water
- 2 tablespoons distilled white vinegar
- 1 tablespoon toasted sesame oil
- 2 teaspoons fresh ginger, finely grated
- 3/4 teaspoon salt
- 1/2 teaspoon sugar
- 1/2 teaspoon crushed red pepper, red
- 3 scallions, sliced
- 1 carrot, peeled and grated

PREPARATION

1. Combine cabbage, garlic and water in a large saucepan and bring to a boil over high heat. Reduce heat to medium-low and cook, stirring once or twice, until tender, 4 to 5 minutes.
2. Meanwhile, whisk vinegar, oil, ginger, salt, sugar and crushed red pepper in a large bowl.
3. Add the cabbage, scallions and carrot to the bowl and toss to combine. Refrigerate for about 25 minutes before serving.

NUTRITION

Per serving: 37 calories; 2 g fat (0 g sat, 1 g mono); 0 mg cholesterol; 4 g carbohydrates; 0 g added sugars;1 g protein; 1 g fiber; 235 mg sodium; 47 mg potassium.
Nutrition Bonus: Vitamin A (50% daily value), Vitamin C (40% dv).
Exchanges: 1 vegetable

Corn & Broccoli Calzones

INGREDIENTS
- 1 1/2 cups chopped broccoli florets
- 1 1/2 cups fresh corn kernels, (about 3 ears; see Tip)
- 1 cup shredded part-skim mozzarella cheese
- 2/3 cup part-skim ricotta cheese
- 4 scallions, thinly sliced
- 1/4 cup chopped fresh basil
- 1/2 teaspoon garlic powder
- 1/4 teaspoon salt
- 1/4 teaspoon freshly ground pepper
- All-purpose flour, for dusting
- 20 ounces prepared whole-wheat pizza dough, (see Tip), thawed if frozen
- 2 teaspoons canola oil

PREPARATION

1. Position racks in upper and lower thirds of oven; preheat to 475°F. Coat 2 baking sheets with cooking spray.
2. Combine broccoli, corn, mozzarella, ricotta, scallions, basil, garlic powder, salt and pepper in a large bowl.
3. On a lightly floured surface, divide dough into 6 pieces. Roll each piece into an 8-inch circle. Place a generous 3/4 cup filling on one half of each circle, leaving a 1-inch border of dough. Brush the border with water and fold the top half over the filling. Fold the edges over and crimp with a fork to seal. Make several small

slits in the top to vent steam; brush each calzone with oil. Transfer the calzones to the prepared baking sheets.
4. Bake the calzones, switching the pans halfway through, until browned on top, about 15 minutes. Let cool slightly before serving.

TIPS & NOTES
- **Tips:** To remove corn kernels from the cob: Stand an uncooked ear of corn on its stem end in a shallow bowl and slice the kernels off with a sharp, thin-bladed knife. This technique produces whole kernels that are good for adding to salads and salsas. If you want to use the corn kernels for soups, fritters or puddings, you can add another step to the process. After cutting the kernels off, reverse the knife and, using the dull side, press it down the length of the ear to push out the rest of the corn and its milk.
- Look for balls of whole-wheat pizza dough at your supermarket, fresh or frozen and without any hydrogenated oils.
- **Healthy Heart Variation:** To reduce saturated fat even further, use nonfat ricotta in place of the reduced-fat ricotta. 334 calories, 2 g saturated fat.

NUTRITION

Per calzone: 350 calories; 7 g fat (3 g sat, 3 g mono); 21 mg cholesterol; 50 g carbohydrates; 17 g protein;4 g fiber; 509 mg sodium; 250 mg potassium.
Nutrition Bonus: Vitamin C (35% daily value), Calcium (25% dv), Vitamin A (20% dv).
Carbohydrate Servings: 3
Exchanges: 3 starch, 1 medium-fat protein

Peanut Noodles with Shredded Chicken & Vegetables

INGREDIENTS
- 1 pound boneless, skinless chicken breasts
- 1/2 cup smooth natural peanut butter
- 2 tablespoons reduced-sodium soy sauce
- 2 teaspoons minced garlic
- 1 1/2 teaspoons chile-garlic sauce, or to taste (see Ingredient note)
- 1 teaspoon minced fresh ginger
- 8 ounces whole-wheat spaghetti
- 1 12-ounce bag fresh vegetable medley, such as carrots, broccoli, snow peas

PREPARATION
1. Put a large pot of water on to boil for cooking pasta.
2. Meanwhile, place chicken in a skillet or saucepan and add enough water to cover; bring to a boil. Cover, reduce heat to low and simmer gently until cooked through and no longer pink in the

middle, 10 to 12 minutes. Transfer the chicken to a cutting board. When cool enough to handle, shred into bite-size strips.
3. Whisk peanut butter, soy sauce, garlic, chile-garlic sauce and ginger in a large bowl.
4. Cook pasta in the boiling water until not quite tender, about 1 minute less than specified in the package directions. Add vegetables and cook until the pasta and vegetables are just tender, 1 minute more. Drain, reserving 1 cup of the cooking liquid. Rinse the pasta and vegetables with cool water to refresh. Stir the reserved cooking liquid into the peanut sauce; add the pasta, vegetables and chicken; toss well to coat. Serve warm or chilled.

TIPS & NOTES
- **Make Ahead Tip**: Cover and refrigerate for up to 2 days. To serve, stir in 2 tablespoons warm water per portion; serve cold or reheat in microwave.
- **Ingredient Note:** Chile-garlic sauce (or chili-garlic sauce, or paste) is a blend of ground chiles, garlic and vinegar and is commonly used to add heat and flavor to Asian soups, sauces and stir-fries. It can be found in the Asian section of large supermarkets and keeps up to 1 year in the refrigerator.

NUTRITION
Per serving: 363 calories; 12 g fat (2 g sat, 0 g mono); 44 mg cholesterol; 36 g carbohydrates; 0 g added sugars; 29 g protein; 7 g fiber; 348 mg sodium; 287 mg potassium.
Nutrition Bonus: Selenium (58% daily value), Fiber (27% dv), Vitamin C (25% dv), Magnesium (19% dv).
Carbohydrate Servings: 2
Exchanges: 2 starch, 1 1/2 vegetable, 3 lean meat

Arugula-Mushroom Salad

INGREDIENTS
- 1 clove garlic, peeled
- 1/4 teaspoon salt
- 1 tablespoon lemon juice
- 1 tablespoon reduced-fat mayonnaise
- 1 tablespoon extra-virgin olive oil
- 1 tablespoon chopped fresh parsley
- Freshly ground pepper, to taste
- 6 cups arugula leaves
- 2 cups sliced mushrooms

PREPARATION
1. Place garlic on a cutting board and crush. Sprinkle with salt and use the flat of a chef's knife blade to mash the garlic to a paste; transfer to a serving bowl. Whisk in lemon juice, mayonnaise, oil and parsley. Season with pepper. Add arugula and mushrooms; toss to coat with the dressing.

NUTRITION
Per serving: 62 calories; 4 g fat (1 g sat, 3 g mono); 1 mg cholesterol; 3 g carbohydrates; 0 g added sugars;2 g protein; 1 g fiber; 188 mg sodium; 235 mg potassium.
Nutrition Bonus: Vitamin C (15% daily value).
Exchanges: 1 vegetable, 1 fat (mono)

Sliced Tomato Salad

INGREDIENTS
- 4 tomatoes, sliced
- 1/4 cup thinly sliced red onion
- 8 anchovies
- 1/2 teaspoon dried oregano
- Salt & freshly ground pepper, to taste
- 2 tablespoons extra-virgin olive oil
- 1 tablespoon white-wine vinegar

PREPARATION
Arrange tomato slices on a platter. Top with onion, anchovies, oregano, salt and pepper. Drizzle with oil and vinegar.

NUTRITION
Per serving: 44 calories; 1 g fat (0 g sat, 0 g mono); 3 mg cholesterol; 8 g carbohydrates; 0 g added sugars; 3 g protein; 2 g fiber; 300 mg sodium; 403 mg potassium.
Nutrition Bonus: Vitamin C (35% daily value), Vitamin A (25% dv).
Carbohydrate Servings: 1/2
Exchanges: 1 vegetable, 1 1/2 fat

Mango Sorbet

INGREDIENTS
- 3 ripe mangoes
- 1/2 cup sugar
- 1/2 cup water
- 1/3 cup coarsely mashed banana, (1 small)
- 2 tablespoons lime juice

PREPARATION

1. Preheat oven to 350°F. Place whole mangoes in a shallow baking pan and roast until very soft, 70 to 90 minutes. Refrigerate until cool, about 1 hour.
2. Meanwhile, combine sugar and water in a small saucepan. Bring to a boil, stirring to dissolve sugar. Remove from heat and refrigerate until cold, about 1 hour.
3. When the mangoes are cool enough to handle, remove skin and coarsely chop pulp, discarding pit. Place the mango pulp and accumulated juices in a food processor. Add banana and lime juice; process until very smooth. Transfer to a large bowl and stir in the sugar syrup. Cover and refrigerate until cold, 40 minutes or overnight.
4. Freeze the mixture in an ice cream maker according to manufacturer's directions. (Alternatively, freeze the mixture in a shallow metal pan until solid, about 6 hours. Break into chunks and process in a food processor until smooth.) Serve immediately or transfer to a storage container and let harden in the freezer for 1 to 1 1/2 hours. Serve in chilled dishes.

TIPS & NOTES

- **Make Ahead Tip**: Store in an airtight container in the freezer for up to 1 week. Let soften in the refrigerator for 1/2 hour before serving. | Equipment: Ice cream maker or food processor

NUTRITION
Per serving: 108 calories; 0 g fat (0 g sat, 0 g mono); 0 mg cholesterol; 28 g carbohydrates; 1 g protein; 2 gfiber; 2 mg sodium; 159 mg potassium.
Nutrition Bonus: Vitamin C (40% daily value).
Carbohydrate Servings: 2
Exchanges: 2 fruit

DAY 27
BREAKFAST

Morning Smoothie
Whole-wheat toast (2 slices)
Plum spread
LUNCH

Skim milk (1 cup)
Tuna & Bean Salad in Pita Pockets or Chicken Parmesan Sub
SNACK

Apple (1 cup, quartered)
DINNER

Turkey Cutlets with Peas & Spring Onions or Edamame Succotash with Shrimp
Brown rice (1/2 cup, cooked)
The Diet House Salad
Berry Frozen Yogurt

DAY 27 RECIPES

Morning Smoothie

INGREDIENTS
- 1 1/4 cups orange juice, preferably calcium-fortified
- 1 banana
- 1 1/4 cups frozen berries, such as raspberries, blackberries, blueberries and/or strawberries
- 1/2 cup low-fat silken tofu, or low-fat plain yogurt
- 1 tablespoon sugar, or Splenda Granular (optional)

PREPARATION
1. Combine orange juice, banana, berries, tofu (or yogurt) and sugar (or Splenda), if using, in a blender; cover and blend until creamy. Serve immediately.

NUTRITION

Per serving: 139 calories; 2 g fat (0 g sat, 0 g mono); 0 mg cholesterol; 33 g carbohydrates; 0 g added sugars; 4 g protein; 4 g fiber; 19 mg sodium; 421 mg potassium.
Nutrition Bonus: Vitamin C (110% daily value), Fiber (16% dv).
Carbohydrate Servings: 2
Exchanges: 2 fruit, 1/2 low-fat milk

Plum spread

INGREDIENTS
- 5 pounds plums, pitted and sliced (14-15 cups)
- 3 Granny Smith apples, washed and quartered (not cored)
- 1/4 cup white grape juice, or other fruit juice
- 2 tablespoons lemon juice
- 3/4 cup sugar, or Splenda Granular
- 1/4 teaspoon ground cinnamon, or ginger (optional)

PREPARATION
1. Place a plate in the freezer for testing consistency later.

2. Combine plums, apples, grape juice (or fruit juice) and lemon juice in a large, heavy-bottomed, nonreactive Dutch oven. Bring to a boil over medium-high heat, stirring. Cover and boil gently, stirring occasionally, until the fruit is softened and juicy, 15 to 20 minutes. Uncover and boil gently, stirring occasionally, until the fruit is completely soft, about 20 minutes. (Adjust heat as necessary to maintain a gentle boil.)
3. Pass the fruit through a food mill to remove the skins and apple seeds.
4. Return the strained fruit to the pot. Add sugar (or Splenda) and cinnamon (or ginger), if using. Cook over medium heat, stirring frequently, until a spoonful of jam dropped onto the chilled plate holds its shape, about 15 minutes longer. (See Tip.) Remove from heat and skim off any foam.

TIPS & NOTES
- **Make Ahead Tip**: Store in an airtight container in the refrigerator for up to 2 months. For longer storage, process in a boiling-water bath (for detailed instructions, refer to www.homecanning.com or call the Home Canner's Hotline at 800-240-3340).
- **To test the consistency of the spread:** Drop a dollop of cooked spread onto a chilled plate. Carefully run your finger through the dollop. If the track remains unfilled, the jam is done.

NUTRITION
Per tablespoon with sugar: 14 calories; 0 g fat (0 g sat, 0 g mono); 0 mg cholesterol; 4 g carbohydrates; 0 g protein; 0 g fiber; 0 mg sodium; 30 mg potassium.
Exchanges: free food
Nutrition Note: Per tablespoon with Splenda: 0 Carbohydrate Servings; 12 calories; 3 g carbohydrate.

Tuna & Bean Salad in Pita Pockets

INGREDIENTS
- 1 clove garlic, crushed and peeled
- 1/4 teaspoon salt and 1 tablespoon lemon juice
- 1 tablespoon extra-virgin olive oil
- 1/4 teaspoon crushed red pepper
- 1 15-ounce can great northern beans, rinsed
- 1 3-ounce can tuna packed in water, drained and flaked (see Note)
- 1 cup arugula leaves, coarsely chopped
- Freshly ground pepper, to taste
- 2 6-inch whole-wheat pita breads
- 2-4 large lettuce leaves
- 1/4 cup thinly sliced red onion

PREPARATION

1. With a chef's knife, mash garlic and salt into a paste. Transfer to a bowl. Whisk in lemon juice, oil and crushed red pepper. Add beans, tuna and arugula; toss to mix. Season with pepper.
2. Cut a quarter off each pita to open the pocket. (Save the trimmings to make pita crisps.) Line the centers with lettuce. Fill with tuna/bean salad and red onion slices

TIPS & NOTES

- **Note:** Chunk light tuna, which comes from the smaller skipjack or yellowfin, has less mercury than canned white albacore tuna. The FDA/EPA advises that women who are or might become pregnant, nursing mothers and young children consume no more than 6 ounces of albacore a week; up to 12 ounces of canned light tuna is considered safe.

NUTRITION
Per serving: 454 calories; 10 g fat (2 g sat, 6 g mono); 13 mg cholesterol; 66 g carbohydrates; 29 g protein;15 g fiber; 782 mg sodium; 842 mg potassium.
Nutrition Bonus: Fiber (59% dv), Folate (48% dv), Potassium (42% dv), Magnesium (33% dv), Iron (30% dv), Calcium (15% dv), Vitamin C (15% dv), Vitamin A. (15% dv).
Carbohydrate Servings: 3
Exchanges: 3 1/2 starch, 1 1/2 vegetable, 3 lean meat

Chicken Parmesan Sub

INGREDIENTS
- 1/4 cup all-purpose flour
- 1/4 teaspoon kosher salt
- 1/2 teaspoon freshly ground pepper
- 2 boneless, skinless chicken breasts, trimmed of fat (8 ounces)
- 3 teaspoons extra-virgin olive oil, divided
- 1 6-ounce bag spinach
- 1/3 cup prepared marinara sauce, (see Tips for Two)
- 2 tablespoons grated Parmesan cheese
- 1/4 cup shredded part-skim mozzarella cheese
- 2 soft whole-wheat sandwich rolls, toasted

PREPARATION

1. Combine flour, salt and pepper in a shallow dish. Place chicken between two large pieces of plastic wrap. Pound with the smooth side of a meat mallet or a

heavy saucepan until the chicken is an even 1/4-inch thickness. Dredge the chicken in the flour mixture.
2. Heat 1 teaspoon oil in a large nonstick skillet over medium-high heat. Add spinach, and cook, stirring often, until wilted, 1 to 2 minutes. Transfer to a small bowl.
3. Add the remaining 2 teaspoons oil to the pan. Add the chicken, and cook until golden on first side, 2 to 3 minutes. Turn the chicken, reduce heat to medium, top with the wilted spinach, marinara sauce and Parmesan. Sprinkle with mozzarella, cover and cook until the cheese is melted and the chicken is cooked through, 2 to 3 minutes. Serve on rolls.

TIPS & NOTES
- **Tips for Two:** Refrigerate marinara sauce for up to 1 week or freeze for up to 3 months. Spread on toasted whole-wheat English muffin halves and top with cheese for a quick snack; use for making lasagna; toss with roasted eggplant or other roasted vegetables.

NUTRITION
Per serving: 458 calories; 16 g fat (4 g sat, 8 g mono); 67 mg cholesterol; 45 g carbohydrates; 39 g protein; 4 g fiber; 693 mg sodium; 672 mg potassium.
Nutrition Bonus: Vitamin A (160% daily value), Vitamin C (45% dv), Folate (42% dv), Magnesium (23% dv).
Carbohydrate Servings: 3
Exchanges: 2 1/2 starch, 1 vegetable, 4 lean meat, 1 fat

Turkey Cutlets with Peas & Spring Onions

INGREDIENTS
- 1/2 cup all-purpose flour
- 1/2 teaspoon salt, divided
- 1/4 teaspoon freshly ground pepper
- 1 pound 1/4-inch-thick turkey breast cutlets, or steaks
- 2 tablespoons extra-virgin olive oil, divided
- 4 ounces shiitake mushrooms, stemmed and sliced (about 1 1/2 cups)
- 1 bunch spring onions, or scallions, sliced, whites and greens separated
- 1 cup reduced-sodium chicken broth
- 1/2 cup dry white wine
- 1 cup peas, fresh or frozen, thawed
- 1 teaspoon freshly grated lemon zest

PREPARATION
1. Whisk flour, 1/4 teaspoon salt and pepper in a shallow dish. Dredge each turkey cutlet (or steak) in the flour mixture. Heat 1 tablespoon oil in a large nonstick

skillet over medium-high heat. Add the turkey and cook until lightly golden, 2 to 3 minutes per side. Transfer to a plate; cover with foil to keep warm.
2. Add the remaining 1 tablespoon oil to the pan and heat over medium-high heat. Add mushrooms and onion (or scallion) whites and cook, stirring often, until the mushrooms are browned and the whites are slightly softened, 2 to 3 minutes. Add broth, wine and the remaining 1/4 teaspoon salt; cook, stirring occasionally, until the sauce is slightly reduced, 2 to 3 minutes. Stir in peas and onion (or scallion) greens and cook, stirring, until heated through, about 1 minute. Stir in lemon zest. Nestle the turkey into the vegetables along with any accumulated juices from the plate. Cook, turning the cutlets once, until heated through, 1 to 2 minutes.

NUTRITION
Per serving: 313 calories; 8 g fat (1 g sat, 5 g mono); 45 mg cholesterol; 23 g carbohydrates; 34 g protein; 3 g fiber; 571 mg sodium; 223 mg potassium.
Nutrition Bonus: Iron (15% daily value), Vitamin A & C (20% dv).
Carbohydrate Servings: 1
Exchanges: 1 starch, 1 vegetable, 4 lean meat, 1 fat

Edamame Succotash with Shrimp

INGREDIENTS
- 2 slices bacon
- 1 tablespoon extra-virgin olive oil
- 1 bunch scallions, sliced, or 1 medium onion, diced
- 1 red bell pepper, diced
- 2 cloves garlic, minced
- 1 1/2 teaspoons chopped fresh thyme
- 1 10-ounce package frozen shelled edamame, (see Tip), thawed
- 1 10-ounce package frozen corn, (about 2 cups), thawed
- 1/2 cup reduced-sodium chicken broth, or vegetable broth
- 1 tablespoon cider vinegar
- 1/4 teaspoon salt
- 1 pound raw shrimp, (26-30 per pound), peeled and deveined
- 1/4 teaspoon lemon pepper

PREPARATION
1. Cook bacon in a large nonstick skillet over medium heat until crisp, about 5 minutes. Leaving the drippings in the pan, use tongs to transfer the bacon to a plate lined with paper towels; let cool.
2. Add oil to the pan. Add scallions (or onion), bell pepper, garlic and thyme and cook, stirring, until softened, about 3 minutes. Stir in edamame, corn, broth,

vinegar and salt. Bring to a simmer; reduce heat to medium-low and cook for 5 minutes.
3. Meanwhile, sprinkle shrimp on both sides with lemon pepper. Scatter the shrimp on top of the vegetables, cover and cook until the shrimp are cooked through, about 5 minutes. Crumble the bacon and sprinkle it on top.

TIPS & NOTES
- **Tip:** Edamame are found in the natural-foods freezer section of large supermarkets and natural-foods stores, sold both in and out of the "pods." For this recipe, you'll need the shelled edamame. One 10-ounce bag contains about 2 cups of shelled beans.

NUTRITION
Per serving: 307 calories; 9 g fat (1 g sat, 4 g mono); 172 mg cholesterol; 26 g carbohydrates; 0 g added sugars; 30 g protein; 7 g fiber; 491 mg sodium; 476 mg potassium.
Nutrition Bonus: Vitamin C (120% daily value), Selenium (53% dv), Vitamin A (40% dv), Iron (30% dv).
Carbohydrate Servings: 1
Exchanges: 1 1/2 starch, 1 vegetable, 3 lean meat

The Diet House Salad

INGREDIENTS
- 4 cups torn green leaf lettuce
- 1 cup sprouts
- 1 cup tomato wedges
- 1 cup peeled, sliced cucumber
- 1 cup shredded carrots
- 1/2 cup chopped radishes
- 1/2 cup Sesame Tamari Vinaigrette (recipe follows), or other dressing

PREPARATION
1. Toss lettuce, sprouts, tomato, cucumber, carrots and radishes in a large bowl with the dressing until the vegetables are coated.

NUTRITION
Per serving: 71 calories; 3 g fat (0 g sat, 1 g mono); 0 mg cholesterol; 11 g carbohydrates; 2 g protein; 3 gfiber; 334 mg sodium; 428 mg potassium.
Nutrition Bonus: Vitamin A (140% daily value), Vitamin C (30% dv), Folate (16% dv).
Carbohydrate Servings: 1
Exchanges: 2 vegetable, 1/2 fat

Berry Frozen Yogurt

INGREDIENTS

- 3 cups fresh or frozen and partially thawed blackberries, or raspberries or a mixture of blackberries, raspberries and blueberries (see Tip)
- 6 tablespoons sugar
- 1 tablespoon lemon juice
- 3/4 cup low-fat plain yogurt

PREPARATION

1. Combine berries, sugar and lemon juice in a food processor; process until smooth. Add yogurt and pulse until mixed in. If using fresh berries, transfer the mixture to a medium bowl, cover and refrigerate until chilled, about 1 hour.
2. Transfer the berry mixture to an ice cream maker and freeze according to manufacturer's directions. (Alternatively, freeze the mixture in a shallow metal pan until solid, about 6 hours. Break into chunks and process in a food processor until smooth and creamy.) Serve immediately or transfer to a storage container and let harden in the freezer for 1 to 1 1/2 hours. Serve in chilled dishes.

TIPS & NOTES

- **Make Ahead Tip**: Store in an airtight container in the freezer for up to 1 week. Let soften in the refrigerator for 1/2 hour before serving. | Equipment: Ice cream maker or food processor
- **Tip:** To freeze fresh berries: Wash berries and pat dry. Spread in a single layer on a tray, cover with plastic wrap and freeze until solid. Pack frozen fruit into ziplock bags, taking care to remove air from the bags. Freeze for up to 1 year.

NUTRITION

Per serving: 106 calories; 1 g fat (0 g sat, 0 g mono); 2 mg cholesterol; 22 g carbohydrates; 3 g protein; 4 gfiber; 22 mg sodium; 192 mg potassium.
Nutrition Bonus: Vitamin C (28% daily value), Fiber (16% dv).
Carbohydrate Servings: 1 1/2
Exchanges: 1 1/2 fruit

DAY 28
BREAKFAST

Sunday Sausage Strata
Skim milk (1 cup)
Orange (1 large)
LUNCH

Chicken Salad Wraps or Lamb Kafta Pockets
Skim milk (1 cup)
SNACK

Fat-free cheese (1 slice)
DINNER

Pizza-Style Meatloaf
Roasted squash (1/2 cup)
Baked potato (1 medium) or Yukon Gold & Sweet Potato Mash
The Wedge
Apricot (1/2 cup, halves)

DAY 28 RECIPES

Sunday Sausage Strata

INGREDIENTS
- 1/2 pound turkey breakfast sausage, (four 2-ounce links), casing removed
- 2 medium onions, chopped (2 cups)
- 1 medium red bell pepper, seeded and diced (1 1/2 cups)
- 12 large eggs
- 4 cups 1% milk
- 1 teaspoon salt, or to taste
- Freshly ground pepper, to taste
- 6 cups cubed, whole-wheat country bread, (about 7 slices, crusts removed)
- 1 tablespoon Dijon mustard
- 1 1/2 cups grated Swiss cheese, (4 ounces)

PREPARATION
1. Coat a 9-by-13-inch baking dish (or similar shallow 3-quart baking dish) with cooking spray.
2. Cook sausage in a large nonstick skillet over medium heat, crumbling with a wooden spoon, until lightly browned, 3 to 4 minutes. Transfer to a plate lined with paper towels to drain. Add onions and bell pepper to the pan and cook, stirring often, until softened, 3 to 4 minutes.
3. Whisk eggs, milk, salt and pepper in a large bowl until blended.

4. Spread bread in the prepared baking dish. Scatter the sausage and the onion mixture evenly over the bread. Brush with mustard. Sprinkle with cheese. Pour in the egg mixture. Cover with plastic wrap and refrigerate for at least 2 hours or overnight.
5. Preheat oven to 350 degrees F. Bake the strata, uncovered, until puffed, lightly browned and set in the center, 55 to 65 minutes. Let cool for about 5 minutes before serving hot.

TIPS & NOTES
- **Make Ahead Tip**: Prepare through Step 4 the night before serving.

NUTRITION

Per serving: 255 calories; 13 g fat (45 g sat, 4 g mono); 229 mg cholesterol; 19 g carbohydrates; 17 gprotein; 2 g fiber; 513 mg sodium; 380 mg potassium.
Nutrition Bonus: Vitamin C (72% daily value), Calcium (23% dv).
Carbohydrate Servings: 1
Exchanges: 2/3 starch, 1/3 milk, 1/2 vegetable, 1 very lean protein, 1 1/3 medium-fat protein

Chicken Salad Wraps

INGREDIENTS
- 1/2 cup lemon juice
- 1/3 cup fish sauce, (see Ingredient note)
- 1/4 cup sugar
- 2 cloves garlic, minced
- 1/4 teaspoon crushed red pepper
- 8 6-inch flour tortillas
- 4 cups shredded romaine lettuce
- 3 cups shredded cooked chicken, (12 ounces)
- 1 large ripe tomato, cut into thin wedges
- 1 cup grated carrots, (2 medium)
- 2/3 cup chopped scallions, and (1 bunch)slivered fresh mint

PREPARATION
1. Whisk lemon juice, fish sauce, sugar, garlic and crushed red pepper in a small bowl until sugar is dissolved.
2. Preheat oven to 325° F. Wrap tortillas in foil and heat in the oven for 10 to 15 minutes, until softened and heated through. Keep warm.
3. Combine lettuce, chicken, tomato, carrots, scallions and mint in a large bowl. Add 1/3 cup of the dressing; toss to coat.

4. Set out the chicken mixture, tortillas and the remaining dressing for diners to assemble wraps at the table. Serve immediately.

TIPS & NOTES
- **Ingredient note:** A pungent, soy sauce-like condiment used throughout Southeast Asia, fish sauce is made from fermented, salted fish. Available in large supermarkets and in Asian markets.
- To warm tortillas in a microwave, stack between two damp paper towels; microwave on high for 30 to 60 seconds, or until heated through.

NUTRITION
Per serving: 439 calories; 9 g fat (2 g sat, 4 g mono); 89 mg cholesterol; 49 g carbohydrates; 40 g protein; 5 g fiber; 1018 mg sodium; 783 mg potassium.
Nutrition Bonus: 140% dv vitamin a, 31 mg vitamin c (50% dv), 179 mcg folate (45% dv), 4 mg iron (25% dv).
Carbohydrate Servings: 3
Exchanges: 3 stach, 1 vegetable, 3 lean meat

Lamb Kafta Pockets

INGREDIENTS
APRICOT SAUCE
- 6 dried apricots
- 1/3 cup orange juice
- 2 tablespoons chopped fresh mint
- 2 tablespoons water
- 1 teaspoon red-wine vinegar

LAMB KAFTA
- 1/3 cup whole-wheat couscous
- 1/3 cup boiling water
- 4 ounces ground lamb
- 1 tablespoon chopped fresh parsley
- 1 teaspoon minced garlic
- 1/4 teaspoon salt
- 1/8 teaspoon ground allspice
- 1 teaspoon extra-virgin olive oil
- 2 whole-wheat pitas, sliced open on top and toasted

PREPARATION

1. To prepare apricot sauce: Combine apricots and orange juice in a small microwave-safe bowl and microwave on High until bubbling, about 1 minute.

Set aside to soften for 10 minutes. Transfer the apricot mixture to a food processor or blender. Add mint, water and vinegar; puree until smooth.
2. To prepare lamb kafta: Place couscous in a medium bowl. Pour boiling water over it and let stand until the water is absorbed, about 5 minutes. Add lamb, parsley, garlic, salt and allspice to the couscous and knead until the mixture is sticky and holds together. Form into 6 balls of equal size.
3. Heat oil in a medium nonstick skillet. Add the meatballs and cook, turning often to prevent scorching, until browned on all sides, about 6 minutes. Pour 1/2 cup water into the skillet, cover and cook until the meatballs are cooked through, about 4 minutes. Using a slotted spoon, transfer the meatballs to a plate. Serve the meatballs inside pitas topped with the apricot sauce.

TIPS & NOTES
- **Make Ahead Tip**: The sauce can be made up to 1 day in advance.

NUTRITION
Per serving: 439 calories; 12 g fat (4 g sat, 5 g mono); 37 mg cholesterol; 75 g carbohydrates; 21 g protein;11 g fiber; 566 mg sodium; 644 mg potassium.
Nutrition Bonus: Vitamin C (40% daily value), Vitamin A (30% dv), Iron (20% dv).
Carbohydrate Servings: 4
Exchanges: 3 1/2 starch, 1 1/2 fruit, 2 medium fat meat

Pizza-Style Meatloaf

INGREDIENTS
- 1 teaspoon extra-virgin olive oil
- 1 medium onion, sliced
- 1 red or yellow bell pepper, sliced
- 4 ounces mushrooms, sliced and 1/4 cup chopped fresh basil
- 1 pound lean ground beef
- 1 clove garlic, minced
- 1/3 cup seasoned (Italian-style) breadcrumbs
- 1/3 cup low-fat milk and 1/2 teaspoon salt
- 1/2 cup prepared marinara sauce
- 1/4 cup shredded sharp Cheddar cheese

PREPARATION
1. Preheat oven to 400°F. Coat a 12-inch pizza pan with cooking spray and place it on a large baking sheet with sides.
2. Heat oil in a large skillet over medium heat. Add onion, bell pepper, mushrooms and basil; cook, stirring, until softened, about 10 minutes.
3. Meanwhile, combine beef, garlic, breadcrumbs, milk and salt in a large bowl. Mix well.

4. Transfer the meat mixture to the prepared pan. With dampened hands, pat into a 10-inch circle. Top with marinara sauce. Spoon the vegetable mixture over the sauce and sprinkle with cheese.

5. Bake until the meat is browned and the cheese has melted, about 30 minutes. Drain off any fat. Cut into wedges and serve.

TIPS & NOTES
- **Make Ahead Tip**: Equipment: Use a perforated pizza pan.

NUTRITION
Per serving: 195 calories; 8 g fat (3 g sat, 2 g mono); 53 mg cholesterol; 11 g carbohydrates; 20 g protein; 2 g fiber; 471 mg sodium; 414 mg potassium.
Nutrition Bonus: Vitamin C (48% daily value), Zinc (27% dv), Selenium (21% dv), Vitamin A (18% dv).
Carbohydrate Servings: 1
Exchanges: 1 other carbohydrate, 21/2 lean meat

Yukon Gold & Sweet Potato Mash

INGREDIENTS
- 1 pound Yukon Gold potatoes, peeled and cut into 1 1/2-inch chunks
- 1 pound sweet potatoes, peeled and cut into 1 1/2-inch chunks
- 1/2 cup low-fat milk
- 2 tablespoons butter
- 1 teaspoon brown sugar
- 3/4 teaspoon salt
- 1/4 teaspoon freshly ground pepper

PREPARATION

1. Place potatoes and sweet potatoes in a large saucepan and add enough water to cover. Bring to a boil over high heat and cook until very tender when pierced with a fork, 20 to 25 minutes.
2. Drain the potatoes, then mash them in the pot to the desired consistency. Place milk and butter in a small bowl and microwave on High until the butter is mostly melted and the milk is warm, 30 to 40 seconds. (Alternatively, place in a small saucepan and heat over medium until the milk is warm.) Stir the milk mixture, sugar, salt and pepper into the mashed potatoes until combined.

NUTRITION
Per serving: 151 calories; 4 g fat (3 g sat, 0 g mono); 11 mg cholesterol; 26 g carbohydrates; 3 g protein; 3 g fiber; 321 mg sodium; 369 mg potassium.
Nutrition Bonus: Vitamin A (190% daily value), Vitamin C (20% dv).

Carbohydrate Servings: 2
Exchanges: 2 starch, 1 fat

The Wedge

INGREDIENTS
- 2 heart of romaine, quartered lengthwise and cores removed
- 1/4 cup chopped fresh chives
- 2 slices cooked bacon, crumbled
- 2 ounces crumbled blue cheese
- 1/2 cup Buttermilk Ranch Dressing, (recipe follows)

PREPARATION
1. Place 2 romaine quarters on each of 4 salad plates. Sprinkle with chives, bacon and blue cheese. Drizzle with Buttermilk Ranch Dressing.

NUTRITION
Per serving: 111 calories; 8 g fat (3 g sat, 2 g mono); 17 mg cholesterol; 5 g carbohydrates; 6 g protein; 1 gfiber; 481 mg sodium; 97 mg potassium.
Nutrition Bonus: Folate, calcium, potassium.
Exchanges: 1 vegetable, 1/2 high-fat meat

1800 CALORIE DIET PLAN

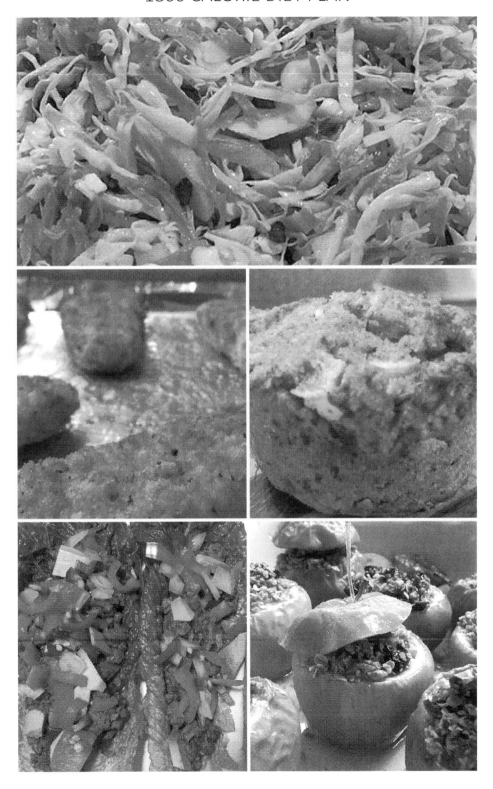

DAY 1
BREAKFAST

Apricot Smoothie
Whole-wheat toast (1 slice)
Plum spread

LUNCH

Grape and Feta Mixed Green Special
Shrimp French Brisque
Whole-wheat toast (1 slice)
Raspberries (1 cup)

SNACK

Apple (1 cup, quartered)
Skim milk (1 cup)

DINNER

Hot and Spicy Halibut or Simple Roast Chicken
Barley & Wild Rice Pilaf or Farro with Pistachios & Herbs
Green Beans with Toasted Nuts
Bread & Tomato Salad
Quick "Cheesecake"

DAY 1 RECIPES

Apricot Smoothie

INGREDIENTS
- 1 cup canned apricot halves in light syrup
- 6 ice cubes
- 1 cup nonfat plain yogurt
- 3 tablespoons sugar

PREPARATION

1. Blend apricot halves, ice cubes, yogurt and sugar in a blender until frothy.

NUTRITION
Per serving: 202 calories; 0 g fat (0 g sat, 0 g mono); 3 mg cholesterol; 49 g carbohydrates; 6 g protein; 2 gfiber; 74 mg sodium; 175 mg potassium.
Carbohydrate Servings: 3
Exchanges: 1 1/2 fruit, 1/2 fat-free milk, 1 other carbohydrate

Plum spread

INGREDIENTS
- 5 pounds plums, pitted and sliced (14-15 cups)
- 3 Granny Smith apples, washed and quartered (not cored)
- 1/4 cup white grape juice, or other fruit juice
- 2 tablespoons lemon juice
- 3/4 cup sugar, or Splenda Granular
- 1/4 teaspoon ground cinnamon, or ginger (optional)

PREPARATION
1. Place a plate in the freezer for testing consistency later.
2. Combine plums, apples, grape juice (or fruit juice) and lemon juice in a large, heavy-bottomed, nonreactive Dutch oven. Bring to a boil over medium-high heat, stirring. Cover and boil gently, stirring occasionally, until the fruit is softened and juicy, 15 to 20 minutes. Uncover and boil gently, stirring occasionally, until the fruit is completely soft, about 20 minutes. (Adjust heat as necessary to maintain a gentle boil.)
3. Pass the fruit through a food mill to remove the skins and apple seeds.
4. Return the strained fruit to the pot. Add sugar (or Splenda) and cinnamon (or ginger), if using. Cook over medium heat, stirring frequently, until a spoonful of jam dropped onto the chilled plate holds its shape, about 15 minutes longer. (See Tip.) Remove from heat and skim off any foam.

TIPS & NOTES
- **Make Ahead Tip**: Store in an airtight container in the refrigerator for up to 2 months. For longer storage, process in a boiling-water bath (for detailed instructions, refer to www.homecanning.com or call the Home Canner's Hotline at 800-240-3340).
- **To test the consistency of the spread:** Drop a dollop of cooked spread onto a chilled plate. Carefully run your finger through the dollop. If the track remains unfilled, the jam is done.

NUTRITION
Per tablespoon with sugar: 14 calories; 0 g fat (0 g sat, 0 g mono); 0 mg cholesterol; 4 g carbohydrates; 0 g protein; 0 g fiber; 0 mg sodium; 30 mg potassium.
Exchanges: free food
Nutrition Note: Per tablespoon with Splenda: 0 Carbohydrate Servings; 12 calories; 3 g carbohydrate.

Grape and Feta Mixed Green Special

INGREDIENTS
DRESSING
- 1/4 cup extra-virgin olive oil
- 2 tablespoons red-wine vinegar
- 1/4 teaspoon salt, or to taste
- Freshly ground pepper, to taste

SALAD
- 8 cups mesclun salad greens, (5 ounces)
- 1 head radicchio, thinly sliced
- 2 cups halved seedless grapes, (about 1 pound), preferably red and green
- 3/4 cup crumbled feta, or blue cheese

PREPARATION
1. To prepare dressing: Whisk (or shake) oil, vinegar, salt and pepper in a small bowl (or jar) until blended.
2. To prepare salad: Just before serving, toss greens and radicchio in a large bowl. Drizzle the dressing on top and toss to coat. Divide the salad among 8 plates. Scatter grapes and cheese over each salad; serve immediately.

TIPS & NOTES
- **Make Ahead Tip**: The dressing will keep, covered, in the refrigerator for up to 2 days.

NUTRITION

Per serving: 133 calories; 10 g fat (3 g sat, 6 g mono); 13 mg cholesterol; 9 g carbohydrates; 3 g protein; 1 g fiber; 239 mg sodium; 183 mg potassium.
Nutrition Bonus: Vitamin C (15% daily value), Folate (9% dv).
Carbohydrate Servings: 1/2
Exchanges: 1/2 fruit, 1 vegetable, 2 fat

Shrimp French Brisque

INGREDIENTS
- 12 ounces shrimp (30-40 per pound), shell-on
- 1 onion, chopped, divided
- 1 carrot, peeled and sliced
- 1 stalk celery (with leaves), sliced
- 1/2 cup dry white wine
- 1/2 teaspoon black peppercorns
- 1 bay leaf

- 3 cups water
- 1 tablespoon extra-virgin olive oil
- 4 ounces mushrooms, wiped clean and sliced (about 1 1/2 cups)
- 1/2 green bell pepper, chopped
- 1/4 cup chopped scallions
- 2 tablespoons chopped fresh parsley
- 1/4 cup all-purpose flour
- 1 1/2 cups low-fat milk
- 1/4 cup reduced-fat sour cream
- 1/4 cup dry sherry
- 1 tablespoon lemon juice
- 1/4 teaspoon salt
- Freshly ground pepper to taste
- Dash of hot sauce

PREPARATION

1. Peel and devein shrimp, reserving the shells. Cut the shrimp into 3/4-inch pieces; cover and refrigerate.
2. Combine the shrimp shells with about half the onion, all the carrot, celery, wine, peppercorns and bay leaf in a large heavy saucepan. Add water and simmer over low heat for about 30 minutes. Strain through a sieve, pressing on the solids to extract all the juices; discard the solids. Measure the shrimp stock and add water, if necessary, to make 1 1/2 cups.
3. Heat oil in the same pan over medium heat. Add mushrooms, bell pepper, scallions, parsley and the remaining onion. Cook, stirring, until the mushrooms are soft, about 5 minutes. Sprinkle with flour and cook, stirring constantly, until it starts to turn golden, 2 to 3 minutes. Slowly stir in milk and the shrimp stock. Cook, stirring to loosen any flour sticking to the bottom of the pot, until the soup returns to a simmer and thickens, about 5 minutes. Add the reserved shrimp and cook until they turn opaque in the center, about 2 minutes more. Add sour cream, sherry and lemon juice; stir over low heat until heated through; do not let it come to a boil. Taste and adjust seasonings with salt, pepper and hot sauce.

TIPS & NOTES
- **Make Ahead Tip**: Cover and refrigerate for up to 1 day.

NUTRITION
Per serving: 163 calories; 5 g fat (2 g sat, 2 g mono); 92 mg cholesterol; 12 g carbohydrates; 13 g protein; 1 g fiber; 241 mg sodium; 255 mg potassium.
Nutrition Bonus: Selenium (30% daily value), Vitamin A (26% dv), Vitamin C (24% dv).
Carbohydrate Servings: 1
Exchanges: 1 starch; 2 very lean meat; 1 fat

Hot and Spicy Halibut

INGREDIENTS
- 1 1/4 pounds halibut, striped bass or tilapia fillet, cut into 4 portions
- 1 teaspoon ground cumin, divided
- 1/4 teaspoon salt
- Freshly ground pepper, to taste
- 1 10-ounce can diced tomatoes with green chiles
- 1/4 cup sliced green olives with pimientos
- 2 tablespoons chopped fresh cilantro
- 1 teaspoon extra-virgin olive oil

PREPARATION
1. Preheat oven to 450°F. Coat a baking sheet with cooking spray. Arrange fish on baking sheet. Season with 1/2 teaspoon cumin, salt and pepper.
2. Combine tomatoes, olives, cilantro, oil and the remaining 1/2 teaspoon cumin in a small bowl. Spoon over the fish.
3. Bake the fish until flaky and opaque in the center, 12 to 15 minutes. Serve immediately.

NUTRITION
Per serving: 188 calories; 7 g fat (1 g sat, 4 g mono); 45 mg cholesterol; 4 g carbohydrates; 30 g protein; 1 g fiber; 758 mg sodium; 638 mg potassium.
Nutrition Bonus: Potassium (18% daily value).
Exchanges: 4 very lean meat, 1 fat (mono)

Simple Roast Chicken

INGREDIENTS
- 1 small onion, peeled and quartered
- 3 cloves garlic, peeled and quartered
- 3 sprigs fresh tarragon
- 3 sprigs fresh thyme
- 1 5-pound chicken, giblets removed
- 2 tablespoons extra-virgin olive oil
- 1 teaspoon kosher salt
- 1/2 teaspoon freshly ground pepper

PREPARATION
1. Preheat oven to 375°F.
2. Place onion, garlic, tarragon and thyme into the cavity of the chicken. Tie the legs together with kitchen string, mostly closing the cavity opening. Pull the wings so the tips overlap on top of the breast; tie in place, wrapping string

around the wings and body. Rub the chicken with oil, salt and pepper. Set in a roasting pan, breast-side down.
3. Roast the chicken for 25 minutes. Turn breast-side up and continue roasting, basting occasionally with pan juices, until a thermometer inserted into the thickest part of the thigh, without touching bone, registers 175°F, 1 1/4 to 1 1/2 hours. Transfer to a cutting board; let rest for 10 minutes. Remove the string before carving.

TIPS & NOTES
- **Make Ahead Tip**: Equipment: Kitchen string
- Roasting Tips
- 1. Very cold meat won't roast evenly. Place it on the counter while preheating the oven.
- 2. Durable cotton kitchen string is sold at kitchenware stores, most gourmet markets and large supermarkets. Do not use sewing thread or yarn, which may contain inedible dyes or unsavory chemicals.
- 3. A heavy-duty, high-sided roasting pan is essential for conducting heat evenly. Never substitute a cookie sheet. A broiler pan will work in a pinch, but the roast will inevitably be somewhat chewier.
- 4. Give it a rest. A roast's internal temperature will rise about 10 degrees while resting. The natural juices will also reincorporate into the meat's fibers and the skin or crust will dry out slightly for a more toothsome yet more succulent dinner.

NUTRITION
Per 3-ounce serving (without skin): 180 calories; 9 g fat (2 g sat, 5 g mono); 64 mg cholesterol; 1 gcarbohydrates; 0 g added sugars; 21 g protein; 0 g fiber; 300 mg sodium; 217 mg potassium.
Nutrition Bonus: Selenium (30% daily value).
Exchanges: 3 lean meat

Barley & Wild Rice Pilaf
INGREDIENTS
- 2 teaspoons extra-virgin olive oil
- 1 medium onion, finely chopped
- 1/2 cup wild rice, rinsed and 1/2 cup pearl barley
- 3 cups reduced-sodium chicken broth, or vegetable broth
- 1/3 cup pine nuts
- 1 cup pomegranate seeds, (1 large fruit; see Tip)
- 2 teaspoons freshly grated lemon zest
- 2 tablespoons chopped flat-leaf parsley

PREPARATION

1. Heat oil in a large saucepan over medium heat. Add onion and cook, stirring often, until softened. Add wild rice and barley; stir for a few seconds. Add broth and bring to a simmer. Reduce heat to low, cover and simmer until the wild rice and barley are tender and most of the liquid has been absorbed, 45 to 50 minutes.
2. Meanwhile, toast pine nuts in a small, dry skillet over medium-low heat, stirring constantly, until light golden and fragrant, 2 to 3 minutes. Transfer to a small bowl to cool.
3. Add pomegranate seeds, lemon zest, parsley and the toasted pine nuts to the pilaf; fluff with a fork. Serve hot.

TIPS & NOTES

- **Make Ahead Tip**: Prepare through Step 2. Cover and refrigerate for up to 2 days. To reheat, place in a baking dish, add 1/4 cup water and cover. Microwave on High for 10 to 15 minutes or bake at 350°F or 25 to 30 minutes.
- **Tip:** To seed a pomegranate and avoid the enduring stains of pomegranate juice, work under water. Fill a large bowl with water. Hold the pomegranate in the water and slice off the crown. Lightly score the fruit into quarters, from crown to stem end. Keeping the fruit under water, break it apart, gently separating the plump seeds from the outer skin and white pith. The seeds will drop to the bottom of the bowl and the pith will float to the surface. Discard the pith. Pour the seeds into a colander. Rinse and pat dry. The seeds can be frozen in an airtight container or sealable bag for up to 3 months.

NUTRITION

Per serving: 209 calories; 7 g fat (1 g sat, 3 g mono); 3 mg cholesterol; 31 g carbohydrates; 0 g added sugars; 7 g protein; 4 g fiber; 75 mg sodium; 250 mg potassium.
Nutrition Bonus: Magnesium (15% dv)
Carbohydrate Servings: 2
Exchanges: 2 starch, 1 fat

Farro with Pistachios & Herbs

INGREDIENTS

- 2 cups farro, (see Tip)
- 4 cups water
- 1 teaspoon kosher salt, divided
- 2 tablespoons plus 1/2 teaspoon extra-virgin olive oil, divided
- 1 large yellow onion, chopped
- 2 cloves garlic, minced

- 4 ounces salted shelled pistachios, (about 1 cup), toasted and chopped (see Tip)
- 1/2 teaspoon freshly ground pepper, divided
- 1/2 cup chopped fresh parsley

PREPARATION
1. Combine farro, water and 3/4 teaspoon salt in a large heavy saucepan and bring to a boil. Stir and reduce the heat to a simmer; cook, uncovered, until the farro is tender, 15 to 20 minutes.
2. Meanwhile, heat 2 tablespoons oil in a medium skillet over medium heat. Add onion and garlic and cook, stirring, until translucent, 4 to 6 minutes. Remove from the heat.
3. Combine pistachios, the remaining 1/2 teaspoon oil and 1/4 teaspoon pepper in a large bowl; toss to combine.
4. Drain the farro and add to the bowl along with the onion mixture and parsley. Season with the remaining 1/4 teaspoon salt and pepper. Toss to combine.

TIPS & NOTES
- **Make Ahead Tip**: Prepare up to 2 hours ahead. Hold at room temperature and reheat over low until warm.
- **Tips:** Farro is a high-fiber whole grain that is an ancestor of modern wheat. It is commonly used in Italian cooking and is becoming more popular in the U.S. Find it in natural-foods stores and amazon.com. Cooked barley can be used as a substitute.
- Toast pistachios in a small dry skillet over medium-low heat, stirring constantly, until fragrant and lightly browned, 4 to 6 minutes.

NUTRITION

Per serving: 220 calories; 9 g fat (1 g sat, 5 g mono); 0 mg cholesterol; 31 g carbohydrates; 8 g protein; 5 gfiber; 163 mg sodium; 160 mg potassium.
Nutrition Bonus: Fiber (20% daily value)
Carbohydrate Servings: 2
Exchanges: 1 1/2 starch, 1 vegetable, 1 1/2 fat

Green Beans with Toasted Nuts

INGREDIENTS
- 1 pound green beans, stem ends trimmed
- 2 teaspoons extra-virgin olive oil
- 2 tablespoons chopped peeled hazelnuts, or walnuts
- 1/4 teaspoon salt
- Freshly ground pepper, to taste

PREPARATION
1. Cook beans in a large pot of boiling salted water until just tender, 5 to 7 minutes. Drain.
2. Heat oil in a large nonstick skillet over low heat. Add nuts and cook, stirring, until golden, about 1 minute. Return the reserved beans to the pot and toss to coat. Season with salt and pepper.

NUTRITION
Per serving: 104 calories; 5 g fat (1 g sat, 3 g mono); 0 mg cholesterol; 9 g carbohydrates; 0 g added sugars; 3 g protein; 4 g fiber; 152 mg sodium; 261 mg potassium.
Nutrition Bonus: Fiber (28% daily value), Vitamin C (22% dv).
Exchanges: 1 vegetable, 1 fat (mono)

Bread & Tomato Salad

INGREDIENTS
- 3 tablespoons extra-virgin olive oil
- 3 tablespoons lemon juice
- 1 small clove garlic, minced
- 1/4 teaspoon salt, or to taste
- Freshly ground pepper, to taste
- 4 cups diced seeded tomatoes, (1 1/2 pounds)
- 2 cups cubed whole-wheat country bread, (5 ounces), crusts removed
- 1/4 cup thinly slivered red onion
- 3 tablespoons chopped fresh basil
- 2 tablespoons capers, rinsed
- 4 4-1/2-ounce cans sardines, (see Ingredient note), optional

PREPARATION
1. Whisk oil, lemon juice, garlic, salt and pepper in a large bowl. Add tomatoes, bread, onion, basil and capers. Toss to combine. Let the salad sit for about 5 minutes to allow it to absorb the dressing's flavors, stirring occasionally. Serve at room temperature.

TIPS & NOTES
- **Ingredient Note:** Our test kitchen is fond of Bela brand sardines from Olhao, Portugal. They are firm, lightly smoked and succulent.

NUTRITION
Per serving: 168 calories; 17 g fat (2 g sat, 9 g mono); 107 mg cholesterol; 19 g carbohydrates; 22 gprotein; 3 g fiber; 657 mg sodium; 666 mg potassium.
Nutrition Bonus: Vitamin C (60% daily value).

Carbohydrate Servings: 1
Exchanges: 1 starch, 1 vegetable, 11/2 fat (mono)

Quick "Cheesecake"

INGREDIENTS
- 4 whole-wheat graham crackers
- 4 tablespoons part-skim ricotta cheese
- 8 teaspoons jam

PREPARATION
1. Spread each graham cracker with 1 tablespoon part-skim ricotta cheese and 2 teaspoons jam.

NUTRITION

Per serving: 239 calories; 6 g fat (2 g sat, 1 g mono); 10 mg cholesterol; 42 g carbohydrates; 7 g protein; 2 g fiber; 259 mg sodium; 39 mg potassium.
Carbohydrate Servings: 3
Exchanges: 3 other carbohydrate, 1 fat

DAY 2
BREAKFAST

Tofu Scrambled Egg
Salsa Cornbread
Strawberries (1 cup)

LUNCH

Spicy Red Lentil Soup
Curried Waldorf Salad
Banana (1 cup, sliced)
Whole-wheat pita bread (1 medium pita)
Skim milk (1 cup)

SNACK

Low-fat vanilla yogurt (8 oz.)

DINNER

Turkey Cutlets with Sage & Lemon or Brazilian Grilled Flank Steak
Glazed Mini Carrots or Cool Fresh Corn Relish
Spinach (1 cup, uncooked)
Light Ranch Dressing
Buttermilk-Herb Mashed Potatoes
Fresh Fruit with Lemon-Mint Cream

DAY 2 RECIPES

Tofu Scrambled Egg

INGREDIENTS
- 1 large egg
- 1/2 teaspoon dried tarragon
- Dash of hot sauce, such as
- Pinch of salt
- Freshly ground pepper, to taste
- 1 teaspoon extra-virgin olive oil, or canola oil
- 2 tablespoons crumbled tofu, (silken or regular)

PREPARATION
Blend egg, tarragon, hot sauce, salt and pepper in a small bowl with a fork. Heat oil in a small nonstick skillet over medium-low heat. Add tofu and cook, stirring, until warmed through, 20 to 30 seconds. Add egg mixture and stir until the egg is set, but still creamy, 20 to 30 seconds. Serve immediately.

NUTRITION
Per serving: 140 calories; 11 g fat (2 g sat, 6 g mono); 212 mg cholesterol; 2 g carbohydrates; 0 g added sugars; 9 g protein; 1 g fiber; 230 mg sodium; 93 mg potassium.
Nutrition Bonus: Selenium (23% daily value).
Exchanges: 1 medium-fat meat. 1 fat (mono)

Salsa Cornbread

INGREDIENTS
- 1 cup all-purpose flour
- 1/2 cup whole-wheat flour
- 1/2 cup cornmeal
- 2 teaspoons baking powder
- 1/2 teaspoon salt
- Freshly ground pepper, to taste
- 3 large eggs, lightly beaten
- 1/2 cup buttermilk, or equivalent buttermilk powder
- 1 tablespoon butter, melted
- 1 tablespoon honey
- 1/2 cup drained canned corn kernels
- 1 small onion, diced
- 1/2 cup chopped tomato
- 1 clove garlic, minced

- 1 jalapeno pepper, seeded and minced
- 1/2 cup grated Cheddar cheese

PREPARATION

1. Preheat oven to 425° F. Place a 9-inch cast-iron skillet (or similar ovenproof skillet, see Tip) in the oven to heat.
2. Whisk all-purpose flour, whole-wheat flour, cornmeal, baking powder, salt and pepper in a large mixing bowl.
3. Whisk eggs, buttermilk, butter and honey in a medium bowl. Add the egg mixture to the dry ingredients; mix with a rubber spatula. Stir in corn, onion, tomato, garlic and jalapeno.
4. Remove the skillet from the oven and coat it with cooking spray. Pour in the batter, spreading evenly. Sprinkle cheese over the top. Bake the cornbread until golden brown and a knife inserted into the center comes out clean, 20 to 25 minutes. Serve warm.

TIPS & NOTES
- **Tip:** If you do not have an ovenproof skillet of the correct size, use an 8-by-8-inch glass baking dish. Do not preheat the empty baking dish in the oven before filling it.

NUTRITION
Per serving: 138 calories; 4 g fat (2 g sat, 1 g mono); 70 mg cholesterol; 20 g carbohydrates; 6 g protein; 1 g fiber; 319 mg sodium; 91 mg potassium.
Carbohydrate Servings: 1
Exchanges: 1 starch, 1 fat

Spicy Red Lentil Soup

INGREDIENTS
- 6 teaspoons extra-virgin olive oil, divided
- 2 onions, chopped (1 1/2 cups)
- 3 cloves garlic, minced
- 2 teaspoons ground cumin
- 8 cups reduced-sodium chicken broth, or vegetable broth
- 1 1/2 cups red lentils, rinsed (see Tip)
- 1/3 cup bulgur
- 2 tablespoons tomato paste and 1 bay leaf
- 3 tablespoons lemon juice
- Freshly ground pepper to taste
- 1 teaspoon paprika
- 1 teaspoon cayenne pepper

PREPARATION
1. Heat 2 teaspoons oil in a soup pot or Dutch oven over medium heat. Add onions and cook, stirring, until softened, 3 to 5 minutes. Add garlic and cumin; cook for 1 minute. Add broth, lentils, bulgur, tomato paste and bay leaf; bring to a simmer, stirring occasionally. Cover and cook over low heat until the lentils and bulgur are very tender, 25 to 30 minutes. Discard the bay leaf.
2. Ladle about 4 cups of the soup into a food processor and puree. Return the pureed soup to the soup pot and heat through. Stir in lemon juice and season with pepper.
3. Just before serving, ladle the soup into bowls. Heat the remaining 4 teaspoons oil in a small skillet and stir in paprika and cayenne. Drizzle about 1/2 teaspoon of the sizzling spice mixture over each bowlful and serve immediately.

TIPS & NOTES
- **Make Ahead Tip**: Prepare through Step 2. Cover and refrigerate for up to 2 days or freeze for up to 2 months.
- **Tip:** You can replace red lentils with brown lentils; add 1/2 cup water and simmer 40 to 45 minutes.

NUTRITION
Per serving: 218 calories; 5 g fat (1 g sat, 3 g mono); 5 mg cholesterol; 31 g carbohydrates; 0 g added sugars; 15 g protein; 7 g fiber; 151 mg sodium; 406 mg potassium.
Nutrition Bonus: Fiber (29% daily value), Iron (15% dv).
Carbohydrate Servings: 2
Exchanges: 1 1/2 starch, 1 vegetable, 1 lean meat

Curried Waldorf Salad

INGREDIENTS
- 1/4 cup nonfat plain yogurt
- 3 tablespoons low-fat mayonnaise
- 1/2 teaspoon curry powder
- 1/8 teaspoon salt
- Pinch of cayenne pepper, or to taste
- 1 orange
- 2 tart-sweet red apples, diced
- 1 cup chopped celery
- 1/3 cup golden raisins
- 1/3 cup coarsely chopped walnuts, toasted (see Tip)

PREPARATION
1. Whisk yogurt, mayonnaise, curry powder, salt and cayenne in a medium bowl. Grate 2 teaspoons zest from the orange and add to the dressing.
2. Using a sharp knife, cut off the peel and white pith from the orange. To make segments, hold the orange over the bowl (to catch the juice) and slice between each segment and its surrounding membranes. Add apples, celery, raisins and walnuts; toss to combine.

TIPS & NOTES
- **Tip:** To toast chopped walnuts, cook in a small dry skillet over medium-low heat, stirring constantly, until fragrant and lightly browned, 2 to 5 minutes.

NUTRITION
Per serving: 136 calories; 5 g fat (0 g sat, 0 g mono); 0 mg cholesterol; 24 g carbohydrates; 0 g added sugars; 2 g protein; 4 g fiber; 134 mg sodium; 222 mg potassium.
Nutrition Bonus: Vitamin C (26% daily value).
Carbohydrate Servings: 1 1/2
Exchanges: 1 1/2 fruit, 1 fat

Turkey Cutlets with Sage & Lemon

INGREDIENTS
- 3 tablespoons all-purpose
- 1 pound turkey breast cutlets
- 1/4 teaspoon salt
- Freshly ground pepper, to taste
- 3 teaspoons extra-virgin olive oil, divided
- 2 cloves garlic, minced
- 2 teaspoons chopped fresh sage
- 1/4 cup dry white wine
- 3/4 cup reduced-sodium chicken broth
- 1 teaspoon lemon juice
- 1 teaspoon butter

PREPARATION
1. Spread flour on a large plate. Cut several small slits in outer edges of the turkey to prevent curling. Pat dry with paper towels and season with salt and pepper. Dredge lightly in flour. Discard any remaining flour.
2. Heat 1 teaspoon oil in a large nonstick skillet over medium-high heat. Add half the turkey and cook until golden outside and no longer pink inside, 1 to 2

minutes per side. Transfer to a platter and tent with foil to keep warm. Saute the remaining turkey in another 1 teaspoon oil until golden; transfer to platter.
3. Add the remaining 1 teaspoon oil to the pan. Add garlic and sage; cook, stirring, until fragrant, about 1 minute. Add wine and cook, scraping up any browned bits, until reduced by half, about 1 minute. Add broth and cook until the liquid is reduced by half, 4 to 5 minutes. Stir in lemon juice and any juices accumulated from the turkey and simmer for 1 minute more. Remove from heat and swirl in butter. Serve, spooning the sauce over the turkey.

NUTRITION
Per serving: 205 calories; 5 g fat (1 g sat, 3 g mono); 48 mg cholesterol; 6 g carbohydrates; 0 g added sugars; 29 g protein; 0 g fiber; 273 mg sodium; 358 mg potassium.
Nutrition Bonus: Selenium (47% daily value).
Exchanges: 4 very lean meat, 1 fat

Brazilian Grilled Flank Steak

INGREDIENTS
STEAK
- 6 cloves garlic, minced
- 1/2 small hot pepper, such as jalapeño or serrano, minced
- 2 teaspoons extra-virgin olive oil
- 1/4 teaspoon kosher salt
- 2 pounds flank steak

SALSA
- 1 14-ounce can hearts of palm, drained, halved lengthwise and thinly sliced
- 4 medium tomatoes, chopped
- 1/2 cup chopped red onion
- 1/2 small hot chile, such as jalapeño or serrano, minced
- 1/4 cup chopped fresh cilantro
- 2 tablespoons red-wine vinegar
- 1/4 teaspoon kosher salt

PREPARATION
1. Preheat grill to high (see Broiling Variation).
2. To prepare steak: Combine garlic, hot pepper, oil and salt in a small bowl. Rub the mixture on both sides of steak.
3. To prepare salsa: Combine hearts of palm, tomatoes, onion, hot pepper, cilantro, vinegar and salt in a medium bowl.

4. Reduce grill heat to medium and grill the steak 4 to 6 minutes per side for medium-rare. Transfer to a cutting board, tent with foil and let rest for 5 minutes. Cut the steak across the grain into thin pieces. Serve with the salsa.

TIPS & NOTES
- **Broiling variation:**
- Instead of grilling, in Step 1 position oven rack 6 inches from the heat source and preheat broiler. In Step 4, cook steak on a broiler pan under the broiler until medium-rare, turning once, about 10 minutes total.

NUTRITION
Per serving: 215 calories; 8 g fat (3 g sat, 4 g mono); 37 mg cholesterol; 7 g carbohydrates; 0 g added sugars; 29 g protein; 2 g fiber; 341 mg sodium; 627 mg potassium.
Nutrition Bonus: Zinc (36% daily value), Vitamin C (25% dv), Iron (20% dv), Potassium (18% dv), Vitamin A (15% dv).
Carbohydrate Servings: 1/2
Exchanges: 1 vegetable, 4 lean meat

Glazed Mini Carrots

INGREDIENTS
- 3 cups mini carrots, (1 pound)
- 1/3 cup water
- 1 tablespoon honey
- 2 teaspoons butter
- 1/4 teaspoon salt, or to taste
- 1 tablespoon lemon juice
- Freshly ground pepper, to taste
- 2 tablespoons chopped fresh parsley

PREPARATION
1. Combine carrots, water, honey, butter and salt in a large skillet. Bring to a simmer over medium-high heat. Cover and cook until tender, 5 to 7 minutes. Uncover and cook, stirring often, until the liquid is a syrupy glaze, 1 to 2 minutes. Stir in lemon juice and pepper. Sprinkle with parsley and serve.

NUTRITION
Per serving: 74 calories; 2 g fat (1 g sat, 1 g mono); 5 mg cholesterol; 14 g carbohydrates; 1 g protein; 2 gfiber; 236 mg sodium; 287 mg potassium.
Nutrition Bonus: Vitamin A (320% daily value), Vitamin C (23% dv).
Carbohydrate Servings: 1

Exchanges: 1 vegetable, 1/2 fat

Cool Fresh Corn Relish

INGREDIENTS
- 5 large ears corn, (about 3 cups kernels)
- 1 1/2 cups finely diced sweet onion
- 3/4 cup finely chopped flat-leaf parsley, (1-2 bunches)
- 3 tablespoons lime juice
- 2 tablespoons extra-virgin olive oil
- 1/4 teaspoon salt

PREPARATION
1. Microwave corn, in the husks, on High until steaming and just tender, 7 to 9 minutes. When cool enough to handle, remove the husks and silk. (Alternatively, bring a large pot of water to a boil. Remove husks and silk from the corn and boil until just tender, about 5 minutes.) Slice the kernels from the corn using a sharp knife.
2. Combine the corn kernels, onion, parsley, lime juice, oil and salt in a medium bowl. Serve at room temperature or cold.

TIPS & NOTES
- **Make Ahead Tip**: Cover and refrigerate for up to 3 days.

NUTRITION
Per serving: 65 calories; 3 g fat (0 g sat, 2 g mono); 0 mg cholesterol; 10 g carbohydrates; 2 g protein; 1 gfiber; 59 mg sodium; 163 mg potassium.
Nutrition Bonus: Vitamin C (15% daily value).
Carbohydrate Servings: 1/2
Exchanges: 1/2 starch, 1/2 fat

Light Ranch Dressing

INGREDIENTS
- 3/4 cup buttermilk
- 1/4 cup reduced-fat mayonnaise
- 1/4 cup chopped scallions
- 3 tablespoons chopped fresh dill
- 1 tablespoon chopped fresh parsley
- 1 tablespoon lemon juice
- 1 tablespoon prepared horseradish
- 1/8 teaspoon salt
- Freshly ground pepper, to taste

PREPARATION
1. Combine buttermilk, mayonnaise, scallions, dill, parsley, lemon juice, horseradish, salt and pepper in a blender. Puree until smooth.

TIPS & NOTES
- **Make Ahead Tip**: Cover and refrigerate for up to 4 days.

NUTRITION

Per tablespoon: 12 calories; 1 g fat (0 g sat, 0 g mono); 1 mg cholesterol; 3 g carbohydrates; 1 g protein; 0 g fiber; 132 mg sodium; 54 mg potassium.

Exchanges: free food

Buttermilk-Herb Mashed Potatoes

INGREDIENTS
- 1 large Yukon Gold potato, peeled and cut into chunks
- 1 clove garlic, peeled
- 1 teaspoon butter
- 2 tablespoons nonfat buttermilk
- 1 1/2 teaspoons chopped fresh herbs
- Salt & freshly ground pepper, to taste

PREPARATION
1. Place potato in a small saucepan and cover with water. Add garlic. Bring to a boil; cook until the potato is tender. Drain; add butter and buttermilk, and mash with a potato masher to the desired consistency. Stir in herbs. Season with salt and freshly ground pepper.

NUTRITION
Per serving: 85 calories; 2 g fat (1 g sat, 0 g mono); 5 mg cholesterol; 14 g carbohydrates; 0 g added sugars; 2 g protein; 1 g fiber; 87 mg sodium; 416 mg potassium.
Carbohydrate Servings: 1
Exchanges: 1 starch

Fresh Fruit with Lemon-Mint Cream

INGREDIENTS
- 3/4 cup nonfat plain yogurt
- 1/4 cup reduced-fat sour cream
- 1/4 cup sugar
- 3 tablespoons lemon juice

- 1 tablespoon finely chopped fresh mint
- 1 cup freshraspberries or other fresh fruit

PREPARATION
1. Whisk yogurt, sour cream, sugar, lemon juice and mint until the sugar dissolves. Chill, covered, for 1 hour. Divide raspberries (or other fruit) between 2 bowls and top with the lemon-mint cream.

NUTRITION
Per serving: 214 calories; 4 g fat (2 g sat, 1 g mono); 14 mg cholesterol; 43 g carbohydrates; 6 g protein; 4 g fiber; 65 mg sodium; 167 mg potassium.
Carbohydrate Servings: 3
Exchanges: 1 fruit, 1 fat-free milk, 1 1/2 carbohydrate, 1 fat

DAY 3
BREAKFAST

Cranberry Muesli
Skim milk (1 cup)
Grapefruit (1/2)

LUNCH

Pasta & Bean Soup
Spinach, Avocado & Mango Salad
Whole-wheat toast (1 slice)
Skim milk (1 cup)
Sesame Carrots

SNACK

Almonds (1 oz)
Apple (1 cup, quartered)

DINNER

Curry-Roasted Shrimp with Oranges or Orange-Rosemary Glazed Chicken
Brown rice (1 cup) or Pesto Latkes
Sesame Green Beans
Snap Pea Salad with Radish & Lime
Strawberries with Sour Cream & Brown Sugar

DAY 3 RECIPES

Cranberry Muesli

INGREDIENTS
- 1/2 cup low-fat plain yogurt
- 1/2 cup unsweetened or fruit-juice-sweetened cranberry juice
- 6 tablespoons old-fashioned rolled oats, (not quick-cooking or steel-cut)
- 2 tablespoons dried cranberries
- 1 tablespoon unsalted sunflower seeds
- 1 tablespoon wheat germ
- 2 teaspoons honey
- 1/4 teaspoon vanilla extract
- 1/8 teaspoon salt

PREPARATION

1. Combine yogurt, juice, oats, cranberries, sunflower seeds, wheat germ, honey, vanilla and salt in a medium bowl; cover and refrigerate for at least 8 hours and up to 1 day.

TIPS & NOTES
- **Make Ahead Tip**: Cover and refrigerate for up to 1 day.

NUTRITION
Per serving: 209 calories; 4 g fat (1 g sat, 1 g mono); 4 mg cholesterol; 37 g carbohydrates; 8 g protein; 3 gfiber; 190 mg sodium; 266 mg potassium.
Nutrition Bonus: Calcium (15% daily value)
Carbohydrate Servings: 2 1/2
Exchanges: 1 starch, 1 fruit, 1/2 other carbohydrate, 1/2 fat

Pasta & Bean Soup

INGREDIENTS
- 4 14-ounce cans reduced-sodium chicken broth
- 6 cloves garlic, crushed and peeled
- 4 4-inch sprigs fresh rosemary, or 1 tablespoon dried
- 1/8-1/4 teaspoon crushed red pepper
- 1 15-1/2-ounce or 19-ounce can cannellini, (white kidney) beans, rinsed, divided
- 1 14-1/2-ounce can diced tomatoes
- 1 cup medium pasta shells, or orecchiette
- 2 cups individually quick-frozen spinach, (6 ounces) (see Ingredient note)
- 6 teaspoons extra-virgin olive oil, (optional)
- 6 tablespoons freshly grated Parmesan cheese

PREPARATION
1. Combine broth, garlic, rosemary and crushed red pepper in a 4- to 6-quart Dutch oven or soup pot; bring to a simmer. Partially cover and simmer over medium-low heat for 20 minutes to intensify flavor. Meanwhile, mash 1 cup beans in a small bowl.
2. Scoop garlic cloves and rosemary from the broth with a slotted spoon (or pass the soup through a strainer and return to the pot). Add mashed and whole beans to the broth, along with tomatoes; return to a simmer. Stir in pasta, cover and cook over medium heat, stirring occasionally, until the pasta is just tender, 10 to 12 minutes.
3. Stir in spinach, cover and cook just until the spinach has thawed, 2 to 3 minutes. Ladle the soup into bowls and garnish each serving with a drizzle of oil, if desired, and a sprinkling of Parmesan. Variation: Substitute chickpeas (garbanzo beans) for the cannellini beans; use a food processor to puree them.

TIPS & NOTES
- **Ingredient Note:** Individually quick-frozen (IQF) spinach is sold in convenient plastic bags. If you have a 10-ounce box of spinach on hand, use just over half of it and cook according to package directions before adding to the soup in Step 3.

NUTRITION
Per serving: 133 calories; 2 g fat (1 g sat, 0 g mono); 6 mg cholesterol; 21 g carbohydrates; 9 g protein; 4 gfiber; 356 mg sodium; 29 mg potassium.
Nutrition Bonus: Vitamin A (35% daily value), Fiber (16% dv).
Carbohydrate Servings: 1
Exchanges: 1 1/ 2 starch, 1 vegetable, 1 lean meat

Spinach, Avocado & Mango Salad
INGREDIENTS
DRESSING
- 1/3 cup orange juice
- 1 tablespoon red-wine vinegar
- 2 tablespoons hazelnut oil, almond oil or canola oil
- 1 teaspoon Dijon mustard
- 1/4 teaspoon salt, or to taste
- Freshly ground pepper, to taste

SALAD
- 10 cups baby spinach leaves, (about 8 ounces)
- 1 1/2 cups radicchio, torn into bite-size pieces
- 8-12 small red radishes, (1 bunch), sliced
- 1 small ripe mango, sliced
- 1 medium avocado, sliced

PREPARATION
1. To prepare dressing: Whisk juice, vinegar, oil, mustard, salt and pepper in a bowl.
2. To prepare salad: Just before serving, combine spinach, radicchio, radishes and mango in a large bowl. Add the dressing; toss to coat. Garnish each serving with avocado slices.

NUTRITION
Per serving: 210 calories; 14 g fat (2 g sat, 2 g mono); 0 mg cholesterol; 10 g carbohydrates; 3 g protein; 6 g fiber; 258 mg sodium; 479 mg potassium.
Nutrition Bonus: Vitamin C (70% daily value), Vitamin A (40% dv), Fiber (26% dv).
Carbohydrate Servings: 1
Exchanges: 3 vegetable, 3 fat (mono)

Sesame Carrots

INGREDIENTS
- 2 cups baby carrots
- 1 tablespoon toasted sesame seeds
- Pinch of dried thyme
- Pinch of kosher salt

PREPARATION
1. Toss carrots with sesame seeds, thyme and kosher salt in a small bowl.

NUTRITION
Per serving: 33 calories; 2 g fat (0 g sat, 1 g mono); 0 mg cholesterol; 8 g carbohydrates; 0 g added sugars; 1 g protein; 2 g fiber; 72 mg sodium; 220 mg potassium.
Nutrition Bonus: Beta carotene, potassium, fiber.
Carbohydrate Servings: 1/2
Exchanges: 1 1/2 vegetable

Curry-Roasted Shrimp with Oranges

INGREDIENTS
- 2 large seedless oranges
- 1/2 teaspoon kosher salt, divided
- 1 1/2 pounds shrimp, (30-40 per pound), peeled and deveined
- 1 tablespoon extra-virgin olive oil
- 1 tablespoon curry powder, preferably Madras (see Note)
- 1/2 teaspoon freshly ground pepper

PREPARATION
1. Preheat oven to 400°F. Line a baking sheet (with sides) with parchment paper. Finely grate the zest of 1 orange; set aside. Using a sharp knife, peel both oranges, removing all the bitter white pith. Thinly slice the oranges crosswise, then cut the slices into quarters. Spread the orange slices on the prepared baking sheet and sprinkle with 1/4 teaspoon salt. Roast until the oranges are slightly dry, about 12 minutes.
2. Meanwhile, toss shrimp with oil, curry powder, pepper, the orange zest and the remaining 1/4 teaspoon salt in a large bowl. Transfer the shrimp to the baking sheet with the oranges and roast until pink and curled, about 6 minutes. Divide the oranges and the shrimp among 4 plates and serve.

TIPS & NOTES
- **Make Ahead Tip**: Refrigerate for up to 4 days. Reheat before serving.
- **Note:** Madras curry powder is made with a hotter blend of spices than standard curry powder.

NUTRITION
Per serving: 253 calories; 7 g fat (1 g sat, 3 g mono); 259 mg cholesterol; 13 g carbohydrates; 0 g added sugars; 35 g protein; 4 g fiber; 548 mg sodium; 338 mg potassium.
Nutrition Bonus: Selenium (93% daily value), Vitamin C (70% dv).
Carbohydrate Servings: 1
Exchanges: 1 fruit, 5 very lean meat, 1 fat (mono)

Orange-Rosemary Glazed Chicken

INGREDIENTS
- 4 bone-in chicken breast halves, (2 1/2-3 pounds total), skin removed, trimmed of fat
- 1/4 teaspoon salt, or to taste
- Freshly ground pepper, to taste
- 1 1/2 teaspoons chopped fresh rosemary, divided
- 3 tablespoons orange marmalade
- 2 tablespoons sherry vinegar, malt vinegar or cider vinegar
- 1 teaspoon extra-virgin olive oil

PREPARATION
1. Preheat oven to 400°F. Coat a roasting pan with cooking spray.
2. Season chicken on both sides with salt and pepper and place, bone-side up, in the prepared pan. Sprinkle with 1 teaspoon rosemary.
3. Bake the chicken for 20 minutes. Meanwhile, combine the remaining 1/2 teaspoon rosemary, marmalade, vinegar and oil in a small bowl.

4. Turn the chicken pieces over and top with the marmalade mixture. Bake until the chicken is no longer pink in the center, 15 to 20 minutes more. Serve immediately, spooning the sauce over the chicken.

NUTRITION

Per serving: 252 calories; 3 g fat (1 g sat, 1 g mono); 107 mg cholesterol; 10 g carbohydrates; 43 g protein;0 g fiber; 274 mg sodium; 477 mg potassium.
Nutrition Bonus: Selenium (47% daily value).
Carbohydrate Servings: 1/2
Exchanges: 1 other carbohydrate, 7 very lean meat

Pesto Latkes

INGREDIENTS
- 2 pounds Yukon Gold potatoes
- 1 medium onion
- 4 cloves garlic, minced
- 3/4 cup packed fresh basil leaves, finely chopped
- 1/3 cup pasteurized egg substitute
- 1/2 cup grated Parmigiano-Reggiano cheese
- 2 tablespoons extra-virgin olive oil
- 1 teaspoon salt
- 1/2 teaspoon freshly ground pepper

PREPARATION
1. Preheat oven to 350°F. Coat a 12-cup muffin pan with cooking spray.
2. Peel potatoes, then grate them through the large holes of a box grater into a large bowl. Squeeze in small batches between your hands over the sink to remove excess moisture. Then grate onion into the bowl through the same holes in the box grater.
3. Stir in garlic, basil, egg substitute, cheese, oil, salt and pepper. Place a generous 1/2 cup of the potato mixture into each muffin cup, packing the mixture firmly.
4. Bake the latkes until lightly browned and firm, 45 to 50 minutes. Cool in the pan on a wire rack for 10 minutes before unmolding.

NUTRITION

Per serving: 215 calories; 7 g fat (2 g sat, 4 g mono); 6 mg cholesterol; 30 g carbohydrates; 8 g protein; 3 gfiber; 519 mg sodium; 927 mg potassium.
Nutrition Bonus: Potassium (26% daily value).
Carbohydrate Servings: 2

Exchanges: 2 starch, 1/2 lean meat

Sesame Green Beans

INGREDIENTS

- 1 pound green beans, trimmed
- 2 teaspoons extra-virgin olive oil
- 2 teaspoons toasted sesame seeds, (see Tip)
- 1 teaspoon sesame oil
- Salt & freshly ground pepper, to taste

PREPARATION

1. Preheat oven to 500°F.
2. Toss green beans with olive oil. Spread in an even layer on a rimmed baking sheet. Roast, turning once halfway through cooking, until tender and beginning to brown, about 10 minutes. Toss with sesame seeds, sesame oil, salt and pepper.

TIPS & NOTES

- **Tip:** To toast sesame seeds: Place in a small dry skillet and cook over medium-low heat, stirring constantly, until fragrant and lightly browned, 2 to 4 minutes.

NUTRITION
Per serving: 67 calories; 4 g fat (1 g sat, 3 g mono); 0 mg cholesterol; 7 g carbohydrates; 0 g added sugars; 2 g protein; 4 g fiber; 73 mg sodium; 280 mg potassium.
Nutrition Bonus: Vitamin C (15% daily value).
Carbohydrate Servings: 1/2
Exchanges: 1 vegetable

Snap Pea Salad with Radish & Lime

INGREDIENTS

- 8 ounces sugar snap peas, trimmed and halved (about 2 cups)
- 7 ounces yellow wax beans, trimmed and cut into 1-inch pieces (about 3 cups)
- 3 tablespoons lime juice
- 2 tablespoons extra-virgin olive oil
- 1/2 cup chopped fresh cilantro
- 1/4 teaspoon salt
- Freshly ground pepper, to taste
- 1 bunch radishes, trimmed and thinly sliced (about 10)

PREPARATION
1. Steam peas over 2 inches of boiling water, stirring once, until crisp-tender, 4 to 5 minutes. Transfer to a baking sheet lined with paper towel. Steam wax beans until crisp-tender, about 5 minutes.
Transfer to the baking sheet. Refrigerate until chilled, about 20 minutes.

2. Whisk lime juice, oil, cilantro, salt and pepper in a large bowl. Add radishes, peas and beans; toss to coat. Serve chilled.

NUTRITION
Per serving: 110 calories; 7 g fat (1 g sat, 5 g mono); 0 mg cholesterol; 9 g carbohydrates; 2 g protein; 3 gfiber; 157 mg sodium; 140 mg potassium.
Nutrition Bonus: Vitamin A (20% daily value).
Carbohydrate Servings: 1/2
Exchanges: 2 vegetable, 1 1/2 fat (mono)

Strawberries with Sour Cream & Brown Sugar

INGREDIENTS
- 2 pints strawberries
- 1/2 cup reduced-fat sour cream
- 1/2 cup light brown sugar

PREPARATION
1. Arrange strawberries on a serving platter. Place sour cream and brown sugar in separate small bowls. To eat, dip a berry into sour cream and then into sugar.

NUTRITION

Per strawberry: 29 calories; 1 g fat (0 g sat, 0 g mono); 2 mg cholesterol; 6 g carbohydrates; 1 g protein; 0 g fiber; 2 mg sodium; 43 mg potassium.
Carbohydrate Servings: 1/2
Exchanges: (per 4 pieces): 1 fruit, 1 carbohydrate, 1 fat

DAY 4
BREAKFAST
Tropical Fruit Smoothie
Whole-wheat toast (1 slice)
Roasted Apple Butter
LUNCH
Lettuce Wraps with Spiced Pork or Turkey & Fontina Melts
Sweet & Tangy Watermelon Salad

Skim milk (1 cup)
Whole-wheat breadsticks (1 8" stick)
   SNACK
Low-fat vanilla yogurt (8 oz.)
Apricot (1 cup, halves)
   DINNER
Chicken Breasts with Roasted Lemons
Arugula-Mushroom Salad
Baked potato (1 medium)
Brussels Sprouts & Chestnuts
Grilled Pineapple with Coconut Black Sticky Rice or Strawberry Cream

DAY 4 RECIPES

Tropical Fruit Smoothie

INGREDIENTS
- 1 cup cubed fresh or canned pineapple
- 1 banana, sliced
- 1/2 cup silken tofu, or low-fat plain yogurt
- 1/3 cup frozen passion fruit concentrate
- 1/2 cup water
- 2 ice cubes and 1 tablespoon wheat bran, or oat bran (optional)

PREPARATION
1. Combine pineapple, banana, tofu (or yogurt), passion fruit concentrate, water, ice cubes and wheat bran (or oat bran), if using, in a blender; cover and blend until creamy. Serve immediately.

NUTRITION
Per serving: 109 calories; 2 g fat (0 g sat, 0 g mono); 0 mg cholesterol; 21 g carbohydrates; 4 g protein; 2 gfiber; 26 mg sodium; 281 mg potassium.
Nutrition Bonus: Vitamin C (40% daily value).
Carbohydrate Servings: 1 1/2
Exchanges: 1 fruit, 1/2 low-fat milk

Roasted Apple Butter

INGREDIENTS
- 8 medium McIntosh apples, (2 3/4 pounds), peeled, cored and quartered
- 2 cups unsweetened apple juice

PREPARATION
1. Preheat oven to 450°F. Arrange apples in a large roasting pan. Pour apple juice over the apples. Bake until tender and lightly browned, about 30 minutes. Using a fork or potato masher, thoroughly mash the apples in the roasting pan.
2. Reduce oven temperature to 350°. Bake the apple puree, stirring occasionally, until very thick and deeply browned, 1 1/2 to 1 3/4 hours. Scrape into a bowl and let cool.

TIPS & NOTES
- **Make Ahead Tip**: Store in an airtight container in the refrigerator for up to 2 weeks or freeze for up to 6 months.

NUTRITION

Per tablespoon: 27 calories; 0 g fat (0 g sat, 0 g mono); 0 mg cholesterol; 7 g carbohydrates; 0 g protein; 1 g fiber; 0 mg sodium; 18 mg potassium.
Carbohydrate Servings: 1/2
Exchanges: 1/2 fruit

Lettuce Wraps with Spiced Pork

INGREDIENTS
SAUCE
- 2 tablespoons oyster sauce
- 2 tablespoons water
- 1 tablespoon hoisin sauce
- 1 tablespoon rice vinegar
- 1 tablespoon dry sherry, or rice wine
- 2 teaspoons cornstarch
- 1 teaspoon brown sugar
- 1 teaspoon reduced-sodium soy sauce
- 1 teaspoon sesame oil

STIR-FRY
- 3 teaspoons canola oil, divided
- 1 pound thin center-cut boneless pork chops, trimmed of fat and cut into thin julienne strips
- 2 cloves garlic, minced
- 1 tablespoon minced fresh ginger
- 1 8-ounce can sliced water chestnuts, rinsed and coarsely chopped
- 1 8-ounce can sliced bamboo shoots, rinsed and coarsely chopped
- 8 ounces shiitake mushrooms, stemmed, cut into julienne strips
- 4 scallions, greens only, sliced
- 1 head iceberg lettuce, leaves separated

PREPARATION
1. To prepare sauce: Combine oyster sauce, water, hoisin sauce, vinegar, sherry (or rice wine), cornstarch, brown sugar, soy sauce and sesame oil in a small bowl.
2. To prepare stir-fry: Heat 2 teaspoons canola oil over medium-high heat in a large nonstick skillet or wok. Add pork; cook, stirring constantly, until no longer pink, about 4 minutes. Transfer to a plate. Wipe out the pan.
3. Add remaining 1 teaspoon oil, garlic and ginger; cook, stirring constantly, until fragrant, 30 seconds. Add water chestnuts, bamboo shoots and mushrooms; cook, stirring often, until the mushrooms have softened, about 4 minutes. Return the pork to the pan and add the sauce. Cook, stirring constantly, until a thick glossy sauce has formed, about 1 minute. Serve sprinkled with scallions and wrapped in lettuce leaves.

TIPS & NOTES
- **Make Ahead Tip**: The sauce will keep, covered, in the refrigerator for up to 2 days.

NUTRITION
Per serving: 350 calories; 16 g fat (5 g sat, 8 g mono); 59 mg cholesterol; 29 g carbohydrates; 25 g protein;7 g fiber; 810 mg sodium; 675 mg potassium.
Nutrition Bonus: Vitamin C (20% daily value), Iron (15% dv).
Carbohydrate Servings: 1
Exchanges: 1/2 other carbohydrate, 2 vegetable, 3 medium-fat meat

Turkey & Fontina Melts

INGREDIENTS
- 2 turkey cutlets, (8 ounces)
- 1 tablespoon all-purpose flour
- 3 teaspoons extra-virgin olive oil, divided
- 1 large shallot, minced
- 1/4 cup dry sherry, (see Note)
- 1 6-ounce bag baby spinach
- 1/4 cup finely shredded Fontina cheese
- 1 teaspoon butter

PREPARATION
1. Position rack in the upper third of the oven; preheat broiler.
2. Sprinkle both sides of turkey with flour. Heat 2 teaspoons oil in a medium ovenproof skillet over medium-high heat. Add the turkey and cook until golden, about 2 minutes per side. Transfer the turkey to a plate.
3. Add the remaining 1 teaspoon oil and shallot to the pan; cook, stirring constantly, until lightly browned, 1 to 2 minutes. Add sherry and spinach; cook,

stirring constantly, until the spinach is wilted, 1 to 2 minutes. Remove from the heat.
   4. Carefully mound equal portions of the spinach on top of the turkey. Transfer the spinach-topped turkey and any accumulated juices to the pan. Top the spinach with cheese and transfer to the oven. Broil until the cheese is melted, 1 to 2 minutes.
   5. Transfer the melts to 2 plates. Add the butter to the pan and whisk into the juices over medium-high heat until melted, about 30 seconds. Drizzle over the melts.

TIPS & NOTES
- **Note:** Sherry is a type of fortified wine originally from southern Spain. Don't use the "cooking sherry" sold in many supermarkets — it can be surprisingly high in sodium. Instead, purchase dry sherry that's sold with other fortified wines in your wine or liquor store.

NUTRITION
Per serving: 332 calories; 14 g fat (5 g sat, 7 g mono); 66 mg cholesterol; 15 g carbohydrates; 34 g protein; 4 g fiber; 347 mg sodium; 89 mg potassium.
Nutrition Bonus: Vitamin A (70% daily value), Iron (25% dv), Vitamin C (20% dv), Calcium (15% dv).
Carbohydrate Servings: 1
Exchanges: 1/2 starch, 2 vegetable, 4 lean meat

Sweet & Tangy Watermelon Salad

INGREDIENTS
- 2 tablespoons rice vinegar
- 2 1/2 teaspoons sugar
- 2 cups diced seeded watermelon
- 2 cups diced cucumber
- 1/2 cup chopped fresh cilantro
- 1/4 cup unsalted dry-roasted peanuts, toasted (see Tip) and coarsely chopped

PREPARATION
   1. Stir together vinegar and sugar in a medium bowl until the sugar almost dissolves. Add watermelon, cucumber and cilantro; toss gently to combine. Just before serving, sprinkle with peanuts.

TIPS & NOTES
- **Tip:** To toast nuts:

- Heat a small dry skillet over medium-low heat. Add nuts and cook, stirring, until lightly browned and fragrant, 2 to 3 minutes. Transfer to a bowl to cool.

NUTRITION
Per serving: 63 calories; 3 g fat (0 g sat, 2 g mono); 0 mg cholesterol; 8 g carbohydrates; 2 g protein; 1 gfiber; 3 mg sodium; 164 mg potassium.
Carbohydrate Servings: 1/2
Exchanges: 1/2 fruit, 1/2 vegetable, 1/2 fat

Chicken Breasts with Roasted Lemons

INGREDIENTS
ROASTED LEMONS
- 3 medium lemons, thinly sliced and seeded
- 1 teaspoon extra-virgin olive oil
- 1/8 teaspoon salt

CHICKEN
- 4 boneless, skinless chicken breast halves, (about 1 pound total), trimmed
- 1/8 teaspoon salt
- Freshly ground pepper, to taste
- 1/4 cup all-purpose flour
- 2 teaspoons extra-virgin olive oil
- 1 1/4 cups reduced-sodium chicken broth
- 2 tablespoons drained capers, rinsed
- 2 teaspoons butter
- 3 tablespoons chopped fresh parsley, divided

PREPARATION
1. To prepare roasted lemons: Preheat oven to 325°F. Line a baking sheet with parchment paper. Arrange lemon slices in a single layer on it. Brush the lemon slices with 1 tablespoon oil and sprinkle with 1/8 teaspoon salt. Roast the lemons until slightly dry and beginning to brown around the edges, 25 to 30 minutes.
2. Meanwhile, prepare chicken: Cover chicken with plastic wrap and pound with a rolling pin or heavy skillet until flattened to about 1/2 inch thick. Sprinkle the chicken with 1/8 teaspoon salt and pepper. Place flour in a shallow dish and dredge the chicken to coat both sides; shake off excess (discard remaining flour).
3. Heat 2 teaspoons oil in a large nonstick skillet over medium-high heat. Add the chicken and cook until golden brown, 2 to 3 minutes per side. Add broth and bring to a boil, scraping up any browned bits. Stir in capers. Boil until the liquid is reduced to syrup consistency, 5 to 8 minutes, turning the chicken halfway. Add the roasted lemons, butter, 2 tablespoons parsley and more pepper, if desired;

simmer until the butter melts and the chicken is cooked through, about 2 minutes. Transfer to a platter. Sprinkle with the remaining 1 tablespoon parsley and serve.

TIPS & NOTES
- **Make Ahead Tip**: Cover and refrigerate the roasted lemons (Step 1) for up to 2 days.

NUTRITION
Per serving: 219 calories; 7 g fat (2 g sat, 3 g mono); 72 mg cholesterol; 6 g carbohydrates; 0 g added sugars; 28 g protein; 1 g fiber; 396 mg sodium; 376 mg potassium.
Nutrition Bonus: Vitamin C (40% daily value).
Carbohydrate Servings: 1/2
Exchanges: 1/2 fruit, 4 very lean meat, 1 fat

Arugula-Mushroom Salad

INGREDIENTS
- 1 clove garlic, peeled
- 1/4 teaspoon salt
- 1 tablespoon lemon juice
- 1 tablespoon reduced-fat mayonnaise
- 1 tablespoon extra-virgin olive oil
- 1 tablespoon chopped fresh parsley
- Freshly ground pepper, to taste
- 6 cups arugula leaves
- 2 cups sliced mushrooms

PREPARATION
1. Place garlic on a cutting board and crush. Sprinkle with salt and use the flat of a chef's knife blade to mash the garlic to a paste; transfer to a serving bowl. Whisk in lemon juice, mayonnaise, oil and parsley. Season with pepper. Add arugula and mushrooms; toss to coat with the dressing.

NUTRITION
Per serving: 62 calories; 4 g fat (1 g sat, 3 g mono); 1 mg cholesterol; 3 g carbohydrates; 0 g added sugars; 2 g protein; 1 g fiber; 188 mg sodium; 235 mg potassium.
Nutrition Bonus: Vitamin C (15% daily value).
Exchanges: 1 vegetable, 1 fat (mono)

Brussels Sprouts & Chestnuts

INGREDIENTS
- 24 fresh chestnuts, (3/4 pound)
- 1 stalk celery
- 1 lemon
- 1 1/2 pounds Brussels sprouts, trimmed
- 1/4 cup reduced-sodium chicken broth
- 1 tablespoon butter
- Salt & freshly ground pepper, to taste

PREPARATION
1. Using a sharp knife, score a cross on the flat side of each chestnut. Dip chestnuts, 4 or 5 at a time, into a saucepan of boiling water. Using a slotted spoon, remove chestnuts and peel away shells and inner brown skins. Place the peeled chestnuts in a large saucepan and add enough boiling water to cover. Add celery stalk and simmer, covered, for 30 to 45 minutes, or until tender. Drain, discarding celery, and refresh with cold water. Set aside.
2. With a vegetable peeler, remove the zest from half the lemon. (Save lemon for another use.) Cut the zest into julienne strips and place in a small saucepan; cover with cold water and bring to a boil. Drain and set aside.
3. With a paring knife, cut a small cross, 1/8 inch deep, in the stem end of each Brussels sprout. Bring a large saucepan of salted water to a boil. Add the Brussels sprouts and cook, uncovered, until tender, 6 to 8 minutes. Drain and refresh with cold water. (The vegetables can be prepared ahead and stored, covered, in the refrigerator for up to 8 hours.)
4. In a large skillet, heat broth and butter. Add the chestnuts and Brussels sprouts and toss over medium heat until heated through. Season with salt and pepper and garnish with the julienned lemon zest.

TIPS & NOTES
- **Make Ahead Tip**: Prepare through Step 3. Cover and refrigerate for up to 8 hours.

NUTRITION
Per serving: 142 calories; 3 g fat (1 g sat, 0 g mono); 4 mg cholesterol; 27 g carbohydrates; 0 g added sugars; 4 g protein; 7 g fiber; 104 mg sodium; 565 mg potassium.
Carbohydrate Servings: 1
Exchanges: 1 starch, 1 1/2 vegetable

Grilled Pineapple with Coconut Black Sticky Rice

INGREDIENTS
- 1 1/2 cups water
- 1 cup black sticky rice, (see Note)
- 1 14-ounce can lite coconut milk
- 1/2 teaspoon ground cardamom
- 3 tablespoons finely chopped palm sugar (see Note) or packed brown sugar
- 1/2 teaspoon salt
- 1 small ripe pineapple, peeled, cored and cut into 1/2-inch-thick slices

PREPARATION
1. Combine water and rice in a medium saucepan. Bring to a boil, reduce heat to maintain a gentle simmer, cover and cook until the rice has absorbed all the water, about 20 minutes. The rice should be cooked yet still somewhat firm.
2. Bring the coconut milk to a boil in another medium saucepan. Reduce heat to medium-low, add cardamom, sugar and salt. Stir until the sugar and salt are dissolved. Set aside 3/4 cup of the seasoned coconut milk. Add the rice to the pan with the remaining seasoned coconut milk, return to a gentle simmer, cover and cook until the rice softens and absorbs almost all the liquid, about 15 minutes.
3. Meanwhile, preheat grill to high. Oil the grill rack (see Tip). Grill the pineapple slices until slightly charred and softened, 1 to 2 minutes per side. Transfer to a cutting board; let stand until cool enough to handle. Chop the pineapple.
4. Serve rice and pineapple with the reserved coconut milk drizzled on top. Serve hot or at room temperature. Variation: White sticky rice can be substituted for the black sticky rice, but the cooking time in Step 1 will be 12 to 15 minutes and, in Step 2, 10 to 15 minutes. Check the rice while it's cooking to prevent scorching.

TIPS & NOTES
- **Notes:** Black sticky rice, often called Forbidden rice, has a sweet, nutty taste, is high in fiber and is a good vegetarian source of iron.
  When cooked the brown-black rice turns a shade of purple-black. It may also be labeled "black glutinous rice" or "black sweet rice." Sushi rice, brown rice or regular white rice cannot be substituted for black sticky rice.

- PALM SUGAR, an unrefined sweetener similar in flavor to brown sugar, is used in sweet and savory Asian dishes. Commonly available in pod-like cakes, but is also sold in paste form at Asian markets. Store as you would other sugar.
- **Tip:** How to oil a grill rack: Oil a folded paper towel, hold it with tongs and rub it over the rack.

NUTRITION

Per serving: 231 calories; 6 g fat (3 g sat, 0 g mono); 0 mg cholesterol; 44 g carbohydrates; 5 g protein; 3 gfiber; 213 mg sodium; 118 mg potassium.
Nutrition Bonus: Vitamin C (60% daily value).
Carbohydrate Servings: 3
Exchanges: 1 1/2 starch, 1 1/2 fruit, 1 fat

Strawberry Cream

INGREDIENTS
CREAM
- 3 tablespoons cold water
- 1 envelope unflavored gelatin
- 4 cups hulled strawberries
- 1/2 cup sugar
- 1 teaspoon vanilla extract
- 3/4 cup reduced-fat sour cream

TOPPING
- 1 cup hulled strawberries, cut into 1/4-inch dice
- 2 teaspoons sugar

PREPARATION

1. To prepare cream: Stir together water and gelatin in a small heatproof cup or bowl. Microwave, uncovered, on High until the gelatin has completely dissolved but the liquid is not boiling, 20 to 30 seconds. (Alternatively, bring 1/2 inch water to a gentle simmer in a small skillet. Set the bowl with the gelatin mixture in the simmering water until the gelatin has dissolved completely.) Stir the mixture until smooth.

2. Place strawberries, sugar and vanilla in a food processor and puree. Add sour cream; pulse to combine. With the motor running, slowly add the dissolved gelatin. Pour the cream into four 8-ounce bowls or wineglasses. Cover and refrigerate until set, about 3 hours.

3. To prepare topping and serve: Toss diced strawberries and sugar in a small bowl; let stand until slightly juicy, about 2 minutes. Divide among the creams.

TIPS & NOTES
- **Make Ahead Tip**: Prepare through Step 2, cover and refrigerate for up to 3 days. Add topping just before serving.

NUTRITION

Per serving: 232 calories; 6 g fat (3 g sat, 2 g mono); 18 mg cholesterol; 43 g carbohydrates; 4 g protein; 4 g fiber; 24 mg sodium; 336 mg potassium.

Nutrition Bonus: Vitamin C (180% daily value)
Carbohydrate Servings: 3
Exchanges: 1 fruit, 2 other carbohydrate, 1 fat

DAY 5
BREAKFAST

Baked Asparagus & Cheese Frittata
Skim milk (1 cup)
Apple (1 cup, quartered)

LUNCH

Broccoli-Cheese Chowder
Chicken Tabbouleh or Spaghetti Squash & Pork Stir-Fry
Skim milk (1 cup)
Ginger-Orange Biscotti
Strawberries (1 cup)

SNACK

Carrot sticks (1 cup)
Roasted Eggplant Dip

DINNER

Grilled Pork Tenderloin with Mustard, Rosemary & Apple Marinade
Salad of Boston Lettuce with Creamy Orange-Shallot Dressing
Brown Rice (1 cup)
Sweet Pea Mash
Roasted Pear Trifle or Pear & Dried Cranberry Strudel

DAY 5 RECIPES

Baked Asparagus & Cheese Frittata

INGREDIENTS
- 2 tablespoons fine dry breadcrumbs
- 1 pound thin asparagus
- 1 1/2 teaspoons extra-virgin olive oil
- 2 onions, chopped
- 1 red bell pepper, chopped
- 2 cloves garlic, minced
- 1/2 teaspoon salt, divided
- 1/2 cup water
- Freshly ground pepper, to taste
- 4 large eggs
- 2 large egg whites

- 1 cup part-skim ricotta cheese
- 1 tablespoon chopped fresh parsley
- 1/2 cup shredded Gruyère cheese

PREPARATION
1. Preheat oven to 325°F. Coat a 10-inch pie pan or ceramic quiche dish with cooking spray. Sprinkle with breadcrumbs, tapping out the excess.
2. Snap tough ends off asparagus. Slice off the top 2 inches of the tips and reserve. Cut the stalks into 1/2-inch-long slices.
3. Heat oil in a large nonstick skillet over medium-high heat. Add onions, bell pepper, garlic and 1/4 teaspoon salt; cook, stirring, until softened, 5 to 7 minutes.
4. Add water and the asparagus stalks to the skillet. Cook, stirring, until the asparagus is tender and the liquid has evaporated, about 7 minutes (the mixture should be very dry). Season with salt and pepper. Arrange the vegetables in an even layer in the prepared pan.
5. Whisk eggs and egg whites in a large bowl. Add ricotta, parsley, the remaining 1/4 teaspoon salt and pepper; whisk to blend. Pour the egg mixture over the vegetables, gently shaking the pan to distribute. Scatter the reserved asparagus tips over the top and sprinkle with Gruyère.
6. Bake the frittata until a knife inserted in the center comes out clean, about 35 minutes. Let stand for 5 minutes before serving.

NUTRITION

Per serving: 195 calories; 11 g fat (5 g sat, 4 g mono); 164 mg cholesterol; 10 g carbohydrates; 15 gprotein; 2 g fiber; 357 mg sodium; 310 mg potassium.
Nutrition Bonus: Vitamin C (70% daily value), Vitamin A (30% dv).
Carbohydrate Servings: 1/2
Exchanges: 2 vegetable, 1 medium-fat meat, 1/2 high-fat meat

Broccoli-Cheese Chowder

INGREDIENTS
- 1 tablespoon extra-virgin olive oil
- 1 large onion, chopped
- 1 large carrot, diced
- 2 stalks celery, diced
- 1 large potato, peeled and diced
- 2 cloves garlic, minced
- 1 tablespoon all-purpose flour
- 1/2 teaspoon dry mustard
- 1/8 teaspoon cayenne pepper

- 2 14-ounce cans vegetable broth, or reduced-sodium chicken broth
- 8 ounces broccoli crowns, (see Ingredient Note), cut into 1-inch pieces, stems and florets separated
- 1 cup shredded reduced-fat Cheddar cheese
- 1/2 cup reduced-fat sour cream
- 1/8 teaspoon salt

PREPARATION
1. Heat oil in a Dutch oven or large saucepan over medium-high heat. Add onion, carrot and celery; cook, stirring often, until the onion and celery soften, 5 to 6 minutes. Add potato and garlic; cook, stirring, for 2 minutes. Stir in flour, dry mustard and cayenne; cook, stirring often, for 2 minutes.
2. Add broth and broccoli stems; bring to a boil. Cover and reduce heat to medium. Simmer, stirring occasionally, for 10 minutes. Stir in florets; simmer, covered, until the broccoli is tender, about 10 minutes more. Transfer 2 cups of the chowder to a bowl and mash; return to the pan.
3. Stir in Cheddar and sour cream; cook over medium heat, stirring, until the cheese is melted and the chowder is heated through, about 2 minutes. Season with salt.

TIPS & NOTES
- **Make Ahead Tip**: Prepare through Step 2. Cover and refrigerate for up to 2 days or freeze for up to 2 months.
- **Ingredient note:** Most supermarkets sell broccoli crowns, which are the tops of the bunches, with the stalks cut off. Although crowns are more expensive than entire bunches, they are convenient and there is considerably less waste.

NUTRITION
Per serving: 205 calories; 9 g fat (4 g sat, 3 g mono); 21 mg cholesterol; 23 g carbohydrates; 9 g protein; 4 g fiber; 508 mg sodium; 436 mg potassium.
Nutrition Bonus: Vitamin C (61% daily value), Vitamin A (64% dv), Calcium (34% dv).
Carbohydrate Servings: 1 1/2
Exchanges: 1 starch, 1 vegetable, 1 high-fat meat

Chicken Tabbouleh

INGREDIENTS
- 3 cups water
- 1 cup bulgur
- 3 cups cubed skinless cooked chicken, (1-inch cubes)
- 1 cup chopped fresh parsley
- 1 cup chopped scallions
- 1/3 cup currants

- 1/4 cup frozen orange juice concentrate
- 2 tablespoons lemon juice
- 1 tablespoon extra-virgin olive oil
- 1 teaspoon ground cumin
- 1/4 teaspoon cayenne pepper, or to taste
- 1/4 teaspoon salt
- Freshly ground pepper, to taste

PREPARATION

1. Bring water to a boil in a large saucepan. Add bulgur and remove from the heat. Let stand until most of the water is absorbed, 20 to 30 minutes.
2. Drain bulgur well, squeezing out excess moisture. Transfer to a large bowl. Add chicken, parsley, scallions and currants.
3. Whisk orange juice concentrate, lemon juice, oil, cumin and cayenne in a small bowl until blended. Toss with the bulgur mixture. Season with salt and pepper and serve.

TIPS & NOTES

- **To poach chicken breasts:** Place boneless, skinless chicken breasts in a medium skillet or saucepan and add lightly salted water to cover; bring to a boil. Cover, reduce heat to low and simmer gently until chicken is cooked through and no longer pink in the middle, 10 to 12 minutes.
- **Ingredient note:** Bulgur is made by parboiling, drying and coarsely grinding or cracking wheat berries. Don't confuse bulgur with cracked wheat, which is simply that—cracked wheat. Since the parboiling step is skipped, cracked wheat must be cooked for up to an hour whereas bulgur simply needs a quick soak in hot water for most uses. Look for it in the natural-foods section of large supermarkets, near other grains, or online at kalustyans.com, lebaneseproducts.com.

NUTRITION
Per serving: 260 calories; 5 g fat (1 g sat, 3 g mono); 60 mg cholesterol; 31 g carbohydrates; 0 g added sugars; 26 g protein; 6 g fiber; 166 mg sodium; 536 mg potassium.
Nutrition Bonus: Vitamin C (60% daily value), Fiber (24% dv), Potassium (15% dv).
Carbohydrate Servings: 1 1/2
Exchanges: 2 starch, 3 very lean meat

Spaghetti Squash & Pork Stir-Fry

INGREDIENTS
- 1 3-pound spaghetti squash
- 1 pound pork tenderloin, trimmed
- 2 teaspoons toasted sesame oil
- 5 medium scallions, thinly sliced
- 2 cloves garlic, minced
- 1 tablespoon minced fresh ginger
- 1/2 teaspoon salt
- 2 tablespoons reduced-sodium soy sauce
- 2 tablespoons rice vinegar
- 1 teaspoon Asian red chile sauce, such as sriracha, or chile oil

PREPARATION
1. Preheat oven to 350°F.
2. Cut squash in half. Scoop out and discard seeds. Place each half, cut-side down, on a baking sheet. Bake until the squash is tender, about 1 hour. Let cool for 10 minutes then shred the flesh with a fork into a bowl. Discard the shell.
3. Slice pork into thin rounds; cut each round into matchsticks.
4. Heat a large wok over medium-high heat. Swirl in oil, then add scallions, garlic, ginger and salt; cook, stirring, until fragrant, 30 seconds. Add the pork; cook, stirring constantly, until just cooked through, 2 to 3 minutes. Add the squash threads and cook, stirring, for 1 minute. Add soy sauce, rice vinegar and chile sauce (or chile oil); cook, stirring constantly, until aromatic, about 30 seconds.

TIPS & NOTES
- **Make Ahead Tip**: Prepare the squash (Steps 1 & 2), cover and refrigerate for up to 2 days.

NUTRITION

Per serving: 236 calories; 6 g fat (1 g sat, 2 g mono); 74 mg cholesterol; 22 g carbohydrates; 27 g protein; 5 g fiber; 707 mg sodium; 878 mg potassium.
Nutrition Bonus: Vitamin C (25% daily value), Potassium (24% dv), Iron (17% dv)
Carbohydrate Servings: 1
Exchanges: 1/2 other carbohydrates, 3 lean meat

Ginger-Orange Biscotti

INGREDIENTS
- 3/4 cup whole-wheat pastry flour
- 3/4 cup all-purpose flour
- 1 cup sugar, or 1/2 cup Splenda Sugar Blend for Baking
- 1/2 cup cornmeal
- 2 teaspoons ground ginger
- 1 teaspoon baking powder
- 1/2 teaspoon baking soda
- 1/4 teaspoon salt
- 2 large eggs
- 2 large egg whites
- 2 teaspoons freshly grated orange zest
- 1 tablespoon orange juice

PREPARATION
1. Preheat oven to 325°F. Line a baking sheet with parchment paper or a silicone baking mat.
2. Whisk whole-wheat flour, all-purpose flour, sugar (or Splenda), cornmeal, ginger, baking powder, baking soda and salt in a medium bowl. Whisk eggs, egg whites, orange zest and orange juice in a large bowl until blended. Stir in the dry ingredients with a wooden spoon until just combined.
3. Divide the dough in half. With dampened hands, form each piece into a 14-by-1 1/2-inch log. Place the logs side by side on the prepared baking sheet
4. Bake until firm, 20 to 25 minutes. Cool on the pan on a wire rack. Reduce oven temperature to 300°.
5. Slice the logs on the diagonal into cookies 1/2 inch thick. Arrange, cut-side down, on 2 ungreased baking sheets. Bake until golden brown and crisp, 15 to 20 minutes. (Rotate the baking sheets if necessary to ensure even browning.) Transfer the biscotti to a wire rack to cool.

TIPS & NOTES
- **Make Ahead Tip**: Store in an airtight container for up to 2 weeks.

NUTRITION

Per biscotti: 34 calories; 0 g fat (0 g sat, 0 g mono); 8 mg cholesterol; 8 g carbohydrates; 1 g protein; 0 gfiber; 34 mg sodium; 9 mg potassium.
Carbohydrate Servings: 1/2
Exchanges: 1/2 other carbohydrate

Nutrition Note: Per biscotti with Splenda: 0 Carbohydrate Servings; 28 calories; 5 g carbohydrate.

Roasted Eggplant Dip

INGREDIENTS
- 1 large head garlic
- 1 eggplant, (1-1 1/4 pounds), cut in half lengthwise
- 1 small onion, cut into 1/2-inch-thick slices
- 1 ripe tomato, cored, sliced in half and seeded
- 3 tablespoons lemon juice
- 2 tablespoons chopped fresh mint
- 1 tablespoon extra-virgin olive oil
- 1/2 teaspoon salt
- Freshly ground pepper, to taste

PREPARATION
1. Set oven racks at the two lowest levels; preheat to 450°F. Peel as much of the papery skin from the garlic as possible and wrap loosely in foil. Bake until the garlic is soft, 30 minutes. Let cool slightly.
2. Meanwhile, coat a baking sheet with cooking spray. Place eggplant halves on the prepared baking sheet, cut-side down. Roast for 10 minutes. Add onion slices and tomato halves to the baking sheet and roast until all the vegetables are soft, 10 to 15 minutes longer. Let cool slightly.
3. Separate the garlic cloves and squeeze the soft pulp into a medium bowl. Mash with the back of a spoon. Slip skins from the eggplant and tomatoes; coarsely chop. Finely chop the onion. Add the chopped vegetables to the garlic pulp and stir in the lemon juice, mint, oil, salt and pepper.

TIPS & NOTES
- **Make Ahead Tip**: Cover and refrigerate for up to 2 days.

NUTRITION
Per tablespoon: 11 calories; 0 g fat (0 g sat, 0 g mono); 0 mg cholesterol; 2 g carbohydrates; 0 g added sugars; 0 g protein; 1 g fiber; 30 mg sodium; 46 mg potassium.
Exchanges: free food

Grilled Pork Tenderloin with Mustard, Rosemary & Apple Marinade

INGREDIENTS
- 1/4 cup frozen apple juice concentrate
- 2 tablespoons plus 1 1/2 teaspoons Dijon mustard

- 2 tablespoons extra-virgin olive oil, divided
- 2 tablespoons chopped fresh rosemary, or thyme
- 4 cloves garlic, minced
- 1 teaspoon crushed peppercorns
- 2 12-ounce pork tenderloins, trimmed of fat
- 1 tablespoon minced shallot
- 3 tablespoons port, or brewed black tea
- 2 tablespoons balsamic vinegar
- 1/4 teaspoon salt, or to taste
- Freshly ground pepper, to taste

PREPARATION
1. Whisk apple juice concentrate, 2 tablespoons mustard, 1 tablespoon oil, rosemary (or thyme), garlic and peppercorns in a small bowl. Reserve 3 tablespoons marinade for basting. Place tenderloins in a shallow glass dish and pour the remaining marinade over them, turning to coat. Cover and marinate in the refrigerator for at least 20 minutes or for up to 2 hours, turning several times.
2. Heat a grill or broiler.
3. Combine shallot, port (or tea), vinegar, salt, pepper and the remaining 1 1/2 teaspoons mustard and 1 tablespoon oil in a small bowl or a jar with a tight-fitting lid; whisk or shake until blended. Set aside.
4. Grill or broil the tenderloins, turning several times and basting the browned sides with the reserved marinade, until just cooked through, 15 to 20 minutes. (An instant-read thermometer inserted in the center should register 155°F. The temperature will increase to 160° during resting.)
5. Transfer the tenderloins to a clean cutting board, tent with foil and let them rest for about 5 minutes before carving them into 1/2-inch-thick slices. Arrange the pork slices on plates and drizzle with the shallot dressing. Serve immediately.

TIPS & NOTES
- **Make Ahead Tip**: The pork can be marinated (Step 1) for up to 2 hours.

NUTRITION
Per serving: 165 calories; 5 g fat (1 g sat, 2 g mono); 63 mg cholesterol; 5 g carbohydrates; 0 g added sugars; 23 g protein; 0 g fiber; 186 mg sodium; 397 mg potassium.
Nutrition Bonus: Vitamin C (20% daily value).
Carbohydrate Servings: 1/2
Exchanges: 1/2 other carbohydrate, 3 lean meat

Salad of Boston Lettuce with Creamy Orange-Shallot Dressing

INGREDIENTS
DRESSING
- 1/4 cup reduced-fat mayonnaise
- 1/2 teaspoon Dijon mustard
- 1/4 cup orange juice
- 2 teaspoons finely chopped shallot
- Freshly ground pepper, to taste

SALAD
- 1 large head Boston lettuce, torn into bite-size pieces (5 cups)
- 1 cup julienned or grated carrot, (1 carrot)
- 1 cup cherry or grape tomatoes, rinsed and cut in half
- 2 tablespoons snipped fresh tarragon, or chives (optional)

PREPARATION

1. To prepare dressing: Whisk mayonnaise and mustard in a small bowl. Slowly whisk in orange juice until smooth. Stir in shallot. Season with pepper.
2. To prepare salad: Divide lettuce among 4 plates and scatter carrot and tomatoes on top. Drizzle the dressing over the salads and sprinkle with tarragon (or chives), if desired. Serve immediately.

NUTRITION
Per serving: 64 calories; 1 g fat (0 g sat, 0 g mono); 0 mg cholesterol; 12 g carbohydrates; 1 g added sugars; 2 g protein; 2 g fiber; 182 mg sodium; 386 mg potassium.
Nutrition Bonus: Vitamin A (120% daily value), Vitamin C (30% dv), Folate (16% dv).
Carbohydrate Servings: 1
Exchanges: 2 vegetable

Sweet Pea Mash

INGREDIENTS
- 3 1/3 cups frozen peas, (1 pound)
- 3 tablespoons water
- 1/4 teaspoon salt
- 2/3 cup reduced-fat sour cream
- 1/4 teaspoon white pepper
- 1/4 cup minced scallion greens, or chives
- 2 slices bacon, cooked and crumbled

PREPARATION
1. Heat peas, water and salt in a medium saucepan over medium-high heat, stirring often, until the peas are heated through, 6 to 10 minutes. Transfer to a food

processor; pulse with sour cream and pepper until a chunky puree forms. Pulse in scallion greens (or chives) and bacon.

NUTRITION
Per serving: 164 calories; 6 g fat (3 g sat, 2 g mono); 19 mg cholesterol; 19 g carbohydrates; 9 g protein; 7 g fiber; 320 mg sodium; 214 mg potassium.
Nutrition Bonus: Vitamin A (60% daily value), Vitamin C (25% dv), Folate (19% dv).
Carbohydrate Servings: 1
Exchanges: 1 starch, 1.5 fat

Roasted Pear Trifle

INGREDIENTS
CUSTARD
- 2 large eggs
- 1/2 cup sugar
- 6 tablespoons cornstarch
- 1/4 teaspoon salt
- 3 1/2 cups low-fat milk, divided
- 2 teaspoons vanilla extract

ROASTED PEARS & TRIFLE
- 8 firm, ripe Bosc pears, (about 3 1/4 pounds), peeled and diced
- 2 tablespoons sugar
- 2 tablespoons lemon juice
- 1/4 cup sliced almonds, (optional)
- 3/4 cup apricot fruit spread, or preserves
- 3 3-ounce packages ladyfingers, (see Note)
- 4 tablespoons amaretto, divided (see Tip)
- 1 pint raspberries, rinsed
- 1 3/4 cups Vanilla Cream, (recipe follows) or "lite" frozen whipped topping, thawed (optional)

PREPARATION
1. To prepare custard: Whisk eggs, 1/2 cup sugar, cornstarch, salt and 1/2 cup milk in a medium bowl until smooth. Heat the remaining 3 cups milk in a large heavy saucepan over medium heat until steaming. Gradually pour the hot milk into the egg mixture, whisking constantly. Return this mixture to the pan and cook over medium heat, whisking constantly, until the custard bubbles and thickens. (Use caution, as hot custard will sputter.) Remove from the heat and stir in vanilla. Transfer the custard to a shallow glass dish. Press plastic wrap directly onto the surface and refrigerate until chilled, at least 1 hour or overnight.

2. To roast pears: Preheat oven to 400°F. Coat a rimmed baking sheet with cooking spray. Toss pears, 2 tablespoons sugar and lemon juice in a large bowl. Spread the pears on the prepared baking sheet. Roast the pears until tender and golden brown in spots, turning occasionally, 45 to 50 minutes.
3. While the pears are roasting, toast almonds, if using, in a small baking pan until fragrant, 4 to 5 minutes. Set aside.
4. To assemble trifle: Melt apricot preserves in a small saucepan over low heat. Arrange 14 to 15 ladyfingers in the bottom of a trifle bowl (8-inch diameter), trimming them if necessary to fit tightly. Drizzle 1 tablespoon amaretto over the ladyfingers and dot with 3 tablespoons of the preserves. Top with one-third of the roasted pears (about 1 1/3 cups) and a scant 1/2 cup raspberries. Spread 3/4 cup custard over. Repeat layering 2 more times with ladyfingers, amaretto, preserves, fruit and custard. Top with 13 to 15 ladyfingers (you may have leftovers); drizzle with remaining amaretto. Spread remaining custard over the top. Cover and refrigerate until cold, at least 1 hour.
5. Meanwhile, make Vanilla Cream, if using.
6. Shortly before serving, spread Vanilla Cream (or whipped topping) on top of the trifle, if desired, and garnish with toasted almonds, if desired, and the remaining raspberries.

TIPS & NOTES
- **Make Ahead Tip**: Refrigerate, without Vanilla Cream, for up to 2 days.
- **Ingredient Note:** Ladyfingers can be found in the in-store bakery of most supermarkets.
- **Tip:** Replace amaretto with 4 tablespoons orange juice mixed with 1/4 teaspoon almond extract.

NUTRITION
Per serving: 197 calories; 1 g fat (1 g sat, 0 g mono); 32 mg cholesterol; 42 g carbohydrates; 4 g protein; 3 g fiber; 65 mg sodium; 116 mg potassium.
Carbohydrate Servings: 3
Exchanges: 1 fruit, 1 other carbohydrate

Pear & Dried Cranberry Strudel

INGREDIENTS
- 3 large Comice or Anjou pears, peeled and thinly sliced
- 1/2 cup dried cranberries
- 1/4 cup plus 1 teaspoon sugar
- 2 teaspoons freshly grated orange zest
- 1 tablespoon orange juice
- 8 sheets phyllo dough, defrosted according to package directions

- 1/4 cup plain dry breadcrumbs
- 1/3 cup walnut oil, (see Ingredient Note) or canola oil
- Confectioners' sugar, for dusting

PREPARATION

1. Preheat oven to 400°F. Coat a baking sheet with cooking spray.
2. Combine pears, dried cranberries, 1/4 cup sugar, orange zest and orange juice in a medium bowl.
3. Unroll phyllo onto a clean, dry surface. Cover with a sheet of wax paper and then a damp kitchen towel. Place a dry kitchen towel with a long edge toward you on the work surface. Sprinkle the towel lightly with breadcrumbs. Lay 1 sheet of phyllo on the towel. (Keep the stack of phyllo sheets covered to prevent them from drying out while you work.) Starting at the center and working toward the edges, lightly brush the phyllo sheet with oil. Sprinkle lightly with breadcrumbs. Lay another sheet of phyllo on top; brush with oil and sprinkle with breadcrumbs. Repeat with 5 of the remaining sheets of phyllo; lay the last sheet on top and brush with oil.
4. Mound the pear filling in a long 3-inch-wide strip on the phyllo stack, leaving a 2-inch border at the bottom and sides. Fold the short edges in and, starting at the long edge nearest you, roll the filling and phyllo into a cylinder, using the towel to help lift as you roll. Roll up firmly but not too tightly, to allow a little room for expansion.
5. Brush the strudel with oil and sprinkle with the remaining 1 teaspoon sugar. Carefully transfer the strudel to the prepared baking sheet, placing it seam-side down. Poke several steam vents in the top using the tip of a sharp knife.
6. Bake the strudel until golden brown, 30 to 35 minutes. Cool on the pan for 5 minutes, then transfer to a wire rack to cool completely. Just before serving, dust with confectioners' sugar.

TIPS & NOTES

- **Make Ahead Tip**: Transfer frozen phyllo dough to the refrigerator to thaw the day before baking.
- **Shopping tip:** The best pears for this strudel are firm yet ripe ones. Remember the cardinal rule for fruit: if it doesn't smell like anything, it won't taste like anything.
- **Ingredient Note:** Walnut oil has a delightful nutty flavor and boasts a high ratio of monounsaturated fats. You can find it in many supermarkets and natural-foods stores. Store it in the refrigerator.

NUTRITION

Per serving: 211 calories; 8 g fat (1 g sat, 2 g mono); 0 mg cholesterol; 34 g carbohydrates; 2 g protein; 3 gfiber; 119 mg sodium; 84 mg potassium.

Carbohydrate Servings: 2
Exchanges: 1 starch, 1 fruit, 1 1/2 fat

DAY 6
BREAKFAST

Jam-Filled Almond Muffins or Berry-Almond Quick Bread
Skim milk (1 cup)
Banana (1 cup)

LUNCH

The Taco
Calabacitas
Real Cornbread

SNACK

Low-fat vanilla yogurt (8 oz.)
Strawberries (1 cup)

DINNER

Sloppy Joes or Turkey Scallopini with Apricot Sauce
Barbecue Bean Salad
Vinegary Coleslaw
Plum Fool

DAY 6 RECIPES

Jam-Filled Almond Muffins

INGREDIENTS
- 1 1/4 cups whole-wheat flour
- 1 cup all-purpose flour
- 1 1/2 teaspoons baking powder
- 1/2 teaspoon baking soda
- 1/4 teaspoon salt
- 2 large eggs
- 1/2 cup packed light brown sugar
- 1 cup buttermilk, (see Tip)
- 1/4 cup orange juice
- 1/4 cup canola oil
- 1 teaspoon vanilla extract
- 1/3 cup blackberry, blueberry, raspberry or cherry jam
- 1/4 teaspoon almond extract
- 1/2 cup sliced almonds
- 1 tablespoon granulated sugar

PREPARATION

1. Preheat oven to 400°F. Coat 12 muffin cups with cooking spray.
2. Whisk whole-wheat flour, all-purpose flour, baking powder, baking soda and salt in a large bowl.
3. Whisk eggs and brown sugar in a medium bowl until smooth. Add buttermilk, orange juice, oil and vanilla; whisk to blend. Add to the dry ingredients and mix with a rubber spatula just until moistened.
4. Scoop half the batter into the prepared pan. Mix jam and almond extract; drop a generous teaspoonful into the center of each muffin. Spoon on the remaining batter, filling each muffin cup completely. Sprinkle with almonds, then sugar.
5. Bake the muffins until the tops are golden brown and spring back when touched lightly, 15 to 25 minutes. Loosen edges and turn muffins out onto a wire rack to cool slightly before serving.

TIPS & NOTES

- **Tip:** You can use buttermilk powder in place of fresh buttermilk. Or make "sour milk": mix 1 tablespoon lemon juice or vinegar to 1 cup milk.

NUTRITION

Per muffin: 229 calories; 8 g fat (1 g sat, 4 g mono); 36 mg cholesterol; 33 g carbohydrates; 6 g protein; 2 gfiber; 182 mg sodium; 77 mg potassium.
Carbohydrate Servings: 2
Exchanges: 2 starch, 1 fat

Berry-Almond Quick Bread

INGREDIENTS

- 1 1/2 cups whole-wheat pastry flour, (see Note) or whole-wheat flour
- 1 cup all-purpose flour
- 1 1/2 teaspoons baking powder
- 1 teaspoon ground cinnamon
- 1/2 teaspoon baking soda
- 1/4 teaspoon salt
- 2 large eggs
- 1 cup nonfat buttermilk, (see Tip)
- 2/3 cup brown sugar
- 2 tablespoons butter, melted
- 2 tablespoons canola oil
- 1 teaspoon vanilla extract
- 1/2 teaspoon almond extract

- 2 cups fresh or frozen berries, (whole blackberries, blueberries, raspberries; diced strawberries)
- 1/2 cup chopped toasted sliced almonds, (see Tip), plus more for topping if desired

PREPARATION
1. Preheat oven to 400°F for muffins, mini loaves and mini Bundts or 375°F for a large loaf. (See pan options, above.) Coat pan(s) with cooking spray.
2. Whisk whole-wheat flour, all-purpose flour, baking powder, cinnamon, baking soda and salt in a large bowl.
3. Whisk eggs, buttermilk, brown sugar, butter, oil, vanilla and almond extract in another large bowl until well combined.
4. Make a well in the center of the dry ingredients, pour in the wet ingredients and stir until just combined. Add berries and almonds. Stir just to combine; do not overmix. Transfer batter to the prepared pan(s). Top with additional almonds, if desired.
5. Bake until golden brown and a wooden skewer inserted into the center comes out clean, 22 to 25 minutes for muffins or mini Bundts, 35 minutes for mini loaves, 1 hour 10 minutes for a large loaf. Let cool in the pan(s) for 10 minutes, then turn out onto a wire rack. Let muffins and mini Bundts cool for 5 minutes more, mini loaves for 30 minutes, large loaves for 40 minutes.

TIPS & NOTES
- **Make Ahead Tip**: Store, individually wrapped, at room temperature for up to 2 days or in the freezer for up to 1 month. | Equipment: Pan options: 1 large loaf (9-by-5-inch pan); 3 mini loaves (6-by-3-inch pan, 2-cup capacity); 6 mini Bundt cakes (6-cup mini Bundt pan, scant 1-cup capacity per cake); 12 muffins (standard 12-cup, 2 1/2-inch muffin pan)
- **Note:** Whole-wheat pastry flour is milled from soft wheat. It contains less gluten than regular whole-wheat flour and helps ensure a tender result in delicate baked goods while providing the nutritional benefits of whole grains. Find it in the baking section of the supermarket or online at King Arthur Flour, (800) 827-6836, bakerscatalogue.com.
- **Tips:** No buttermilk? Mix 1 tablespoon lemon juice into 1 cup milk.
- **To toast sliced almonds:** cook in a small dry skillet over medium-low heat, stirring constantly, until fragrant and lightly browned, 2 to 4 minutes.

NUTRITION
Per serving: 220 calories; 7 g fat (2 g sat, 3 g mono); 41 mg cholesterol; 33 g carbohydrates; 6 g protein; 3 g fiber; 183 mg sodium; 81 mg potassium.
Carbohydrate Servings: 2
Exchanges: 1 starch, 1 other carb, 1 fat

The Taco

INGREDIENTS
HOMEMADE TACO SHELLS
- 12 6-inch corn tortillas
- Canola oil cooking spray
- 3/4 teaspoon chili powder, divided
- 1/4 teaspoon salt, divided

TACO MEAT
- 8 ounces 93%-lean ground beef
- 8 ounces 99%-lean ground turkey breast
- 1/2 cup chopped onion
- 1 10-ounce can diced tomatoes with green chiles, preferably Rotel brand (see Tip), or 1 1/4 cups petite-diced tomatoes
- 1/2 teaspoon ground cumin
- 1/2 teaspoon ground chipotle chile or 1 teaspoon chili powder
- 1/2 teaspoon dried oregano

TOPPINGS
- 3 cups shredded romaine lettuce
- 3/4 cup shredded reduced-fat Cheddar cheese
- 3/4 cup diced tomatoes
- 3/4 cup prepared salsa
- 1/4 cup diced red onion

PREPARATION
1. To prepare taco shells: Preheat oven to 375°F.
2. Working with 6 tortillas at a time, wrap in a barely damp cloth or paper towel and microwave on High until steamed, about 30 seconds. Lay the tortillas on a clean work surface and coat both sides with cooking spray; sprinkle a little chili powder and salt on one side. Carefully drape each tortilla over two bars of the oven rack. Bake until crispy, 7 to 10 minutes. Repeat with the remaining 6 tortillas.
3. To prepare taco meat: Place beef, turkey and onion in a large nonstick skillet over medium heat. Cook, breaking up the meat with a wooden spoon, until cooked through, about 10 minutes. Transfer to a colander to drain off fat. Wipe out the pan. Return the meat to the pan and add tomatoes, cumin, ground

chipotle (or chili powder) and oregano. Cook over medium heat, stirring occasionally, until most of the liquid has evaporated, 3 to 6 minutes.
4. To assemble tacos: Fill each shell with a generous 3 tablespoons taco meat, 1/4 cup lettuce, 1 tablespoon each cheese, tomato and salsa and 1 teaspoon onion.

TIPS & NOTES
- **Make Ahead Tip**: Store taco shells in an airtight container for up to 2 days. Reheat at 375°F for 1 to 2 minutes before serving. Cover and refrigerate taco meat for up to 1 day. Reheat just before serving.
- **Tip:** Look for Rotel brand diced tomatoes with green chiles—original or mild, depending on your spice preference—and set the heat level with either ground chipotle chile (adds smoky heat) or chili powder (adds rich chili taste without extra spice).

NUTRITION
Per serving: 252 calories; 5 g fat (1 g sat, 1 g mono); 38 mg cholesterol; 30 g carbohydrates; 0 g added sugars; 24 g protein; 5 g fiber; 576 mg sodium; 254 mg potassium.
Nutrition Bonus: Vitamin A (49% daily value), Vitamin C & Zinc (17% dv)
Carbohydrate Servings: 2
Exchanges: 1 1/2 starch, 1 vegetable, 3 lean meat

Calabacitas

INGREDIENTS
- 1 tablespoon extra-virgin olive oil
- 1 medium onion, chopped
- 1 poblano or Anaheim chile pepper, seeded and diced
- 2 cups diced zucchini
- 2 cups diced summer squash
- 1/2 teaspoon salt
- 2 tablespoons chopped fresh cilantro, (optional)

PREPARATION
1. Heat oil in a large nonstick skillet over medium heat. Add onion and chile; cook, stirring, until soft, about 4 minutes. Add zucchini, summer squash and salt; cover and cook, stirring once or twice, until tender, about 3 minutes. Remove from the heat and stir in cilantro (if using).

NUTRITION

Per serving: 40 calories; 2 g fat (0 g sat, 2 g mono); 0 mg cholesterol; 4 g carbohydrates; 0 g added sugars; 1 g protein; 1 g fiber; 199 mg sodium; 201 mg potassium.
Nutrition Bonus: Vitamin C (30% dv).
Exchanges: 1 vegetable, 1/2 fat

Real Cornbread

INGREDIENTS
- 3 tablespoons canola oil
- 2 cups yellow or white cornmeal
- 1 teaspoon baking powder
- 1/2 teaspoon salt
- 1 large egg, beaten
- 1 1/2 cups nonfat milk or nonfat buttermilk

PREPARATION
1. Preheat oven to 450°F. Place oil in a 9-inch cast-iron skillet or similar-size glass baking dish and transfer to the preheating oven.
2. Mix cornmeal, baking powder and salt in a medium bowl. Add egg and milk (or buttermilk); stir until just combined. Remove the pan from the oven and swirl the oil to coat the bottom and a little way up the sides. Very carefully pour the excess hot oil into the cornmeal mixture; stir until just combined. Pour the batter into the hot pan.
3. Bake until the bread is firm in the middle and lightly golden, about 20 minutes. Let cool for 5 minutes before slicing. Serve warm.

TIPS & NOTES
- **Make Ahead Tip:** The cornbread can be made up to 3 hours in advance. Reheat, wrapped in foil, in a warm oven.

NUTRITION

Per serving: 172 calories; 7 g fat (1 g sat, 3 g mono); 27 mg cholesterol; 24 g carbohydrates; 0 g added sugars; 5 g protein; 3 g fiber; 228 mg sodium; 85 mg potassium.
Carbohydrate Servings: 1 1/2
Exchanges: 1 1/2 starch, 1 1/2 fat

Sloppy Joes

INGREDIENTS
- 12 ounces 90%-lean ground beef
- 1 large onion, finely diced

- 2 cups finely chopped cremini mushrooms, (about 4 ounces)
- 5 plum tomatoes, diced
- 2 tablespoons all-purpose flour
- 1/2 cup water
- 1/4 cup cider vinegar
- 1/4 cup chili sauce, such as Heinz
- 1/4 cup ketchup
- 8 whole-wheat hamburger buns, toasted if desired

PREPARATION
1. Crumble beef into a large nonstick skillet; cook over medium heat until it starts to sizzle, about 1 minute. Add onion and mushrooms and cook, stirring occasionally, breaking up the meat with a wooden spoon, until the vegetables are soft and the moisture has evaporated, 8 to 10 minutes.
2. Add tomatoes and flour; stir to combine. Stir in water, vinegar, chili sauce and ketchup and bring to a simmer, stirring often. Reduce heat to a low simmer and cook, stirring occasionally, until the sauce is thickened and the onion is very tender, 8 to 10 minutes. Serve warm on buns.

TIPS & NOTES
- **Make Ahead Tip**: The filling will keep in the freezer for up to 1 month.

NUTRITION

Per serving: 233 calories; 6 g fat (2 g sat, 2 g mono); 28 mg cholesterol; 31 g carbohydrates; 14 g protein; 5 g fiber; 436 mg sodium; 504 mg potassium.
Nutrition Bonus: Zinc (20% daily value), Vitamin C (15% dv).
Carbohydrate Servings: 2
Exchanges: 2 starch, 1 1/2 very lean meat

Turkey Scallopini with Apricot Sauce

INGREDIENTS
- 2 tablespoons all-purpose flour
- 1/4 teaspoon salt
- 1/4 teaspoon freshly ground pepper
- 8 ounces turkey cutlets
- 2 teaspoons canola oil
- 1 1/2 tablespoons minced shallot, or onion
- 1 1/2 teaspoons minced fresh ginger
- 1/3 cup apricot or peach nectar, (see Tips for Two)
- 1/3 cup reduced-sodium chicken broth, (see Tips for Two)
- 1 tablespoon cider vinegar, or white-wine vinegar

- 1/2 teaspoon brown sugar
- 2 tablespoons chopped dried apricots
- 1 teaspoon chopped fresh mint, or 1/4 teaspoon dried

PREPARATION
1. Combine flour, salt and pepper in a shallow dish. Dredge turkey in the flour mixture.
2. Heat oil in a medium nonstick skillet over medium-high heat. Add the turkey and cook until golden and cooked through, 2 to 3 minutes per side. Transfer to a plate and cover with foil to keep warm.
3. Add shallot (or onion) and ginger to the pan. Cook, stirring, until fragrant, about 30 seconds. Add nectar, broth, vinegar and sugar; bring to a boil, stirring. Add apricots and cook until the apricots are tender and the sauce has reduced slightly, 2 to 3 minutes. Remove from the heat and stir in mint. Spoon the sauce over the turkey.

TIPS & NOTES
- **Tips for Two:** Refrigerate leftover nectar for up to 1 week. Add to smoothies; whisk into salad dressing; combine with sparkling water for a refreshing nonalcoholic beverage.
- Store leftover canned broth up to 5 days in the refrigerator or up to 3 months in your freezer. Leftover broth in aseptic packages keeps for up to 1 week in the refrigerator. Add to soups, sauces, stews; use for cooking rice and grains; add a little when reheating leftovers to prevent them from drying out.

NUTRITION
Per serving: 239 calories; 5 g fat (0 g sat, 3 g mono); 46 mg cholesterol; 18 g carbohydrates; 30 g protein; 1 g fiber; 329 mg sodium; 189 mg potassium.
Nutrition Bonus: Vitamin A (20% daily value), Vitamin C (15% dv).
Carbohydrate Servings: 1
Exchanges: 1 fruit, 4 very lean meat, 1 fat

Barbecue Bean Salad

INGREDIENTS
- 1/3 cup prepared spicy barbecue sauce
- 3 tablespoons cider vinegar
- 2 teaspoons molasses
- 1 15-ounce can pinto beans, rinsed
- 2 medium tomatoes, seeded and coarsely chopped
- 1 bunch scallions, trimmed and chopped (1 cup)
- Freshly ground pepper, to taste and Hot sauce, to taste

PREPARATION

1. Whisk barbecue sauce, vinegar and molasses in a large bowl. Add beans, tomatoes and scallions; toss to coat. Season with pepper and hot sauce. If not serving immediately, cover and refrigerate for up to 2 days. Serve at room temperature.

NUTRITION

Per serving: 142 calories; 1 g fat (0 g sat, 0 g mono); 0 mg cholesterol; 31 g carbohydrates; 6 g protein; 7 gfiber; 555 mg sodium; 604 mg potassium.
Nutrition Bonus: Potassium (17% daily value).
Carbohydrate Servings: 1 1/2
Exchanges: 1 starch, 1 vegetable, 1 very lean meat.

Vinegary Coleslaw

INGREDIENTS
- 2 tablespoons white-wine vinegar
- 1 tablespoon canola oil
- 1 teaspoon sugar
- 1 teaspoon Dijon mustard
- Pinch of celery seed
- Pinch of salt
- 1 1/2 cups shredded cabbage
- 1 carrot, peeled and grated
- 1/4 cup slivered red onion

PREPARATION

1. Whisk vinegar, oil, sugar, mustard, celery seed and salt in a medium bowl. Add cabbage, carrot and onion and toss to coat.

NUTRITION

Per serving: 101 calories; 7 g fat (1 g sat, 4 g mono); 0 mg cholesterol; 9 g carbohydrates; 2 g added sugars; 1 g protein; 2 g fiber; 138 mg sodium; 248 mg potassium.
Nutrition Bonus: Vitamin A (100% daily value), Vitamin C (35% dv).
Carbohydrate Servings: 1
Exchanges: 1 vegetable, 1 1/2 fat

Plum Fool

INGREDIENTS
- 1 pound plums, pitted and sliced (about 2 1/2 cups)
- 1/4-1/2 cup sugar, or Splenda Granular
- 1/2 teaspoon grated fresh ginger
- 1/2 teaspoon ground cinnamon
- 1 1/2 cups low-fat vanilla yogurt and 1/3 cup whipping cream

PREPARATION
1. Set aside a few plum slices for garnish. Combine the remaining plum slices, 1/4 cup sugar (or Splenda), ginger and cinnamon in a small heavy saucepan. Bring to a simmer, stirring, over medium heat. Cook until the mixture has softened into a chunky puree, 15 to 20 minutes. Taste and add more sugar (or Splenda), if desired. Transfer to a bowl and chill until cool, about 1 hour.
2. Meanwhile, set a fine-mesh stainless-steel sieve over a bowl. Spoon in yogurt and let drain in the refrigerator until reduced to 1 cup, about 1 hour.
3. Whip cream to soft peaks in a chilled bowl. Gently fold in the drained yogurt with a rubber spatula. Fold this mixture into the fruit puree, leaving distinct swirls. Spoon into 6 dessert dishes and cover with plastic wrap. Refrigerate for at least 1 hour or up to 2 days. Garnish with the reserved plum slices before serving.

NUTRITION
Per serving: 156 calories; 5 g fat (3 g sat, 2 g mono); 18 mg cholesterol; 25 g carbohydrates; 4 g protein; 1 g fiber; 45 mg sodium; 259 mg potassium.
Nutrition Bonus: Calcium (12% daily value), Vitamin C (12% dv).
Carbohydrate Servings: 1 1/2
Exchanges: 11/2 fruit, 1 fat
Nutrition Note: Per serving with Splenda: 1 Carbohydrate Serving, 128 calories, 18 g carbohydrate.

DAY 7
BREAKFAST

Crustless Crab Quiche
Strawberries (1 cup)
Whole-wheat toast (1 slice)
LUNCH

Curried Corn Bisque
Grilled Chicken Caesar Salad or Chopped Salad al Tonno
Skim milk (1 cup)
Apple (1 cup)

SNACK

Almonds (1 oz)
Skim milk (1 cup)

DINNER

Tofu with Peanut-Ginger Sauce or Mock Ceviche
Brown rice (1 cup, cooked)
Spinach Salad with Black Olive Vinaigrette
Tropical Fruit Ice

DAY 7 RECIPES

Crustless Crab Quiche

INGREDIENTS
- 2 teaspoons extra-virgin olive oil, divided
- 1 onion, chopped
- 1 red bell pepper, chopped
- 12 ounces mushrooms, wiped clean and sliced (about 4 1/2 cups)
- 2 large eggs
- 2 large egg whites
- 1 1/2 cups low-fat cottage cheese
- 1/2 cup low-fat plain yogurt
- 1/4 cup all-purpose flour
- 1/4 cup freshly grated Parmesan cheese
- 1/4 teaspoon cayenne pepper
- 1/4 teaspoon salt
- 1/4 teaspoon freshly ground pepper
- 8 ounces cooked lump crabmeat, (fresh or frozen and thawed), drained and picked over (about 1 cup)
- 1/2 cup grated sharp Cheddar cheese, (2 ounces)
- 1/4 cup chopped scallions

PREPARATION
1. Preheat oven to 350°F. Coat a 10-inch pie pan or ceramic quiche dish with cooking spray.
2. Heat 1 teaspoon oil in large nonstick skillet over medium-high heat. Add onion and bell pepper; cook, stirring, until softened, about 5 minutes; transfer to a large bowl. Add the remaining 1 teaspoon oil to the skillet and heat over high heat. Add mushrooms and cook, stirring, until they have softened and most of their liquid has evaporated, 5 to 7 minutes. Add to the bowl with the onion mixture.

3. Place eggs, egg whites, cottage cheese, yogurt, flour, Parmesan, cayenne, salt and pepper in a food processor or blender; blend until smooth. Add to the vegetable mixture, along with crab, Cheddar and scallions; mix with a rubber spatula. Pour into the prepared baking dish.
4. Bake the quiche until a knife inserted in the center comes out clean, 40 to 50 minutes. Let stand for 5 minutes before serving.

NUTRITION
Per serving: 225 calories; 10 g fat (4 g sat, 3 g mono); 122 mg cholesterol; 14 g carbohydrates; 27 gprotein; 2 g fiber; 661 mg sodium; 355 mg potassium.
Nutrition Bonus: Vitamin C (70% daily value), Calcium (25% dv), Vitamin A (20% dv).
Carbohydrate Servings: 1
Exchanges: 2 1/2 vegetable, 1 1/2 very lean meat, 1 high-fat meat

Curried Corn Bisque

INGREDIENTS
- 2 teaspoons canola oil
- 1 cup fresh or frozen chopped onions
- 1 tablespoon curry powder
- 1/2 teaspoon hot sauce, or to taste
- 1/4 teaspoon salt, or to taste
- 1/4 teaspoon freshly ground pepper
- 2 16-ounce packages frozen corn, or 3 10-ounce boxes
- 2 cups reduced-sodium chicken broth
- 2 cups water
- 1 cup "lite" coconut milk, (see Ingredient note)

PREPARATION
1. Heat oil in a large saucepan over medium-high heat. Add onions and cook, stirring occasionally, until soft, about 3 minutes. Add curry powder, hot sauce, salt and pepper and stir to coat the onions. Stir in corn, broth and water; increase the heat to high and bring the mixture to a boil. Remove from the heat and puree in a blender or food processor (in batches, if necessary) into a homogeneous mixture that still has some texture. Pour the soup into a clean pot, add coconut milk and heat through. Serve hot or cold. Make Curried Sweet Pea Bisque by substituting frozen peas for the corn.

TIPS & NOTES
- **Make Ahead Tip:** Cover and refrigerate for up to 2 days or freeze for up to 2 months.
- **Ingredient Note:** Look for reduced-fat coconut milk (labeled "lite") in the Asian section of your market.

NUTRITION

Per serving: 138 calories; 4 g fat (2 g sat, 1 g mono); 1 mg cholesterol; 24 g carbohydrates; 0 g added sugars; 5 g protein; 3 g fiber; 121 mg sodium; 291 mg potassium.
Nutrition Bonus: Fiber (13% daily value).
Carbohydrate Servings: 1 1/2
Exchanges: 1 1/2 starch, 1 fat

Grilled Chicken Caesar Salad

INGREDIENTS
- 1 pound boneless, skinless chicken breasts, trimmed of fat
- 1 teaspoon canola oil
- 1/4 teaspoon salt, or to taste
- Freshly ground pepper, to taste
- 8 cups washed, dried and torn romaine lettuce
- 1 cup fat-free croutons
- 1/2 cup Caesar Salad Dressing, (recipe follows)
- 1/2 cup Parmesan curls, (see Tip)
- Lemon wedges

PREPARATION
1. Prepare a grill or preheat broiler.
2. Rub chicken with oil and season with salt and pepper. Grill or broil chicken until browned and no trace of pink remains in the center, 3 to 4 minutes per side.
3. Combine lettuce and croutons in a large bowl. Toss with Caesar Salad Dressing and divide among 4 plates. Cut chicken into 1/2-inch slices and fan over salad. Top with Parmesan curls. Serve immediately, with lemon wedges.

TIPS & NOTES
- **Tip:** To make parmesan curls, start with a piece of cheese that is at least 4 ounces. Use a swivel-bladed vegetable peeler to shave off curls.

NUTRITION

Per serving: 278 calories; 6 g fat (2 g sat, 2 g mono); 74 mg cholesterol; 14 g carbohydrates; 34 g protein; 1 g fiber; 662 mg sodium; 308 mg potassium.
Carbohydrate Servings: 1
Exchanges: 1/2 starch, 2 vegetable, 4 very lean meat, For Caesar Salad Dressing, free food

Chopped Salad al Tonno

INGREDIENTS
- 1/4 cup lemon juice
- 3 tablespoons extra-virgin olive oil
- 1/2 teaspoon garlic, salt
- Freshly ground pepper, to taste
- 8 cups chopped hearts of romaine
- 2 medium tomatoes, diced
- 1/2 cup sliced pimiento-stuffed green olives
- 2 6-ounce cans chunk light tuna, drained (see Note)

PREPARATION
1. Whisk lemon juice, oil, garlic salt and pepper in a large bowl. Add romaine, tomatoes and olives; toss to coat. Add tuna and toss again.

TIPS & NOTES
- **Note:** Chunk light tuna, which comes from the smaller skipjack or yellowfin, has less mercury than canned white albacore tuna. The FDA/EPA advises that women who are or might become pregnant, nursing mothers and young children consume no more than 6 ounces of albacore a week; up to 12 ounces of canned light tuna is considered safe.

NUTRITION
Per serving: 258 calories; 13 g fat (2 g sat, 9 g mono); 53 mg cholesterol; 8 g carbohydrates; 0 g added sugars; 26 g protein; 3 g fiber; 428 mg sodium; 406 mg potassium.
Nutrition Bonus: Vitamin A (110% daily value), Vitamin C (60% dv), Folate (32% dv).
Carbohydrate Servings: 1/2
Exchanges: 2 vegetable, 3 very lean meat, 2 1/2 fat

Tofu with Peanut-Ginger Sauce

INGREDIENTS
SAUCE
- 5 tablespoons water
- 4 tablespoons smooth natural peanut butter
- 1 tablespoon rice vinegar, (see Ingredient note) or white vinegar
- 2 teaspoons reduced-sodium soy sauce
- 2 teaspoons honey
- 2 teaspoons minced ginger
- 2 cloves garlic, minced

TOFU & VEGETABLES

- 14 ounces extra-firm tofu, preferably water-packed
- 2 teaspoons extra-virgin olive oil
- 4 cups baby spinach, (6 ounces)
- 1 1/2 cups sliced mushrooms, (4 ounces)
- 4 scallions, sliced (1 cup)

PREPARATION
1. To prepare sauce: Whisk water, peanut butter, rice vinegar (or white vinegar), soy sauce, honey, ginger and garlic in a small bowl.
2. To prepare tofu: Drain and rinse tofu; pat dry. Slice the block crosswise into eight 1/2-inch-thick slabs. Coarsely crumble each slice into smaller, uneven pieces.
3. Heat oil in a large nonstick skillet over high heat. Add tofu and cook in a single layer, without stirring, until the pieces begin to turn golden brown on the bottom, about 5 minutes. Then gently stir and continue cooking, stirring occasionally, until all sides are golden brown, 5 to 7 minutes more.
4. Add spinach, mushrooms, scallions and the peanut sauce and cook, stirring, until the vegetables are just cooked, 1 to 2 minutes more.

TIPS & NOTES
- **Ingredient Note:** Rice vinegar (or rice-wine vinegar) is mild, slightly sweet vinegar made from fermented rice. Find it in the Asian section of supermarkets and specialty stores.

NUTRITION

Per serving: 221 calories; 14 g fat (2 g sat, 3 g mono); 0 mg cholesterol; 15 g carbohydrates; 3 g added sugars; 12 g protein; 4 g fiber; 231 mg sodium; 262 mg potassium.
Nutrition Bonus: Calcium (16% daily value), Iron (16% dv).
Carbohydrate Servings: 1
Exchanges: 2 vegetable, 2 medium-fat meat

Mock Ceviche

INGREDIENTS
- 1 pound tilapia fillets, cut into 2-inch pieces
- 1-2 jalapeño peppers, minced
- 1/2 cup lime juice
- 1/2 cup chopped fresh cilantro, divided
- 1 teaspoon chopped fresh oregano
- 1/4 teaspoon salt
- 1 large green bell pepper, halved crosswise and thinly sliced

- 1 large tomato, chopped
- 1/2 cup very thinly sliced white onion
- 1/4 cup quartered green olives
- 1 avocado, chopped

PREPARATION
1. Place tilapia in a medium skillet. Cover with water. Bring to a boil over high heat, remove from the heat, cover and let stand for 5 minutes.
2. Meanwhile, place jalapeño to taste in a small bowl and whisk in lime juice, 2 tablespoons cilantro, oregano and salt. Transfer the tilapia to a large, shallow, nonreactive dish with a slotted spoon and pour the lime juice mixture over the top. Add bell pepper, tomato, onion and olives; gently mix to combine. (It's OK if the tilapia breaks apart.) Cover and chill for at least 20 minutes.
3. Sprinkle with the remaining cilantro and avocado just before serving.

TIPS & NOTES
- **Make Ahead Tip**: Cover and refrigerate for up to 2 hours.

NUTRITION

Per serving: 236 calories; 11 g fat (2 g sat, 7 g mono); 57 mg cholesterol; 13 g carbohydrates; 0 g added sugars; 25 g protein; 5 g fiber; 378 mg sodium; 831 mg potassium.
Nutrition Bonus: Vitamin C (80% daily value), Potassium (24% dv), Folate (22% dv), Vitamin A (15% dv).
Carbohydrate Servings: 1/2
Exchanges: 1 vegetable, 3 very lean meat, 2 fat

Spinach Salad with Black Olive Vinaigrette

INGREDIENTS
- 3 tablespoons extra-virgin olive oil
- 1 1/2 tablespoons red-wine vinegar, or lemon juice
- 6 pitted Kalamata olives, finely chopped
- 1/4 teaspoon salt
- Freshly ground pepper, to taste
- 6 cups torn spinach leaves
- 1/2 cucumber, seeded and sliced
- 1/2 red onion, thinly sliced

PREPARATION
1. Whisk oil, vinegar (or lemon juice) and olives in a salad bowl. Season with salt and pepper. Add spinach, cucumbers and onions; toss well. Serve immediately.

NUTRITION
Per serving: 128 calories; 12 g fat (2 g sat, 9 g mono); 0 mg cholesterol; 3 g carbohydrates; 2 g protein; 1 gfiber; 271 mg sodium; 284 mg potassium.
Nutrition Bonus: Vitamin A (80% daily value), Folate (22% dv), Vitamin C (20% dv).
Exchanges: 1 vegetable, 2 fat

Tropical Fruit Ice

INGREDIENTS
- 1 11-1/2-ounce can frozen passion fruit concentrate, (see Ingredient note)
- 2 cups water
- 2 tablespoons lime juice

PREPARATION
1. Combine passion fruit concentrate, water and lime juice in a medium bowl.
2. Pour the juice mixture into an ice cream maker and freeze according to manufacturer's directions. (Alternatively, freeze the mixture in a shallow metal pan until solid, about 6 hours. Break into chunks and process in a food processor until smooth.) Serve immediately or transfer to a storage container and let harden in the freezer for 1 to 1 1/2 hours. Serve in chilled dishes.

TIPS & NOTES
- **Make Ahead Tip**: Store in an airtight container in the freezer for up to 2 days. Let soften in the refrigerator for 1/2 hour before serving. | Equipment: Ice cream maker or food processor
- **Ingredient Note:** Welch's frozen passion-fruit cocktail concentrate can be found in supermarkets. Substitute the same size can of your favorite frozen juice concentrate for endless variations.

NUTRITION
Per serving: 84 calories; 1 g fat (0 g sat, 0 g mono); 0 mg cholesterol; 15 g carbohydrates; 0 g added sugars; 2 g protein; 0 g fiber; 31 mg sodium; 311 mg potassium.
Nutrition Bonus: Vitamin A (35% daily value), Vitamin C (25% dv).
Carbohydrate Servings: 1
Exchanges: 1 fruit

DAY 8
BREAKFAST

Overnight Oatmeal
Apricot (1 cup, halves)
Low-fat vanilla yogurt (8 oz.)

LUNCH

Chicken, Escarole & Rice Soup
Strawberry, Melon & Avocado Salad
Whole-wheat toast (1 slice)

SNACK

Skim milk (1 cup)
Banana (1 cup, sliced)

DINNER

Southwestern Steak & Peppers or Roasted Pork Tenderloin with Cherry & Tomato Chutney
Oven "Fries"
Broccoli with Caramelized Onions & Pine Nuts
Rustic Berry Tart or Dried Fruit Compote

DAY 8 RECIPES

Overnight Oatmeal

INGREDIENTS
- 8 cups water
- 2 cups steel-cut oats, (see Ingredient note)
- 1/3 cup dried cranberries
- 1/3 cup dried apricots, chopped
- 1/4 teaspoon salt, or to taste

PREPARATION
1. Combine water, oats, dried cranberries, dried apricots and salt in a 5- or 6-quart slow cooker. Turn heat to low. Put the lid on and cook until the oats are tender and the porridge is creamy, 7 to 8 hours. Stovetop Variation Halve the above recipe to accommodate the size of most double boilers: Combine 4 cups water, 1 cup steel-cut
oats, 3 tablespoons dried cranberries, 3 tablespoons dried apricots and 1/8 teaspoon salt in the top of a double boiler. Cover and cook over boiling water for about 1 1/2 hours, checking the water level in the bottom of the double boiler from time to time.

TIPS & NOTES

- **Ingredient Note:** Steel-cut oats, sometimes labeled "Irish oatmeal," look like small pebbles. They are toasted oat groats—the oat kernel that has been removed from the husk that have been cut in 2 or 3 pieces. Do not substitute regular rolled oats, which have a shorter cooking time, in the slow-cooker oatmeal recipe.
- For easy cleanup, try a slow-cooker liner. These heat-resistant, disposable liners fit neatly inside the insert and help prevent food from sticking to the bottom and sides of your slow cooker.

NUTRITION

Per serving: 193 calories; 3 g fat (0 g sat, 1 g mono); 0 mg cholesterol; 34 g carbohydrates; 0 g added sugars; 6 g protein; 9 g fiber; 77 mg sodium; 195 mg potassium.
Nutrition Bonus: Fiber (36% daily value).
Carbohydrate Servings: 2
Exchanges: 2 starch, 1/2 fruit

Chicken, Escarole & Rice Soup

INGREDIENTS

- 1 tablespoon extra-virgin olive oil
- 1 large onion, chopped
- 2 cloves garlic, minced
- 1 head escarole, trimmed and thinly sliced
- 3 14-ounce cans reduced-sodium chicken broth
- 1 14-ounce can diced tomatoes
- 1/2 cup long-grain white rice
- 1 pound boneless, skinless chicken breasts, trimmed and cut into 1/2-inch pieces
- Freshly ground pepper, to taste
- 6 tablespoons freshly grated Romano or Parmesan cheese

PREPARATION

1. Heat oil in a large pot over medium-high heat. Add onion and garlic; cook, stirring frequently, until they soften and begin to brown, 5 to 7 minutes. Add escarole and cook, stirring occasionally, until wilted, 2 to 3 minutes. Add broth, tomatoes and rice; bring to a boil. Reduce heat to low, cover and simmer until the rice is almost tender, 12 to 15 minutes.
2. Add chicken and simmer until it is no longer pink in the center and the rice is tender, about 5 minutes. Season with pepper. Serve hot, sprinkled with Romano (or Parmesan).

TIPS & NOTES
- **Make Ahead Tip**: Cover and refrigerate for up to 2 days or freeze for up to 2 months.

NUTRITION
Per serving: 157 calories; 4 g fat (1 g sat, 2 g mono); 30 mg cholesterol; 15 g carbohydrates; 16 g protein; 2 g fiber; 166 mg sodium; 337 mg potassium.
Nutrition Bonus: Folate (21% daily value), Vitamin A (20% dv).
Carbohydrate Servings: 1
Exchanges: 1 starch, 1 1/2 lean meat

Strawberry, Melon & Avocado Salad

INGREDIENTS
- 1/4 cup honey
- 2 tablespoons sherry vinegar, or red-wine vinegar
- 2 tablespoons finely chopped fresh mint
- 1/4 teaspoon freshly ground pepper
- Pinch of salt
- 4 cups baby spinach
- 1 small avocado, (4-5 ounces), peeled, pitted and cut into 16 slices
- 16 thin slices cantaloupe, (about 1/2 small cantaloupe), rind removed
- 1 1/2 cups hulled strawberries, sliced
- 2 teaspoons sesame seeds, toasted (see Tip)

PREPARATION
1. Whisk honey, vinegar, mint, pepper and salt in a small bowl.
2. Divide spinach among 4 salad plates. Arrange alternating slices of avocado and cantaloupe in a fan on top of the spinach. Top each salad with strawberries, drizzle with dressing and sprinkle with sesame seeds.

TIPS & NOTES
- **Make Ahead Tip**: The dressing will keep, covered, in the refrigerator for up to 1 day.
- **Tip:** To toast sesame seeds, heat a small dry skillet over low heat. Add sesame seeds and stir constantly until golden and fragrant, about 2 minutes. Transfer to a small bowl and let cool.

NUTRITION
Per serving: 202 calories; 8 g fat (1 g sat, 1 g mono); 0 mg cholesterol; 24 g carbohydrates; 3 g protein; 7 gfiber; 90 mg sodium; 503 mg potassium.

Nutrition Bonus: Vitamin C (100% daily value), Vitamin A (60% dv), Folate (18% dv).
Carbohydrate Servings: 2
Exchanges: 1 vegetable, 2 fruit, 1 1/2 fat (mono)

Southwestern Steak & Peppers

INGREDIENTS
- 1/2 teaspoon ground cumin
- 1/2 teaspoon ground coriander
- 1/2 teaspoon chili powder
- 1/4 teaspoon salt, or to taste
- 3/4 teaspoon coarsely ground pepper, plus more to taste
- 1 pound boneless top sirloin steak, trimmed of fat
- 3 cloves garlic, peeled, 1 halved and 2 minced
- 3 teaspoons canola oil, or extra-virgin olive oil, divided
- 2 red bell peppers, thinly sliced
- 1 medium white onion, halved lengthwise and thinly sliced
- 1 teaspoon brown sugar
- 1/2 cup brewed coffee, or prepared instant coffee
- 1/4 cup balsamic vinegar
- 4 cups watercress sprigs

PREPARATION
1. Mix cumin, coriander, chili powder, salt and 3/4 teaspoon pepper in a small bowl. Rub steak with the cut garlic. Rub the spice mix all over the steak.
2. Heat 2 teaspoons oil in a large heavy skillet, preferably cast iron, over medium-high heat. Add the steak and cook to desired doneness, 4 to 6 minutes per side for medium-rare. Transfer to a cutting board and let rest.
3. Add remaining 1 teaspoon oil to the skillet. Add bell peppers and onion; cook, stirring often, until softened, about 4 minutes. Add minced garlic and brown sugar; cook, stirring often, for 1 minute. Add coffee, vinegar and any accumulated meat juices; cook for 3 minutes to intensify flavor. Season with pepper.
4. To serve, mound 1 cup watercress on each plate. Top with the sauteed peppers and onion. Slice the steak thinly across the grain and arrange on the vegetables. Pour the sauce from the pan over the steak. Serve immediately.

NUTRITION
Per serving: 226 calories; 12 g fat (3 g sat, 5 g mono); 60 mg cholesterol; 12 g carbohydrates; 1 g added sugars; 26 g protein; 3 g fiber; 216 mg sodium; 606 mg potassium.
Nutrition Bonus: Vitamin C (210% daily value), Vitamin A (60% dv), Iron (25% dv).

Carbohydrate Servings: 1
Exchanges: 2 vegetable, 3 lean meat

Roasted Pork Tenderloin with Cherry & Tomato Chutney

INGREDIENTS

CHUTNEY
- 1 1/2 cups fresh or frozen (thawed; see Tip) dark sweet cherries, pitted and chopped
- 1/3 cup chopped onion
- 1/3 cup sugar
- 1/3 cup cider vinegar
- 1 tablespoon minced fresh ginger
- 1 1/2 teaspoons yellow mustard seed
- 1/2 teaspoon ground cinnamon
- 1/2 teaspoon ground allspice
- 1/2 teaspoon salt
- 1/2 teaspoon coarsely ground pepper
- 1 1/3 cups chopped tomatoes, slightly underripe

PORK
- 2 pork tenderloins, 1 pound each, trimmed of fat
- 1/3 cup reduced-sodium chicken broth
- 2 tablespoons canola oil, divided
- 1/2 teaspoon salt
- 1/2 teaspoon freshly ground pepper
- 1/2 teaspoon dried thyme leaves
- Fresh cilantro sprigs, for garnish (optional)

PREPARATION

1. To prepare chutney: Combine cherries, onion, sugar, vinegar, ginger, mustard seed, cinnamon, allspice, salt and pepper in a medium nonreactive saucepan (see Note). Bring to a boil over medium-high heat and cook, stirring occasionally, for 5 minutes. Stir in tomatoes and continue to simmer until they are cooked through and the liquid is slightly thickened, 3 to 4 minutes. Remove from the heat; cool, stirring occasionally, for 30 minutes.
2. To marinate pork: Place pork in a heavy-duty sealable plastic bag. Add 3/4 cup of the cooled chutney, chicken broth and 1 tablespoon oil. Seal the bag and turn to coat the pork with the marinade. Refrigerate the pork overnight. Refrigerate the remaining chutney.
3. To roast pork: Preheat oven to 425°F. Remove the pork from the marinade, shaking off excess (discard marinade). Pat the pork dry with paper towels and season with salt, pepper and thyme.

4. Heat the remaining 1 tablespoon oil over high heat in a large ovenproof skillet until hot but not smoking. Add the pork and cook, turning until browned on all sides, 3 to 5 minutes.
5. Transfer the pan to the oven and roast the pork until just cooked through and an instant-read thermometer registers 155°F in the center of the pork, 15 to 17 minutes. Transfer the pork to a cutting board and let rest for 5 minutes before slicing. Garnish the pork with cilantro, if using, and serve with the reserved chutney.

TIPS & NOTES

- **Make Ahead Tip**: Cover and refrigerate the chutney (Step 1) for up to 3 weeks.
- **Tip:** Be sure to measure frozen cherries while still frozen, then thaw. (Drain before using.)
- **Note:** A nonreactive pan or container—stainless steel, enamel-coated or glass—is necessary when preparing acidic foods, such as cherries, to prevent the food from reacting with the pan or container. Reactive pans, such as aluminum or cast-iron, can impart an off color and/or off flavor in acidic foods.

NUTRITION
Per serving: 228 calories; 8 g fat (2 g sat, 4 g mono); 63 mg cholesterol; 15 g carbohydrates; 23 g protein; 1 g fiber; 344 mg sodium; 507 mg potassium.
Nutrition Bonus: Selenium (56% daily value), Zinc (15% dv).
Carbohydrate Servings: 1
Exchanges: 1 other carb, 3 lean meat

Oven "Fries"
INGREDIENTS
- 2 large Yukon Gold potatoes, cut into wedges
- 4 teaspoons extra-virgin olive oil
- 1/2 teaspoon salt
- 1/2 teaspoon dried thyme, (optional)

PREPARATION
1. Preheat oven to 450°F.
2. Toss potato wedges with oil, salt and thyme (if using). Spread the wedges out on a rimmed baking sheet.
3. Bake until browned and tender, turning once, about 20 minutes total.

NUTRITION

Per serving: 102 calories; 5 g fat (1 g sat, 4 g mono); 0 mg cholesterol; 13 g carbohydrates; 0 g added sugars; 2 g protein; 1 g fiber; 291 mg sodium; 405 mg potassium.
Carbohydrate Servings: 1
Exchanges: 1 starch, 1 fat

Broccoli with Caramelized Onions & Pine Nuts

INGREDIENTS

- 3 tablespoons pine nuts, or chopped slivered almonds
- 2 teaspoons extra-virgin olive oil
- 1 cup chopped onion, (about 1 medium)
- 1/4 teaspoon salt, or to taste
- 4 cups broccoli florets
- 2 teaspoons balsamic vinegar
- Freshly ground pepper, to taste

PREPARATION

1. Toast pine nuts (or almonds) in a medium dry skillet over medium-low heat, stirring constantly, until lightly browned and fragrant, 2 to 3 minutes. Transfer to a small bowl to cool.
2. Add oil to the pan and heat over medium heat. Add onion and salt; cook, stirring occasionally, adjusting heat as necessary, until soft and golden brown, 15 to 20 minutes.
3. Meanwhile, steam broccoli until just tender, 4 to 6 minutes. Transfer to a large bowl. Add the nuts, onion, vinegar and pepper; toss to coat. Serve immediately.

NUTRITION

Per serving: 102 calories; 7 g fat (1 g sat, 3 g mono); 0 mg cholesterol; 9 g carbohydrates; 0 g added sugars; 3 g protein; 3 g fiber; 166 mg sodium; 328 mg potassium.
Nutrition Bonus: 69 mg vitamin c (110% dv), 45% dv vitamin a, 62 mcg folate (16% dv).
Carbohydrate Servings: 1/2
Exchanges: 1 1/2 vegetable, 1 fat

Rustic Berry Tart

INGREDIENTS
CRUST

- 3/4 cup whole-wheat pastry flour, (see Ingredient note)
- 3/4 cup all-purpose flour
- 2 tablespoons sugar, plus 1 teaspoon for sprinkling

- 1/4 teaspoon salt
- 4 tablespoons cold butter, (1/2 stick), cut into small pieces
- 1 tablespoon canola oil
- 1/4 cup ice water, plus more as needed
- 1 large egg, separated (see Tip; save the white to glaze the pastry)
- 1 teaspoon lemon juice, or white vinegar

FILLING & GLAZE
- 1/4 cup slivered almonds, (1 ounce)
- 1/4 cup whole-wheat flour, (regular or pastry flour)
- 1/4 cup plus 3 tablespoons sugar, or Splenda Granular
- 4 cups mixed berries, such as blackberries, raspberries and blueberries
- 2 teaspoons lemon juice
- 1 tablespoon water
- 2 tablespoons raspberry, blueberry or blackberry jam

PREPARATION
1. To prepare crust: Whisk whole-wheat flour, all-purpose flour, 2 tablespoons sugar and salt in a medium bowl. Cut in butter with a pastry blender or your fingers until the mixture resembles coarse crumbs with a few larger pieces. Add oil and stir with a fork to blend. Mix 1/4 cup water, egg yolk and 1 teaspoon lemon juice (or vinegar) in a measuring cup. Add just enough of the egg yolk mixture to the flour mixture, stirring with a fork, until the dough clumps together. (Add a little water if the dough seems too dry.) Turn the dough out onto a lightly floured surface and knead several times. Form the dough into a ball, then flatten into a disk. Wrap in plastic wrap and refrigerate for at least 1 hour.
2. Preheat oven to 425°F. Line a baking sheet with parchment paper or foil and coat with cooking spray.
3. To prepare filling & assemble tart: Spread almonds in a small baking pan. Bake until light golden and fragrant, about 5 minutes. Let cool. Combine whole-wheat flour, 1/4 cup sugar (or Splenda) and the toasted almonds in a food processor or blender; process until the almonds are ground.
4. Roll the dough into a rough 13- to 14-inch circle on a lightly floured surface, about 1/4 inch thick. Roll it back over the rolling pin, brush off excess flour, and transfer to the prepared baking sheet. Spread the almond mixture over the pastry, leaving a 2-inch border all around. Toss berries with the remaining 3 tablespoons sugar (or Splenda) and 2 teaspoons lemon juice in a large bowl; spoon over the almond mixture. Fold the border up and over the filling, pleating as necessary. Blend the reserved egg white and 1 tablespoon water with a fork; brush lightly over the tart rim. Sprinkle with the remaining 1 teaspoon sugar.

5. Bake the tart for 15 minutes. Reduce oven temperature to 350°F and bake until the crust is golden and the juices are bubbling, 30 to 40 minutes. Leaving the tart on the parchment (or foil), carefully slide it onto a wire rack. Let cool.
6. Shortly before serving, melt jam in a small saucepan over low heat; brush over the berries. Cut the tart into wedges.

TIPS & NOTES
- **Make Ahead Tip**: Prepare crust through Step 1; wrap in plastic wrap and refrigerate for up to 2 days or freeze for up to 3 months.
- **Ingredient Note:** Whole-wheat pastry flour is milled from soft wheat. It contains less gluten than regular whole-wheat flour and helps ensure a tender result in delicate baked goods while providing the nutritional benefits of whole grains. Available in large supermarkets and in natural-foods stores. Store in the freezer.
- **Tip:** To separate eggs safely: Use an egg separator, an inexpensive gadget found in cookware stores; separating eggs by passing the yolk back and forth between pieces of eggshell or your hands can expose the eggs to bacteria.

NUTRITION

Per serving: 200 calories; 7 g fat (3 g sat, 2 g mono); 28 mg cholesterol; 31 g carbohydrates; 3 g protein; 4 g fiber; 55 mg sodium; 89 mg potassium.
Nutrition Bonus: Fiber (16% daily value), Vitamin C (15% dv).
Carbohydrate Servings: 2
Exchanges: 2 other carbohydrate, 1 fat

Dried Fruit Compote

INGREDIENTS
- 2 cups water
- 1/2 cup sugar
- 1/2 teaspoon ground cinnamon
- 1/4 teaspoon ground cloves
- 1/4 teaspoon salt
- 4 ounces dried apricots, (3/4 cup)
- 4 ounces pitted prunes, (3/4 cup)
- 4 ounces dried pear halves, cut in half (3/4 cup)

PREPARATION
1. Stir water, sugar, cinnamon, cloves and salt in a large saucepan over medium-high heat until the sugar dissolves. Add apricots, prunes and pears and bring to a simmer. Cover, reduce heat and simmer slowly for 30 minutes.

2. Uncover and continue simmering slowly until thickened, about 10 minutes. Let cool completely before serving. Serve at room temperature or chilled.

TIPS & NOTES
- **Make Ahead Tip**: Store, covered, in a plastic or glass container in the refrigerator for up to 5 days.

NUTRITION
Per serving: 214 calories; 0 g fat (0 g sat, 0 g mono); 0 mg cholesterol; 54 g carbohydrates; 1 g protein; 4 gfiber; 102 mg sodium; 486 mg potassium.
Nutrition Bonus: Vitamin A (20% daily value), Fiber (16% dv).
Carbohydrate Servings: 3 1/2
Exchanges: 2 1/2 fruit, 1 other carbohydrate

DAY 9
BREAKFAST
Nonfat plain yogurt (8 oz.)
Whole-wheat toast (1 slice)
Pear Butter
LUNCH
Creamy Tomato Bisque with Mozzarella Crostini
Tuna & White Bean Salad
Skim milk (1 cup)
Whole-wheat pita bread (1 medium pita)
SNACK
Pumpkin Popovers or Avocado Tea Sandwiches
Blueberries (1 cup)
DINNER
Korean-Style Steak & Lettuce Wraps
Shredded carrots (1 cup)
Broccoli with Black Bean-Garlic Sauce
Brown Rice (1 cup)
Strawberry Bruschetta or Cookie Cups with Lemon Thyme-Scented Berry Compote

DAY 9 RECIPES

Pear Butter

INGREDIENTS
- 4 ripe but firm Bartlett pears, (1-1 1/4 pounds), peeled, cored and cut into 1-inch chunks
- 3/4 cup pear nectar

PREPARATION

1. Place pears and pear nectar in a heavy medium saucepan; bring to a simmer. Cover and simmer over medium-low heat, stirring occasionally, until the pears are very tender, 30 to 35 minutes. Cooking time will vary depending on the ripeness of the pears.
2. Mash the pears with a potato masher. Cook, uncovered, over medium-low heat, stirring often, until the puree has cooked down to a thick mass (somewhat thicker than applesauce), 20 to 30 minutes. Stir almost constantly toward the end of cooking. Scrape the pear butter into a bowl or storage container and let cool.

TIPS & NOTES
- **Make Ahead Tip**: Store in an airtight container in the refrigerator for up to 2 weeks or freeze for up to 6 months.

NUTRITION
Per tablespoon: 22 calories; 0 g fat (0 g sat, 0 g mono); 0 mg cholesterol; 6 g carbohydrates; 0 g protein; 1 g fiber; 1 mg sodium; 33 mg potassium.
Carbohydrate Servings: 1/2
Exchanges: 1/2 fruit

Creamy Tomato Bisque with Mozzarella Crostini

INGREDIENTS
- 2 tablespoons extra-virgin olive oil
- 1 large onion, chopped
- 4 cloves garlic, crushed and peeled
- 1 14-ounce can reduced-sodium chicken broth
- 2 cups water and 1/4 cup white rice
- 1 28-ounce can crushed tomatoes
- 1/2 cup silken tofu
- 1 tablespoon rice vinegar
- 6 3/4-inch-thick slices baguette, preferably whole-grain
- 3 tablespoons shredded part-skim mozzarella cheese

PREPARATION
1. Heat oil in a Dutch oven over medium heat. Add onion and garlic and cook, stirring occasionally, until beginning to soften, about 3 minutes. Stir in broth, water and rice; bring to a boil. Reduce heat to a simmer and cook, stirring occasionally, until the rice is very tender, about 15 minutes.
2. Preheat oven to 450°F.
3. Stir tomatoes, tofu and vinegar into the soup. Remove from the heat and puree, in batches, in a blender. (Use caution when pureeing hot liquids.) Return the soup to the pot and reheat over medium-high heat, stirring often.
4. Meanwhile, top slices of baguette with mozzarella and place on a baking sheet. Bake until the cheese is melted and bubbly, about 5 minutes. Ladle soup into bowls and top each serving with a cheesy crostini.

TIPS & NOTES
- **Make Ahead Tip**: Prepare the soup (Steps 1 & 3), cover and refrigerate for up to 2 days. When ready to serve, make crostini and reheat the soup (Steps 2 & 4).

NUTRITION
Per serving: 218 calories; 8 g fat (1 g sat, 4 g mono); 3 mg cholesterol; 31 g carbohydrates; 8 g protein; 4 gfiber; 355 mg sodium; 478 mg potassium.
Nutrition Bonus: Vitamin C (25% daily value), Vitamin A (20% dv), Iron (15% dv).
Carbohydrate Servings: 2
Exchanges: 1 starch, 1 vegetable, 1 medium-fat meat

Tuna & White Bean Salad

INGREDIENTS
- 3 tablespoons lemon juice
- 2 tablespoons extra-virgin olive oil
- 1 clove garlic, minced
- 1/8 teaspoon salt
- Freshly ground pepper, to taste
- 1 19-ounce can cannellini (white kidney) beans, rinsed
- 1 6-ounce can chunk light tuna in water, drained and flaked (see Note)
- 1/4 cup chopped red onion
- 3 tablespoons chopped fresh parsley
- 3 tablespoons chopped fresh basil

PREPARATION
1. Whisk lemon juice, oil, garlic, salt and pepper in a medium bowl. Add beans, tuna, onion, parsley and basil; toss to coat well.

TIPS & NOTES
- **Make Ahead Tip**: Cover and refrigerate for up to 2 days.
- **Note:** Chunk light tuna, which comes from the smaller skipjack or yellowfin, has less mercury than canned white albacore tuna. The FDA/EPA advises that women who are or might become pregnant, nursing mothers and young children consume no more than 6 ounces of albacore a week; up to 12 ounces of canned light tuna is considered safe.

NUTRITION
Per serving: 226 calories; 8 g fat (1 g sat, 5 g mono); 13 mg cholesterol; 21 g carbohydrates; 0 g added sugars; 16 g protein; 6 g fiber; 498 mg sodium; 157 mg potassium.
Nutrition Bonus: Fiber (24% daily value), Iron (16% dv), Vitamin C (15% dv).
Carbohydrate Servings: 1
Exchanges: 1 starch, 2 very lean meat, 1 fat (mono)

Pumpkin Popovers

INGREDIENTS
- 1/4 cup canned pumpkin puree
- 3 large eggs
- 3 large egg whites
- 2 cups nonfat milk
- 2 tablespoons canola oil
- 2 cups all-purpose flour
- 1/2 teaspoon salt
- 1/4 teaspoon pumpkin-pie spice
- 1/8 teaspoon cayenne

PREPARATION
1. Preheat the oven to 400°F. Place a 12-cup muffin pan on a baking sheet in the oven to preheat.
2. Whisk together pumpkin puree, eggs, egg whites, milk and oil in a medium bowl until smooth. 3. Combine flour, salt, pie spice and cayenne in a large bowl. Add the pumpkin mixture to the dry ingredients and whisk until smooth.
3. Remove the muffin pan from the oven and coat it with cooking spray. Divide the batter among the prepared cups. Bake the popovers until they are puffed and browned, about 25 minutes. Remove the popovers from the oven and reduce the oven temperature to 350°. With a small knife cut small slits into the sides of the popovers, about 3 or 4 per popover. Bake an additional 7 to 10 minutes. Serve hot.

TIPS & NOTES
- **Make Ahead Tip**: Prepare up to 8 hours in advance. Reheat at 325° for 7 minutes.

NUTRITION
Per serving: 134 calories; 4 g fat (1 g sat, 1 g mono); 54 mg cholesterol; 19 g carbohydrates; 6 g protein; 1 g fiber; 146 mg sodium; 128 mg potassium.
Nutrition Bonus: Selenium (20% daily value), Vitamin A (19% dv), Folate (17% dv).
Carbohydrate Servings: 1
Exchanges: 1 starch, 1 fat

Avocado Tea Sandwiches

INGREDIENTS
- 1 avocado, ripe, sliced
- 1 tablespoon reduced-fat mayonnaise
- 1/2 teaspoon lemon juice
- 1/8 teaspoon cracked black pepper
- 8 very thin slices wheat bread
- 2 ounces thinly sliced smoked salmon
- 12 thin slices European cucumber

PREPARATION
1. Combine mayonnaise, lemon juice and pepper in a small bowl. Thinly spread on bread and top with salmon, avocado and cucumber.

NUTRITION

Per serving: 143 calories; 6 g fat (4 g sat, 3 g mono); 3 mg cholesterol; 17 g carbohydrates; 6 g protein; 4 gfiber; 303 mg sodium; 129 mg potassium.
Nutrition Bonus: Protein, fiber, vitamin C.
Carbohydrate Servings: 1
Exchanges: 1 starch, 1/2 very lean meat, 1 fat

Korean-Style Steak & Lettuce Wraps

INGREDIENTS
- 1 pound flank steak
- 1/4 teaspoon salt
- 1/4 teaspoon freshly ground pepper
- 1 cup diced peeled cucumber
- 6 cherry tomatoes, halved
- 1/4 cup thinly sliced shallot

- 1 tablespoon finely chopped fresh mint
- 1 tablespoon finely chopped fresh basil
- 1 tablespoon finely chopped fresh cilantro
- 1 tablespoon brown sugar
- 2 tablespoons reduced-sodium soy sauce
- 2 tablespoons lime juice
- 1/2 teaspoon crushed red pepper
- 1 head Bibb lettuce, leaves separated

PREPARATION
1. Preheat grill to medium-high.
2. Sprinkle steak with salt and pepper. Oil the grill rack (see Tip). Grill the steak for 6 to 8 minutes per side for medium. Transfer to a cutting board and let rest for 5 minutes. Cut across the grain into thin slices.
3. Combine the sliced steak, cucumber, tomatoes, shallot, mint, basil and cilantro in a large bowl. Mix sugar, soy sauce, lime juice and crushed red pepper in a small bowl. Drizzle over the steak mixture; toss well to coat. To serve, spoon a portion of the steak mixture into a lettuce leaf and roll into a "wrap."

TIPS & NOTES

- **Make Ahead Tip**: The steak mixture will keep, covered, in the refrigerator for up to 1 day.
- **To oil a grill rack:** Oil a folded paper towel, hold it with tongs and rub it over the rack. Do not use cooking spray on a hot grill.

NUTRITION

Per serving: 199 calories; 7 g fat (3 g sat, 3 g mono); 45 mg cholesterol; 9 g carbohydrates; 3 g added sugars; 24 g protein; 1 g fiber; 465 mg sodium; 542 mg potassium.
Nutrition Bonus: Vitamin A (35% daily value), Vitamin C (20% dv), Iron (15% dv).
Carbohydrate Servings: 1/2
Exchanges: 1 1/2 vegetable, 3 lean meat

Broccoli with Black Bean-Garlic Sauce
INGREDIENTS
- 1 teaspoon sesame seeds
- 1/2 cup water, divided
- 1 teaspoon rice-wine vinegar, or white-wine vinegar
- 1 teaspoon cornstarch

- 2 teaspoons black bean-garlic sauce, (see Ingredient note)
- 2 teaspoons canola oil
- 1 clove garlic, minced
- 4 cups broccoli florets

PREPARATION
1. Toast sesame seeds in a small dry skillet over medium-low heat, stirring constantly, until lightly browned and fragrant, 2 to 3 minutes. Transfer to a bowl to cool.
2. Mix 1/4 cup water, vinegar and cornstarch in a small bowl. Add black bean sauce and stir until smooth.
3. Heat oil in a large nonstick skillet or stir-fry pan over medium-high heat. Add garlic and stir-fry until fragrant, about 30 seconds. Add broccoli and stir to coat. Add the remaining 1/4 cup water; cover and steam just until the broccoli is tender-crisp, 1 to 3 minutes. Push broccoli to the sides and pour the sauce mixture in the center. Stir until the sauce begins to thicken, about 1 minute. Stir in the broccoli to coat. Serve immediately, sprinkled with the sesame seeds.

TIPS & NOTES
- **Ingredient Note:** Black bean-garlic sauce, made from pureed salted and fermented black soybeans, is a widely used condiment in Chinese cooking and can be found with the Asian food in most supermarkets.

NUTRITION
Per serving: 53 calories; 3 g fat (0 g sat, 2 g mono); 0 mg cholesterol; 6 g carbohydrates; 0 g added sugars; 2 g protein; 2 g fiber; 133 mg sodium; 247 mg potassium.
Nutrition Bonus: Vitamin C (110% daily value), Vitamin A (45% dv), Folate (13% dv).
Carbohydrate Servings: 1/2
Exchanges: 1 vegetable, 1/2 fat (mono)

Strawberry Bruschetta

INGREDIENTS
- 4 thick slices whole-wheat bread
- 6 tablespoons light brown sugar
- 1 teaspoon grated lemon zest
- 2 teaspoons lemon juice
- 3 cups sliced or diced hulled strawberries
- 4 tablespoons mascarpone, (Italian cream cheese)

PREPARATION
1. Toast bread in a toaster.
2. Meanwhile, heat a large skillet over high heat. Add sugar, lemon zest and lemon juice and cook, stirring, until the sugar melts and the mixture begins to bubble, 30 seconds to 1 minute. Add strawberries and stir until juices begin to exude and the berries are heated through, 30 seconds to 1 minute more.
3. Spread 1 tablespoon mascarpone on each piece of toast. Top with the warm berries.

TIPS & NOTES

- **Make Ahead Tip**: Prepare the sauce (Step 2), cover and refrigerate for up to 2 days or freeze for up to 1 month. To reheat, microwave on High for about 1 minute (defrost first, if necessary).

NUTRITION
Per serving: 203 calories; 5 g fat (2 g sat, 1 g mono); 9 mg cholesterol; 40 g carbohydrates; 4 g protein; 4 gfiber; 152 mg sodium; 240 mg potassium.
Nutrition Bonus: Vitamin C (108% daily value), Selenium (16% dv).
Carbohydrate Servings: 2 1/2
Exchanges: 1 starch, 1 1/2 fruit, 1 fat (sat)

Cookie Cups with Lemon Thyme-Scented Berry Compote
INGREDIENTS

Cookie cups with lemon thyme-scented berry compote
- 6 tablespoons all-purpose flour
- 1/2 teaspoon ground cinnamon
- Pinch of salt
- 2 large egg whites
- 1/3 cup sugar
- 1 tablespoon butter, melted
- 1 tablespoon canola oil
- 1/4 teaspoon vanilla extract

Compote
- 4 teaspoons fresh lemon thyme leaves
- 3 cups mixed fresh berries, (raspberries, blueberries, blackberries)
- 2 tablespoons creme de cassis, or black currant syrup
- 1 tablespoon fresh lemon juice
- 1 tablespoon sugar

- 1 1/2 cups reduced-fat vanilla ice cream, lemon sorbet or raspberry sorbet, slightly softened before serving
- Lemon thyme sprigs for garnish

PREPARATION
1. Preheat oven to 325°F. Line 2 baking sheets with parchment paper. Coat parchment with cooking spray.
2. To prepare cookie cups: Whisk flour, cinnamon and salt in a small bowl. Whisk egg whites, sugar, butter, oil and vanilla in a medium bowl until smooth. Add dry ingredients and whisk until blended.
3. For each cookie cup, spoon 1 1/2 tablespoons batter onto a prepared baking sheet, allowing 2 cookies per baking sheet. With an offset metal spatula, spread each mound of batter into a 5 1/2- to 6-inch circle.
4. Bake cookies, one sheet at a time, until golden brown around the edges, 8 to 12 minutes. Have ready two 12-ounce custard cups (or similar bowls with a 3-inch base). As soon as the cookies are done, loosen from parchment with a wide metal spatula, then set inside the cups. Gently press each cookie into the bottom of the cup and pleat the sides to form a tulip shape. (If cookies become too brittle to shape, return them to the oven for a minute or two to soften.)
5. To prepare compote: Place lemon thyme in a mortar or small bowl; bruise with a pestle or wooden spoon to release its fragrance. Transfer to a medium bowl. Add 1/4 cup berries and mash with a fork. Add creme de cassis (or black currant syrup), lemon juice and sugar, stirring until sugar has dissolved. Add remaining berries and stir gently to coat with sauce.
6. To assemble desserts: Place cookie cups on individual plates. Fill each with a scoop of ice cream (or sorbet), spoon on compote and garnish with lemon thyme sprigs.

TIPS & NOTES
- **Make Ahead Tip**: The cookies will keep in an airtight container for up to 4 days. If cookies soften, crisp in a 325°F oven for about 5 minutes.
- The cookies are pliable only while hot, so work quickly. Have a wide metal spatula and two 12-ounce custard cups (or similar bowls) ready before baking.

NUTRITION
Per serving: 217 calories; 6 g fat (2 g sat, 2 g mono); 14 mg cholesterol; 38 g carbohydrates; 4 g protein; 4 g fiber; 68 mg sodium; 192 mg potassium.
Carbohydrate Servings: 2 1/2
Exchanges: 1 1/2 starch, 1 fruit, 1 fat

DAY 10
BREAKFAST

Eggs Baked Over a Spicy Vegetable Ragout
Honey Oat Quick Bread
Skim milk (1 cup)

LUNCH

Asian Chicken Salad or Smoked Salmon Salad Niçoise
Roasted Tomato Soup
Skim milk (1 cup)
Whole-wheat toast (1 slice)
Strawberries (1 cup)

SNACK

White Bean Spread
Wasa crispbread (1 cracker)

DINNER

Grilled Lamb with Fresh Mint Chutney or Raspberry-Balsamic Chicken with Shallots
Green Beans with Poppy Seed Dressing
Whole-wheat couscous (1 cup, cooked)
Orange Slices with Warm Raspberries

DAY 10 RECIPES

Eggs Baked Over a Spicy Vegetable Ragout

INGREDIENTS

- 3 teaspoons extra-virgin olive oil, divided
- 1 small eggplant, cut into 1/2-inch cubes
- 1 medium onion, chopped
- 1 large red bell pepper, diced
- 6 cloves garlic, minced
- 2 teaspoons ground cumin
- 1/8-1/4 teaspoon hot sauce, such as Hot pepper
- 1 medium summer squash, halved lengthwise and thinly sliced
- 1 14-ounce can diced tomatoes
- 1/4 cup water
- 3 tablespoons chopped fresh parsley, divided
- 1/8 teaspoon salt
- Freshly ground pepper to taste
- 4 large large eggs

PREPARATION
1. Preheat oven to 400°F. Coat a shallow 2-quart baking dish with cooking spray.
2. Heat 2 teaspoons oil in a large nonstick skillet over medium-high heat. Add eggplant and cook, stirring frequently, until browned and softened, 5 to 7 minutes. Transfer to a plate.
3. Heat the remaining 1 teaspoon oil in a Dutch oven or large deep sauté pan over medium heat. Add onion and cook, stirring occasionally, until softened, 3 to 5 minutes. Add bell pepper and cook, stirring occasionally, until softened, 3 to 5 minutes. Add garlic, cumin and hot sauce and cook until fragrant, 15 to 30 seconds. Stir in squash, tomatoes, water and the eggplant. Cover and simmer for 10 minutes. Stir in 2 tablespoons parsley, salt and pepper.
4. Spread the vegetable ragout in the prepared baking dish. Make 4 shallow wells in the ragout and gently crack 1 egg into each well, being careful not to break yolks.
5. Bake, uncovered, until the eggs are barely set, 10 to 12 minutes. (Caution: Eggs can overcook very quickly. Check them often and remove from the oven when they still look a little underdone; they will continue to cook in the hot ragout. If the baking dish is ceramic, the cooking time will be closer to 12 minutes. A glass dish will cook eggs much faster.) Sprinkle with the remaining 1 tablespoon parsley. Serve immediately.

TIPS & NOTES
- **Make Ahead Tip**: Prepare through Step 3, cover and refrigerate for up to 2 days. Reheat before continuing.

NUTRITION
Per serving: 201 calories; 9 g fat (2 g sat, 5 g mono); 212 mg cholesterol; 23 g carbohydrates; 0 g added sugars; 10 g protein; 6 g fiber; 282 mg sodium; 471 mg potassium.
Nutrition Bonus: Vitamin C (170% daily value), Vitamin A (45% dv), Fiber (24% dv), Folate (17% dv), Iron (15% dv).
Carbohydrate Servings: 1
Exchanges: 4 vegetable; 1 medium-fat meat; 1/2 fat (mono)

Honey Oat Quick Bread

INGREDIENTS
- 2 tablespoons plus 1 cup old-fashioned rolled oats, or quick-cooking (not instant) oats, divided
- 1 1/3 cups whole-wheat flour, or white whole-wheat flour (see Tip)
- 1 cup all-purpose flour
- 2 1/4 teaspoons baking powder

- 1/4 teaspoon baking soda
- 1 1/4 teaspoons salt
- 8 ounces (scant 1 cup) nonfat or low-fat plain yogurt
- 1 large egg
- 1/4 cup canola oil
- 1/4 cup clover honey, or other mild honey
- 3/4 cup nonfat or low-fat milk

PREPARATION
1. Position rack in middle of oven; preheat to 375°F. Generously coat a 9-by-5-inch (or similar size) loaf pan with cooking spray. Sprinkle 1 tablespoon oats in the pan. Tip the pan back and forth to coat the sides and bottom with oats.
2. Thoroughly stir together whole-wheat flour, all-purpose flour, baking powder, baking soda and salt in a large bowl. Using a fork, beat the remaining 1 cup oats, yogurt, egg, oil and honey in a medium bowl until well blended. Stir in milk. Gently stir the yogurt mixture into the flour mixture just until thoroughly incorporated but not overmixed (excess mixing can cause toughening). Immediately scrape the batter into the pan, spreading evenly to the edges. Sprinkle the remaining 1 tablespoon oats over the top.
3. Bake the loaf until well browned on top and a toothpick inserted in the center comes out clean, 40 to 50 minutes. (It's normal for the top to crack.) Let stand in the pan on a wire rack for 15 minutes. Run a table knife around and under the loaf to loosen it and turn it out onto the rack. Let cool until barely warm, about 45 minutes.

TIPS & NOTES
- **Make Ahead Tip**: Store cooled bread, tightly wrapped, for up to 1 day at room temperature. If desired, warm (wrapped in foil) at 375°F before serving.
- **Tip:** White whole-wheat flour, made from a special variety of white wheat, is light in color and flavor but has the same nutritional properties as regular whole-wheat flour. Two companies that distribute the flour nationally are King Arthur Flour (kingarthurflour.com) and Bob's Red Mill (bobsredmill.com).

NUTRITION
Per slice: 193 calories; 6 g fat (1 g sat, 3 g mono); 18 mg cholesterol; 31 g carbohydrates; 6 g protein; 3 gfiber; 396 mg sodium; 100 mg potassium.
Nutrition Bonus: Iron (15% daily value).
Carbohydrate Servings: 2
Exchanges: 2 starch, 1 fat

Asian Chicken Salad

INGREDIENTS

DRESSING

- 1/4 cup reduced-sodium soy sauce
- 3 tablespoons rice-wine vinegar
- 1 1/2 tablespoons brown sugar and 1 1/2 teaspoons sesame oil
- 1 1/2 teaspoons chile-garlic sauce, (see Ingredient notes)
- 3 tablespoons canola oil
- 1 tablespoon minced fresh ginger and 2 cloves garlic, minced
- 1 tablespoon tahini paste
- 3/4 cup reduced-sodium chicken broth, or reserved chicken-poaching liquid

SALAD

- 2 tablespoons sesame seeds
- 8 cups shredded napa cabbage, (1 small head; see Ingredient notes)
- 1 1/2 cups grated carrots, (2-3 medium)
- 5 radishes, sliced (about 1 cup)
- 1/2 cup chopped scallions
- 3 1/2 cups shredded skinless cooked chicken, (about 1 1/2 pounds boneless, skinless chicken breast) (see Tip)

PREPARATION

1. To prepare dressing: Combine soy sauce, vinegar, brown sugar, sesame oil and chile-garlic sauce in a glass measuring cup; stir to blend. Heat canola oil in a small saucepan over medium-high heat. Add ginger and garlic; cook, stirring, until fragrant, 1 to 2 minutes. Add the soy sauce mixture to the pan; bring to a simmer. Whisk in tahini and broth (or poaching liquid); cook until reduced slightly, 3 to 4 minutes. Let cool.
2. To prepare salad: Heat a small dry skillet over medium-low heat. Add sesame seeds and cook, stirring, until lightly browned and fragrant, 1 to 2 minutes. Transfer to a small plate to cool.
3. Combine cabbage, carrots, radishes, scallions and chicken in a large shallow bowl. Stir dressing to recombine and drizzle over the salad; toss to coat. Sprinkle the sesame seeds on top.

TIPS & NOTES

- **Make Ahead Tip**: Cover and refrigerate the dressing (Step 1) for up to 2 days.
- **Ingredient Notes:** Chile-garlic sauce is a spicy blend of chiles, garlic and other seasonings; it is found in the Asian section of the market.
- Napa cabbage has an elongated head and is pale green in color with tender, tapered white ribs. Its tightly packed, crinkled leaves have a crisp texture. Discard the cone-shaped core. One small head yields about 8 cups shredded.

- **Tip:** To poach chicken: Combine two 14-ounce cans reduced-sodium chicken broth, 2 chopped scallions, 2 slivers fresh ginger and 2 cloves garlic in a large skillet; bring to a simmer. Add 11/2 pounds boneless, skinless chicken breast and cook over medium heat until no longer pink inside, 10 to 15 minutes. The flavorful poaching liquid will keep, tightly covered, in the refrigerator for up to 2 days or in the freezer for up to 6 months.

NUTRITION
Per serving: 289 calories; 14 g fat (2 g sat, 7 g mono); 64 mg cholesterol; 14 g carbohydrates; 3 g added sugars; 28 g protein; 3 g fiber; 518 mg sodium; 355 mg potassium.
Nutrition Bonus: Vitamin A (100% daily value), Vitamin C (60% dv).
Carbohydrate Servings: 1
Exchanges: 1 1/2 vegetable, 3 lean meat, 2 fat

Smoked Salmon Salad Niçoise

INGREDIENTS
- 8 ounces small red potatoes, scrubbed and halved
- 6 ounces green beans, preferably thin haricots verts, trimmed and halved
- 2 tablespoons reduced-fat mayonnaise
- 1 tablespoon white-wine vinegar
- 1 teaspoon lemon juice
- 1 teaspoon Worcestershire sauce
- 1 teaspoon Dijon mustard
- 1/2 teaspoon dried dill
- 1/4 teaspoon freshly ground pepper
- 6 cups mixed salad greens
- 1/2 small cucumber, halved, seeded and thinly sliced
- 12 small cherry or grape tomatoes, halved
- 4 ounces smoked salmon, cut into 2-inch pieces

PREPARATION
1. Place a large bowl of ice water next to the stove. Bring 1 inch of water to a boil in a large saucepan. Place potatoes in a steamer basket over the boiling water, cover and steam until tender when pierced with a fork, 10 to 15 minutes. Transfer the potatoes with a slotted spoon to the ice water. Add green beans to the steamer, cover and steam until tender-crisp, 4 to 5 minutes. Transfer the green beans with a slotted spoon to the ice water. Transfer the potatoes and beans to a towel-lined baking sheet to drain.
2. Meanwhile, whisk mayonnaise, vinegar, lemon juice, Worcestershire sauce, mustard, dill and pepper in a large bowl. Add the potatoes and green beans, salad greens, cucumber and tomatoes; toss gently to coat.

3. Divide the salad and smoked salmon between 2 plates.

TIPS & NOTES
- **Make Ahead Tip**: Store the potatoes and beans (Step 1) in an airtight container in the refrigerator for up to 2 days.

NUTRITION
Per serving: 291 calories; 7 g fat (1 g sat, 2 g mono); 17 mg cholesterol; 40 g carbohydrates; 19 g protein; 9 g fiber; 651 mg sodium; 1092 mg potassium.
Nutrition Bonus: Vitamin A & Vitamin C (120% daily value), Potassium (31% dv), Iron (25% dv), Calcium (15% dv), high omega-3s.
Carbohydrate Servings: 2 1/2
Exchanges: 1 starch, 3 vegetable, 1 1/2 lean meat

Roasted Tomato Soup

INGREDIENTS
- 1 1/2 pounds large tomatoes, such as beefsteak, cut in half crosswise
- 1 medium sweet onion, such as Vidalia, peeled and cut in half crosswise
- 3 large cloves garlic, unpeeled
- 1 tablespoon plus 1 teaspoon extra-virgin olive oil, divided
- 1/4 teaspoon salt, or to taste
- Freshly ground pepper, to taste
- 2 cups reduced-sodium chicken broth, or vegetable broth, divided
- 1/4 cup tomato juice
- 1 teaspoon tomato paste
- 1/4 teaspoon Worcestershire sauce
- 1 tablespoon fresh basil, chopped
- Brown sugar, to taste (optional)
- 1/2 cup corn kernels, (fresh, from 1 ear, see Tip) or frozen, thawed

PREPARATION

1. Preheat oven to 400°F. Coat a baking sheet with cooking spray.
2. Toss tomatoes, onion and garlic in a mixing bowl with 1 tablespoon oil. Season with salt and pepper. Spread on the prepared baking sheet and roast until the vegetables are soft and caramelized, about 30 minutes. Let cool.
3. Peel and seed the tomatoes. Trim off the onion ends. Peel the garlic. Place the vegetables in a food processor or blender with 1 cup broth and the remaining 1 teaspoon oil. Pulse to desired thickness and texture.
4. Transfer the vegetable puree to a large heavy pot or Dutch oven. Add the remaining 1 cup broth, tomato juice, tomato pate, Worcestershire sauce, basil

and brown sugar (if using). Bring to a simmer over medium heat, stirring often. Ladle into 6 soup bowls, garnish with corn and serve.

TIPS & NOTES
- **Make Ahead Tip**: Cover and refrigerate for up to 2 days or freeze for up to 2 months.
- **Tip:** Removing Corn from the Cob: Stand an uncooked ear of corn on its stem end in a shallow bowl and slice the kernels off with a sharp, thin-bladed knife. This technique produces whole kernels that are good for adding to salads and salsas. If you want to use the corn kernels for soups, fritters or puddings, you can add another step to the process. After cutting the kernels off, reverse the knife and, using the dull side, press it down the length of the ear to push out the rest of the corn and its milk.

NUTRITION
Per serving: 95 calories; 4 g fat (1 g sat, 2 g mono); 1 mg cholesterol; 15 g carbohydrates; 0 g added sugars; 3 g protein; 3 g fiber; 340 mg sodium; 406 mg potassium.
Nutrition Bonus: Vitamin C (35% daily value), Vitamin A (20% dv).
Carbohydrate Servings: 1
Exchanges: 2 vegetable, 1 fat

White Bean Spread

INGREDIENTS
- 2 15-ounce cans cannellini beans, (white kidney beans), rinsed
- 1/4 cup extra-virgin olive oil
- 2 tablespoons lemon juice
- Pinch of cayenne pepper
- 1/8 teaspoon salt
- Freshly ground pepper, to taste
- 1/4 cup chopped scallions
- 2 tablespoons chopped fresh dill

PREPARATION
1. Combine beans, oil, lemon juice, cayenne, salt and black pepper in a food processor; process until smooth. Scrape into a bowl; stir in scallions and dill.

TIPS & NOTES
- **Make Ahead Tip:** Cover and refrigerate for up to 4 days.

NUTRITION
Per tablespoon: 25 calories; 1 g fat (0 g sat, 1 g mono); 0 mg cholesterol; 3 g carbohydrates; 0 g added sugars; 1 g protein; 1 g fiber; 44 mg sodium; 2 mg potassium.
Exchanges: free food

Grilled Lamb with Fresh Mint Chutney

INGREDIENTS
- Fresh Mint Chutney, (recipe follows)
- 8 rib lamb chops, (about 3 ounces each), trimmed
- 1 clove garlic, cut in half
- 1 teaspoon extra-virgin olive oil, or canola oil
- 1/4 teaspoon kosher salt
- Freshly ground pepper, to taste

PREPARATION
1. Prepare Fresh Mint Chutney.
2. Heat gas grill. Rub lamb chops with garlic, then brush with oil and season with salt and pepper. Grill the chops until cooked to desired doneness, 4 to 5 minutes per side for medium-rare. Serve with Fresh Mint Chutney.

NUTRITION
Per serving: 296 calories; 13 g fat (4 g sat, 6 g mono); 112 mg cholesterol; 6 g carbohydrates; 36 g protein; 1 g fiber; 653 mg sodium; 486 mg potassium.
Nutrition Bonus: Selenium (57% daily value), Vitamin C (50% dv), Zinc (36% dv).
Carbohydrate Servings: 1/2
Exchanges: 1 vegetable, 5 lean meat

Raspberry-Balsamic Chicken with Shallots

INGREDIENTS
- 3/4 cup seedless all-fruit raspberry jam
- 1/4 cup balsamic vinegar
- 1/2 teaspoon salt
- 1/4 teaspoon freshly ground pepper
- 4 4- to 5-ounce boneless, skinless chicken breasts, tenders removed (see Tip)
- 2 1/2 teaspoons extra-virgin olive oil
- 1/2 cup chopped shallots, (2-3 large)
- 1 1/2 teaspoons minced fresh thyme

PREPARATION
1. Combine jam and vinegar in a small pan over medium-low heat. Cook, stirring often, until the jam is dissolved, 3 to 4 minutes. Remove from heat, stir in salt

and pepper and let cool slightly. Reserve 1/2 cup of the sauce. Place chicken breasts and the rest of the sauce in a large sealable plastic bag. Seal and shake gently to coat. Marinate in the refrigerator for 1 to 1 1/2 hours.
2. Heat oil in a large nonstick skillet over medium-high heat. Add shallots and thyme and cook, stirring often, until the shallots begin to soften, about 1 minute. Remove the chicken from the marinade (discard marinade). Add the chicken to the pan and cook until just beginning to brown, 2 minutes on each side. Add the reserved raspberry sauce; stir to melt the jam and coat the chicken. Reduce heat to low, cover and cook until the chicken is cooked through and no longer pink in the center, 6 to 10 minutes. Serve immediately.

TIPS & NOTES
- **Make Ahead Tip**: Cover and refrigerate the sauce for up to 1 week.
- **Tip:** Chicken tenders, virtually fat-free, are a strip of rib meat typically found attached to the underside of the chicken breast, but they can also be purchased separately. Four 1-ounce tenders will yield a 3-ounce cooked portion. Tenders are perfect for quick stir-fries, chicken satay or kid-friendly breaded "chicken fingers."
- Boneless, skinless chicken breasts, arguably the most versatile cut of chicken, are very low in fat, only 1 to 2 grams of fat per serving. Conveniently, one 4- to 5-ounce breast, tender removed, yields a perfect 3-ounce cooked portion. When preparing, trim any excess fat from the outer edge of the breast.

NUTRITION
Per serving: 296 calories; 4 g fat (1 g sat, 3 g mono); 66 mg cholesterol; 36 g carbohydrates; 0 g added sugars; 27 g protein; 0 g fiber; 371 mg sodium; 370 mg potassium.
Nutrition Bonus: Selenium (28% daily value).
Carbohydrate Servings: 2 1/2
Exchanges: 2 1/2 other carbohydrate, 4 very lean meat

Green Beans with Poppy Seed Dressing

INGREDIENTS
- 1 teaspoon poppy seeds
- 2 tablespoons extra-virgin olive oil
- 1 tablespoon white-wine vinegar, or rice-wine vinegar
- 1 teaspoon Dijon mustard
- 1/2 teaspoon honey
- 1 tablespoon minced shallot
- 1/8 teaspoon salt, or to taste
- Freshly ground pepper, to taste
- 1 pound green beans, stem ends trimmed

PREPARATION

1. To prepare dressing: Heat a small dry skillet over medium-low heat. Add poppy seeds and toast, stirring, until fragrant, about 1 minute. Transfer to a small bowl (or jar) and let cool. Add oil, vinegar, mustard, honey, shallot, salt and pepper; whisk (or shake) until blended.
2. To prepare beans: Cook beans in a large pot of boiling water until just tender, 5 to 7 minutes. Drain. Warm the dressing in a large skillet over medium heat. Add beans and toss to coat.

TIPS & NOTES

- **Make Ahead Tip**: Cover and refrigerate the dressing (step 1) for up to 2 days.

NUTRITION

Per serving: 113 calories; 8 g fat (1 g sat, 5 g mono); 0 mg cholesterol; 11 g carbohydrates; 1 g added sugars; 3 g protein; 4 g fiber; 104 mg sodium; 185 mg potassium.
Nutrition Bonus: Vitamin C (20% daily value), Fiber (15% dv), Vitamin A (15% dv).
Carbohydrate Servings: 1
Exchanges: 1 1/2 vegetable, 1 1/2 fat (mono)

Orange Slices with Warm Raspberries

INGREDIENTS

- 4 seedless oranges, such as navel oranges
- 2 tablespoons sugar, or Splenda Granular
- 1 tablespoon lemon juice
- 1/4 teaspoon ground cinnamon
- 2 cups frozen unsweetened raspberries, (not thawed)

PREPARATION

1. With a sharp knife, remove and discard the skin and white pith from oranges; slice the oranges crosswise and arrange on 4 dessert plates.
2. Combine sugar (or Splenda), lemon juice and cinnamon in a small saucepan; stir over low heat until bubbling. Add raspberries and stir gently until the berries are just thawed. Spoon over the orange slices and serve immediately.

NUTRITION

Per serving: 122 calories; 0 g fat (0 g sat, 0 g mono); 0 mg cholesterol; 30 g carbohydrates; 2 g protein; 5 gfiber; 2 mg sodium; 237 mg potassium.
Nutrition Bonus: Vitamin C (157% daily value), Fiber (20% dv).
Carbohydrate Servings: 1 1/2
Exchanges: 2 fruit

Nutrition Note: Per serving with Splenda: 1 Carbohydrate Serving; 100 calories; 25 g carbohydrate.

DAY 11
BREAKFAST
Spiced Apple Butter Bran Muffins
Skim milk (1 cup)
Grapefruit (1/2)
LUNCH
Honey-Mustard Turkey Burgers or Grilled Lobster Rolls
Broccoli Slaw
Fat-free cheese (1 slice)
Oatmeal Chocolate Chip Cookies
Skim milk (1 cup)
SNACK
Frosted Grapes
Almonds (1 oz.)
DINNER
Herbed Scallop Kebabs or Five-Spice Roasted Duck Breasts
Whole-Wheat Couscous with Parmesan & Peas
Steamed cauliflower (1 cup)
Sliced Fennel Salad
Almond Cream with Strawberries

DAY 11 RECIPES

Spiced Apple Butter Bran Muffins
INGREDIENTS
- 1/2 cup raisins
- 3/4 cup whole-wheat flour
- 3/4 cup all-purpose flour
- 2 1/2 teaspoons baking powder
- 1/4 teaspoon salt
- 1/2 teaspoon ground cinnamon
- 3/4 cup unprocessed wheat bran, or oat bran
- 1 large egg, lightly beaten
- 1/2 cup low-fat milk
- 1/2 cup spiced apple butter
- 1/2 cup packed light brown sugar, or 1/4 cup Splenda Sugar Blend for Baking
- 1/4 cup canola oil

- 3 tablespoons molasses
- 1 cup finely diced peeled apple

PREPARATION

1. Preheat oven to 375°F. Coat 12 standard 2 1/2-inch muffin cups with cooking spray. Place raisins in a small bowl and cover with hot water. Set aside.
2. Whisk whole-wheat flour, all-purpose flour, baking powder, salt and cinnamon in a large bowl. Stir in bran.
3. Whisk egg, milk, apple butter, brown sugar (or Splenda), oil and molasses in a large bowl until blended. Make a well in the dry ingredients and pour in the wet ingredients. Drain the raisins; add them and the diced apple to the bowl. Stir until just combined. Scoop the batter into the prepared pan (the cups will be very full).
4. Bake the muffins until the tops spring back when touched lightly, 18 to 22 minutes. Let cool in the pan for 5 minutes. Loosen the edges and turn the muffins out onto a wire rack to cool slightly before serving.

TIPS & NOTES

- Wrap leftover muffins individually in plastic wrap, place in a plastic storage container or ziplock bag and freeze for up to 1 month. To thaw, remove plastic wrap, wrap in a paper towel and microwave on Defrost for about 2 minutes.

NUTRITION
Per muffin: 197 calories; 6 g fat (1 g sat, 3 g mono); 18 mg cholesterol; 38 g carbohydrates; 4 g protein; 4 gfiber; 148 mg sodium; 221 mg potassium.
Nutrition Bonus: Fiber (16% daily value).
Carbohydrate Servings: 2
Exchanges: 2 starch, 1 fat
Nutrition Note: Per muffin with Splenda: 2 Carbohydrate Servings; 187 calories, 31 g carbohydrate

Honey-Mustard Turkey Burgers

INGREDIENTS
- 1/4 cup coarse-grained mustard
- 2 tablespoons honey
- 1 pound ground turkey breast and 1/4 teaspoon salt
- 1/4 teaspoon freshly ground pepper
- 2 teaspoons canola oil
- 4 whole-wheat hamburger rolls, split and toasted
- Lettuce, tomato slices and red onion slices, for garnish

PREPARATION
1. Prepare a grill.
2. Whisk mustard and honey in a small bowl until smooth.
3. Combine turkey, 3 tablespoons of the mustard mixture, salt and pepper in a bowl; mix well. Form into four 1-inch-thick burgers.
4. Lightly brush the burgers on both sides with oil. Grill until no pink remains in center, 5 to 7 minutes per side. Brush the burgers with the remaining mustard mixture. Serve on rolls with lettuce, tomato and onion slices.

NUTRITION

Per serving: 317 calories; 11 g fat (3 g sat, 2 g mono); 65 mg cholesterol; 31 g carbohydrates; 26 g protein;3 g fiber; 593 mg sodium; 387 mg potassium.
Nutrition Bonus: Folate (20% daily value), Iron (20% dv), Calcium (15% dv).
Carbohydrate Servings: 2
Exchanges: 2 starch, 4 lean meat

Grilled Lobster Rolls

INGREDIENTS
- 2 10- to 12-ounce lobster tails, thawed if frozen (see Tip)
- 2 teaspoons extra-virgin olive oil
- 4 whole-wheat hot-dog buns
- 1 cup snow peas, trimmed
- 1/4 cup minced celery
- 1/4 cup reduced-fat mayonnaise
- 1 tablespoon plus 2 teaspoons lemon juice
- 1 tablespoon minced shallot
- 2 teaspoons Dijon mustard
- 1 teaspoon chopped fresh tarragon
- 1/2 teaspoon freshly ground pepper
- 1/8 teaspoon salt, or more to taste
- 1/4 teaspoon garlic powder

PREPARATION
1. Preheat grill to medium-high.
2. Lay lobster tails on a cutting board with the soft side of the shell facing up. Cut the tails in half lengthwise through the shell using kitchen shears, starting from the fan (see Kitchen Notes). Run your fingertips along the inside of the shell to loosen the meat in the shell. Brush the meat with oil.
3. Lay the tails on the grill, cut-side down, and cook until the meat is lightly charred and the shell is beginning to turn red, 5 to 6 minutes. Turn and continue grilling

until the meat is opaque and cooked through and the shell is completely red, 2 to 4 minutes more. Transfer the lobster to a cutting board. Meanwhile, toast buns over indirect heat, 3 to 5 minutes.
4. While the lobster cools, bring a small pan of water to a boil. Cook snow peas until bright green, 1 minute. Drain, refresh under cold water and slice very thinly (almost shredded). When the lobster is cool enough to handle, remove the shell and coarsely chop the meat.
5. Mix celery, mayonnaise, lemon juice, shallot, mustard, tarragon, pepper, salt and garlic powder in a large bowl. Stir in the chopped lobster and snow peas. Divide the salad among the toasted buns.

TIPS & NOTES
- **Tip:** To defrost frozen lobster tails or crab legs, let thaw in the refrigerator overnight.
- **Kitchen Note:** How to Shell a Lobster:
- 1. Grasp claw at the knuckle, near the body. With a firm twist, remove the claw from the body. Repeat with the second claw.
- 2. To remove claw meat, crack through the claw shell using a pair of kitchen shears. (Alternatively, crack with a lobster cracker.)
- 3. Holding the body in one hand and firmly grasping the tail in the other, twist and gently pull the tail from the body. (Discard the body.)
- 4. Cut the tail in half lengthwise with kitchen shears, starting from the underside. Serve halves in the shell or remove the meat.

NUTRITION
Per serving: 310 calories; 8 g fat (1 g sat, 3 g mono); 86 mg cholesterol; 30 g carbohydrates; 30 g protein; 4 g fiber; 665 mg sodium; 386 mg potassium.
Nutrition Bonus: Zinc (53% daily value), Magnesium (23% dv), Vitamin C (20% dv), Iron (15% dv).
Carbohydrate Servings: 2
Exchanges: 2 starch, 3 very lean meat, 1 1/2 fat

Broccoli Slaw

INGREDIENTS
- 4 slices turkey bacon
- 1 12- to 16-ounce bag shredded broccoli slaw, or 1 large bunch broccoli (about 1 1/2 pounds)
- 1/4 cup low-fat or nonfat plain yogurt
- 1/4 cup reduced-fat mayonnaise
- 3 tablespoons cider vinegar
- 2 teaspoons sugar
- 1/2 teaspoon salt, or to taste

- Freshly ground pepper, to taste
- 1 8-ounce can low-sodium sliced water chestnuts, rinsed and coarsely chopped
- 1/2 cup finely diced red onion, (1/2 medium)

PREPARATION
1. Cook bacon in a large skillet over medium heat, turning frequently, until crisp, 5 to 8 minutes. (Alternatively, microwave on High for 2 1/2 to 3 minutes.) Drain bacon on paper towels. Chop coarsely.
2. If using whole broccoli, trim about 3 inches off the stems. Chop the rest into 1/4-inch pieces.
3. Whisk yogurt, mayonnaise, vinegar, sugar, salt and pepper in a large bowl. Add water chestnuts, onion, bacon and broccoli; toss to coat. Chill until serving time.

TIPS & NOTES
- **Make Ahead Tip**: Cover and chill for up to 2 days.

NUTRITION
Per serving: 80 calories; 3 g fat (1 g sat, 1 g mono); 5 mg cholesterol; 9 g carbohydrates; 1 g added sugars; 3 g protein; 3 g fiber; 271 mg sodium; 181 mg potassium.
Nutrition Bonus: Vitamin C (70% daily value).
Carbohydrate Servings: 1/2
Exchanges: 2 vegetable, 1 fat

Oatmeal Chocolate Chip Cookies

INGREDIENTS
- 2 cups rolled oats, (not quick-cooking)
- 1/2 cup whole-wheat pastry flour, (see Ingredient Note)
- 1/2 cup all-purpose flour
- 1 teaspoon ground cinnamon
- 1/2 teaspoon baking soda
- 1/2 teaspoon salt
- 1/2 cup tahini, (see Ingredient Note)
- 4 tablespoons cold unsalted butter, cut into pieces
- 2/3 cup granulated sugar
- 2/3 cup packed light brown sugar
- 1 large egg
- 1 large egg white
- 1 tablespoon vanilla extract
- 1 cup semisweet or bittersweet chocolate chips
- 1/2 cup chopped walnuts

PREPARATION
1. Position racks in upper and lower thirds of oven; preheat to 350°F. Line 2 baking sheets with parchment paper.
2. Whisk oats, whole-wheat flour, all-purpose flour, cinnamon, baking soda and salt in a medium bowl. Beat tahini and butter in a large bowl with an electric mixer until blended into a paste. Add granulated sugar and brown sugar; continue beating until well combined; the mixture will still be a little grainy. Beat in egg, then egg white, then vanilla. Stir in the oat mixture with a wooden spoon until just moistened. Stir in chocolate chips and walnuts.
3. With damp hands, roll 1 tablespoon of the batter into a ball, place it on a prepared baking sheet and flatten it until squat, but don't let the sides crack. Continue with the remaining batter, spacing the flattened balls 2 inches apart.
4. Bake the cookies until golden brown, about 16 minutes, switching the pans back to front and top to bottom halfway through. Cool on the pans for 2 minutes, then transfer the cookies to a wire rack to cool completely. Let the pans cool for a few minutes before baking another batch.

TIPS & NOTES

- **Make Ahead Tip**: Store in an airtight container for up to 2 days or freeze for longer storage.
- **Ingredient notes:** Whole-wheat pastry flour, lower in protein than regular whole-wheat flour, has less gluten-forming potential, making it a better choice for tender baked goods. You can find it in the natural-foods section of large super markets and natural-foods stores. Store in the freezer.
- Tahini is a paste made from ground sesame seeds. Look for it in natural-foods stores and some supermarkets.

NUTRITION
Per cookie: 102 calories; 5 g fat (2 g sat, 1 g mono); 7 mg cholesterol; 14 g carbohydrates; 2 g protein; 1 gfiber; 45 mg sodium; 53 mg potassium.
Carbohydrate Servings: 1
Exchanges: 1 other carbohydrate, 1 fat

Frosted Grapes

INGREDIENTS
- 2 cups seedless grapes

PREPARATION
1. Wash and pat dry grapes. Freeze 45 minutes. Let stand for 2 minutes at room temperature before serving.

NUTRITION
Per serving: 55 calories; 0 g fat (0 g sat, 0 g mono); 0 mg cholesterol; 14 g carbohydrates; 1 g protein; 1 gfiber; 2 mg sodium; 153 mg potassium.
Carbohydrate Servings: 1
Exchanges: 1 fruit

Herbed Scallop Kebabs

INGREDIENTS
- 3 tablespoons lemon juice
- 1 1/2 tablespoons chopped fresh thyme
- 2 teaspoons extra-virgin olive oil
- 2 teaspoons freshly grated lemon zest
- 1 teaspoon freshly ground pepper
- 1/4 teaspoon salt, or to taste
- 1 1/4 pounds sea scallops, trimmed
- 1 lemon, cut into 8 wedges

PREPARATION
1. Preheat grill to medium-high. Place a fine-mesh nonstick grill topper on grill to heat.
2. Whisk lemon juice, thyme, oil, lemon zest, pepper and salt in a small bowl.
3. Toss scallops with 2 tablespoons of the lemon mixture; reserve the remaining mixture for basting the kebabs. Thread the scallops and the lemon wedges onto four 10-inch-long skewers (see Tip), placing 6 to 7 scallops and 2 lemon wedges on each skewer.
4. Lightly oil the grill rack (see Tip). Cook the kebabs, turning from time to time and basting with the reserved lemon mixture, until the scallops are opaque in the center, 8 to 12 minutes. Serve immediately.

TIPS & NOTES
- If using wooden skewers, soak them in water for 20 to 30 minutes first to prevent them from scorching.
- **To oil a grill rack:** Oil a folded paper towel, hold it with tongs and rub it over the rack. Do not use cooking spray on a hot grill.

NUTRITION
Per serving: 152 calories; 3 g fat (0 g sat, 2 g mono); 47 mg cholesterol; 5 g carbohydrates; 0 g added sugars; 24 g protein; 0 g fiber; 374 mg sodium; 478 mg potassium.
Nutrition Bonus: Selenium (44% daily value), Vitamin C (20% dv).
Exchanges: 31/2 very lean meat

Five-Spice Roasted Duck Breasts

INGREDIENTS
- 2 pounds boneless duck breast, (see Note)
- 1 teaspoon five-spice powder, (see Note)
- 1/2 teaspoon kosher salt
- Zest & juice of 2 oranges and 2 teaspoons honey
- 1 tablespoon reduced-sodium soy sauce
- 1/4 teaspoon cornstarch, dissolved in 1 teaspoon water

PREPARATION
1. Preheat oven to 375°F.
2. Place duck skin-side down on a cutting board. Trim off all excess skin that hangs over the sides. Turn over, and make three parallel, diagonal cuts in the skin of each breast, cutting through the fat but not into the meat. Sprinkle both sides with five-spice powder and salt.
3. Place the duck skin-side down in an ovenproof skillet over medium-low heat. Cook until the fat is melted and the skin is golden brown, about 10 minutes. Transfer the duck to a plate; pour off all the fat from the pan. Return the duck to the pan skin-side up and transfer to the oven.
4. Roast the duck for 10 to 15 minutes for medium, depending on the size of the breast, until a thermometer inserted into the thickest part registers 150°F. Transfer to a cutting board; let rest for 5 minutes.
5. Pour off any fat remaining in the pan (take care, the handle will still be hot); place the pan over medium-high heat and add orange juice and honey. Bring to a simmer, stirring to scrape up any browned bits. Add orange zest and soy sauce and continue to cook until the sauce is slightly reduced, about 1 minute. Stir cornstarch mixture then whisk into the sauce; cook, stirring, until slightly thickened, 1 minute. Remove the duck skin and thinly slice the breast meat. Drizzle with the orange sauce.

TIPS & NOTES
- **Notes:** Boneless duck breast halves range widely in weight, from about 1/2 to 1 pound, depending on the breed of duck. They can be found in most supermarkets in the poultry or specialty-meat sections or online at mapleleaffarms.com or dartagnan.com.

- Often a blend of cinnamon, cloves, fennel seed, star anise and Szechuan peppercorns, five-spice powder was originally considered a cure-all miracle blend encompassing the five elements (sour, bitter, sweet, pungent, salty). Look for it in the supermarket spice section.

NUTRITION

Per 3-oz. serving: 152 calories; 2 g fat (0 g sat, 1 g mono); 122 mg cholesterol; 8 g carbohydrates; 2 gadded sugars; 24 g protein; 0 g fiber; 309 mg sodium; 86 mg potassium.
Nutrition Bonus: Vitamin C (45% daily value), Selenium (36% dv), Iron (25% dv).
Carbohydrate Servings: 1
Exchanges: 1 fruit, 3 very lean meat

Whole-Wheat Couscous with Parmesan & Peas

INGREDIENTS
- 1 14-ounce can reduced-sodium chicken broth, or vegetable broth
- 1/4 cup water
- 2 teaspoons extra-virgin olive oil
- 1 cup whole-wheat couscous
- 1 1/2 cups frozen peas
- 2 tablespoons chopped fresh dill
- 1 teaspoon freshly grated lemon zest
- Salt & freshly ground pepper, to taste
- 1/2 cup freshly grated Parmesan cheese

PREPARATION
1. Combine broth, water and oil in a large saucepan; bring to a boil. Stir in couscous and remove from heat. Cover and let plump for 5 minutes.
2. Meanwhile, cook peas on the stovetop or in the microwave according to package directions.
3. Add the peas, dill, lemon zest, salt and pepper to the couscous; mix gently and fluff with a fork. Serve hot, sprinkled with cheese.

NUTRITION

Per serving: 208 calories; 4 g fat (1 g sat, 2 g mono); 6 mg cholesterol; 35 g carbohydrates; 0 g added sugars; 10 g protein; 7 g fiber; 186 mg sodium; 45 mg potassium.
Carbohydrate Servings: 2
Exchanges: 2 starch

Sliced Fennel Salad

INGREDIENTS
- 1 large fennel bulb
- 1 tablespoon extra-virgin olive oil
- 1 tablespoon lemon juice
- 1/8 teaspoon salt and Freshly ground pepper, to taste

PREPARATION
1. Trim base from fennel bulb. Remove and discard the fennel stalks; reserve some of the feathery leaves for garnish. Pull off and discard any discolored parts from the bulb. Stand the bulb upright and cut vertically into very thin slices. Arrange the slices on 4 salad plates.
2. Whisk oil, lemon juice and salt in a small bowl. Drizzle the mixture over the fennel and garnish with a grinding of pepper and a few fennel leaves.

NUTRITION
Per serving: 51 calories; 4 g fat (0 g sat, 3 g mono); 0 mg cholesterol; 5 g carbohydrates; 0 g added sugars;1 g protein; 2 g fiber; 103 mg sodium; 247 mg potassium.
Nutrition Bonus: Vitamin C (15% daily value).
Exchanges: vegetable, 1 fat (mono)

Almond Cream with Strawberries
INGREDIENTS
- 1/4 cup slivered almonds
- 2 cups strawberries, rinsed
- 1 cup part-skim ricotta
- 2 tablespoons sugar or Splenda Granular
- 1/4 teaspoon almond extract

PREPARATION
1. Toast almonds in a small dry skillet over medium-low heat, stirring constantly, until golden and fragrant, 2 to 3 minutes. Transfer to a plate to cool.
2. Hull strawberries, slice and divide among 4 dessert plates. Mix ricotta with sugar (or Splenda) and almond extract until smooth. Spoon over the berries and sprinkle with the toasted almonds.

NUTRITION
Per serving: 189 calories; 9 g fat (3 g sat, 4 g mono); 19 mg cholesterol; 16 g carbohydrates; 9 g protein; 2 g fiber; 78 mg sodium; 237 mg potassium.
Nutrition Bonus: Vitamin C (82% daily value), Calcium (19% dv).
Carbohydrate Servings: 1
Exchanges: 1 fruit, 1 medium-fat meat
Nutrition Note: Per serving with Splenda: 1; 168 calories, 12 g carbohydrate

DAY 12
BREAKFAST
Oatbran Bagel
Skim milk (1 cup)
Vegetable Cream Cheese

LUNCH
Pasta, Tuna & Roasted Pepper Salad
Whole-wheat pita bread (1 medium pita)
Banana (1 cup, sliced)
Skim milk (1 cup)

SNACK
Lima Bean Spread with Cumin & Herbs
Toasted Pita Crisps

DINNER
Pampered Chicken or Ham & Swiss Rosti
Carrot Saute with Ginger & Orange
Baked potato (1 medium) or Parsley Tabbouleh
Feta-Herb Spread
Squash Pie

DAY 12 RECIPES

Vegetable Cream Cheese

INGREDIENTS
- 8 ounces light cream cheese
- 1/4 cup chopped scallions
- 1/4 cup finely chopped carrots
- 1/4 cup finely chopped daikon radish
- 2 tablespoons chopped fresh dill
- 1/4 teaspoon freshly ground pepper

PREPARATION
1. Blend all ingredients in a small bowl.

NUTRITION
Per tablespoon: 30 calories; 2 g fat (1 g sat, 1 g mono); 7 mg cholesterol; 2 g carbohydrates; 1 g protein; 1 g fiber; 56 mg sodium; 10 mg potassium.
Exchanges: 1/2 fat

Pasta, Tuna & Roasted Pepper Salad

INGREDIENTS

- 1 6-ounce can chunk light tuna in water, drained (see Note)
- 1 7-ounce jar roasted red peppers, rinsed and sliced (2/3 cup), divided
- 1/2 cup finely chopped red onion or scallions
- 2 tablespoons capers, rinsed, coarsely chopped if large
- 2 tablespoons nonfat plain yogurt
- 2 tablespoons chopped fresh basil
- 1 tablespoon extra-virgin olive oil
- 1 1/2 teaspoons lemon juice
- 1 small clove garlic, crushed and peeled
- 1/8 teaspoon salt, or to taste
- Freshly ground pepper, to taste
- 6 ounces whole-wheat penne or rigatoni, (1 3/4 cups)

PREPARATION

1. Put a large pot of lightly salted water on to boil.
2. Combine tuna, 1/3 cup red peppers, onion (or scallions) and capers in a large bowl.
3. Combine yogurt, basil, oil, lemon juice, garlic, salt, pepper and the remaining 1/3 cup red peppers in a blender or food processor. Puree until smooth.
4. Cook pasta until just tender, 10 to 14 minutes or according to package directions. Drain and rinse under cold water. Add to the tuna mixture along with the red pepper sauce; toss to coat.

TIPS & NOTES

- **Note:** Chunk light tuna, which comes from the smaller skipjack or yellowfin, has less mercury than canned white albacore tuna. The FDA/EPA advises that women who are or might become pregnant, nursing mothers and young children consume no more than 6 ounces of albacore a week; up to 12 ounces of canned light tuna is considered safe.

NUTRITION
Per serving: 270 calories; 5 g fat (1 g sat, 3 g mono); 13 mg cholesterol; 39 g carbohydrates; 0 g added sugars; 18 g protein; 6 g fiber; 539 mg sodium; 234 mg potassium.
Nutrition Bonus: Vitamin C (30% daily value), Fiber (23% dv), Magnesium (19% dv).
Carbohydrate Servings: 2
Exchanges: 2 starch, 2 very lean meat

Lima Bean Spread with Cumin & Herbs

INGREDIENTS
- 1 10-ounce package frozen lima beans
- 4 cloves garlic, crushed and peeled
- 1/4 teaspoon crushed red pepper
- 2 tablespoons extra-virgin olive oil
- 4 teaspoons lemon juice
- 1 teaspoon ground cumin
- 1/2 teaspoon salt, or to taste
- Freshly ground pepper, to taste
- 1 tablespoon chopped fresh mint
- 1 tablespoon chopped fresh cilantro
- 1 tablespoon chopped fresh dill

PREPARATION
1. Bring a large saucepan of lightly salted water to a boil. Add lima beans, garlic and crushed red pepper; cook until the beans are tender, about 10 minutes. Remove from heat and let cool in the liquid.
2. Drain the beans and garlic. Transfer to a food processor. Add oil, lemon juice, cumin, salt and pepper; process until smooth. Scrape into a bowl, stir in mint, cilantro and dill.

TIPS & NOTES
- **Make Ahead Tip**: Cover and refrigerate for up to 4 days or freeze for up to 6 months.

NUTRITION
Per tablespoon: 25 calories; 1 g fat (0 g sat, 1 g mono); 0 mg cholesterol; 3 g carbohydrates; 0 g added sugars; 1 g protein; 1 g fiber; 56 mg sodium; 62 mg potassium.
Exchanges: Free food

Toasted Pita Crisps

INGREDIENTS
- 4 whole-wheat pita breads
- Olive oil cooking spray, or extra-virgin olive oil

PREPARATION
1. Preheat oven to 425°F.

2. Cut pitas into 4 triangles each. Separate each triangle into 2 halves at the fold. Arrange, rough side up, on a baking sheet. Spritz lightly with cooking spray or brush lightly with oil. Bake until crisp, 8 to 10 minutes.

TIPS & NOTES
- **Make Ahead Tip**: Store in an airtight container at room temperature for up to 1 week or in the freezer for up to 2 months.

NUTRITION

Per crisp: 23 calories; 0 g fat (0 g sat, 0 g mono); 0 mg cholesterol; 4 g carbohydrates; 0 g added sugars; 1 g protein; 1 g fiber; 43 mg sodium; 14 mg potassium.
Exchanges: 1/3 starch

Pampered Chicken

INGREDIENTS
- 4 boneless, skinless chicken breast halves, (about 1 pound), trimmed of fat
- 4 slices Monterey Jack cheese, (2 ounces)
- 2 egg whites
- 1/3 cup seasoned (Italian-style) breadcrumbs
- 2 tablespoons freshly grated Parmesan cheese
- 2 tablespoons chopped fresh parsley
- 1/4 teaspoon salt, or to taste
- 1/2 teaspoon freshly ground pepper
- 2 teaspoons extra-virgin olive oil
- Lemon wedges, for garnish

PREPARATION
1. Preheat oven to 400°F. Place a chicken breast, skinned-side down, on a cutting board. Keeping the blade of a sharp knife parallel to the board, make a horizontal slit along the thinner, long edge of the breast, cutting nearly through to the opposite side. Open the breast so it forms two flaps, hinged at the center. Place a slice of cheese on one flap, leaving a 1/2-inch border at the edge. Press remaining flap down firmly over the cheese and set aside. Repeat with the remaining breasts.
2. Lightly beat egg whites with a fork in a medium bowl. Mix breadcrumbs, Parmesan, parsley, salt and pepper in a shallow dish. Holding a stuffed breast together firmly, dip it in the egg whites and then roll in the breadcrumbs. Repeat with the remaining breasts.

3. Heat oil in a large ovenproof skillet over medium-high heat. Add the stuffed breasts and cook until browned on one side, about 2 minutes. Turn the breasts over and place the skillet in the oven.
4. Bake the chicken until no longer pink in the center, about 20 minutes. Serve with lemon wedges.

NUTRITION
Per serving: 255 calories; 11 g fat (4 g sat, 4 g mono); 78 mg cholesterol; 7 g carbohydrates; 31 g protein; 1 g fiber; 518 mg sodium; 268 mg potassium.
Nutrition Bonus: Selenium (40% daily value), Calcium (15% dv).
Carbohydrate Servings: 1/2
Exchanges: 1/2 starch, 4 very lean meat, 1 medium-fat meat

Ham & Swiss Rosti

INGREDIENTS
- 1 large egg
- 1 cup diced ham, (about 5 ounces)
- 1 cup shredded part-skim Jarlsberg, or Swiss cheese, divided
- 1 shallot, minced
- 1 teaspoon chopped fresh rosemary, or 1/4 teaspoon dried
- 1/2 teaspoon freshly ground pepper
- 1/4 teaspoon salt
- 4 cups frozen hash brown potatoes
- 2 tablespoons extra-virgin olive oil, divided

PREPARATION
1. Beat egg in a large bowl. Stir in ham, 1/2 cup cheese, shallot, rosemary, pepper and salt. Add frozen potatoes and stir to combine.
2. Heat 1 tablespoon oil in a large nonstick skillet over medium heat. Pat the potato mixture into an even round in the pan. Cover and cook until browned and crispy on the bottom, 4 to 6 minutes.
3. Remove the pan from the heat. Place a rimless baking sheet on top. Wearing oven mitts, grasp the pan and baking sheet together and carefully invert, unmolding the rösti onto the baking sheet. Wipe out any browned bits from the pan. Return it to the heat and add the remaining 1 tablespoon oil. Slide the rösti back into the pan. Top with the remaining 1/2 cup cheese, cover and cook the second side until crispy and browned, 4 to 6 minutes. Slide onto a platter, cut into wedges and serve.

NUTRITION
Per serving: 262 calories; 13 g fat (3 g sat, 8 g mono); 94 mg cholesterol; 15 g carbohydrates; 0 g added sugars; 21 g protein; 2 g fiber; 276 mg sodium; 174 mg potassium.
Nutrition Bonus: Selenium (34% daily value), Calcium (25% dv), Zinc (15% dv).
Carbohydrate Servings: 1
Exchanges: 1 starch, 3 lean meat

Carrot Saute with Ginger & Orange

INGREDIENTS
- 2 teaspoons canola oil
- 3 cups grated carrots, (6 medium-large)
- 2 teaspoons minced fresh ginger
- 1/2 cup orange juice
- 1/4 teaspoon salt, or to taste
- Freshly ground pepper, to taste

PREPARATION
1. Heat oil in a large nonstick skillet over medium-high heat. Add carrots and ginger; cook, stirring often, until wilted, about 2 minutes. Stir in orange juice and salt; simmer, uncovered, until the carrots are tender and most of the liquid has evaporated, 1 to 2 minutes. Season with pepper and serve.

NUTRITION
Per serving: 69 calories; 3 g fat (0 g sat, 1 g mono); 0 mg cholesterol; 6 g carbohydrates; 0 g added sugars;1 g protein; 2 g fiber; 20 mg sodium; 330 mg potassium.
Nutrition Bonus: Vitamin A (200% daily value), Vitamin C (35% dv).
Carbohydrate Servings: 1
Exchanges: 2 vegetable, 1/2 fat (mono)

Parsley Tabbouleh

INGREDIENTS
- 1 cup water
- 1/2 cup bulgur
- 1/4 cup lemon juice
- 2 tablespoons extra-virgin olive oil
- 1/2 teaspoon minced garlic
- 1/4 teaspoon salt
- Freshly ground pepper, to taste
- 2 cups finely chopped flat-leaf parsley, (about 2 bunches)
- 1/4 cup chopped fresh mint

- 2 tomatoes, diced
- 1 small cucumber, peeled, seeded and diced
- 4 scallions, thinly sliced

PREPARATION
1. Combine water and bulgur in a small saucepan. Bring to a full boil, remove from heat, cover and let stand until the water is absorbed and the bulgur is tender, 25 minutes or according to package directions. If any water remains, drain bulgur in a fine-mesh sieve. Transfer to a large bowl and let cool for 15 minutes.
2. Combine lemon juice, oil, garlic, salt and pepper in a small bowl. Add parsley, mint, tomatoes, cucumber and scallions to the bulgur. Add the dressing and toss. Serve at room temperature or chill for at least 1 hour to serve cold.

TIPS & NOTES
- **Make Ahead Tip**: Cover and refrigerate for up to 1 day.

NUTRITION
Per serving: 165 calories; 8 g fat (1 g sat, 6 g mono); 0 mg cholesterol; 22 g carbohydrates; 0 g added sugars; 4 g protein; 6 g fiber; 175 mg sodium; 555 mg potassium.
Nutrition Bonus: Vitamin C (100% daily value), Vitamin A (70% dv), Folate (21% dv), Iron (20% dv).
Carbohydrate Servings: 1
Exchanges: 1 starch, 1 vegetable, 1 1/2 fat

Feta-Herb Spread

INGREDIENTS
- 1 32-ounce container low-fat or nonfat plain yogurt
- 1 clove garlic, crushed and peeled
- 1/2 teaspoon salt, or to taste
- 1 cup crumbled feta cheese, (about 4 ounces)
- 1 tablespoon extra-virgin olive oil
- 2 teaspoons chopped fresh parsley
- 1 teaspoon dried oregano

PREPARATION
1. Line a sieve with cheesecloth and spoon in yogurt. Set the sieve over a bowl, leaving at least 1 inch clearance at the bottom. Cover and refrigerate for at least 8 hours or overnight.
2. Place garlic on a cutting board, sprinkle with salt and mash into a paste with the side of a chef's knife. Transfer to a medium bowl. Add the drained yogurt (discard whey) and whisk until smooth. Stir in feta cheese, oil, parsley and oregano.

TIPS & NOTES
- **Make Ahead Tip**: Cover and refrigerate for up to 4 days.

NUTRITION
Per serving: 65 calories; 3 g fat (1 g sat, 1 g mono); 7 mg cholesterol; 4 g carbohydrates; 0 g added sugars; 4 g protein; 0 g fiber; 248 mg sodium; 83 mg potassium.
Exchanges: 1/2 low-fat milk

Squash Pie

INGREDIENTS
CRUST
- 3/4 cup whole-wheat pastry flour, (see Ingredient Note)
- 3/4 cup all-purpose flour
- 1 tablespoon sugar
- 1/4 teaspoon salt
- 2 tablespoons unsalted butter
- 1/3 cup almond oil, (see Ingredient Note) or canola oil
- 1/4 teaspoon distilled white vinegar
- 3-4 tablespoons ice water

FILLING
- 2 cups Pureed Roasted Winter Squash, (recipe follows)
- 1 1/2 cups evaporated low-fat or fat-free milk
- 1/4 cup honey
- 2 large egg yolks, lightly beaten
- 1 large egg, lightly beaten
- 1/3 cup sugar
- 1 teaspoon ground cinnamon
- 1/2 teaspoon freshly grated nutmeg
- 1/4 teaspoon salt

PREPARATION
1. To prepare crust: Mix whole-wheat flour, all-purpose flour, 1 tablespoon sugar and 1/4 teaspoon salt in a medium bowl. Using a pastry cutter or two forks, cut in butter until the pieces are roughly the size of peas. Stir in oil and vinegar with a fork, then stir in just enough water so the dough gathers into a ball.
2. Dust a large piece of wax paper with flour, then turn the dough out onto it. Dust a rolling pin with flour and roll the dough into a 14-inch circle. Invert into a 9-inch pie pan, gently pressing the dough into the bottom of the pan. Trim any uneven edges, leaving 1/2 inch of dough hanging over the rim. Fold the edges

under and crimp into a decorative design. Cover with plastic wrap; refrigerate for at least 30 minutes.
3. Preheat oven to 350°F.
4. Prick the crust with a fork several times; line with parchment paper and add enough pie weights or dried beans to cover the bottom. Set the pie pan on a baking sheet. Bake until the crust is firm but not colored, about 20 minutes.
5. Meanwhile, to prepare filling & bake pie: Whisk squash, evaporated milk, honey, egg yolks and egg in a large bowl until smooth. Stir in 1/3 cup sugar, cinnamon, nutmeg and 1/4 teaspoon salt. Pour the filling into the crust (it will be very full). Place the pie pan on the baking sheet.
6. Bake the pie until the crust edges are nicely browned, about 40 minutes. Cover the edges with foil and continue to bake until a knife inserted into the center comes out clean, 25 to 40 minutes more. Cool the pie on a wire rack before slicing, at least 2 hours.

TIPS & NOTES

- **Make Ahead Tip**: Prepare crust through Step 2; wrap in plastic wrap and refrigerate for up to 2 days or freeze for up to 2 months (do not thaw before baking).
- **Ingredient Notes:** Milled from soft wheat, whole-wheat pastry flour contains less gluten than regular whole-wheat flour. It helps ensure a tender result in baked goods while providing the nutritional benefits of whole grains. It is available in natural-foods stores and large supermarkets. Store it in an airtight container in the refrigerator or freezer.
- Almond oil is an unrefined oil pressed from almonds. You can find it in many supermarkets and health-food stores. Store it in the refrigerator.

NUTRITION
Per serving: 225 calories; 9 g fat (2 g sat, 5 g mono); 58 mg cholesterol; 36 g carbohydrates; 6 g protein; 3 g fiber; 145 mg sodium; 343 mg potassium.
Nutrition Bonus: Vitamin A (30% daily value), Calcium (10% dv).
Carbohydrate Servings: 2
Exchanges: 2 other carbohydrate, 2 fat

DAY 13
BREAKFAST

Healthy Pancakes
Strawberries (1 cup)
Low-fat vanilla yogurt (8 oz.)

LUNCH

Chicken & White Bean Soup
Whole-wheat toast (1 slice)
Fat-free cheese (1 slice)
Orange (1 large)
Skim milk (1 cup)

SNACK

Nectarine (1 small)

DINNER

Oven-Fried Fish Fillets or Golden Baked Pork Cutlets
Tarragon Tartar Sauce or Blueberry Ketchup
Roasted Asparagus with Pine Nuts
Brown rice (1 cup, cooked)
Endive & Watercress Salad with Pomegranate Dressing
Watermelon-Yogurt Ice

DAY 13 RECIPES

Healthy Pancakes

INGREDIENTS
- 2 1/2 cups whole-wheat flour
- 1 cup buttermilk powder, (see Note)
- 5 tablespoons dried egg whites, such as Just Whites (see Note)
- 1/4 cup sugar
- 1 1/2 tablespoons baking powder
- 2 teaspoons baking soda
- 1 teaspoon salt
- 1 cup flaxseed meal, (see Note)
- 1 cup nonfat dry milk
- 1/2 cup wheat bran, or oat bran
- 1 1/2 cups nonfat milk
- 1/4 cup canola oil
- 1 teaspoon vanilla extract

PREPARATION
1. Whisk flour, buttermilk powder, dried egg whites, sugar, baking powder, baking soda and salt in a large bowl. Stir in flaxseed meal, dry milk and bran. (Makes 6 cups dry mix.)
2. Combine milk, oil and vanilla in a glass measuring cup.
3. Place 2 cups pancake mix in a large bowl. (Refrigerate the remaining pancake mix in an airtight container for up to 1 month or freeze for up to 3 months.) Make a well in the center of the pancake mix. Whisk in the milk mixture until just blended; do not overmix. (The batter will seem quite thin, but will thicken up as it stands.) Let stand for 5 minutes.
4. Coat a nonstick skillet or griddle with cooking spray and place over medium heat. Whisk the batter. Using 1/4 cup batter for each pancake, cook pancakes until the edges are dry and bubbles begin to form, about 2 minutes. Turn over and cook until golden brown, about 2 minutes longer. Adjust heat as necessary for even browning.

TIPS & NOTES
- **Notes:** Buttermilk powder, such as Saco Buttermilk Blend, is a useful substitute for fresh buttermilk. Look in the baking section or with the powdered milk in most markets.
- **Dried egg whites:** Dried egg whites are convenient in recipes calling for egg whites because there is no waste. Look for brands like Just Whites in the baking or natural-foods section of most supermarkets or online at bakerscatalogue.com.
- **Flaxseed meal:** You can find flaxseed meal in the natural-foods section of large supermarkets. You can also start with whole flaxseeds: Grind 2/3 cup whole flaxseeds to yield 1 cup.
- **Variations:** Chocolate-Chocolate Chip Pancakes: Fold 1/2 cup cocoa powder and 3 ounces chocolate chips into the batter. Blueberry: Fold 1 cup frozen blueberries into the batter. Banana-Nut: Fold 1 cup thinly sliced bananas and 4 tablespoons finely chopped toasted pecans into the batter.

NUTRITION
Per serving: 272 calories; 13 g fat (2 g sat, 6 g mono); 8 mg cholesterol; 27 g carbohydrates; 12 g protein; 5 g fiber; 471 mg sodium; 336 mg potassium.
Nutrition Bonus: Calcium (24% daily value), Fiber (20% dv)
Carbohydrate Servings: 1/2
Exchanges: 2 starch, 1 very lean meat, 2 fat (mono)

Chicken & White Bean Soup

INGREDIENTS
- 2 teaspoons extra-virgin olive oil
- 2 leeks, white and light green parts only, cut into 1/4-inch rounds
- 1 tablespoon chopped fresh sage, or 1/4 teaspoon dried
- 2 14-ounce cans reduced-sodium chicken broth
- 2 cups water
- 1 15-ounce can cannellini beans, rinsed
- 1 2-pound roasted chicken, skin discarded, meat removed from bones and shredded (4 cups)

PREPARATION
1. Heat oil in a Dutch oven over medium-high heat. Add leeks and cook, stirring often, until soft, about 3 minutes. Stir in sage and continue cooking until aromatic, about 30 seconds. Stir in broth and water, increase heat to high, cover and bring to a boil. Add beans and chicken and cook, uncovered, stirring occasionally, until heated through, about 3 minutes. Serve hot.

TIPS & NOTES
- **Make Ahead Tip**: Cover and refrigerate for up to 2 days.

NUTRITION
Per serving: 172 calories; 4 g fat (1 g sat, 2 g mono); 54 mg cholesterol; 10 g carbohydrates; 0 g added sugars; 24 g protein; 3 g fiber; 350 mg sodium; 389 mg potassium.
Carbohydrate Servings: 1/2
Exchanges: 1 starch, 3 lean meat

Oven-Fried Fish Fillets

INGREDIENTS
- 1/3 cup fine, dry, unseasoned breadcrumbs
- 1/4 teaspoon salt
- Freshly ground pepper, to taste
- 1 pound Pacific sole fillets
- 1 tablespoon extra-virgin olive oil
- 1/2 cup Tarragon Tartar Sauce, (recipe follows)
- Lemon wedges

PREPARATION
1. Preheat oven to 450°F. Coat a baking sheet with cooking spray.

2. Place breadcrumbs, salt and pepper in a small dry skillet over medium heat. Cook, stirring, until toasted, about 5 minutes. Remove from heat. Brush both sides of each fish fillet with oil and dredge in the breadcrumb mixture. Place on the prepared baking sheet.
3. Bake the fish until opaque in the center, 5 to 6 minutes.
4. Meanwhile, make Tarragon Tartar Sauce.
5. To serve, carefully transfer the fish to plates using a spatula. Garnish with a dollop of the sauce and serve with lemon wedges.

NUTRITION
Per serving: 229 calories; 10 g fat (2 g sat, 4 g mono); 59 mg cholesterol; 11 g carbohydrates; 23 g protein;1 g fiber; 444 mg sodium; 472 mg potassium.
Nutrition Bonus: Selenium (57% daily value).
Carbohydrate Servings: 1
Exchanges: 1/2 starch, 3 lean meat

Golden Baked Pork Cutlets

INGREDIENTS
- 1 pound pork tenderloin, trimmed
- 1/2 cup dry breadcrumbs, preferably whole-wheat (see Tip)
- 1 teaspoon sugar
- 1/2 teaspoon paprika
- 1/2 teaspoon onion powder
- 1/2 teaspoon salt
- 4 teaspoons canola oil
- 1 large egg white, lightly beaten
- 4 teaspoons cornstarch

PREPARATION
1. Preheat oven to 400°F. Coat a rimmed baking sheet with cooking spray.
2. Holding a chef's knife at a 45° angle and perpendicular to the tenderloin, slice the pork into 4 long, thin "fillets."
3. Mix breadcrumbs, sugar, paprika, onion powder and salt in a shallow dish. Drizzle with oil and mash with a fork until the oil is thoroughly incorporated. Lightly beat egg white with a fork in another shallow dish. Sprinkle cornstarch over the pork slices and pat to coat evenly on both sides. Dip the pork into the egg, then press into the breading mixture until evenly coated on both sides. (Discard leftover mixture.)
4. Place the pork on the prepared baking sheet. Bake until just barely pink in the center and an instant-read thermometer registers 145°F, 14 to 16 minutes.

TIPS & NOTES

- **Tip:** To make fresh breadcrumbs, trim crusts from whole-wheat bread. Tear bread into pieces and process in a food processor until coarse crumbs form. One slice of bread makes about 1/2 cup fresh crumbs. For dry breadcrumbs, spread the fresh crumbs on a baking sheet and bake at 250°F until crispy, about 15 minutes. One slice of fresh bread makes about 1/3 cup dry crumbs. Or use prepared coarse dry breadcrumbs. We like Ian's brand labeled "Panko breadcrumbs." Find them in the natural-foods section of large supermarkets.

NUTRITION

Per serving: 220 calories; 7 g fat (1 g sat, 4 g mono); 74 mg cholesterol; 11 g carbohydrates; 1 g added sugars; 26 g protein; 1 g fiber; 377 mg sodium; 475 mg potassium.
Nutrition Bonus: Selenium (50% daily value).
Carbohydrate Servings: 1
Exchanges: 1 starch, 3 lean meat

Tarragon Tartar Sauce

INGREDIENTS

- 1/2 cup nonfat or low-fat plain yogurt
- 1/2 cup reduced-fat mayonnaise
- 1 teaspoon sugar
- 1/2 teaspoon Dijon mustard
- 1/2 teaspoon lemon juice
- 1/4 cup finely chopped dill pickle
- 1 tablespoon drained capers, minced
- 2 tablespoons chopped fresh parsley
- 2 teaspoons chopped fresh tarragon, or 1/2 teaspoon dried
- 1 clove garlic, minced

PREPARATION

1. Whisk yogurt, mayonnaise, sugar, mustard and lemon juice in a small bowl. Stir in pickle, capers, parsley, tarragon and garlic.

TIPS & NOTES

- **Make Ahead Tip:** The sauce will keep, covered, in the refrigerator for up to 4 days.

NUTRITION

Per tablespoon: 22 calories; 2 g fat (0 g sat, 0 g mono); 2 mg cholesterol; 2 g carbohydrates; 0 g protein; 0 g fiber; 71 mg sodium; 6 mg potassium.

Exchanges: Per tablespoon: free food

Blueberry Ketchup

INGREDIENTS
- 2 1/2 cups fresh blueberries
- 1 medium shallot, minced (about 2 tablespoons)
- 1 1/4 cups sugar
- 1/2 cup red-wine vinegar
- 2 tablespoons minced fresh ginger
- 1 tablespoon lime juice
- 1/4 teaspoon salt
- 1/4 teaspoon freshly ground pepper

PREPARATION
1. Place blueberries, sugar, vinegar, ginger, lime juice, salt and pepper in a large saucepan over medium-high heat. Stir until the sugar dissolves, about 5 minutes. Bring to a simmer, reduce heat to medium-low and simmer, stirring occasionally, until the blueberries have mostly broken down and the sauce has thickened, 20 to 30 minutes. Spoon into glass jars or a large bowl and refrigerate until chilled and thickened, about 4 hours.

TIPS & NOTES
- **Make Ahead Tip**: Cover and refrigerate for up to 2 weeks or freeze for up to 1 month.
- To oil a grill rack, oil a folded paper towel, hold it with tongs and rub it over the rack. (Do not use cooking spray on a hot grill.)

NUTRITION

Per tablespoon: 25 calories; 0 g fat (0 g sat, 0 g mono); 0 mg cholesterol; 6 g carbohydrates; 0 g protein; 0 g fiber; 13 mg sodium; 9 mg potassium.
Nutrition Bonus: Blueberries are a good source of the phytochemicals anthocyanidins and ellagic acid.
Carbohydrate Servings: 1/2
Exchanges: 1/2 fruit

Roasted Asparagus with Pine Nuts

INGREDIENTS
- 2 tablespoons pine nuts
- 1 1/2 pounds asparagus
- 1 large shallot, thinly sliced
- 2 teaspoons extra-virgin olive oil

- 1/4 teaspoon salt, divided
- Freshly ground pepper, to taste
- 1/4 cup balsamic vinegar

PREPARATION
1. Preheat oven to 350° F. Spread pine nuts in a small baking pan and toast in the oven until golden and fragrant, 7 to 10 minutes. Transfer to a small bowl to cool.
2. Increase oven temperature to 450° F. Snap off the tough ends of asparagus. Toss the asparagus with shallot, oil, 1/8 teaspoon salt and pepper. Spread in a single layer on a large baking sheet with sides. Roast, turning twice, until the asparagus is tender and browned, 10 to 15 minutes.
3. Meanwhile, bring vinegar and the remaining 1/8 teaspoon salt to a simmer in a small skillet over medium-high heat. Reduce heat to medium-low and simmer, swirling the pan occasionally, until slightly syrupy and reduced to 1 tablespoon, about 5 minutes. To serve, toss the asparagus with the reduced vinegar and sprinkle with the pine nuts.

NUTRITION
Per serving: 112 calories; 5 g fat (1 g sat, 3 g mono); 0 mg cholesterol; 12 g carbohydrates; 0 g added sugars; 5 g protein; 4 g fiber; 150 mg sodium; 491 mg potassium.
Nutrition Bonus: Vitamin C (30% daily value), Vitamin A (20% dv).
Carbohydrate Servings: 1
Exchanges: 2 vegetable, 1 fat (mono)

Endive & Watercress Salad with Pomegranate Dressing

INGREDIENTS
- 1/4 cup pomegranate juice
- 2 tablespoons walnut oil
- 2 tablespoons white-wine vinegar
- 1/2 teaspoon sugar
- Salt & freshly ground pepper to taste
- 1 ounce ounce walnut, or pecan halves
- 4 heads Belgian endive, trimmed, leaves separated and broken into 1 1/2-inch lengths
- 1 bunch watercress, large stems removed, leaves washed and dried
- 1 small red onion, thinly sliced
- 1/2 cup pomegranate seeds or raspberries

PREPARATION
1. Whisk or shake pomegranate juice, oil, vinegar, sugar, salt and pepper together in a small bowl or a jar.

2. Preheat oven to 350°F. Spread walnuts or pecans on a pie plate and toast for about 10 minutes, or until lightly browned and fragrant. Let cool and chop coarsely.
3. Combine endives, watercress and red onions in a salad bowl. Drizzle the dressing over and toss. Taste and adjust seasonings. Sprinkle pomegranate seeds or raspberries and the toasted nuts over top and serve.

NUTRITION
Per serving: 113 calories; 6 g fat (1 g sat, 1 g mono); 0 mg cholesterol; 13 g carbohydrates; 0 g added sugars; 4 g protein; 8 g fiber; 97 mg sodium; 893 mg potassium.
Nutrition Bonus: Vitamin A (117% daily value), Folate (93% dv), Vitamin C (35% dv), Potassium (26% dv), Calcium (15% dv).
Exchanges: 2 vegetable, 1 fat

Watermelon-Yogurt Ice

INGREDIENTS
- 1/4 cup water
- 1/4 cup sugar
- 4 cups diced seedless watermelon, (about 3 pounds with the rind)
- 1 cup low-fat vanilla yogurt
- 1 tablespoon lime juice

PREPARATION
1. Combine water and sugar in a small saucepan. Cook, stirring, over high heat until the sugar is dissolved. Transfer to a glass measuring cup and let cool slightly.
2. Puree watermelon in a food processor or blender, in 2 batches, pulsing until smooth. Transfer to a large bowl. Whisk in the cooled sugar syrup, yogurt and lime juice until combined. Pour the mixture through a fine-mesh sieve into another large bowl, whisking to release all juice. Discard pulp. Pour the extracted juices into an ice cream maker and freeze according to manufacturer's directions. (Alternatively, pour into a shallow metal pan and freeze until solid, about 6 hours or overnight. Remove from freezer to defrost slightly, 5 minutes. Break into small chunks and process in a food processor, in batches, until smooth and creamy.) Serve immediately or transfer to a storage container and freeze for up to 2 hours.

TIPS & NOTES
- **Make Ahead Tip**: If frozen longer than 2 hours, break into chunks and puree in a food processor until smooth before serving.

NUTRITION

Per serving: 74 calories; 1 g fat (0 g sat, 0 g mono); 2 mg cholesterol; 16 g carbohydrates; 2 g protein; 0 gfiber; 21 mg sodium; 155 mg potassium.
Carbohydrate Servings: 1
Exchanges: 1 fruit

DAY 14
BREAKFAST

Sunday Sausage Strata
Skim milk (1 cup)
Grapefruit (1/2)

LUNCH

Barbecued Chicken Burritos or Turkey Sausage & Arugula Pasta
Roasted Corn, Black Bean & Mango Salad
Orange (1 large)

SNACK

Melon (1 cup, cubes)
Low-fat vanilla yogurt (8 oz.)

DINNER

Roasted Vegetable Pasta or Five-Spice Turkey & Lettuce Wraps
Spinach Salad with Black Olive Vinaigrette
Blueberries with Lemon Cream

DAY 14 RECIPES

Sunday Sausage Strata

INGREDIENTS
- 1/2 pound turkey breakfast sausage, (four 2-ounce links), casing removed
- 2 medium onions, chopped (2 cups)
- 1 medium red bell pepper, seeded and diced (1 1/2 cups)
- 12 large eggs
- 4 cups 1% milk
- 1 teaspoon salt, or to taste
- Freshly ground pepper, to taste
- 6 cups cubed, whole-wheat country bread, (about 7 slices, crusts removed)
- 1 tablespoon Dijon mustard
- 1 1/2 cups grated Swiss cheese, (4 ounces)

PREPARATION
1. Coat a 9-by-13-inch baking dish (or similar shallow 3-quart baking dish) with cooking spray.
2. Cook sausage in a large nonstick skillet over medium heat, crumbling with a wooden spoon, until lightly browned, 3 to 4 minutes. Transfer to a plate lined with paper towels to drain. Add onions and bell pepper to the pan and cook, stirring often, until softened, 3 to 4 minutes.
3. Whisk eggs, milk, salt and pepper in a large bowl until blended.
4. Spread bread in the prepared baking dish. Scatter the sausage and the onion mixture evenly over the bread. Brush with mustard. Sprinkle with cheese. Pour in the egg mixture. Cover with plastic wrap and refrigerate for at least 2 hours or overnight.
5. Preheat oven to 350 degrees F. Bake the strata, uncovered, until puffed, lightly browned and set in the center, 55 to 65 minutes. Let cool for about 5 minutes before serving hot.

TIPS & NOTES
- **Make Ahead Tip**: Prepare through Step 4 the night before serving.

NUTRITION
Per serving: 255 calories; 13 g fat (45 g sat, 4 g mono); 229 mg cholesterol; 19 g carbohydrates; 17 gprotein; 2 g fiber; 513 mg sodium; 380 mg potassium.
Nutrition Bonus: Vitamin C (72% daily value), Calcium (23% dv).
Carbohydrate Servings: 1
Exchanges: 2/3 starch, 1/3 milk, 1/2 vegetable, 1 very lean protein, 1 1/3 medium-fat protein

Barbecued Chicken Burritos

INGREDIENTS
- 1 2-pound roasted chicken, skin discarded, meat removed from bones and shredded (4 cups)
- 1/2 cup prepared barbecue sauce
- 1 cup canned black beans, rinsed
- 1/2 cup frozen corn, thawed, or canned corn, drained
- 1/4 cup reduced-fat sour cream
- 4 leaves romaine lettuce
- 4 10-inch whole-wheat tortillas
- 2 limes, cut in wedges

PREPARATION

1. Place a large nonstick skillet over medium-high heat. Add chicken, barbecue sauce, beans, corn and sour cream; stir to combine. Cook until hot, 4 to 5 minutes.
2. Assemble the wraps by placing a lettuce leaf in the center of each tortilla and topping with one-fourth of the chicken mixture; roll as you would a burrito. Slice in half diagonally and serve warm, with lime wedges.

TIPS & NOTES

- Eat neat: Keeping the filling inside a wrap or burrito can be a challenge, especially if you're on the go. That's why we recommend wrapping your burrito in foil so you can pick it up and eat it without losing the filling, peeling back the foil as you go.

NUTRITION

Per serving: 404 calories; 8 g fat (2 g sat, 1 g mono); 80 mg cholesterol; 48 g carbohydrates; 32 g protein; 6 g fiber; 600 mg sodium; 531 mg potassium.
Nutrition Bonus: Fiber (24% daily value), Iron (20% dv).
Carbohydrate Servings: 2 1/2
Exchanges: 2 1/2 starch, 1 vegetable, 4 very lean meat

Turkey Sausage & Arugula Pasta

INGREDIENTS

- 12 ounces whole-wheat short pasta, such as shells or twists
- 8 ounces hot Italian turkey sausage links, removed from casings
- 3 cloves garlic, chopped
- 8 cups arugula, or baby spinach
- 2 cups halved cherry tomatoes
- 1/2 cup finely shredded Pecorino Romano, or Parmesan cheese
- 1 teaspoon freshly ground pepper and 1/4 teaspoon salt
- 1 tablespoon extra-virgin olive oil

PREPARATION

1. Bring a large pot of water to a boil. Cook pasta until just tender, 9 to 11 minutes, or according to package directions.
2. Meanwhile, cook sausage in a large nonstick skillet over medium-high heat, breaking it up into small pieces with a wooden spoon, until cooked through, about 5 minutes. Stir in garlic, arugula (or spinach) and tomatoes. Cook, stirring often, until the greens wilt and the tomatoes begin to break down, about 3 minutes. Remove from heat; cover and keep warm.

3. Combine 1/2 cup cheese, pepper and salt in a large bowl. Measure out 1/2 cup of the cooking liquid; drain the pasta. Whisk the cooking liquid and oil into the cheese mixture; add the pasta and toss to combine. Serve the pasta topped with the sausage mixture and an extra sprinkle of cheese, if desired.

NUTRITION
Per serving: 352 calories; 9 g fat (3 g sat, 2 g mono); 26 mg cholesterol; 47 g carbohydrates; 0 g added sugars; 18 g protein; 6 g fiber; 382 mg sodium; 379 mg potassium.
Nutrition Bonus: Vitamin A (30% daily value), Fiber (26% dv), Vitamin C (20% dv), Calcium (15% dv).
Carbohydrate Servings: 2 1/2
Exchanges: 2.5 starch, 2 vegetable, 2 medium-fat meat

Roasted Corn, Black Bean & Mango Salad

INGREDIENTS
- 2 teaspoons canola oil
- 1 clove garlic, minced
- 1 1/2 cups corn kernels, (from 3 ears)
- 1 large ripe mango, (about 1 pound), peeled and diced
- 1 15-ounce or 19-ounce can black beans, rinsed
- 1/2 cup chopped red onion
- 1/2 cup diced red bell pepper
- 3 tablespoons lime juice
- 1 small canned chipotle pepper in adobo sauce, (see Ingredient Note), drained and chopped
- 1 1/2 tablespoons chopped fresh cilantro
- 1/4 teaspoon ground cumin
- 1/4 teaspoon salt

PREPARATION
1. Heat oil in a large nonstick skillet over medium-high heat. Add garlic and cook, stirring, until fragrant, about 30 seconds. Stir in corn and cook, stirring occasionally, until browned, about 8 minutes. Transfer the corn mixture to a large bowl. Stir in mango, beans, onion, bell pepper, lime juice, chipotle, cilantro, cumin and salt.

TIPS & NOTES
- **Make Ahead Tip**: Cover and refrigerate for up to 8 hours. Serve at room temperature.

- **Ingredient Note:** Chipotle peppers are smoked jalapenos with a fiery taste that are canned in adobo sauce. Look for them in the Hispanic section of large supermarkets and in specialty stores.

NUTRITION
Per serving: 125 calories; 2 g fat (0 g sat, 1 g mono); 0 mg cholesterol; 26 g carbohydrates; 0 g added sugars; 4 g protein; 4 g fiber; 245 mg sodium; 223 mg potassium.
Nutrition Bonus: Vitamin C (70% daily value), Fiber (18% dv).
Carbohydrate Servings: 2
Exchanges: 1 starch, 1 fruit

Roasted Vegetable Pasta

INGREDIENTS
- 1 medium zucchini, diced
- 1 red or yellow bell pepper, seeded and diced
- 1 large onion, thinly sliced
- 2 tablespoons extra-virgin olive oil, divided
- Salt & freshly ground pepper, to taste
- 2 large tomatoes, chopped
- 1/4 cup chopped fresh basil
- 2 cloves garlic, minced
- 12 ounces whole-wheat pasta
- 1/2 cup crumbled feta cheese

PREPARATION

1. Preheat oven to 450°F. Put a large pot of lightly salted water on to boil.
2. Toss zucchini, bell pepper and onion with 1 tablespoon oil in a large roasting pan or a large baking sheet with sides. Season with salt and pepper. Roast the vegetables, stirring every 5 minutes, until tender and browned, 10 to 20 minutes.
3. Meanwhile, combine tomatoes, basil, garlic and the remaining 1 tablespoon oil in a large bowl. Season with salt and pepper.
4. Cook pasta until just tender, 8 to 10 minutes. Drain and transfer to the bowl with the tomatoes. Add the roasted vegetables and toss well. Adjust seasoning with salt and pepper. Serve, passing feta cheese separately.

NUTRITION
Per serving: 288 calories; 12 g fat (4 g sat, 6 g mono); 17 mg cholesterol; 75 g carbohydrates; 17 g protein;6 g fiber; 226 mg sodium; 619 mg potassium.

Nutrition Bonus: Vitamin C (90% daily value), Fiber (34% dv), Vitamin A (25% dv).
Carbohydrate Servings: 2 1/2
Exchanges: 3 starch, 1 vegetable, 1 fat

Five-Spice Turkey & Lettuce Wraps

INGREDIENTS
- 1/2 cup water
- 1/2 cup instant brown rice
- 2 teaspoons sesame oil
- 1 pound 93%-lean ground turkey
- 1 tablespoon minced fresh ginger
- 1 large red bell pepper, finely diced
- 1 8-ounce can water chestnuts, rinsed and chopped
- 1/2 cup reduced-sodium chicken broth
- 2 tablespoons hoisin sauce, (see Note)
- 1 teaspoon five-spice powder, (see Note)
- 1/2 teaspoon salt
- 2 heads Boston lettuce, leaves separated
- 1/2 cup chopped fresh herbs, such as cilantro, basil, mint and/or chives
- 1 large carrot, shredded

PREPARATION
1. Bring water to a boil in a small saucepan. Add rice; reduce heat to low, cover and cook for 5 minutes. Remove from the heat.
2. Meanwhile, heat oil in a large nonstick pan over medium-high heat. Add turkey and ginger; cook, crumbling with a wooden spoon, until the turkey is cooked through, about 6 minutes. Stir in the cooked rice, bell pepper, water chestnuts, broth, hoisin sauce, five-spice powder and salt; cook until heated through, about 1 minute.
3. To serve, divide lettuce leaves among plates, spoon some of the turkey mixture into each leaf, top with herbs and carrot and roll into wraps.

TIPS & NOTES
- **Make Ahead Tip**: Prepare the filling (through Step 2), cover and refrigerate for up to 1 day. Serve cold or reheat in the microwave.
- **Notes:** Hoisin sauce is a spicy, sweet sauce made from soybeans, chiles, garlic and spices. It will keep in the refrigerator for at least a year.
- Often a blend of cinnamon, cloves, fennel seed, star anise and Szechuan peppercorns, five-spice powder was originally considered a cure-all miracle blend encompassing the five elements (sour, bitter, sweet, pungent, salty). Look for it in the supermarket spice section.

NUTRITION

Per serving: 276 calories; 11 g fat (3 g sat, 1 g mono); 66 mg cholesterol; 24 g carbohydrates; 0 g added sugars; 26 g protein; 5 g fiber; 543 mg sodium; 390 mg potassium.
Nutrition Bonus: Vitamin A (150% daily value), Vitamin C (140% dv), Iron (25% dv), Folate (20% dv).
Carbohydrate Servings: 1
Exchanges: 1/2 starch, 2 vegetable, 3 lean meat

Spinach Salad with Black Olive Vinaigrette

INGREDIENTS
- 3 tablespoons extra-virgin olive oil
- 1 1/2 tablespoons red-wine vinegar, or lemon juice
- 6 pitted Kalamata olives, finely chopped
- 1/4 teaspoon salt
- Freshly ground pepper, to taste
- 6 cups torn spinach leaves
- 1/2 cucumber, seeded and sliced
- 1/2 red onion, thinly sliced

PREPARATION
1. Whisk oil, vinegar (or lemon juice) and olives in a salad bowl. Season with salt and pepper. Add spinach, cucumbers and onions; toss well. Serve immediately.

NUTRITION

Per serving: 128 calories; 12 g fat (2 g sat, 9 g mono); 0 mg cholesterol; 3 g carbohydrates; 2 g protein; 1 gfiber; 271 mg sodium; 284 mg potassium.
Nutrition Bonus: Vitamin A (80% daily value), Folate (22% dv), Vitamin C (20% dv).
Exchanges: 1 vegetable, 2 fat

Blueberries with Lemon Cream

INGREDIENTS
- 4 ounces reduced-fat cream cheese (Neufchâtel)
- 3/4 cup low-fat vanilla yogurt
- 1 teaspoon honey
- 2 teaspoons freshly grated lemon zest
- 2 cups fresh blueberries

PREPARATION
1. Using a fork, break up cream cheese in a medium bowl. Drain off any liquid from the yogurt; add yogurt to the bowl along with honey. Using an electric mixer, beat at high speed until light and creamy. Stir in lemon zest.
2. Layer the lemon cream and blueberries in dessert dishes or wineglasses. If not serving immediately, cover and refrigerate for up to 8 hours.

TIPS & NOTES
- **Make Ahead Tip**: Cover and refrigerate for up to 8 hours.

NUTRITION
Per serving: 156 calories; 7 g fat (4 g sat, 0 g mono); 22 mg cholesterol; 19 g carbohydrates; 6 g protein; 2 g fiber; 151 mg sodium; 189 mg potassium.
Nutrition Bonus: Vitamin C (15% daily value).
Carbohydrate Servings: 1
Exchanges: 1 fruit, 1 fat (saturated)

DAY 15
BREAKFAST

Morning Smoothie
Whole-Wheat Irish Soda Bread
Pear Butter
LUNCH

Romaine Salad with Chicken, Apricots & Mint
Whole-wheat pita bread (1 medium pita)
Raspberries (1 cup)
Skim milk (1 cup)
SNACK

Low-fat cottage cheese (1 cup)
Melon (1 cup, cubes)
DINNER

Pacific Sole with Oranges & Pecans or Saute of Chicken with Apples & Leeks
Roasted Snap Peas with Shallots or Chard with Shallots, Pancetta & Walnuts
Rice Pilaf with Lime & Cashews
Polenta Biscotti

DAY 15 RECIPES

Morning Smoothie

INGREDIENTS
- 1 1/4 cups orange juice, preferably calcium-fortified
- 1 banana
- 1 1/4 cups frozen berries, such as raspberries, blackberries, blueberries and/or strawberries
- 1/2 cup low-fat silken tofu, or low-fat plain yogurt
- 1 tablespoon sugar, or Splenda Granular (optional)

PREPARATION
1. Combine orange juice, banana, berries, tofu (or yogurt) and sugar (or Splenda), if using, in a blender; cover and blend until creamy. Serve immediately.

NUTRITION

Per serving: 139 calories; 2 g fat (0 g sat, 0 g mono); 0 mg cholesterol; 33 g carbohydrates; 0 g added sugars; 4 g protein; 4 g fiber; 19 mg sodium; 421 mg potassium.
Nutrition Bonus: Vitamin C (110% daily value), Fiber (16% dv).
Carbohydrate Servings: 2
Exchanges: 2 fruit, 1/2 low-fat milk

Whole-Wheat Irish Soda Bread

INGREDIENTS
- 2 cups whole-wheat flour
- 2 cups all-purpose flour, plus more for dusting
- 1 teaspoon baking soda
- 1 teaspoon salt
- 2 1/4 cups buttermilk

PREPARATION
1. Preheat oven to 450°F. Coat a baking sheet with cooking spray and sprinkle with a little flour.
2. Whisk whole-wheat flour, all-purpose flour, baking soda and salt in a large bowl. Make a well in the center and pour in buttermilk. Using one hand, stir in full circles (starting in the center of the bowl working toward the outside of the bowl) until all the flour is incorporated. The dough should be soft but not too wet and sticky. When it all comes together, in a matter of seconds, turn it out onto a well-floured surface. Clean dough off your hand.

3. Pat and roll the dough gently with floury hands, just enough to tidy it up and give it a round shape. Flip over and flatten slightly to about 2 inches. Transfer the loaf to the prepared baking sheet. Mark with a deep cross using a serrated knife and prick each of the four quadrants.
4. Bake the bread for 20 minutes. Reduce oven temperature to 400° and continue to bake until the loaf is brown on top and sounds hollow when tapped, 30 to 35 minutes more. Transfer the loaf to a wire rack and let cool for about 30 minutes.

NUTRITION

Per slice: 165 calories; 1 g fat (0 g sat, 0 g mono); 2 mg cholesterol; 37 g carbohydrates; 8 g protein; 3 gfiber; 347 mg sodium; 179 mg potassium.
Nutrition Bonus: Fiber (13% daily value).
Carbohydrate Servings: 2
Exchanges: 2 starch

Pear Butter

INGREDIENTS
- 4 ripe but firm Bartlett pears, (1-1 1/4 pounds), peeled, cored and cut into 1-inch chunks
- 3/4 cup pear nectar

PREPARATION
1. Place pears and pear nectar in a heavy medium saucepan; bring to a simmer. Cover and simmer over medium-low heat, stirring occasionally, until the pears are very tender, 30 to 35 minutes. Cooking time will vary depending on the ripeness of the pears.
2. Mash the pears with a potato masher. Cook, uncovered, over medium-low heat, stirring often, until the puree has cooked down to a thick mass (somewhat thicker than applesauce), 20 to 30 minutes. Stir almost constantly toward the end of cooking. Scrape the pear butter into a bowl or storage container and let cool.

TIPS & NOTES

- **Make Ahead Tip:** Store in an airtight container in the refrigerator for up to 2 weeks or freeze for up to 6 months.

NUTRITION

Per tablespoon: 22 calories; 0 g fat (0 g sat, 0 g mono); 0 mg cholesterol; 6 g carbohydrates; 0 g protein; 1 g fiber; 1 mg sodium; 33 mg potassium.
Carbohydrate Servings: 1/2

Exchanges: 1/2 fruit

Romaine Salad with Chicken, Apricots & Mint

INGREDIENTS
MARINADE & DRESSING
- 1/2 cup dried apricots
- 1 cup hot water
- 2 cups loosely packed mint leaves, (about 1 bunch)
- 1 teaspoon freshly grated orange zest
- 1/2 cup orange juice
- 2 tablespoons honey
- 4 teaspoons Dijon mustard
- 4 teaspoons red-wine vinegar
- 1/2 teaspoon salt, or to taste
- Freshly ground pepper, to taste
- 1/4 cup extra-virgin olive oil

SALAD
- 1 pound boneless, skinless chicken breast, trimmed of fat
- 1 large head romaine lettuce, torn into bite-size pieces (10 cups)
- 6 fresh apricots, or plums, pitted and cut into wedges
- 1 cup loosely packed mint leaves, (about 1/2 bunch), roughly chopped
- 1/2 cup sliced almonds, toasted (see Tip)

PREPARATION
1. Preheat grill.
2. To prepare marinade & dressing: Soak dried apricots in hot water for 10 minutes. Drain and transfer apricots to a food processor. Add 2 cups mint, orange zest, orange juice, honey, mustard, vinegar, salt and pepper. Process until smooth. With the motor running, gradually drizzle in oil. Reserve 1 cup for the dressing.
3. To prepare salad: Transfer the remaining marinade to a large sealable plastic bag. Add chicken, seal and turn to coat. Marinate in the refrigerator for 20 minutes.
4. Lightly oil the grill rack (hold a piece of oil-soaked paper towel with tongs and rub it over the grate). Grill the chicken over medium-high heat until no longer pink in the center, 6 to 8 minutes per side. (Discard the marinade.)
5. Meanwhile, combine lettuce, apricot (or plum) wedges and chopped mint in a large bowl. Add the reserved dressing and toss to coat. Divide the salad among 4 plates. Slice the chicken and arrange over the salads. Sprinkle with almonds and serve.

TIPS & NOTES
- **Make Ahead Tip**: The dressing will keep, covered, in the refrigerator for up to 2 days.
- **Tip**: To toast almonds: Spread on a baking sheet and bake at 350°F until golden brown and fragrant, 5 to 7 minutes. Toasted almonds will keep, tightly covered, at room temperature for up to 1 week.

NUTRITION
Per serving: 456 calories; 20 g fat (3 g sat, 13 g mono); 66 mg cholesterol; 33 g carbohydrates; 34 gprotein; 10 g fiber; 433 mg sodium; 1281 mg potassium.
Nutrition Bonus: Vitamin A (230% daily value), Vitamin C (110% dv), Fiber (41% dv).
Carbohydrate Servings: 2
Exchanges: 1 fruit, 3 vegetable, 4 lean meat, 1fat (mono)

Pacific Sole with Oranges & Pecans

INGREDIENTS
- 1 orange
- 10 ounces Pacific sole, (see Note) or tilapia fillets
- 1/4 teaspoon salt
- 1/4 teaspoon freshly ground pepper
- 2 teaspoons unsalted butter
- 1 medium shallot, minced
- 2 tablespoons white-wine vinegar
- 2 tablespoons chopped pecans, toasted (see Cooking Tip)
- 2 tablespoons chopped fresh dill

PREPARATION
1. Using a sharp paring knife, remove the skin and white pith from orange. Hold the fruit over a medium bowl and cut between the membranes to release individual orange sections into the bowl, collecting any juice as well. Discard membranes, pith and skin.
2. Sprinkle both sides of fillets with salt and pepper. Coat a large nonstick skillet with cooking spray and place over medium heat. Add the fillets and cook 1 minute for sole or 3 minutes for tilapia. Gently flip and cook until the fish is opaque in the center and just cooked through, 1 to 2 minutes for sole or 3 to 5 minutes for tilapia. Divide between 2 serving plates; tent with foil.
3. Add butter to the pan and melt over medium heat. Add shallot and cook, stirring, until soft, about 30 seconds. Add vinegar and the orange sections and juice; loosen any browned bits on the bottom of the pan and cook for 30 seconds. Spoon the sauce over the fish and sprinkle each portion with pecans and dill. Serve immediately. Makes 2 servings.

TIPS & NOTES
- **Ingredient Note:** The term "sole" is widely used for many types of flatfish from both the Atlantic and Pacific. Flounder and Atlantic halibut are included in the group that is often identified as sole or grey sole. The best choices are Pacific, Dover or English sole. Other sole and flounder are overfished.
- **Cooking Tip:** To toast chopped nuts or seeds: Cook in a small dry skillet over medium-low heat, stirring constantly, until fragrant and lightly browned, 2 to 4 minutes.

NUTRITION
Per serving: 234 calories; 9 g fat (3 g sat, 3 g mono); 70 mg cholesterol; 11 g carbohydrates; 0 g added sugars; 28 g protein; 2 g fiber; 401 mg sodium; 556 mg potassium.
Nutrition Bonus: Vitamin C (70% daily value); Calcium (20% dv).
Carbohydrate Servings: 1
Exchanges: 1 fruit, 4 very lean meat, 1 fat

Saute of Chicken with Apples & Leeks

INGREDIENTS
- 4 boneless, skinless chicken breast halves (1-1 1/4 pounds), trimmed
- 3 teaspoons extra-virgin olive oil, divided
- 1/4 teaspoon salt
- Freshly ground pepper to taste
- 2 large leeks, white parts only, washed and cut into julienne strips (2 cups)
- 2 large cloves garlic, minced
- 1 tablespoon sugar
- 2 teaspoons minced fresh rosemary, or 1/2 teaspoon dried
- 1/4 cup cider vinegar
- 2 firm tart apples, such as York or Granny Smith, peeled, cored and thinly sliced
- 1 cup reduced-sodium chicken broth

PREPARATION
1. Place chicken breasts between 2 sheets of plastic wrap. Use a rolling pin or a small heavy pot to pound them to a thickness of 1/2 inch.
2. Heat 1 1/2 teaspoons oil in a large nonstick skillet over medium-high heat. Season the chicken breasts with salt and pepper and add to the pan. Cook until browned on both sides, 4 to 5 minutes per side. Transfer to a plate and keep warm.
3. Reduce the heat to low. Add the remaining 1 1/2 teaspoons oil and leeks. Cook, stirring, until the leeks are soft, about 5 minutes. Add garlic, sugar and rosemary and cook until fragrant, about 2 minutes more. Increase the heat to medium-high, stir in vinegar and cook until most of the liquid has evaporated.

4. Add apples and broth and cook, stirring once or twice, until the apples are tender, about 3 minutes. Reduce the heat to low and return the chicken and any juices to the pan. Simmer gently until the chicken is heated through. Serve immediately.

NUTRITION
Per serving: 235 calories; 7 g fat (1 g sat, 4 g mono); 64 mg cholesterol; 19 g carbohydrates; 0 g added sugars; 25 g protein; 2 g fiber; 245 mg sodium; 346 mg potassium.
Nutrition Bonus: Selenium (30% daily value), Vitamin A (16% dv).
Carbohydrate Servings: 1
Exchanges: 1 fruit, 4 very lean meat, 1 fat

Roasted Snap Peas with Shallots

INGREDIENTS
- 1 pound sugar snap peas, trimmed (about 4 cups)
- 1 large shallot, halved and thinly sliced (about 1/4 cup)
- 2 teaspoons extra-virgin olive oil
- 1/4 teaspoon salt
- Freshly ground pepper to taste
- 2 pieces cooked bacon, crumbled (optional)

PREPARATION
1. Preheat oven to 475°F.
2. Toss peas, shallot, oil, salt and pepper in a medium bowl. Transfer to a baking sheet and spread in a single layer. Roast in the oven, stirring once halfway through, until the peas are tender and beginning to brown slightly, 12 to 14 minutes. Serve warm, sprinkled with bacon if desired.

NUTRITION
Per serving: 83 calories; 2 g fat (0 g sat, 2 g mono); 0 mg cholesterol; 11 g carbohydrates; 3 g protein; 3 gfiber; 147 mg sodium; 212 mg potassium.
Nutrition Bonus: Vitamin C (20% daily value).
Carbohydrate Servings: 1
Exchanges: 1 1/2 vegetable, 1/2 fat

Chard with Shallots, Pancetta & Walnuts

INGREDIENTS
- 2 thin slices pancetta, (1 1/2 ounces), diced (see Tip)
- 2 medium shallots, thinly sliced
- 1 pound chard, stems and leaves separated, chopped (see Note)

- 1 teaspoon chopped fresh thyme
- 1/4 cup water
- 1 tablespoon lemon juice
- 2 tablespoons chopped walnuts, toasted (see Tip)
- 1/4 teaspoon freshly ground pepper

PREPARATION
1. Cook pancetta in a Dutch oven over medium heat, stirring, until it begins to brown, 4 to 6 minutes. Using a slotted spoon, transfer to a plate lined with paper towels.
2. Add shallots, chard stems and thyme to the pan drippings and cook, stirring, until the shallots begin to brown, 4 to 5 minutes. Add chard leaves, water and lemon juice and cook, stirring, until wilted, about 2 minutes. Cover and cook until tender, 2 to 4 minutes more. Remove from the heat; stir in the pancetta, walnuts and pepper.

TIPS & NOTES
- **Tips:** Pancetta is an unsmoked Italian bacon usually found in the deli section of large supermarkets and specialty food stores. Regular or turkey bacon may be substituted.
- **To toast chopped walnuts:** Cook in a small dry skillet over medium-low heat, stirring constantly, until fragrant and lightly browned, 2 to 4 minutes.
- **Note:** After washing the chard, allow some of the water to cling to the leaves. It helps steam the chard and prevents a dry dish.

NUTRITION
Per serving: 62 calories; 4 g fat (1 g sat, 1 g mono); 5 mg cholesterol; 5 g carbohydrates; 0 g added sugars; 3 g protein; 2 g fiber; 252 mg sodium; 452 mg potassium.
Nutrition Bonus: Vitamin K (346% daily value), Vitamin A (90% dv), Vitamin C (25% dv), Magnesium (18% dv).
Exchanges: 1 vegetable, 1 fat

Rice Pilaf with Lime & Cashews

INGREDIENTS
- 1 cup basmati rice
- 1 1/2 cups cold water
- 1 tablespoon canola oil
- 1 teaspoon black or yellow mustard seeds
- 2 tablespoons coarsely chopped cashews
- 2-3 tablespoons lime juice

- 2 tablespoons finely chopped fresh cilantro, or 12 fresh kari leaves (see Ingredient Note), chopped
- 2-3 fresh Thai, cayenne or serrano chiles, or 1 jalapeno pepper, seeded and minced
- 1/4 teaspoon turmeric
- 1/4 teaspoon salt

PREPARATION

1. Place rice in a medium saucepan with enough water to cover by about 1 inch. Gently swish grains in the pan with your fingertips until the water becomes cloudy; drain. Repeat 3 or 4 times, until the water remains almost clear. Cover with 1 1/2 cups cold water; let soak for 30 minutes.
2. Bring the rice and water to a boil over medium-high heat. Cook, uncovered, stirring occasionally, until most of the liquid evaporates from the surface, 4 to 6 minutes. Cover the pan and reduce the heat to the lowest setting; cook for 5 minutes. Remove from the heat and let sit undisturbed for 5 minutes.
3. Meanwhile, heat oil in a small skillet over medium-high heat; add mustard seeds. When the seeds begin to pop, cover the pan until the popping stops. Reduce heat to medium; add cashews and cook, stirring, until golden brown, 30 seconds to 1 minute. Remove from the heat; add lime juice, cilantro (or kari leaves), chiles (or jalapeno), turmeric and salt. Add the mixture to the cooked rice; mix well. Brown-Rice Variation: If using brown basmati rice, rinse as directed in Step 1 then soak in 2 cups water. In Step 2, bring rice and water to a boil over medium-high heat. Reduce the heat to low, cover and simmer until the water is absorbed and the rice is tender, 25 to 30 minutes. Remove from the heat and let sit for 5 minutes. Proceed with Step 3.

TIPS & NOTES

- **Ingredient Note:** Olive-green kari leaves (also called curry leaves), a distant cousin to the citrus family, have a delicate aroma and flavor and are available in the produce section of Indian grocery stores. They last up to 3 weeks in the refrigerator or in the freezer for up to a month. Do not use the dried (and highly insipid) version of these leaves, substitute cilantro instead.

NUTRITION

Per serving: 161 calories; 4 g fat (1 g sat, 2 g mono); 0 mg cholesterol; 29 g carbohydrates; 3 g protein; 0 gfiber; 101 mg sodium; 36 mg potassium.
Carbohydrate Servings: 2
Exchanges: 1 1/2 starch, 1/2 fat

Polenta Biscotti

INGREDIENTS
- 2 cups all-purpose flour
- 1 cup sugar
- 1/2 cup fine cornmeal, or polenta (see Note)
- 1 teaspoon baking powder
- 1/4 teaspoon salt
- 3 large eggs
- 2 tablespoons mild-flavored olive oil, or canola oil
- 1 teaspoon vanilla extract

PREPARATION
1. Position racks in the upper and lower thirds of oven; preheat to 325°F. Coat 2 large baking sheets with cooking spray.
2. Whisk flour, sugar, cornmeal (or polenta), baking powder and salt in a large bowl. Whisk eggs, oil and vanilla in another bowl until frothy and well combined. Add the egg mixture to the flour mixture and stir with a spoon until a soft dough forms.
3. Turn the dough out onto a well-floured work surface. Divide it in half and shape each half into a log 12 inches long by 2 inches wide. Brush off excess flour and place the logs on one baking sheet.
4. Bake the logs on the upper rack until almost firm when pressed on top, 20 to 25 minutes. Remove from the oven and let cool on the pan for 20 minutes; reduce the oven temperature to 300°F.
5. Place the logs on a cutting board and slice diagonally into 1/2-inch-thick slices using a serrated knife. Divide the biscotti between the 2 baking sheets, standing them up about 1 inch apart.
6. Return the biscotti to the oven and bake until lightly colored and dry, 20 to 25 minutes. Transfer to wire racks to cool (the biscotti will crisp as they cool).

TIPS & NOTES
- **Make Ahead Tip**: Store in an airtight container for up to 4 days.
- **Note:** Imported varieties of coarsely ground cornmeal may be labeled "polenta"—that's what you need for this recipe. Porridge made from the cornmeal is also called polenta, so it can be confusing.
- Storage smarts: To extend the life of your baked goods, store them in an airtight container in a single layer or between layers of parchment paper to prevent sticking.

NUTRITION
Per biscotti: 48 calories; 1 g fat (0 g sat, 1 g mono); 13 mg cholesterol; 9 g carbohydrates; 1 g protein; 0 gfiber; 28 mg sodium; 10 mg potassium.

Carbohydrate Servings: 1/2
Exchanges: 1/2 other carbohydrate

DAY 16
BREAKFAST
Cocoa-Date Oatmeal
Skim milk (1 cup)
Melon (1 cup, cubes)
LUNCH
Skim milk (1 cup)
Five-Spice Chicken & Orange Salad or Light Salade aux Lardons
Apricot (1 cup, halves)
Whole-wheat pita bread (1 medium pita)
SNACK
White Bean Spread
Carrot sticks (1 cup)
DINNER
Pork Medallions with a Port-&-Cranberry Pan Sauce or Bistro Beef Tenderloin
Quick-cooking barley (1 cup)
Roasted Florets
Grape and Feta Mixed Green Special
Honeyed Couscous Pudding

DAY 16 RECIPES

Cocoa-Date Oatmeal

INGREDIENTS
- 1/4 cup chopped pitted dates, (10-12 dates)
- 1 cup old-fashioned rolled oats
- 2 tablespoons cocoa
- Pinch of salt
- 2 cups water

PREPARATION
1. Combine dates, oats, cocoa and salt in a 1-quart microwavable container. Slowly stir in the water. Partially cover with plastic wrap. Microwave on Medium for 4 or 5 minutes, then stir. Microwave on Medium again for 3 or 4 minutes, then stir. Continue cooking and stirring until the cereal is creamy.

TIPS & NOTES
- **Note:** The cooking times will vary considerably depending on the power of your microwave. New microwaves tend to cook much faster than older models.

NUTRITION
Per serving: 142 calories; 4 g fat (1 g sat, 1 g mono); 0 mg cholesterol; 61 g carbohydrates; 0 g added sugars; 8 g protein; 9 g fiber; 81 mg sodium; 497 mg potassium.
Nutrition Bonus: Fiber (16% daily value).
Carbohydrate Servings: 2
Exchanges: 11/2 starch, 1/2 fruit
Nutrition Note: Chocolate contains compounds called flavonoids, which can function as antioxidants and also seem to keep blood from clotting. Cocoa is unusually rich in two kinds of flavonoids, flavonols and proanthocyanidins, which appear to be especially potent. To get

Five-Spice Chicken & Orange Salad

INGREDIENTS
- 6 teaspoons extra-virgin olive oil, divided
- 1 teaspoon five-spice powder, (see Note)
- 1 teaspoon kosher salt, divided
- 1/2 teaspoon freshly ground pepper, plus more to taste
- 1 pound boneless, skinless chicken breasts, trimmed
- 3 oranges
- 12 cups mixed Asian or salad greens
- 1 red bell pepper, cut into thin strips
- 1/2 cup slivered red onion
- 3 tablespoons cider vinegar
- 1 tablespoon Dijon mustard

PREPARATION
1. Preheat oven to 450°F. Combine 1 teaspoon oil, five-spice powder, 1/2 teaspoon salt and 1/2 teaspoon pepper in a small bowl. Rub the mixture into both sides of the chicken breasts.
2. Heat 1 teaspoon oil in a large ovenproof nonstick skillet over medium-high heat. Add chicken breasts; cook until browned on one side, 3 to 5 minutes. Turn them over and transfer the pan to the oven. Roast until the chicken is just cooked through (an instant-read thermometer inserted into the center should read 165°F), 6 to 8 minutes. Transfer the chicken to a cutting board; let rest for 5 minutes.

3. Meanwhile, peel and segment two of the oranges (see Tip), collecting segments and any juice in a large bowl. (Discard membranes, pith and skin.) Add the greens, bell pepper and onion to the bowl. Zest and juice the remaining orange. Place the zest and juice in a small bowl; whisk in vinegar, mustard, the remaining 4 teaspoons oil, remaining 1/2 teaspoon salt and freshly ground pepper to taste. Pour the dressing over the salad; toss to combine. Slice the chicken and serve on the salad.

TIPS & NOTES

- **Make Ahead Tip**: Prepare through Step 2. Store the chicken in an airtight container in the refrigerator for up to 2 days. Slice and serve chilled.
- **Note:** Often a blend of cinnamon, cloves, fennel seed, star anise and Szechuan peppercorns, five-spice powder was originally considered a cure-all miracle blend encompassing the five elements (sour, bitter, sweet, pungent, salty). Look for it in the supermarket spice section.
- **Tip:** To segment citrus: With a sharp knife, remove the skin and white pith from the fruit. Working over a bowl, cut the segments from their surrounding membranes. Squeeze juice into the bowl before discarding the membranes.

NUTRITION
Per serving: 278 calories; 10 g fat (2 g sat, 6 g mono); 63 mg cholesterol; 23 g carbohydrates; 0 g added sugars; 26 g protein; 7 g fiber; 491 mg sodium; 450 mg potassium.
Nutrition Bonus: Vitamin C (170% daily value), Vitamin A (140% dv), Selenium (30% dv), Iron (15% dv).
Carbohydrate Servings: 1
Exchanges: 1 fruit, 1 1/2 vegetable, 3 lean meat, 1 1/2 fat

Light Salade aux Lardons

INGREDIENTS

- 3 tablespoons extra-virgin olive oil, divided
- 8 ounces Canadian bacon, cut into 1/2-inch dice (1 3/4 cups)
- 2 medium heads frisée, or curly-leaf endive lettuce, torn (8 cups)
- 1 large shallot, minced
- 3 tablespoons white-wine vinegar
- 1 teaspoon Dijon mustard
- 1/4 teaspoon salt
- 1/4 teaspoon freshly ground pepper, plus more to taste
- 4 large eggs

PREPARATION
1. Heat 1 tablespoon oil in a skillet over medium-high heat. Add bacon; cook, stirring, until brown and crisp, about 8 minutes.
2. Use a slotted spoon to transfer the bacon to a large bowl. Add lettuce to the bowl. Add shallot to the pan and cook over medium heat, stirring, until softened, about 2 minutes. Remove from the heat and stir in the remaining 2 tablespoons oil, vinegar, mustard, salt and pepper. Pour this mixture onto the lettuce; toss to coat.
3. Meanwhile, bring about 1 inch of water to a boil in a medium skillet. Crack each egg into a small bowl and slip them one at a time into the boiling water, taking care not to break the yolks. Reduce heat to low. Cover the pan and poach the eggs until the yolks are just set, 4 to 5 minutes.
4. Divide the salad among 4 plates. Top each serving with a poached egg. Grind pepper over the top and serve immediately.

NUTRITION

Per serving: 263 calories; 18 g fat (4 g sat, 11 g mono); 232 mg cholesterol; 8 g carbohydrates; 17 gprotein; 3 g fiber; 902 mg sodium; 589 mg potassium.
Nutrition Bonus: Vitamin A (50% daily value), Folate (43% dv), Selenium (36% dv), Potassium (17% dv), Iron (15% dv), Vitamin C (15% dv).
Carbohydrate Servings: 1/2
Exchanges: 2 vegetable, 2 lean protein, 2 fat

White Bean Spread

INGREDIENTS
- 2 15-ounce cans cannellini beans, (white kidney beans), rinsed
- 1/4 cup extra-virgin olive oil
- 2 tablespoons lemon juice
- Pinch of cayenne pepper
- 1/8 teaspoon salt
- Freshly ground pepper, to taste
- 1/4 cup chopped scallions
- 2 tablespoons chopped fresh dill

PREPARATION
1. Combine beans, oil, lemon juice, cayenne, salt and black pepper in a food processor; process until smooth. Scrape into a bowl; stir in scallions and dill.

TIPS & NOTES
- **Make Ahead Tip**: Cover and refrigerate for up to 4 days.

NUTRITION
Per tablespoon: 25 calories; 1 g fat (0 g sat, 1 g mono); 0 mg cholesterol; 3 g carbohydrates; 0 g added sugars; 1 g protein; 1 g fiber; 44 mg sodium; 2 mg potassium.
Exchanges: free food

Pork Medallions with a Port-&-Cranberry Pan Sauce

INGREDIENTS
- 1/4 cup dried cranberries
- 1/4 cup port
- 1 pound pork tenderloin, trimmed
- Salt & freshly ground pepper to taste
- 1 teaspoon extra-virgin olive oil
- 2 cloves cloves garlic, peeled and halved
- 1 teaspoon balsamic vinegar
- 2 sage leaves
- 1/2 cup reduced-sodium chicken broth

PREPARATION
1. Combine cranberries and port in a small bowl. Set aside. Slice tenderloin into medallions 1 1/2 inches thick. Place between 2 layers of plastic wrap, and pound the medallions with the bottom of a saucepan until they are 1/2 inch thick. Season both sides with salt and pepper.
2. Heat oil in a nonstick skillet over medium-high heat. Sear medallions on one side until golden brown, 2 to 3 minutes. Turn and sear on the other side for 4 to 5 minutes; turn medallions again and continue cooking until golden brown and no longer pink in the center, 2 to 3 minutes. Remove to a serving platter and cover loosely to keep warm.
3. Add garlic to the pan and return to medium-high heat. Cook, stirring, 1 minute. Add port with cranberries, vinegar and sage leaves; cook for 1 minute, scraping skillet for browned bits. Pour in broth, swirl the pan and bring to a boil again. Continue cooking until sauce thickens and is reduced by half, about 3 minutes. Remove the garlic and sage. Season the sauce to taste with salt and pepper. Spoon over the pork and serve.

NUTRITION
Per serving: 194 calories; 5 g fat (2 g sat, 2 g mono); 64 mg cholesterol; 9 g carbohydrates; 0 g added sugars; 23 g protein; 0 g fiber; 137 mg sodium; 370 mg potassium.
Nutrition Bonus: Selenium (55% daily value).
Carbohydrate Servings: 1/2
Exchanges: 1/2 fruit, 4 1/2 lean meat

Bistro Beef Tenderloin

INGREDIENTS
- 1 3-pound beef tenderloin, trimmed of fat
- 2 tablespoons extra-virgin olive oil
- 1 teaspoon kosher salt
- 1/2 teaspoon freshly ground pepper
- 2/3 cup chopped mixed fresh herbs, such as chives, parsley, chervil, tarragon, thyme
- 2 tablespoons Dijon mustard

PREPARATION
1. Preheat oven to 400 degrees F.
2. Tie kitchen string around tenderloin in three places so it doesn't flatten while roasting. Rub the tenderloin with oil; pat on salt and pepper. Place in a large roasting pan.
3. Roast until a thermometer inserted into the thickest part of the tenderloin registers 140 degrees F for medium-rare, about 45 minutes, turning two or three times during roasting to ensure even cooking. Transfer to a cutting board; let rest for 10 minutes. Remove the string.
4. Place herbs on a large plate. Coat the tenderloin evenly with mustard; then roll in the herbs, pressing gently to adhere. Slice and serve.

TIPS & NOTES
- **Make Ahead Tip**: Equipment: Kitchen string
- Roasting Tips
- 1. Very cold meat won't roast evenly. Place it on the counter while preheating the oven.
2. Durable cotton kitchen string is sold at kitchenware stores, most gourmet markets and large supermarkets. Do not use sewing thread or yarn, which may contain inedible dyes or unsavory chemicals.
- 3. A heavy-duty, high-sided roasting pan is essential for conducting heat evenly. Never substitute a cookie sheet. A broiler pan will work in a pinch, but the roast will inevitably be somewhat chewier.
- 4. Give it a rest. A roast's internal temperature will rise about 10 degrees while resting. The natural juices will also reincorporate into the meat's fibers and the skin or crust will dry out slightly for a more toothsome yet more succulent dinner.

NUTRITION

Per 3-oz. serving: 185 calories; 9 g fat (3 g sat, 4 g mono); 67 mg cholesterol; 1 g carbohydrates; 0 g added sugars; 24 g protein; 0 g fiber; 178 mg sodium; 214 mg potassium.
Nutrition Bonus: Selenium (40% daily value), Zinc (30% dv).
Exchanges: 3 lean meat

Roasted Florets

INGREDIENTS
- 8 cups bite-size cauliflower florets, or broccoli florets (about 1 head), sliced
- 2 tablespoons extra-virgin olive oil
- 1/2 teaspoon salt, or to taste
- Freshly ground pepper, to taste
- Lemon wedges, (optional)

PREPARATION
1. Preheat oven to 450°F. Place florets in a large bowl with oil, salt and pepper and toss to coat. Spread out on a baking sheet. Roast the vegetables, stirring once, until tender-crisp and browned in spots, 15 to 25 minutes. Serve hot or warm with lemon wedges, if desired.

NUTRITION

Per serving (cauliflower): 113 calories; 7 g fat (1 g sat, 5 g mono); 0 mg cholesterol; 7 g carbohydrates; 4 gprotein; 4 g fiber; 327 mg sodium; 433 mg potassium.
Carbohydrate Servings: 1/2
Exchanges: 2 vegetable, 11/2 fat (mono)
Nutrition Note: Per serving (broccoli): 101 calories; 7 g fat (1 g sat, 5 g mono); 0 mg cholesterol; 7 g carbohydrate; 4 g protein; 4 g fiber; 327 mg sodium.

Grape and Feta Mixed Green Special

INGREDIENTS
DRESSING
- 1/4 cup extra-virgin olive oil
- 2 tablespoons red-wine vinegar
- 1/4 teaspoon salt, or to taste
- Freshly ground pepper, to taste

SALAD
- 8 cups mesclun salad greens, (5 ounces)
- 1 head radicchio, thinly sliced
- 2 cups halved seedless grapes, (about 1 pound), preferably red and green
- 3/4 cup crumbled feta, or blue cheese

PREPARATION
1. To prepare dressing: Whisk (or shake) oil, vinegar, salt and pepper in a small bowl (or jar) until blended.
2. To prepare salad: Just before serving, toss greens and radicchio in a large bowl. Drizzle the dressing on top and toss to coat. Divide the salad among 8 plates. Scatter grapes and cheese over each salad; serve immediately.

TIPS & NOTES
- **Make Ahead Tip**: The dressing will keep, covered, in the refrigerator for up to 2 days.

NUTRITION
Per serving: 133 calories; 10 g fat (3 g sat, 6 g mono); 13 mg cholesterol; 9 g carbohydrates; 3 g protein; 1 g fiber; 239 mg sodium; 183 mg potassium.
Nutrition Bonus: Vitamin C (15% daily value), Folate (9% dv).
Carbohydrate Servings: 1/2
Exchanges: 1/2 fruit, 1 vegetable, 2 fat

Honeyed Couscous Pudding

INGREDIENTS
- 3/4 cup chopped pitted dates
- 3 cups low-fat milk
- 1/4 cup honey
- 1 cinnamon stick
- 1 teaspoon freshly grated orange zest
- 1 cup plain or whole-wheat couscous
- 1 teaspoon vanilla extract
- Ground cinnamon for dusting pudding
- 2 tablespoons chopped skinned pistachios, (optional)

PREPARATION
1. Put dates in a small bowl. Add boiling water to cover. Cover the bowl and set aside.
2. Heat milk, honey, cinnamon stick and orange zest in a saucepan over medium high heat until nearly simmering. Stir in couscous and vanilla, remove from the heat and cover. Let stand until most of the milk has been absorbed, about 20 minutes. Remove the cinnamon stick.
3. Drain the dates and stir them into the couscous. To serve, spoon into bowls and sprinkle with ground cinnamon and pistachios, if using. Variation: Instead of oatmeal for breakfast, make Honeyed Couscous Pudding with half the honey. Garnish with some nonfat yogurt or a spoonful of orange marmalade.

NUTRITION
Per serving: 239 calories; 3 g fat (2 g sat, 1 g mono); 10 mg cholesterol; 49 g carbohydrates; 7 g protein; 4 g fiber; 51 mg sodium; 339 mg potassium.
Nutrition Bonus: Calcium (16% daily value).
Carbohydrate Servings: 3
Exchanges: 1/2 milk, 3 other carbohydrate

DAY 17
BREAKFAST
Savory Breakfast Muffins
Greek Potato & Feta Omelet or Tomato & Ham Breakfast Melt
Grapefruit (1/2)
LUNCH
Steak Salad-Stuffed Pockets or Winter Squash & Chicken Tzimmes
Skim milk (1 cup)
Strawberries (1 cup)
SNACK
Low-fat cottage cheese (1 cup)
Nectarine(1 small)
DINNER
Chicken Tabbouleh
Sliced Tomato Salad
Baked Apples

DAY 17 RECIPES

Savory Breakfast Muffins
INGREDIENTS
- 2 cups whole-wheat flour
- 1 cup all-purpose flour
- 1 tablespoon baking powder
- 1/2 teaspoon baking soda
- 1/2 teaspoon freshly ground pepper
- 1/4 teaspoon salt
- 2 eggs
- 1 1/3 cups buttermilk
- 3 tablespoons extra-virgin olive oil
- 2 tablespoons butter, melted
- 1 cup thinly sliced scallions, (about 1 bunch)
- 3/4 cup diced Canadian bacon, (3 ounces)

- 1/2 cup grated Cheddar cheese
- 1/2 cup finely diced red bell pepper

PREPARATION

1. Preheat oven to 400°F. Coat 12 muffin cups with cooking spray.
2. Combine whole-wheat flour, all-purpose flour, baking powder, baking soda, pepper and salt in a large bowl.
3. Whisk eggs, buttermilk, oil and butter in a medium bowl. Fold in scallions, bacon, cheese and bell pepper. Make a well in the center of the dry ingredients. Add the wet ingredients and mix with a rubber spatula until just moistened. Scoop the batter into the prepared pan (the cups will be very full).
4. Bake the muffins until the tops are golden brown, 20 to 22 minutes. Let cool in the pan for 5 minutes. Loosen the edges and turn the muffins out onto a wire rack to cool slightly before serving.

TIPS & NOTES
- **Make Ahead Tip**: Individually wrap in plastic and refrigerate for up to 3 days or freeze for up to 1 month. To reheat, remove plastic, wrap in a paper towel and microwave on High for 30 to 60 seconds.
- Reheat & Run
- Bake muffins on weekends and enjoy the leftovers for grab-and-go weekday breakfasts. Wrap leftover muffins individually in plastic wrap, place in a plastic storage container or ziplock bag and freeze for up to 1 month. To thaw, remove plastic wrap, wrap in a paper towel and microwave on High for 30 to 60 seconds.
- Storage smarts: For long-term freezer storage, wrap your food in a layer of plastic wrap followed by a layer of foil. The plastic will help prevent freezer burn while the foil will help keep off-odors from seeping into the food.

NUTRITION

Per muffin: 217 calories; 9 g fat (3 g sat, 4 g mono); 50 mg cholesterol; 24 g carbohydrates; 9 g protein; 3 gfiber; 339 mg sodium; 113 mg potassium.
Nutrition Bonus: Vitamin C (25% daily value), Fiber (13% dv).
Carbohydrate Servings: 1 1/2
Exchanges: 1 1/2 starch, 1/2 meat, 1 fat

Greek Potato & Feta Omelet

INGREDIENTS
- 2 teaspoons extra-virgin olive oil, divided
- 1 cup frozen hash brown potatoes, or cooked potatoes cut into 1/2-inch cubes
- 1/3 cup chopped scallions

- 4 large eggs
- 1/8 teaspoon salt
- Freshly ground pepper to taste
- 1/4 cup crumbled feta cheese

PREPARATION
1. Heat 1 teaspoon oil in a medium nonstick skillet over medium-high heat. Add potatoes and cook, shaking the pan and tossing the potatoes, until golden brown, 4 to 5 minutes. Add scallions and cook for 1 minute longer. Transfer to a plate. Wipe out the pan.
2. Blend eggs, salt and pepper in a medium bowl. Stir in feta and the potato mixture.
3. Preheat broiler. Brush the pan with the remaining 1 teaspoon oil; heat over medium heat. Add the egg mixture and tilt to distribute evenly. Reduce heat to medium-low and cook until the bottom is light golden, lifting the the edges to allow uncooked egg to flow underneath, 3 to 4 minutes. Place the pan under the broiler and cook until the top is set, 1 1/2 to 2 1/2 minutes. Slide the omelet onto a plate and cut into wedges.

NUTRITION

Per serving: 294 calories; 17 g fat (5 g sat, 7 g mono); 380 mg cholesterol; 18 g carbohydrates; 16 gprotein; 3 g fiber; 433 mg sodium; 442 mg potassium.
Nutrition Bonus: Vitamin A (15% daily value), Vitamin C (15% dv).
Carbohydrate Servings: 1
Exchanges: 1 starch; 2 medium-fat meat; 1 1/2 fat (mono)

Tomato & Ham Breakfast Melt

INGREDIENTS
- 2 slices thin multigrain bread, toasted
- 4 thin slices tomato
- 4 thin slices ham
- 2 slices reduced-fat Cheddar cheese

PREPARATION
1. Top toasted bread with tomato, ham and cheese. Toast in a toaster oven or under the broiler until the cheese is melted.

NUTRITION

Per serving: 298 calories; 9 g fat (4 g sat, 3 g mono); 48 mg cholesterol; 25 g carbohydrates; 31 g protein; 7 g fiber; 1124 mg sodium; 521 mg potassium.

Nutrition Bonus: Calcium (30% daily value), Selenium (25% dv), Zinc (24% dv), Vitamin C (20% dv), Magnesium (17% dv), Iron & Vitamin A (15% dv).
Carbohydrate Servings: 1
Exchanges: 1 1/2 starch, 1 vegetable, 4 lean meat

Steak Salad-Stuffed Pockets

INGREDIENTS
- 1/4 cup lemon juice
- 3 tablespoons extra-virgin olive oil
- 2 teaspoons Dijon mustard
- 1/4 teaspoon salt, or to taste
- Freshly ground pepper, to taste
- 1 pound top round steak, 1 1/2 inches thick, trimmed
- 4 cups romaine lettuce, chopped
- 1 medium cucumber, diced
- 1 large tomato, diced
- 8 4-inch whole-wheat pitas, or four 8-inch pitas, split open (see Tip)

PREPARATION
1. Position rack in upper third of oven; preheat broiler.
2. Whisk lemon juice, oil, mustard, salt and pepper in a large bowl. Place steak in a shallow dish and pour half the dressing over it. Let marinate at room temperature, turning once, for 10 minutes.
3. Meanwhile, prepare the salad by adding lettuce, cucumber and tomato to the remaining dressing in the bowl; toss to coat.
4. Transfer the meat to a broiling pan. Broil for 5 minutes on each side for medium-rare, or until it reaches desired doneness. Transfer to a cutting board, let rest for 3 minutes, then slice thinly against the grain. Mix the meat with the salad and fill each pita. Serve immediately.

TIPS & NOTES
- **Tip:** Warm pitas on the bottom rack of the oven while the steak is broiling.

NUTRITION
Per serving: 408 calories; 16 g fat (3 g sat, 8 g mono); 71 mg cholesterol; 36 g carbohydrates; 0 g added sugars; 32 g protein; 6 g fiber; 534 mg sodium; 774 mg potassium.
Nutrition Bonus: Vitamin A (70% daily value), Selenium (66% dv), Vitamin C (45% dv), Folate (29% dv), Iron (25% dv), Magnesium (20% dv).
Carbohydrate Servings: 2
Exchanges: 2 starch, 1 vegetable, 4 lean meat, 2 fat

Winter Squash & Chicken Tzimmes

INGREDIENTS
- 9 cups cubed peeled butternut, buttercup or hubbard squash, (1-inch cubes; see Tip)
- 1 cup small pitted prunes
- 3 cloves garlic, minced
- 2 medium shallots, thinly sliced and separated into rings
- 1 teaspoon ground cinnamon
- 1 teaspoon dried, oregano
- 1 teaspoon dried thyme
- 1 teaspoon salt, divided
- 1/2 teaspoon freshly ground pepper
- 8 skinless, bone-in chicken thighs, (about 3 1/2 pounds), trimmed
- 1 cup reduced-sodium chicken broth, or vegetable broth
- 1 teaspoon freshly grated orange zest
- 1/4 cup orange juice

PREPARATION
1. Preheat oven to 350°F.
2. Place squash, prunes, garlic, shallots, cinnamon, oregano, thyme, 1/2 teaspoon salt and pepper in a large bowl and mix well. Transfer to a 9-by-13-inch baking dish. Sprinkle chicken with the remaining 1/2 teaspoon salt and place on top of the vegetables. Mix broth, orange zest and juice in a small bowl and pour over the chicken. Cover the baking dish with foil.
3. Bake for 40 minutes. Uncover and continue baking until the vegetables are tender and the chicken is cooked through, basting often, about 1 hour more.

TIPS & NOTES
- **Tip:** For quicker prep, look for cubed butternut squash in your market's produce section.

NUTRITION
Per serving: 398 calories; 11 g fat (3 g sat, 4 g mono); 101 mg cholesterol; 46 g carbohydrates; 0 g added sugars; 32 g protein; 7 g fiber; 404 mg sodium; 1330 mg potassium.
Nutrition Bonus: Vitamin A (580% daily value), Vitamin C (100% dv), Potassium (38% dv), Magnesium (31% dv).
Carbohydrate Servings: 2 1/2
Exchanges: 2 starch, 1 fruit, 4 lean meat

Chicken Tabbouleh

INGREDIENTS
- 3 cups water
- 1 cup bulgur
- 3 cups cubed skinless cooked chicken, (1-inch cubes)
- 1 cup chopped fresh parsley
- 1 cup chopped scallions
- 1/3 cup currants
- 1/4 cup frozen orange juice concentrate
- 2 tablespoons lemon juice
- 1 tablespoon extra-virgin olive oil
- 1 teaspoon ground cumin
- 1/4 teaspoon cayenne pepper, or to taste
- 1/4 teaspoon salt
- Freshly ground pepper, to taste

PREPARATION
1. Bring water to a boil in a large saucepan. Add bulgur and remove from the heat. Let stand until most of the water is absorbed, 20 to 30 minutes.
2. Drain bulgur well, squeezing out excess moisture. Transfer to a large bowl. Add chicken, parsley, scallions and currants.
3. Whisk orange juice concentrate, lemon juice, oil, cumin and cayenne in a small bowl until blended. Toss with the bulgur mixture. Season with salt and pepper and serve.

TIPS & NOTES
- **To poach chicken breasts:** Place boneless, skinless chicken breasts in a medium skillet or saucepan and add lightly salted water to cover; bring to a boil. Cover, reduce heat to low and simmer gently until chicken is cooked through and no longer pink in the middle, 10 to 12 minutes.
- **Ingredient note:** Bulgur is made by parboiling, drying and coarsely grinding or cracking wheat berries. Don't confuse bulgur with cracked wheat, which is simply that—cracked wheat. Since the parboiling step is skipped, cracked wheat must be cooked for up to an hour whereas bulgur simply needs a quick soak in hot water for most uses. Look for it in the natural-foods section of large supermarkets, near other grains, or online at kalustyans.com, lebaneseproducts.com.

NUTRITION
Per serving: 260 calories; 5 g fat (1 g sat, 3 g mono); 60 mg cholesterol; 31 g carbohydrates; 0 g added sugars; 26 g protein; 6 g fiber; 166 mg sodium; 536 mg potassium.

Nutrition Bonus: Vitamin C (60% daily value), Fiber (24% dv), Potassium (15% dv).
Carbohydrate Servings: 1 1/2
Exchanges: 2 starch, 3 very lean meat

Sliced Tomato Salad

INGREDIENTS
- 4 tomatoes, sliced
- 1/4 cup thinly sliced red onion
- 8 anchovies
- 1/2 teaspoon dried oregano
- Salt & freshly ground pepper, to taste
- 2 tablespoons extra-virgin olive oil
- 1 tablespoon white-wine vinegar

PREPARATION
1. Arrange tomato slices on a platter. Top with onion, anchovies, oregano, salt and pepper. Drizzle with oil and vinegar.

NUTRITION
Per serving: 44 calories; 1 g fat (0 g sat, 0 g mono); 3 mg cholesterol; 8 g carbohydrates; 0 g added sugars; 3 g protein; 2 g fiber; 300 mg sodium; 403 mg potassium.
Nutrition Bonus: Vitamin C (35% daily value), Vitamin A (25% dv).
Carbohydrate Servings: 1/2
Exchanges: 1 vegetable, 1 1/2 fat

Baked Apples

INGREDIENTS
- 2 apples, cored
- 4 teaspoons dried fruit, chopped, such as cranberries, raisins or dates
- 4 teaspoons toasted nuts, chopped, such as pecans, walnuts or almonds
- 1 teaspoon honey
- Pinch of cinnamon
- 1/2 cup apple cider
- 1/4 cup plain yogurt

PREPARATION
1. Preheat oven to 350°F.
2. Combine fruit, nuts, honey and cinnamon; spoon into the apples. Place the apples in a small baking dish and pour apple cider around them. Cover with foil. Bake until tender, about 45 minutes. Serve topped with yogurt.

NUTRITION

Per serving: 165 calories; 4 g fat (0 g sat, 2 g mono); 0 mg cholesterol; 35 g carbohydrates; 1 g protein; 4 gfiber; 2 mg sodium; 215 mg potassium.
Nutrition Bonus: Fiber (16% daily value).
Carbohydrate Servings: 2
Exchanges: 2 fruit, 1 fat

DAY 18
BREAKFAST
Overnight Oatmeal
Low-fat vanilla yogurt (8 oz.)
Grapefruit (1/2)
LUNCH
Skim milk (1 cup)
Grilled Chicken Caesar Salad or Endive & Pomegranate Salad
Whole-wheat pita bread (1 medium pita)
Orange (1 large)
SNACK
Apricot (1 cup, halves)
Almonds (1 oz.)
DINNER
Chicken-Sausage & Kale Stew or Turkey with Blueberry Pan Sauce
Mexican Coleslaw
Brown rice (1 cup, cooked)
Strawberry Frozen Yogurt

DAY 18 RECIPES

Overnight Oatmeal

INGREDIENTS
- 8 cups water
- 2 cups steel-cut oats, (see Ingredient note)
- 1/3 cup dried cranberries
- 1/3 cup dried apricots, chopped
- 1/4 teaspoon salt, or to taste

PREPARATION
1. Combine water, oats, dried cranberries, dried apricots and salt in a 5- or 6-quart slow cooker. Turn heat to low. Put the lid on and cook until the oats are tender and the porridge is creamy, 7 to 8 hours. Stovetop Variation Halve the above

recipe to accommodate the size of most double boilers: Combine 4 cups water, 1 cup steel-cut oats, 3 tablespoons dried cranberries, 3 tablespoons dried apricots and 1/8 teaspoon salt in the top of a double boiler. Cover and cook over boiling water for about 1 1/2 hours, checking the water level in the bottom of the double boiler from time to time.

TIPS & NOTES
- **Ingredient Note:** Steel-cut oats, sometimes labeled "Irish oatmeal," look like small pebbles. They are toasted oat groats—the oat kernel that has been removed from the husk that have been cut in 2 or 3 pieces. Do not substitute regular rolled oats, which have a shorter cooking time, in the slow-cooker oatmeal recipe.
- For easy cleanup, try a slow-cooker liner. These heat-resistant, disposable liners fit neatly inside the insert and help prevent food from sticking to the bottom and sides of your slow cooker.

NUTRITION
Per serving: 193 calories; 3 g fat (0 g sat, 1 g mono); 0 mg cholesterol; 34 g carbohydrates; 0 g added sugars; 6 g protein; 9 g fiber; 77 mg sodium; 195 mg potassium.
Nutrition Bonus: Fiber (36% daily value).
Carbohydrate Servings: 2
Exchanges: 2 starch, 1/2 fruit

Grilled Chicken Caesar Salad
INGREDIENTS
- 1 pound boneless, skinless chicken breasts, trimmed of fat
- 1 teaspoon canola oil
- 1/4 teaspoon salt, or to taste
- Freshly ground pepper, to taste
- 8 cups washed, dried and torn romaine lettuce
- 1 cup fat-free croutons
- 1/2 cup Caesar Salad Dressing, (recipe follows)
- 1/2 cup Parmesan curls, (see Tip)
- Lemon wedges

PREPARATION
1. Prepare a grill or preheat broiler.
2. Rub chicken with oil and season with salt and pepper. Grill or broil chicken until browned and no trace of pink remains in the center, 3 to 4 minutes per side.

3. Combine lettuce and croutons in a large bowl. Toss with Caesar Salad Dressing and divide among 4 plates. Cut chicken into 1/2-inch slices and fan over salad. Top with Parmesan curls. Serve immediately, with lemon wedges.

TIPS & NOTES
- **Tip:** To make parmesan curls, start with a piece of cheese that is at least 4 ounces. Use a swivel-bladed vegetable peeler to shave off curls.

NUTRITION

Per serving: 278 calories; 6 g fat (2 g sat, 2 g mono); 74 mg cholesterol; 14 g carbohydrates; 34 g protein; 1 g fiber; 662 mg sodium; 308 mg potassium.
Carbohydrate Servings: 1
Exchanges: 1/2 starch, 2 vegetable, 4 very lean meat, For Caesar Salad Dressing, free food

Endive & Pomegranate Salad

INGREDIENTS
DRESSING
- 6 tablespoons pomegranate juice
- 3 tablespoons canola oil
- 2 teaspoons Dijon mustard
- 1 small clove garlic, minced
- 1/4 teaspoon salt
- Freshly ground pepper, to taste

SALAD
- 2 large navel oranges
- 2 Belgian endives
- 1 cup watercress
- 1 avocado
- 12 medium cooked shrimp, (about 8 ounces), optional
- 1 cup pomegranate seeds, (1 large fruit; see Tip)

PREPARATION
1. To prepare dressing: Whisk dressing ingredients in a small bowl.
2. To prepare salad: Peel oranges with a paring knife, removing the white pith. Quarter and slice the oranges. Wipe endives with a damp cloth (do not soak as they tend to absorb water); cut into 1/4-inch-thick slices. Wash and dry watercress. Peel and pit avocado; cut into thin slices lengthwise.

3. To assemble salads: Alternate avocado slices and orange sections in a fan shape on each of 4 salad plates. Top with endive, watercress and shrimp, if using. Drizzle with dressing, sprinkle with pomegranate seeds and serve.

TIPS & NOTES

- **Make Ahead Tip**: Cover and refrigerate the dressing (Step 1) for up to 2 days.
- **Ingredient note:** Look for pomegranate juice with other bottled juices or in the produce section of well-stocked supermarkets and natural-foods stores.
- **Tip:** To avoid the enduring stains of pomegranate juice, work under water! Fill a large bowl with water. Hold the pomegranate in the water and slice off the crown. Lightly score the fruit into quarters, from crown to stem end. Keeping the fruit under water, break it apart, gently separating the plump arils from the outer skin and white pith. The seeds will drop to the bottom of the bowl and the pith will float to the surface. Discard the pith. Pour the seeds into a colander. Rinse and pat dry. The seeds can be frozen in an airtight container or sealable bag for up to 3 months.

NUTRITION
Per serving: 292 calories; 19 g fat (2 g sat, 11 g mono); 0 mg cholesterol; 32 g carbohydrates; 0 g added sugars; 5 g protein; 13 g fiber; 244 mg sodium; 1336 mg potassium.
Nutrition Bonus: Vitamin A & C (120% daily value), Folate (108% dv), Potassium (38% dv), Calcium (20% dv), Magnesium & Zinc (16% dv), Iron (15% dv).
Carbohydrate Servings: 1
Exchanges: 1 1/2 fruit, 2 vegetable, 3 1/2 fat (without shrimp)

Chicken-Sausage & Kale Stew

INGREDIENTS

- 1 tablespoon extra-virgin olive oil and 1 large onion, diced
- 4 cups kale, torn into bite-size pieces and rinsed
- 2 14-ounce cans reduced-sodium chicken broth
- 4 plum tomatoes, chopped
- 2 cups diced cooked potatoes, (see Note), preferably red-skinned
- 1 teaspoon chopped fresh rosemary
- 1/2 teaspoon freshly ground pepper
- 1 12-ounce package cooked chicken sausages, halved lengthwise and sliced
- 1 tablespoon cider vinegar

PREPARATION
1. Heat oil in a Dutch oven over medium-high heat. Add onion and kale and cook, stirring often, until the onion starts to soften, 5 to 7 minutes.
2. Stir in broth, tomatoes, potatoes, rosemary and pepper. Cover, increase heat to high and bring to a boil, stirring occasionally. Reduce heat and simmer, covered, until the vegetables are just tender, about 15 minutes. Stir in sausage and vinegar and continue to cook, stirring often, until heated through, about 2 minutes more.

TIPS & NOTES
- **Make Ahead Tip**: Cover and refrigerate for up to 2 days.
- **Note:** Convenient cooked and diced potatoes can be found in the refrigerated section of the produce and/or dairy department of the supermarket.

NUTRITION
Per serving: 214 calories; 7 g fat (1 g sat, 2 g mono); 40 mg cholesterol; 25 g carbohydrates; 0 g added sugars; 14 g protein; 3 g fiber; 346 mg sodium; 689 mg potassium.
Nutrition Bonus: Vitamin A (140% daily value), Vitamin C (120% dv), Potassium (20% dv).
Carbohydrate Servings: 2
Exchanges: 1 1/2 starch, 1 vegetable, 2 lean meat

Turkey with Blueberry Pan Sauce

INGREDIENTS
- 1/4 cup all-purpose flour
- 3/4 teaspoon salt, divided
- 1/2 teaspoon freshly ground pepper
- 1 pound turkey tenderloin, (see Ingredient note)
- 1 tablespoon extra-virgin olive oil
- 1/4 cup chopped shallots
- 1 tablespoon chopped fresh thyme
- 2 cups blueberries
- 3 tablespoons balsamic vinegar

PREPARATION
1. Preheat oven to 450°F. Whisk flour, 1/2 teaspoon salt and pepper in a shallow dish. Dredge turkey in the mixture. (Discard any leftover flour.)
2. Heat oil in a large ovenproof skillet over high heat. Add the turkey; cook until golden brown on one side, 3 to 5 minutes. Turn the turkey over and transfer the pan to the oven. Roast until the turkey is just cooked through and no longer pink

in the middle, 15 to 20 minutes. Transfer the turkey to a plate and tent with foil to keep warm.
3. Place the skillet over medium heat. (Take care, the handle will still be very hot.) Add shallots and thyme and cook, stirring constantly, until the shallots begin to brown, 30 seconds to 1 minute. Add blueberries, vinegar and the remaining 1/4 teaspoon salt; continue cooking, stirring occasionally and scraping up any brown bits, until the blueberries burst and release their juices and the mixture becomes thick and syrupy, 4 to 5 minutes. Slice the turkey and serve with the blueberry pan sauce.

TIPS & NOTES
- **Ingredient Note:** A turkey tenderloin is an all-white piece that comes from the rib side of the breast. Tenderloins typically weigh between 7 and 14 ounces each and can be found with other turkey products in the meat section of most supermarkets.

NUTRITION
Per serving: 215 calories; 5 g fat (1 g sat, 3 g mono); 45 mg cholesterol; 15 g carbohydrates; 0 g added sugars; 29 g protein; 2 g fiber; 273 mg sodium; 104 mg potassium.
Nutrition Bonus: Vitamin C (15% daily value).
Carbohydrate Servings: 1
Exchanges: 1 fruit, 4 very lean meat

Mexican Coleslaw

INGREDIENTS
- 6 cups very thinly sliced green cabbage, (about 1/2 head) (see Tip)
- 1 1/2 cups peeled and grated carrots, (2-3 medium)
- 1/3 cup chopped cilantro
- 1/4 cup rice vinegar
- 2 tablespoons extra-virgin olive oil
- 1/4 teaspoon salt

PREPARATION
1. Place cabbage and carrots in a colander; rinse thoroughly with cold water to crisp. Let drain for 5 minutes.
2. Meanwhile, whisk cilantro, vinegar, oil and salt in a large bowl. Add cabbage and carrots; toss well to coat.

TIPS & NOTES

- **Make Ahead Tip**: Cover and refrigerate for up to 1 day. Toss again to refresh just before serving.
- **Tip:** To make this coleslaw even faster, use a coleslaw mix containing cabbage and carrots from the produce section of the supermarket.

NUTRITION

Per serving: 53 calories; 4 g fat (1 g sat, 3 g mono); 0 mg cholesterol; 5 g carbohydrates; 0 g added sugars;1 g protein; 2 g fiber; 97 mg sodium; 199 mg potassium.
Nutrition Bonus: Vitamin A (50% daily value), Vitamin C (30% dv), phytochemicals sulforaphane and indoles.
Exchanges: 1 vegetable, 1/2 fat (mono

Strawberry Frozen Yogurt

INGREDIENTS

- 4 cups strawberries, hulled
- 1/3 cup sugar
- 2 tablespoons orange juice
- 1/2 cup nonfat or low-fat plain yogurt

PREPARATION

1. Place berries in a food processor and process until smooth, scraping down the sides as necessary. Add sugar and orange juice; process for a few seconds. Add yogurt and pulse several times until blended. Transfer to a bowl. Cover and refrigerate until chilled, about 1 hour or overnight.
2. Pour the strawberry mixture into an ice cream maker and freeze according to manufacturer's directions. Serve immediately or transfer to a storage container and let harden in the freezer for 1 to 1 1/2 hours. Serve in chilled dishes.

TIPS & NOTES

- **Make Ahead Tip**: Freeze for up to 1 week. Let soften in the refrigerator for 1/2 hour before serving. | Equipment: Ice cream maker

NUTRITION

Per serving: 82 calories; 0 g fat (0 g sat, 0 g mono); 0 mg cholesterol; 20 g carbohydrates; 1 g protein; 2 gfiber; 12 mg sodium; 170 mg potassium.
Nutrition Bonus: Vitamin C (100% daily value).
Carbohydrate Servings: 1
Exchanges: 1 fruit

DAY 19
BREAKFAST
Tofu Scrambled Egg
Salsa Cornbread
Strawberries (1 cup)

LUNCH
Turkey & Balsamic Onion Quesadillas
Salad of Boston Lettuce with Creamy Orange-Shallot Dressing
Banana (1 cup, sliced)

SNACK
Low-fat vanilla yogurt (8 oz.)

DINNER
Salmon on a Bed of Lentils or Pork Fajitas
Sesame Green Beans
Whole-wheat couscous (1 cup, cooked) or Easy Black Beans
Japanese Cucumber Salad
Plum Fool

DAY 19 RECIPES

Tofu Scrambled Egg
INGREDIENTS
- 1 large egg
- 1/2 teaspoon dried tarragon
- Dash of hot sauce, such as
- Pinch of salt
- Freshly ground pepper, to taste
- 1 teaspoon extra-virgin olive oil, or canola oil
- 2 tablespoons crumbled tofu, (silken or regular)

PREPARATION
1. Blend egg, tarragon, hot sauce, salt and pepper in a small bowl with a fork. Heat oil in a small nonstick skillet over medium-low heat. Add tofu and cook, stirring, until warmed through, 20 to 30 seconds. Add egg mixture and stir until the egg is set, but still creamy, 20 to 30 seconds. Serve immediately.

NUTRITION
Per serving: 140 calories; 11 g fat (2 g sat, 6 g mono); 212 mg cholesterol; 2 g carbohydrates; 0 g added sugars; 9 g protein; 1 g fiber; 230 mg sodium; 93 mg potassium.
Nutrition Bonus: Selenium (23% daily value).

Exchanges: 1 medium-fat meat. 1 fat (mono)

Salsa Cornbread

INGREDIENTS
- 1 cup all-purpose flour
- 1/2 cup whole-wheat flour
- 1/2 cup cornmeal
- 2 teaspoons baking powder
- 1/2 teaspoon salt
- Freshly ground pepper, to taste
- 3 large eggs, lightly beaten
- 1/2 cup buttermilk, or equivalent buttermilk powder
- 1 tablespoon butter, melted
- 1 tablespoon honey
- 1/2 cup drained canned corn kernels
- 1 small onion, diced
- 1/2 cup chopped tomato
- 1 clove garlic, minced
- 1 jalapeno pepper, seeded and minced
- 1/2 cup grated Cheddar cheese

PREPARATION
1. Preheat oven to 425° F. Place a 9-inch cast-iron skillet (or similar ovenproof skillet, see Tip) in the oven to heat.
2. Whisk all-purpose flour, whole-wheat flour, cornmeal, baking powder, salt and pepper in a large mixing bowl.
3. Whisk eggs, buttermilk, butter and honey in a medium bowl. Add the egg mixture to the dry ingredients; mix with a rubber spatula. Stir in corn, onion, tomato, garlic and jalapeno.
4. Remove the skillet from the oven and coat it with cooking spray. Pour in the batter, spreading evenly. Sprinkle cheese over the top. Bake the cornbread until golden brown and a knife inserted into the center comes out clean, 20 to 25 minutes. Serve warm.

TIPS & NOTES
- **Tip:** If you do not have an ovenproof skillet of the correct size, use an 8-by-8-inch glass baking dish. Do not preheat the empty baking dish in the oven before filling it.

NUTRITION

Per serving: 138 calories; 4 g fat (2 g sat, 1 g mono); 70 mg cholesterol; 20 g carbohydrates; 6 g protein; 1 g fiber; 319 mg sodium; 91 mg potassium.
Carbohydrate Servings: 1
Exchanges: 1 starch, 1 fat

Turkey & Balsamic Onion Quesadillas

INGREDIENTS
- 1 small red onion, thinly sliced
- 1/4 cup balsamic vinegar
- 4 10-inch whole-wheat tortillas
- 1 cup shredded sharp Cheddar cheese
- 8 slices deli turkey, preferably smoked (8 ounces)

PREPARATION
1. Combine onion and vinegar in a bowl; let marinate for 5 minutes. Drain, reserving the vinegar for another use, such as salad dressing.
2. Warm 2 tortillas in a large nonstick skillet over medium-high heat for about 45 seconds, then flip. Pull the tortillas up the edges of the pan so they are no longer overlapping. Working on one half of each tortilla, sprinkle one-fourth of the cheese, cover with 2 slices of turkey and top with one-fourth of the onion. Fold the tortillas in half, flatten gently with a spatula and cook until the cheese starts to melt, about 2 minutes. Flip and cook until the second side is golden, 1 to 2 minutes more. Transfer to a plate and cover to keep warm. Make 2 more quesadillas with the remaining ingredients.

NUTRITION

Per serving: 328 calories; 12 g fat (6 g sat, 0 g mono); 56 mg cholesterol; 30 g carbohydrates; 24 g protein; 2 g fiber; 871 mg sodium; 33 mg potassium.
Nutrition Bonus: Calcium (30% daily value).
Carbohydrate Servings: 1 1/2
Exchanges: 1 1/2 starch, 3 lean meat

Salad of Boston Lettuce with Creamy Orange-Shallot Dressing

INGREDIENTS
DRESSING
- 1/4 cup reduced-fat mayonnaise
- 1/2 teaspoon Dijon mustard
- 1/4 cup orange juice
- 2 teaspoons finely chopped shallot

- Freshly ground pepper, to taste

SALAD
- 1 large head Boston lettuce, torn into bite-size pieces (5 cups)
- 1 cup julienned or grated carrot, (1 carrot)
- 1 cup cherry or grape tomatoes, rinsed and cut in half
- 2 tablespoons snipped fresh tarragon, or chives (optional)

PREPARATION
1. To prepare dressing: Whisk mayonnaise and mustard in a small bowl. Slowly whisk in orange juice until smooth. Stir in shallot. Season with pepper.
2. To prepare salad: Divide lettuce among 4 plates and scatter carrot and tomatoes on top. Drizzle the dressing over the salads and sprinkle with tarragon (or chives), if desired. Serve immediately.

NUTRITION
Per serving: 64 calories; 1 g fat (0 g sat, 0 g mono); 0 mg cholesterol; 12 g carbohydrates; 1 g added sugars; 2 g protein; 2 g fiber; 182 mg sodium; 386 mg potassium.
Nutrition Bonus: Vitamin A (120% daily value), Vitamin C (30% dv), Folate (16% dv).
Carbohydrate Servings: 1
Exchanges: 2 vegetable

Salmon on a Bed of Lentils

INGREDIENTS
- 2 teaspoons extra-virgin olive oil
- 1 tablespoon finely chopped shallots
- 2 teaspoons minced garlic
- 2 1/2 cups reduced-sodium chicken broth
- 1 cup green or brown lentils, rinsed
- 1 small onion, peeled and studded with a clove
- 1 1/2 teaspoons chopped fresh thyme, or 1/2 teaspoon dried
- 1/4 teaspoon salt
- Freshly ground pepper, to taste
- 2 carrots, peeled and finely chopped
- 2 small white turnips, peeled and finely chopped
- 1 pound salmon fillet, skin removed, cut into 4 portions
- 2 tablespoons chopped fresh parsley
- 1 lemon, quartered

PREPARATION
1. Heat oil in a Dutch oven or deep sauté pan over medium heat. Add shallots and garlic and cook, stirring, until softened, about 30 seconds. Add broth, lentils, onion, thyme, salt and pepper. Bring to a boil, reduce heat to low and simmer, covered, until the lentils are tender, 25 minutes.
2. Add carrots and turnips; simmer until the vegetables are tender, about 10 minutes more. Remove the onion. Add more broth if necessary; the mixture should be slightly soupy. Taste and adjust seasonings. Lay salmon fillets on top, cover the pan and cook until the salmon is opaque in the center, 8 to 10 minutes.
3. Serve in shallow bowls, garnished with parsley and lemon wedges.

NUTRITION
Per serving: 382 calories; 11 g fat (2 g sat, 4 g mono); 65 mg cholesterol; 35 g carbohydrates; 0 g added sugars; 36 g protein; 9 g fiber; 342 mg sodium; 1142 mg potassium.
Nutrition Bonus: Vitamin A (80% daily value), Potassium (56% dv), Fiber (36% dv), Vitamin C(20% dv), Iron (20% dv).
Carbohydrate Servings: 2
Exchanges: 1 1/2 starch, 1 vegetable, 4 lean meat

Pork Fajitas

INGREDIENTS
- 1 pepper plus 1 teaspoon sauce from a can of chipotle chile in adobo (see Tips)
- 1 clove garlic, minced
- 1/2 cup orange juice
- 3 tablespoons lime juice
- 1 tablespoon red-wine vinegar
- 1 teaspoon dried oregano
- 1/2 teaspoon ground cumin
- 1/4 teaspoon salt
- 1/4 teaspoon freshly ground pepper
- 8 ounces pork tenderloin (see Tips), trimmed
- 1 small green bell pepper, cut into 1-inch-wide strips
- 1 small red bell pepper, cut into 1-inch-wide strips
- 1 small red onion, cut into 1/2-inch-thick rounds
- 2 teaspoons canola oil
- 4 6-inch or two 10-inch flour tortillas, preferably whole-wheat, warmed (see Tips)
- 1/4 cup nonfat sour cream
- 1/4 cup prepared salsa

PREPARATION

1. Combine chipotle chile and sauce, garlic, orange juice, lime juice, vinegar, oregano, cumin, salt and pepper in a blender or mini food processor; blend or process until the chipotle is chopped and the mixture is relatively smooth. Pour into a sealable plastic bag, add pork and seal, squeezing out any excess air from the bag. Turn to coat with the marinade. Refrigerate at least 1 hour and up to 8 hours.
2. Preheat grill to high or heat a large indoor grill pan over high heat. Remove the pork from the marinade (discard marinade). Grill the pork, turning occasionally, until an instant-read thermometer inserted diagonally into the center of the meat registers 145°F, 12 to 15 minutes. Transfer the pork to a cutting board and let rest for 5 minutes before slicing.
3. Lightly brush bell peppers and onion with oil. Grill until lightly browned and soft, turning once, 3 to 7 minutes. (If using a grill pan, you may need to grill the vegetables in two batches.) Let cool on a cutting board.
4. Thinly slice the pork and chop the onion. Toss the onion, peppers and pork together in a large bowl. Serve the fajita filling in tortillas with sour cream and salsa.

TIPS & NOTES

- **Make Ahead Tip**: Marinate the pork (Step 1) in the refrigerator for up to 8 hours.
- **Tips:** Chipotle chiles in adobo sauce are smoked jalapenos packed in a flavorful sauce. Look for the small cans with the Mexican foods in large supermarkets. Once opened, they'll keep up to 2 weeks in the refrigerator or 6 months in the freezer.
- One pork tenderloin typically weighs about 1 pound, enough for 4 servings. You can marinate a whole pound in the same amount of marinade used to marinate the 8 ounces in this recipe and have enough cooked tenderloin for 2 dinners (for 2 people). Or freeze half for up to 3 months.
- To warm tortillas, wrap in foil and bake at 300°F until steaming, about 5 minutes. Or wrap in barely damp paper towels and microwave on High for 30 to 45 seconds.

NUTRITION

Per serving: 311 calories; 8 g fat (1 g sat, 4 g mono); 77 mg cholesterol; 36 g carbohydrates; 1 g added sugars; 29 g protein; 5 g fiber; 592 mg sodium; 889 mg potassium.
Nutrition Bonus: Vitamin C (143% daily value), Vitamin A (30% dv), Potassium (25% dv), Zinc (21% dv), Iron (19% dv)
Carbohydrate Servings: 2
Exchanges: 1 1/2 starch, 2 vegetable, 3 lean meat, 1 fat

Sesame Green Beans

INGREDIENTS
- 1 pound green beans, trimmed
- 2 teaspoons extra-virgin olive oil
- 2 teaspoons toasted sesame seeds, (see Tip)
- 1 teaspoon sesame oil
- Salt & freshly ground pepper, to taste

PREPARATION
1. Preheat oven to 500°F.
2. Toss green beans with olive oil. Spread in an even layer on a rimmed baking sheet. Roast, turning once halfway through cooking, until tender and beginning to brown, about 10 minutes. Toss with sesame seeds, sesame oil, salt and pepper.

TIPS & NOTES
- **Tip:** To toast sesame seeds: Place in a small dry skillet and cook over medium-low heat, stirring constantly, until fragrant and lightly browned, 2 to 4 minutes.

NUTRITION
Per serving: 67 calories; 4 g fat (1 g sat, 3 g mono); 0 mg cholesterol; 7 g carbohydrates; 0 g added sugars;2 g protein; 4 g fiber; 73 mg sodium; 280 mg potassium.
Nutrition Bonus: Vitamin C (15% daily value).
Carbohydrate Servings: 1/2
Exchanges: 1 vegetable

Easy Black Beans

INGREDIENTS
- 2 teaspoons extra-virgin olive oil
- 1 medium yellow onion, diced (about 1 1/2 cups)
- 2 cloves garlic, minced
- 2 teaspoons ground ancho chile pepper, (see Note)
- 1/2 teaspoon ground cumin
- 1/2 teaspoon dried oregano
- 2 15-ounce cans black beans, rinsed
- 1 cup water
- 1 tablespoon tomato paste

PREPARATION
1. Heat oil in a medium saucepan over medium-high heat. Add onion and cook, stirring, until translucent, 4 to 5 minutes. Add garlic and cook, stirring constantly, for 30 seconds. Add ground chile, cumin and oregano and cook, stirring, until fragrant, about 30 seconds more. Add beans, water and tomato paste; stir to combine. Bring to a simmer, reduce heat to medium-low and cook, stirring occasionally, until the beans are heated through and the sauce is slightly thickened, 8 to 10 minutes. Serve warm.

TIPS & NOTES
- **Make Ahead Tip**: Cover and refrigerate for up to 2 days. Reheat in a saucepan with 2 tablespoons water over medium-low heat, stirring occasionally, for about 5 minutes.
- **Ingredient Note**: Ancho chile peppers, one of the most popular dried chiles used in Mexico, are dried poblano peppers. They have a mild, sweet, spicy flavor. Ground ancho chile pepper can be found in the specialty-spice section of large supermarkets, or substitute ground chili powder with a pinch of cayenne.

NUTRITION
Per serving: 117 calories; 1 g fat (0 g sat, 1 g mono); 0 mg cholesterol; 21 g carbohydrates; 0 g added sugars; 6 g protein; 5 g fiber; 84 mg sodium; 69 mg potassium.
Nutrition Bonus: Folate (41% daily value), Magnesium (19% dv), Iron (15% dv).
Carbohydrate Servings: 1
Exchanges: 1 starch, 1 very lean meat

Japanese Cucumber Salad

INGREDIENTS
- 2 medium cucumbers, or 1 large English cucumber
- 1/4 cup rice vinegar
- 1 teaspoon sugar
- 1/4 teaspoon salt
- 2 tablespoons sesame seeds, toasted (see Tip)

PREPARATION
1. Peel cucumbers to leave alternating green stripes. Slice the cucumbers in half lengthwise; scrape the seeds out with a spoon. Using a food processor or sharp knife, cut into very thin slices. Place in a double layer of paper towel and squeeze gently to remove any excess moisture.
2. Combine vinegar, sugar and salt in a medium bowl, stirring to dissolve. Add the cucumbers and sesame seeds; toss well to combine. Serve immediately.

TIPS & NOTES
- **Tip:** To toast sesame seeds, heat a small dry skillet over low heat. Add sesame seeds and stir constantly until golden and fragrant, about 2 minutes. Transfer to a small bowl and let cool.

NUTRITION

Per serving: 46 calories; 2 g fat (0 g sat, 0 g mono); 0 mg cholesterol; 4 g carbohydrates; 1 g protein; 1 gfiber; 147 mg sodium; 137 mg potassium.
Nutrition Bonus: Iron (35% daily value).
Exchanges: 1 vegetable, 1/2 fat

Plum Fool

INGREDIENTS
- 1 pound plums, pitted and sliced (about 2 1/2 cups)
- 1/4-1/2 cup sugar, or Splenda Granular
- 1/2 teaspoon grated fresh ginger
- 1/2 teaspoon ground cinnamon
- 1 1/2 cups low-fat vanilla yogurt
- 1/3 cup whipping cream

PREPARATION
1. Set aside a few plum slices for garnish. Combine the remaining plum slices, 1/4 cup sugar (or Splenda), ginger and cinnamon in a small heavy saucepan. Bring to a simmer, stirring, over medium heat. Cook until the mixture has softened into a chunky puree, 15 to 20 minutes. Taste and add more sugar (or Splenda), if desired. Transfer to a bowl and chill until cool, about 1 hour.
2. Meanwhile, set a fine-mesh stainless-steel sieve over a bowl. Spoon in yogurt and let drain in the refrigerator until reduced to 1 cup, about 1 hour.
3. Whip cream to soft peaks in a chilled bowl. Gently fold in the drained yogurt with a rubber spatula. Fold this mixture into the fruit puree, leaving distinct swirls. Spoon into 6 dessert dishes and cover with plastic wrap. Refrigerate for at least 1 hour or up to 2 days. Garnish with the reserved plum slices before serving.

NUTRITION

Per serving: 156 calories; 5 g fat (3 g sat, 2 g mono); 18 mg cholesterol; 25 g carbohydrates; 4 g protein; 1 g fiber; 45 mg sodium; 259 mg potassium.
Nutrition Bonus: Calcium (12% daily value), Vitamin C (12% dv).
Carbohydrate Servings: 1 1/2
Exchanges: 11/2 fruit, 1 fat

Nutrition Note: Per serving with Splenda: 1 Carbohydrate Serving, 128 calories, 18 g carbohydrate.

DAY 20
BREAKFAST

Cranberry Muesli
Skim milk (1 cup)
Grapefruit (1/2)
LUNCH

Skim milk (1 cup)
Penne with Braised Squash & Greens
Tangy Cauliflower Salad or Peas & Lettuce
Strawberries (1 cup)
SNACK

Apple (1 cup, quartered)
Oatmeal Chocolate Chip Cookies
DINNER

Pampered Chicken or Cider-Brined Pork Chops
Sliced Fennel Salad
Quick-cooking barley (1 cup)
Steamed cauliflower (1/2 cup)
Pina Colada Yogurt Parfait

DAY 20 RECIPES

Cranberry Muesli

INGREDIENTS
- 1/2 cup low-fat plain yogurt
- 1/2 cup unsweetened or fruit-juice-sweetened cranberry juice
- 6 tablespoons old-fashioned rolled oats, (not quick-cooking or steel-cut)
- 2 tablespoons dried cranberries
- 1 tablespoon unsalted sunflower seeds
- 1 tablespoon wheat germ
- 2 teaspoons honey
- 1/4 teaspoon vanilla extract
- 1/8 teaspoon salt

PREPARATION

1. Combine yogurt, juice, oats, cranberries, sunflower seeds, wheat germ, honey, vanilla and salt in a medium bowl; cover and refrigerate for at least 8 hours and up to 1 day.

TIPS & NOTES

- **Make Ahead Tip**: Cover and refrigerate for up to 1 day.

NUTRITION

Per serving: 209 calories; 4 g fat (1 g sat, 1 g mono); 4 mg cholesterol; 37 g carbohydrates; 8 g protein; 3 gfiber; 190 mg sodium; 266 mg potassium.
Nutrition Bonus: Calcium (15% daily value)
Carbohydrate Servings: 2 1/2
Exchanges: 1 starch, 1 fruit, 1/2 other carbohydrate, 1/2 fat

Penne with Braised Squash & Greens

INGREDIENTS

- 2 teaspoons extra-virgin olive oil
- 4 ounces cubed smoked tofu
- 1 medium onion, chopped
- 3 cloves garlic, minced
- Pinch of crushed red pepper
- 1 1/2 cups vegetable broth
- 1 pound butternut squash, peeled and cut into 3/4-inch cubes (3 cups)
- 1 small bunch Swiss chard, stems removed, leaves cut into 1-inch pieces
- 8 ounces whole-wheat penne, rigatoni or fusilli
- 1/2 cup freshly grated Parmesan cheese
- 1/4 teaspoon salt, or to taste
- Freshly ground pepper, to taste

PREPARATION

1. Put a large pot of water on to boil for cooking pasta.
2. Heat oil in a large nonstick skillet over medium heat. Add tofu and cook, stirring, until lightly browned, 3 to 5 minutes. Transfer to a plate. Add onion to the pan; cook, stirring often, until softened and golden, 2 to 3 minutes. Add garlic and crushed red pepper; cook, stirring, for 30 seconds. Return the tofu to the pan and add broth and squash; bring to a simmer. Cover and cook for 10 minutes. Add chard and stir to immerse. Cover and cook until the squash and chard are tender, about 5 minutes.
3. Meanwhile, cook pasta until just tender, 8 to 10 minutes or according to package directions. Drain and return to the pot. Add the squash mixture, Parmesan, salt and pepper; toss to coat.

NUTRITION

Per serving: 386 calories; 5 g fat (2 g sat, 1 g mono); 18 mg cholesterol; 63 g carbohydrates; 16 g protein; 9 g fiber; 660 mg sodium; 755 mg potassium.
Nutrition Bonus: Vitamin A (340% daily value), Vitamin C (80% dv), Calcium (25% dv), Potassium (22% dv).
Carbohydrate Servings: 4
Exchanges: 4 starch, 1 vegetable, 1 medium-fat meat, 1/2 fat

Tangy Cauliflower Salad

INGREDIENTS
- 1 small clove garlic, minced
- 2 tablespoons capers
- 2 tablespoons extra-virgin olive oil
- 2 tablespoons white-wine vinegar
- 1/4 teaspoon crushed red pepper
- 1 lemon, zested (2 teaspoons) and juiced (2 tablespoons)
- 8 cups bite-size cauliflower florets, (about 1 head), cooked until tender-crisp (see Tip)

PREPARATION
1. Whisk garlic, capers, oil, vinegar, crushed red pepper, lemon zest and juice in a large bowl. Add cauliflower to the bowl and toss to coat. Chill the salad for 30 minutes, or overnight. Serve cold.

TIPS & NOTES
- **Make Ahead Tip**: Refrigerate for up to 2 days.

- **Tip:** To cook florets: In a steamer basket, cover and steam 8 to 10 minutes for tender-crisp or 15 minutes for very tender. Or microwave, covered, with 1/4 cup water for 2 to 4 minutes for tender-crisp or 3 to 5 minutes for tender. A 2-pound head of cauliflower yields about 8 cups bite-size florets.

NUTRITION

Per serving: 113 calories; 8 g fat (1 g sat, 5 g mono); 0 mg cholesterol; 9 g carbohydrates; 0 g added sugars; 4 g protein; 6 g fiber; 158 mg sodium; 294 mg potassium.
Nutrition Bonus: Cauliflower is a good source of vitamin C, a powerful antioxidant, and has a modest amount of calcium.
Carbohydrate Servings: 1/2
Exchanges: 1 1/2 vegetable, 1 1/2 fat

Peas & Lettuce

INGREDIENTS
- 4 teaspoons extra-virgin olive oil
- 2 cups shelled fresh peas, (3 pounds unshelled)
- 1 tablespoon finely chopped fresh mint
- 4 cups thinly sliced Boston lettuce, (about 1 small head)
- 1/4 teaspoon salt
- Freshly ground pepper, to taste

PREPARATION
1. Heat oil in a large nonstick skillet over medium-low heat. Add peas and stir to coat with oil. Cover and cook, stirring once or twice, until beginning to brown, about 4 minutes. Stir in mint and cook for 30 seconds. Add lettuce, cover and cook, stirring once or twice, until wilted, 1 to 2 minutes. Remove from the heat and season with salt and pepper.

NUTRITION
Per serving: 113 calories; 5 g fat (1 g sat, 4 g mono); 0 mg cholesterol; 13 g carbohydrates; 0 g added sugars; 5 g protein; 5 g fiber; 206 mg sodium; 225 mg potassium.
Nutrition Bonus: Vitamin A (70% daily value), Folate (22% dv), Vitamin C (15% dv).
Carbohydrate Servings: 1
Exchanges: 1 starch, 1/2 vegetable, 1 fat

Oatmeal Chocolate Chip Cookies

INGREDIENTS
- 2 cups rolled oats, (not quick-cooking)
- 1/2 cup whole-wheat pastry flour, (see Ingredient Note)
- 1/2 cup all-purpose flour
- 1 teaspoon ground cinnamon
- 1/2 teaspoon baking soda
- 1/2 teaspoon salt
- 1/2 cup tahini, (see Ingredient Note)
- 4 tablespoons cold unsalted butter, cut into pieces
- 2/3 cup granulated sugar
- 2/3 cup packed light brown sugar
- 1 large egg
- 1 large egg white
- 1 tablespoon vanilla extract
- 1 cup semisweet or bittersweet chocolate chips
- 1/2 cup chopped walnuts

PREPARATION
1. Position racks in upper and lower thirds of oven; preheat to 350°F. Line 2 baking sheets with parchment paper.
2. Whisk oats, whole-wheat flour, all-purpose flour, cinnamon, baking soda and salt in a medium bowl. Beat tahini and butter in a large bowl with an electric mixer until blended into a paste. Add granulated sugar and brown sugar; continue beating until well combined; the mixture will still be a little grainy. Beat in egg, then egg white, then vanilla. Stir in the oat mixture with a wooden spoon until just moistened. Stir in chocolate chips and walnuts.
3. With damp hands, roll 1 tablespoon of the batter into a ball, place it on a prepared baking sheet and flatten it until squat, but don't let the sides crack. Continue with the remaining batter, spacing the flattened balls 2 inches apart.
4. Bake the cookies until golden brown, about 16 minutes, switching the pans back to front and top to bottom halfway through. Cool on the pans for 2 minutes, then transfer the cookies to a wire rack to cool completely. Let the pans cool for a few minutes before baking another batch.

TIPS & NOTES
- **Make Ahead Tip**: Store in an airtight container for up to 2 days or freeze for longer storage.
- **Ingredient notes:** Whole-wheat pastry flour, lower in protein than regular whole-wheat flour, has less gluten-forming potential, making it a better choice for tender baked goods. You can find it in the natural-foods section of large super markets and natural-foods stores. Store in the freezer.
- Tahini is a paste made from ground sesame seeds. Look for it in natural-foods stores and some supermarkets.

NUTRITION
Per cookie: 102 calories; 5 g fat (2 g sat, 1 g mono); 7 mg cholesterol; 14 g carbohydrates; 2 g protein; 1 gfiber; 45 mg sodium; 53 mg potassium.
Carbohydrate Servings: 1
Exchanges: 1 other carbohydrate, 1 fat

Pampered Chicken

INGREDIENTS
- 4 boneless, skinless chicken breast halves, (about 1 pound), trimmed of fat
- 4 slices Monterey Jack cheese, (2 ounces)
- 2 egg whites
- 1/3 cup seasoned (Italian-style) breadcrumbs
- 2 tablespoons freshly grated Parmesan cheese
- 2 tablespoons chopped fresh parsley

- 1/4 teaspoon salt, or to taste
- 1/2 teaspoon freshly ground pepper
- 2 teaspoons extra-virgin olive oil
- Lemon wedges, for garnish

PREPARATION
1. Preheat oven to 400°F. Place a chicken breast, skinned-side down, on a cutting board. Keeping the blade of a sharp knife parallel to the board, make a horizontal slit along the thinner, long edge of the breast, cutting nearly through to the opposite side. Open the breast so it forms two flaps, hinged at the center. Place a slice of cheese on one flap, leaving a 1/2-inch border at the edge. Press remaining flap down firmly over the cheese and set aside. Repeat with the remaining breasts.
2. Lightly beat egg whites with a fork in a medium bowl. Mix breadcrumbs, Parmesan, parsley, salt and pepper in a shallow dish. Holding a stuffed breast together firmly, dip it in the egg whites and then roll in the breadcrumbs. Repeat with the remaining breasts.
3. Heat oil in a large ovenproof skillet over medium-high heat. Add the stuffed breasts and cook until browned on one side, about 2 minutes. Turn the breasts over and place the skillet in the oven.
4. Bake the chicken until no longer pink in the center, about 20 minutes. Serve with lemon wedges.

NUTRITION
Per serving: 255 calories; 11 g fat (4 g sat, 4 g mono); 78 mg cholesterol; 7 g carbohydrates; 31 g protein; 1 g fiber; 518 mg sodium; 268 mg potassium.
Nutrition Bonus: Selenium (40% daily value), Calcium (15% dv).
Carbohydrate Servings: 1/2
Exchanges: 1/2 starch, 4 very lean meat, 1 medium-fat meat

Cider-Brined Pork Chops

INGREDIENTS
BRINE
- 2 cups apple cider
- 1 cup water
- 1/4 cup kosher salt
- 1/4 cup honey
- 1/8 teaspoon ground cinnamon
- 2 cups ice

PORK CHOPS & SAUTEED APPLES

- 2 bone-in pork rib chops, (about 1 3/4 pounds, 1-1 1/4 inch thick), trimmed
- 1 teaspoon fresh sage, chopped
- 1 teaspoon freshly ground pepper
- 1/4 teaspoon ground ginger, divided
- 2 teaspoons extra-virgin olive oil
- 1 teaspoon butter
- 1/2 cup onion, thinly sliced
- 1/2 cup white wine
- 1 tart apple, peeled and thinly sliced
- 1/2 cup apple cider

PREPARATION
1. To prepare cider brine: Pour cider and water into a bowl and stir in salt until dissolved, then stir in honey and cinnamon until the honey is dissolved. Stir in ice and check to see that the mixture registers 45°F or lower on an instant-read thermometer.
2. To prepare chops & apples: Place chops in a large sealable plastic bag. Carefully add the brine to the bag, seal, then place the bag in a bowl in case of any leaks. Refrigerate for at least 3 hours or up to 8 hours.
3. Combine sage, pepper and 1/8 teaspoon ginger in a small bowl. Remove the chops from the brine. (Discard bag and brine.) Sprinkle both sides of the chops with the sage mixture.
4. Heat a large heavy skillet over medium heat. Add oil and the chops. Cook until lightly browned, 2 to 3 minutes per side. Transfer the chops to a plate.
5. Melt butter in the pan; add onion, stir to coat, cover and cook, stirring often, until starting to turn translucent and brown, 2 to 3 minutes. Add wine and stir, scraping up any browned bits; cook for 1 minute. Stir in apple, cider and 1/8 teaspoon ginger; bring to a boil. Nestle the chops into the sauce, reduce heat to a simmer, cover and cook for 3 minutes. Turn the chops, cover and cook until an instant-read thermometer inserted into the center of the chops registers 145°F, 3 to 5 minutes. Transfer the chops to a warm platter and tent with foil.
6. Bring the sauce in the pan to a boil and cook until it is syrupy, 3 to 4 minutes. Spoon the sauce over the chops and serve.

TIPS & NOTES
- **Make Ahead Tip**: Brine chops (Steps 1-2) for up to 8 hours.

NUTRITION
Per serving: 261 calories; 12 g fat (4 g sat, 6 g mono); 74 mg cholesterol; 8 g carbohydrates; 22 g protein; 1 g fiber; 369 mg sodium; 490 mg potassium.
Nutrition Bonus: Selenium (51% daily value), Zinc (22% dv), Potassium (14% dv).

Carbohydrate Servings: 1/2
Exchanges: 1/2 fruit, 3 lean meat

Sliced Fennel Salad

INGREDIENTS
- 1 large fennel bulb
- 1 tablespoon extra-virgin olive oil
- 1 tablespoon lemon juice
- 1/8 teaspoon salt
- Freshly ground pepper, to taste

PREPARATION
1. Trim base from fennel bulb. Remove and discard the fennel stalks; reserve some of the feathery leaves for garnish. Pull off and discard any discolored parts from the bulb. Stand the bulb upright and cut vertically into very thin slices. Arrange the slices on 4 salad plates.
2. Whisk oil, lemon juice and salt in a small bowl. Drizzle the mixture over the fennel and garnish with a grinding of pepper and a few fennel leaves.

NUTRITION
Per serving: 51 calories; 4 g fat (0 g sat, 3 g mono); 0 mg cholesterol; 5 g carbohydrates; 0 g added sugars;1 g protein; 2 g fiber; 103 mg sodium; 247 mg potassium.
Nutrition Bonus: Vitamin C (15% daily value).
Exchanges: vegetable, 1 fat (mono)

Pina Colada Yogurt Parfait

INGREDIENTS
- 1/3 cup reduced-fat vanilla yogurt
- 1/2 cup crushed canned pineapple, or canned mandarin oranges
- 1 tablespoon toasted coconut, (see Tip)

PREPARATION
1. Top yogurt with pineapple (or canned mandarin oranges) and coconut.

TIPS & NOTES
- **Tip:** To toast coconut: Place coconut in a small dry skillet and cook, stirring often, until golden, about 5 minutes or spread in a shallow baking dish and bake at 350°F until light golden and fragrant, 5 to 10 minutes.

NUTRITION
Per serving (with pineapple): 155 calories; 3 g fat (3 g sat, 0 g mono); 4 mg cholesterol; 28 gcarbohydrates; 5 g protein; 2 g fiber; 57 mg sodium; 325 mg potassium.
Carbohydrate Servings: 2
Exchanges: pineapple: 1/2 low-fat milk, 1 fruit, oranges: 1/2 low-fat milk, 1 fruit
Nutrition Note: Per serving (with oranges): 133 calories; 3 g fat (3 g sat, 0 g mono); 4 mg cholesterol; 22 g carbohydrate; 5 g protein; 1 g fiber; 60 mg sodium; 333 mg potassium.1 1/2 Carbohydrate Servings
Exchanges: 1/2 low-fat milk, 1 fruit

DAY 21
BREAKFAST

Skim milk (1 cup)
Cranberry Muesli
Banana (1 cup, sliced)

LUNCH

Curried Tofu Salad or Grilled Smoky Eggplant Salad
Whole-wheat pita bread (1 medium pita)
Roasted Corn, Black Bean & Mango Salad

SNACK

Low-fat vanilla yogurt (8 oz.)
Nectarine (1 small)

DINNER

Roast Salmon with Salsa
Brown rice (1 cup, cooked)
North African Spiced Carrots
Rainbow Chopped Salad
Grilled Apples with Cheese & Honey or Summer Berry Pudding

DAY 21 RECIPES

Cranberry Muesli

INGREDIENTS
- 1/2 cup low-fat plain yogurt
- 1/2 cup unsweetened or fruit-juice-sweetened cranberry juice
- 6 tablespoons old-fashioned rolled oats, (not quick-cooking or steel-cut)
- 2 tablespoons dried cranberries
- 1 tablespoon unsalted sunflower seeds
- 1 tablespoon wheat germ

- 2 teaspoons honey
- 1/4 teaspoon vanilla extract
- 1/8 teaspoon salt

PREPARATION

1. Combine yogurt, juice, oats, cranberries, sunflower seeds, wheat germ, honey, vanilla and salt in a medium bowl; cover and refrigerate for at least 8 hours and up to 1 day.

TIPS & NOTES

- **Make Ahead Tip**: Cover and refrigerate for up to 1 day.

NUTRITION

Per serving: 209 calories; 4 g fat (1 g sat, 1 g mono); 4 mg cholesterol; 37 g carbohydrates; 8 g protein; 3 gfiber; 190 mg sodium; 266 mg potassium.
Nutrition Bonus: Calcium (15% daily value)
Carbohydrate Servings: 2 1/2
Exchanges: 1 starch, 1 fruit, 1/2 other carbohydrate, 1/2 fat

Curried Tofu Salad

INGREDIENTS

- 3 tablespoons low-fat plain yogurt
- 2 tablespoons reduced-fat mayonnaise
- 2 tablespoons prepared mango chutney
- 2 teaspoons hot curry powder, preferably Madras
- 1/4 teaspoon salt
- Freshly ground pepper, to taste
- 1 14-ounce package extra-firm water-packed tofu, drained, rinsed and finely crumbled (see Ingredient note)
- 2 stalks celery, diced
- 1 cup red grapes, sliced in half
- 1/2 cup sliced scallions
- 1/4 cup chopped walnuts

PREPARATION

1. Whisk yogurt, mayonnaise, chutney, curry powder, salt and pepper in a large bowl. Stir in tofu, celery, grapes, scallions and walnuts.

TIPS & NOTES

- **Make Ahead Tip**: Cover and refrigerate for up to 2 days.

- **Ingredient Note:** We prefer water-packed tofu from the refrigerated section of the supermarket. Crumbling it into uneven pieces creates more surface area, improving the texture and avoiding the blocky look that turns many people away.

NUTRITION
Per serving: 140 calories; 8 g fat (1 g sat, 2 g mono); 2 mg cholesterol; 13 g carbohydrates; 3 g added sugars; 7 g protein; 2 g fiber; 241 mg sodium; 271 mg potassium.
Nutrition Bonus: Calcium (15% daily value).
Carbohydrate Servings: 1
Exchanges: 1 other carb, 1 medium-fat meat

Grilled Smoky Eggplant Salad

INGREDIENTS
- 2 small eggplants, (about 1 pound total)
- 3/4 teaspoon kosher salt, divided
- Olive oil cooking spray
- 1/4 cup extra-virgin olive oil
- 1 tablespoon sherry vinegar
- 1 small plum tomato, diced
- 1 small clove garlic, chopped
- 1 1/2 teaspoons smoked paprika, (see Note)
- 3 cups mixed baby salad greens
- 2 ounces Manchego cheese, cut into thin curls with a vegetable peeler (see Note)

PREPARATION
1. Preheat grill to medium.
2. Cut stripes in each eggplant's peel by running a vegetable peeler down the length of it and repeating at about 1-inch intervals. Slice the eggplants into rounds 1/3 to 1/2 inch thick. Lay them on a baking sheet and sprinkle lightly with 1/2 teaspoon salt. Let stand for about 5 minutes.
3. Blot the eggplant slices with paper towels and lightly coat both sides with olive oil cooking spray. Grill the eggplant, flipping halfway through, until soft and browned on both sides, 9 to 11 minutes total.
4. Puree oil, vinegar, tomato, garlic, paprika and the remaining 1/4 teaspoon salt in a blender until well combined.
5. Toss salad greens with half the vinaigrette in a medium bowl. Arrange the eggplant slices on 6 salad plates. Drizzle with the remaining vinaigrette. Place

the salad greens over and between the eggplant slices, then scatter the cheese curls on top of each salad. Serve warm or at room temperature.

TIPS & NOTES

- **Make Ahead Tip**: Prepare eggplant and vinaigrette (Steps 1-4), cover and refrigerate separately for up to 1 day. Bring to room temperature before serving.
- **Note:** To experience the full flavor of this salad, it's worth seeking out the two signature Spanish ingredients: mild- flavored, smooth sheep-milk Manchego cheese and smoked paprika. If you can't find them, substitute Parmigiano-Reggiano and Hungarian paprika.

NUTRITION

Per serving: 141 calories; 12 g fat (3 g sat, 7 g mono); 7 mg cholesterol; 6 g carbohydrates; 3 g protein; 3 gfiber; 280 mg sodium; 287 mg potassium.
Nutrition Bonus: Vitamin A (25% daily value), Vitamin C (15% dv)
Carbohydrate Servings: 1/2
Exchanges: 1 vegetable, 2 fat

Roasted Corn, Black Bean & Mango Salad

INGREDIENTS

- 2 teaspoons canola oil
- 1 clove garlic, minced
- 1 1/2 cups corn kernels, (from 3 ears)
- 1 large ripe mango, (about 1 pound), peeled and diced
- 1 15-ounce or 19-ounce can black beans, rinsed
- 1/2 cup chopped red onion
- 1/2 cup diced red bell pepper
- 3 tablespoons lime juice
- 1 small canned chipotle pepper in adobo sauce, (see Ingredient Note), drained and chopped
- 1 1/2 tablespoons chopped fresh cilantro
- 1/4 teaspoon ground cumin
- 1/4 teaspoon salt

PREPARATION

1. Heat oil in a large nonstick skillet over medium-high heat. Add garlic and cook, stirring, until fragrant, about 30 seconds. Stir in corn and cook, stirring occasionally, until browned, about 8 minutes. Transfer the corn mixture to a large bowl. Stir in mango, beans, onion, bell pepper, lime juice, chipotle, cilantro, cumin and salt.

TIPS & NOTES
- **Make Ahead Tip**: Cover and refrigerate for up to 8 hours. Serve at room temperature.
- **Ingredient Note:** Chipotle peppers are smoked jalapenos with a fiery taste that are canned in adobo sauce. Look for them in the Hispanic section of large supermarkets and in specialty stores.

NUTRITION
Per serving: 125 calories; 2 g fat (0 g sat, 1 g mono); 0 mg cholesterol; 26 g carbohydrates; 0 g added sugars; 4 g protein; 4 g fiber; 245 mg sodium; 223 mg potassium.
Nutrition Bonus: Vitamin C (70% daily value), Fiber (18% dv).
Carbohydrate Servings: 2
Exchanges: 1 starch, 1 fruit

Roast Salmon with Salsa

INGREDIENTS
- 2 medium plum tomatoes, chopped
- 1 small onion, roughly chopped
- 1 clove garlic, peeled and quartered
- 1 fresh jalapeno pepper, seeded and chopped
- 2 teaspoons cider vinegar
- 1 teaspoon chili powder
- 1/2 teaspoon ground cumin
- 1/2 teaspoon salt
- 2-4 dashes hot sauce
- 1 1/2 pounds salmon fillet, skinned and cut into 6 portions

PREPARATION
1. Preheat oven to 400°F.
2. Place tomatoes, onion, garlic, jalapeno, vinegar, chili powder, cumin, salt and hot sauce to taste in a food processor; process until finely diced and uniform.
3. Place salmon in a large roasting pan; spoon the salsa on top. Roast until the salmon is flaky on the outside but still pink inside, about 15 minutes.

NUTRITION
Per serving: 227 calories; 13 g fat (3 g sat, 5 g mono); 65 mg cholesterol; 3 g carbohydrates; 0 g added sugars; 23 g protein; 1 g fiber; 269 mg sodium; 474 mg potassium.
Nutrition Bonus: Good source of omega-3s
Exchanges: 1/2 vegetable, 3.5 lean meat

North African Spiced Carrots

INGREDIENTS
- 1 tablespoon extra-virgin olive oil
- 4 cloves garlic, minced
- 2 teaspoons paprika
- 1 teaspoon ground cumin
- 1 teaspoon ground coriander
- 3 cups sliced carrots, (4 medium-large)
- 1 cup water
- 3 tablespoons lemon juice
- 1/8 teaspoon salt, or to taste
- 1/4 cup chopped fresh parsley

PREPARATION

1. Heat oil in a large nonstick skillet over medium heat. Add garlic, paprika, cumin and coriander; cook, stirring, until fragrant but not browned, about 20 seconds. Add carrots, water, lemon juice and salt; bring to a simmer. Reduce heat to low, cover and cook until almost tender, 5 to 7 minutes. Uncover and simmer, stirring often, until the carrots are just tender and the liquid is syrupy, 2 to 4 minutes. Stir in parsley. Serve hot or at room temperature.

NUTRITION

Per serving: 51 calories; 3 g fat (0 g sat, 2 g mono); 0 mg cholesterol; 7 g carbohydrates; 0 g added sugars;1 g protein; 2 g fiber; 86 mg sodium; 186 mg potassium.
Nutrition Bonus: Vitamin A (210% daily value), Vitamin C (15% dv).
Carbohydrate Servings: 1/2
Exchanges: 1 vegetable, 1/2 fat (mono)

Rainbow Chopped Salad

INGREDIENTS
ORANGE-OREGANO DRESSING
- 1/2 teaspoon orange zest
- 1/2 cup orange juice, preferably freshly squeezed
- 1/4 cup cider vinegar
- 1 tablespoon extra-virgin olive oil
- 2 teaspoons fresh oregano, chopped, or 3/4 teaspoon dried
- 1 teaspoon Dijon mustard

- 1/2 teaspoon salt
- 1/2 teaspoon freshly ground pepper

SALAD
- 1 1/2 cups bell peppers, chopped
- 1 1/2 cups broccoli florets, chopped
- 1 cup shredded carrots
- 1/2 cup radishes, diced
- 1 tablespoon red onion, minced
- 1/2 cup Orange-Oregano Dressing

PREPARATION

1. To prepare dressing: Place orange zest and juice, vinegar, oil, oregano, mustard, salt and pepper in a jar. Cover and shake to combine. (Makes about 1 cup.)
2. To prepare salad: Combine bell peppers, broccoli, carrots, radishes and onion in a medium bowl. Add 1/2 cup of the dressing and toss to coat. Refrigerate until ready to serve. (Refrigerate extra dressing for up to 1 week.)

TIPS & NOTES
- **Make Ahead Tip**: Cover and refrigerate dressing for up to 1 week.

NUTRITION

Per serving: 52 calories; 1 g fat (0 g sat, 1 g mono); 0 mg cholesterol; 9 g carbohydrates; 0 g added sugars; 2 g protein; 3 g fiber; 111 mg sodium; 350 mg potassium.
Nutrition Bonus: Vitamin C (173% daily value), Vitamin A (143% dv)
Carbohydrate Servings: 1/2
Exchanges: 1 1/2 vegetable, 1/2 fat

Grilled Apples with Cheese & Honey

INGREDIENTS
- 1 large or 2 small tart apples, peeled and sliced into 1/2-inch-thick rounds
- 2 teaspoons almond or canola oil
- 1 teaspoon confectioners' sugar
- 1 ounce sharp Cheddar or Parmigiano-Reggiano cheese
- 2 tablespoons chopped pecans, toasted
- 4 teaspoons honey

PREPARATION

1. Preheat grill or grill pan to medium heat. Toss apple slices with oil and sugar in a large bowl. Grill the apple slices until just tender and lightly marked, turning once, about 6 minutes total. Shave cheese into thin strips with a vegetable peeler. Top the apple slices with a sprinkling of cheese and nuts and drizzle with honey.

TIPS & NOTES

- **Make Ahead Tip**: Let your cheese come to room temperature before serving for the best flavor.

NUTRITION

Per serving: 250 calories; 14 g fat (3 g sat, 6 g mono); 15 mg cholesterol; 30 g carbohydrates; 5 g protein; 3 g fiber; 93 mg sodium; 174 mg potassium.
Carbohydrate Servings: 2
Exchanges: 2 fruit, 3 fat

Summary Berry Pudding

INGREDIENTS

- 4 small slices firm white bread, crusts removed
- 1 cup sliced fresh strawberries
- 1 cup fresh blueberries
- 1 cup fresh raspberries
- 2 tablespoons sugar
- 2 tablespoons water
- Pinch of salt

PREPARATION

1. Place a 1-cup (8-ounce) ramekin or similar-size dish on top of a slice of bread and cut around it to trim the bread to fit the dish. Repeat with the remaining 3 slices of bread.
2. Combine berries, sugar, water and salt in a medium saucepan and cook over medium-high heat until the berries break down, 5 to 6 minutes. Reserve 1/3 cup for garnish; cover and refrigerate.
3. Place 1 tablespoon of the remaining berry mixture in the bottom of each ramekin. Top with a slice of bread. Divide the remaining berry mixture between each, then top with another slice of bread.
4. Put the puddings on a large plate to catch any overflowing juices. Cover each with plastic wrap, then place a 15-ounce weight, such as a can of beans, on top of each pudding. Refrigerate for at least 6 hours or up to 2 days.

5. To unmold, remove the weight and plastic wrap, run a knife around the inside of the ramekin, and invert onto a dessert plate. Spoon the reserved berry mixture over the puddings.

TIPS & NOTES
- **Make Ahead Tip**: Cover and refrigerate for up to 2 days. | Equipment: Two 1-cup (8-ounce) ramekins or similar-size dishes

NUTRITION
Per serving: 252 calories; 2 g fat (0 g sat, 0 g mono); 0 mg cholesterol; 56 g carbohydrates; 5 g protein; 8 gfiber; 299 mg sodium; 277 mg potassium.
Nutrition Bonus: Vitamin C (120% daily value), rich in antioxidants (anthocyanidins, ellagic acid).
Carbohydrate Servings: 3
Exchanges: 1 starch, 1 1/2 fruit, 1 other carbohydrate

DAY 22
BREAKFAST
Oatbran Bagel
Skim milk (1 cup)
Vegetable Cream Cheese
LUNCH
Skim milk (1 cup)
Bistro Beef Salad or King Crab & Potato Salad
Whole-wheat pita bread (1 medium pita)
Apricot (1 cup, halves)
SNACK
Carrot sticks (1 cup)
Black Bean Dip
DINNER
Chicken, Broccoli Rabe & Feta on Toast or The Cobb Salad
Green Tea Rice
Mixed Berry Sundaes

DAY 22 RECIPES

Vegetable Cream Cheese

INGREDIENTS
- 8 ounces light cream cheese
- 1/4 cup chopped scallions
- 1/4 cup finely chopped carrots
- 1/4 cup finely chopped daikon radish
- 2 tablespoons chopped fresh dill
- 1/4 teaspoon freshly ground pepper

PREPARATION
1. Blend all ingredients in a small bowl.

NUTRITION
Per tablespoon: 30 calories; 2 g fat (1 g sat, 1 g mono); 7 mg cholesterol; 2 g carbohydrates; 1 g protein; 1 g fiber; 56 mg sodium; 10 mg potassium.
Exchanges: 1/2 fat

Bistro Beef Salad

INGREDIENTS
- 4 red potatoes, scrubbed and cut into quarters (1 pound)
- Salt, to taste
- 2 tablespoons chopped shallots
- 2 tablespoons white-wine vinegar
- 1 tablespoon Dijon mustard
- 1 tablespoon chopped fresh parsley
- 1 tablespoon chopped fresh tarragon, or 1 teaspoon dried
- 2 tablespoons cold water
- 1 tablespoon extra-virgin olive oil
- Freshly ground black pepper, to taste
- 1 large head red leaf lettuce, torn (8 cups)
- 2 cups red or yellow cherry tomatoes, cut in half
- 12 ounces cooked roast beef, or steak, thinly sliced

PREPARATION
1. Place potatoes in a medium saucepan and cover with lightly salted water by 1 inch. Bring to a boil over medium heat and cook until tender, about 15 minutes.
2. Meanwhile, whisk shallots, vinegar, mustard, parsley, tarragon and water in a small bowl. Slowly whisk in oil. Season with salt and pepper.

3. Drain the potatoes and rinse with cold water. Divide lettuce among 4 plates; arrange the potatoes, tomatoes and beef on top. Drizzle with the dressing and serve.

NUTRITION
Per serving: 355 calories; 15 g fat (5 g sat, 7 g mono); 69 mg cholesterol; 25 g carbohydrates; 28 g protein;3 g fiber; 283 mg sodium; 615 mg potassium.
Nutrition Bonus: Vitamin A (100% daily value), Vitamin C (70% dv), Zinc (44% dv), Selenium (29% dv), Iron (25% dv).
Carbohydrate Servings: 2
Exchanges: 2 starch, 2 vegetable, 3 lean meat, 1 fat

King Crab & Potato Salad

INGREDIENTS
- 3/4 pound green beans, trimmed
- 1 1/2 pounds small red-skinned potatoes, cut into eighths
- 1 3/4 pounds cooked king crab legs, thawed if frozen (see Tip), meat removed and cut into 1-inch pieces
- 3 stalks celery, thinly sliced
- 6 radishes, halved and thinly sliced
- 1 small red onion, diced
- 1 clove garlic, crushed
- 3 tablespoons lemon juice
- 2 tablespoons white-wine vinegar
- 1 tablespoon Dijon mustard
- 5 tablespoons extra-virgin olive oil
- 2 tablespoons minced fresh basil
- 1/2 teaspoon salt
- 1/2 teaspoon freshly ground pepper

PREPARATION
1. Bring a large pot of water to a boil. Add beans and cook until bright green, 2 to 3 minutes. Transfer to a colander using a slotted spoon; refresh under cold water.
2. Add potatoes to the boiling water. Cook until tender when pierced with a fork, 8 to 10 minutes. Drain in a colander; refresh under cold water until room temperature.
3. Toss the green beans and potatoes with crab, celery, radishes and onion in a large bowl.
4. Whisk garlic, lemon juice, vinegar and mustard in a small bowl; slowly whisk in oil. Whisk in basil, salt and pepper. Discard the garlic; pour the dressing over the salad and toss to coat.

TIPS & NOTES
- **Make Ahead Tip**: Cover and refrigerate for up to 1 day.
- **Tip:** To defrost frozen lobster tails or crab legs, let thaw in the refrigerator overnight.

NUTRITION
Per serving: 330 calories; 16 g fat (2 g sat, 11 g mono); 67 mg cholesterol; 28 g carbohydrates; 0 g added sugars; 18 g protein; 4 g fiber; 483 mg sodium; 428 mg potassium.
Nutrition Bonus: Vitamin C (70% daily value), Selenium (41% dv), Zinc (20% dv).
Carbohydrate Servings: 2
Exchanges: 1 1/2 starch, 1 vegetable, 2 lean meat, 2 fat

Black Bean Dip

INGREDIENTS
- 1 19-ounce or 15-ounce can black beans, rinsed
- 1/2 cup prepared salsa, hot or mild
- 2 tablespoons fresh lime juice
- 2 tablespoons chopped fresh cilantro
- 1/4 teaspoon ground cumin
- Salt & freshly ground pepper, to taste

PREPARATION
1. Combine black beans, salsa, lime juice, cilantro and cumin in a food processor. Process until smooth. Season with salt and pepper.

TIPS & NOTES
- **Make Ahead Tip**: Cover and refrigerate for up to 2 days.

NUTRITION
Per tablespoon: 17 calories; 0 g fat (0 g sat, 0 g mono); 0 mg cholesterol; 3 g carbohydrates; 0 g added sugars; 1 g protein; 1 g fiber; 53 mg sodium; 2 mg potassium.
Exchanges: free food

Chicken, Broccoli Rabe & Feta on Toast

INGREDIENTS
- 4 thick slices whole-wheat country bread
- 1 clove garlic, peeled (optional), plus 1/4 cup chopped garlic
- 4 teaspoons extra-virgin olive oil, divided
- 1 pound chicken tenders, cut crosswise into 1/2-inch pieces

- 1 bunch broccoli rabe, stems trimmed, cut into 1-inch pieces, or 2 bunches broccolini, chopped (see Ingredient note)
- 2 cups cherry tomatoes, halved
- 1 tablespoon red-wine vinegar
- 1/8 teaspoon salt
- Freshly ground pepper, to taste
- 3/4 cup crumbled feta cheese

PREPARATION
1. Grill or toast bread. Lightly rub with peeled garlic clove, if desired. Discard the garlic.
2. Heat 2 teaspoons oil in a large nonstick skillet over high heat until shimmering but not smoking. Add chicken; cook, stirring occasionally, until just cooked through and no longer pink in the middle, 4 to 5 minutes. Transfer the chicken and any juices to a plate; cover to keep warm.
3. Add the remaining 2 teaspoons oil to the pan. Add chopped garlic and cook, stirring constantly, until fragrant but not brown, about 30 seconds. Add broccoli rabe (or broccolini) and cook, stirring often, until bright green and just wilted, 2 to 4 minutes. Stir in tomatoes, vinegar, salt and pepper; cook, stirring occasionally, until the tomatoes are beginning to break down, 2 to 4 minutes. Return the chicken and juices to the pan, add feta cheese and stir to combine. Cook until heated through, 1 to 2 minutes. Serve warm over garlic toasts.

TIPS & NOTES
- **Ingredient Note:** Pleasantly pungent and mildly bitter, broccoli rabe, or rapini, is a member of the cabbage family and commonly used in Mediterranean cooking. Broccolini (a cross between broccoli and Chinese kale) is sweet and tender - the florets and stalks are edible.

NUTRITION

Per serving: 313 calories; 11 g fat (5 g sat, 5 g mono); 85 mg cholesterol; 26 g carbohydrates; 35 g protein;4 g fiber; 653 mg sodium; 423 mg potassium.
Nutrition Bonus: Vitamin C (160% daily value), Vitamin A (140% dv), Selenium (28% dv), Calcium (20% dv).
Carbohydrate Servings: 2
Exchanges: 1 starch, 2 vegetable, 4 lean meat

The Cobb Salad

INGREDIENTS

- 3 tablespoons white-wine vinegar
- 2 tablespoons finely minced shallot
- 1 tablespoon Dijon mustard
- 1 teaspoon freshly ground pepper and 1/4 teaspoon salt
- 3 tablespoons extra-virgin olive oil
- 10 cups mixed salad greens
- 8 ounces shredded cooked chicken breast, (about 1 large breast half; see Tip)
- 2 large eggs, hard-boiled (see Tip), peeled and chopped
- 2 medium tomatoes, diced
- 1 large cucumber, seeded and sliced
- 1 avocado, diced
- 2 slices cooked bacon, crumbled
- 1/2 cup crumbled blue cheese, (optional)

PREPARATION

1. Whisk vinegar, shallot, mustard, pepper and salt in a small bowl to combine. Whisk in oil until combined. Place salad greens in a large bowl. Add half of the dressing and toss to coat.
2. Divide the greens among 4 plates. Arrange equal portions of chicken, egg, tomatoes, cucumber, avocado, bacon and blue cheese (if using) on top of the lettuce. Drizzle the salads with the remaining dressing.

TIPS & NOTES

- **Tips:** To poach chicken breasts, place boneless, skinless chicken breasts in a medium skillet or saucepan and add lightly salted water to cover; bring to a boil. Cover, reduce heat to low and simmer gently until chicken is cooked through and no longer pink in the middle, 10 to 15 minutes. To shred the chicken, use two forks to pull it apart into long shreds.
- To hard-boil eggs, place in a single layer in a saucepan; cover with water. Bring to a simmer over medium-high heat. Reduce heat to low and cook at the barest simmer for 10 minutes. Remove from heat, pour out hot water and fill the pan with a mixture of cold water and ice cubes; let stand until the eggs are completely cooled.

NUTRITION

Per serving: 352 calories; 24 g fat (4 g sat, 15 g mono); 134 mg cholesterol; 18 g carbohydrates; 21 gprotein; 8 g fiber; 445 mg sodium; 788 mg potassium.

Nutrition Bonus: Vitamin A (117% daily value), Vitamin C (27% dv), Potassium (20% dv), Folate (18% dv), Iron (15% dv).
Carbohydrate Servings: 1/2
Exchanges: 2 vegetable, 3 lean meat, 3 fat

Green Tea Rice

INGREDIENTS
- 1 1/2 cups short-grain rice, preferably Japanese (see Substitution Note)
- 2 cups cold water
- 2 tablespoons sake
- 1 tablespoon green tea leaves, preferably sencha
- 3/4 teaspoon kosher salt
- 2 tablespoons sesame seeds, toasted (see Tip)

PREPARATION
1. Place rice in a fine-mesh sieve and rinse under cold water, using your hand to gently stir the rice until the milky-white liquid runs clear, about 2 minutes.
2. Transfer the rice to a heavy medium saucepan and add water and sake. Let soak for at least 1 hour.
3. Using a mortar and pestle or spice grinder, grind tea leaves and salt to make a powder. Stir it into the rice.
4. Bring the rice to a boil. Reduce heat to very low and cook, covered, for 10 minutes. Remove from the heat and let the rice rest, covered, for 10 minutes more, so it can settle and finish cooking.
5. Remove the lid and gently stir the rice. Sprinkle each serving with some toasted sesame seeds.

TIPS & NOTES
- **Substitution note:** Although brown rice is not used in traditional Japanese cooking, you can use short-grain brown rice instead of white rice in this recipe. Rinse and soak the rice as directed in Steps 1 and 2. In Step 4, increase water to 2 1/2 cups and cook the brown rice for 22 minutes, then let rest for 10 minutes.
- **Tip:** To toast sesame seeds: Heat a small dry skillet over medium-low heat. Add sesame seeds and cook, stirring, until they are lightly browned, 2 to 3 minutes.

NUTRITION
Per serving: 229 calories; 2 g fat (0 g sat, 1 g mono); 0 mg cholesterol; 45 g carbohydrates; 4 g protein; 2 gfiber; 448 mg sodium; 58 mg potassium.
Nutrition Bonus: Folate (23% daily value), Selenium (16% dv), Iron (15% dv).
Carbohydrate Servings: 3
Exchanges: 3 starch

Mixed Berry Sundaes
INGREDIENTS
- 3 cups mixed fresh berries, such as raspberries, blueberries, blackberries, sliced strawberries, divided
- 2 tablespoons crème de cassis, or black currant juice
- 1 tablespoon lemon juice
- 1 tablespoon sugar
- 1 pint nonfat raspberry sorbet, or lemon sorbet, slightly softened

PREPARATION
1. Crush 1/4 cup berries in a bowl with a fork. Add crème de cassis (or juice), lemon juice and sugar, stirring until sugar is dissolved. Add the remaining 2 3/4 cups berries; stir gently to coat. Place a scoop of sorbet in each dish and top with the berry mixture.

NUTRITION
Per serving: 191 calories; 0 g fat (0 g sat, 0 g mono); 0 mg cholesterol; 47 g carbohydrates; 1 g protein; 7 gfiber; 1 mg sodium; 146 mg potassium.
Nutrition Bonus: Vitamin C (45% daily value), Fiber (25% dv).
Carbohydrate Servings: 3
Exchanges: 1 fruit, 2 carbohydrate

DAY 23
BREAKFAST

Skim Milk
Cocoa-Date Oatmeal
Banana (1 cup, sliced)
LUNCH

Bacony Barley Salad with Marinated Shrimp or Barbecued Raspberry-Hoisin Chicken
Whole-wheat pita bread (1 medium pita)
Apricot (1 cup, halves)
Broccoli-Cheese Chowder
SNACK

Almonds (1 oz.)
Celery sticks (1 cup)
DINNER

Rosemary & Garlic Crusted Pork Loin with Butternut Squash & Potatoes or Fennel-Crusted Salmon on White Beans
Steamed cauliflower (1 cup)

Blueberries with Lemon Cream

DAY 23 RECIPES

Cocoa-Date Oatmeal

INGREDIENTS
- 1/4 cup chopped pitted dates, (10-12 dates)
- 1 cup old-fashioned rolled oats
- 2 tablespoons cocoa
- Pinch of salt
- 2 cups water

PREPARATION

1. Combine dates, oats, cocoa and salt in a 1-quart microwavable container. Slowly stir in the water. Partially cover with plastic wrap. Microwave on Medium for 4 or 5 minutes, then stir. Microwave on Medium again for 3 or 4 minutes, then stir. Continue cooking and stirring until the cereal is creamy.

TIPS & NOTES
- **Note:** The cooking times will vary considerably depending on the power of your microwave. New microwaves tend to cook much faster than older models.

NUTRITION
Per serving: 142 calories; 4 g fat (1 g sat, 1 g mono); 0 mg cholesterol; 61 g carbohydrates; 0 g added sugars; 8 g protein; 9 g fiber; 81 mg sodium; 497 mg potassium.
Nutrition Bonus: Fiber (16% daily value).
Carbohydrate Servings: 2
Exchanges: 11/2 starch, 1/2 fruit
Nutrition Note: Chocolate contains compounds called flavonoids, which can function as antioxidants and also seem to keep blood from clotting. Cocoa is unusually rich in two kinds of flavonoids, flavonols and proanthocyanidins, which appear to be especially potent. To get

Bacony Barley Salad with Marinated Shrimp

INGREDIENTS
- 3 strips bacon, chopped
- 1 1/3 cups water
- 1/2 teaspoon salt

- 2/3 cup quick-cooking barley
- 1 pound peeled cooked shrimp, (21-25 per pound; thawed if frozen), tails removed, coarsely chopped
- 1/3 cup lime juice
- 2 cups cherry tomatoes, halved
- 1/2 cup finely diced red onion
- 1/2 cup chopped fresh cilantro
- 2 tablespoons extra-virgin olive oil
- Freshly ground pepper, to taste
- 1 avocado, peeled and diced

PREPARATION

1. Cook bacon in a small saucepan over medium heat, stirring often, until crispy, about 4 minutes. Drain on paper towel; discard fat.
2. Add water and salt to the pan and bring to a boil. Add barley and return to a simmer. Reduce heat to low, cover and simmer until all the liquid is absorbed, 10 to 12 minutes.
3. Combine shrimp and lime juice in a large bowl. Add the cooked barley; toss to coat. Let stand for 10 minutes, stirring occasionally, to allow the barley to absorb some of the lime juice. Add tomatoes, onion, cilantro and the bacon; toss to coat. Add oil and pepper and toss again. Stir in avocado and serve.

TIPS & NOTES
- **Make Ahead Tip**: Prepare without avocado, cover and refrigerate for up to 2 days. Stir in the avocado just before serving.

NUTRITION

Per serving: 393 calories; 19 g fat (3 g sat, 11 g mono); 235 mg cholesterol; 3 g carbohydrates; 35 gprotein; 7 g fiber; 752 mg sodium; 859 mg potassium.
Nutrition Bonus: Vitamin C (50% daily value), Fiber (29% dv), Iron (25% dv), Folate (15% dv).
Carbohydrate Servings: 1 1/2
Exchanges: 1 starch, 1 vegetable, 4 very lean meat, 3 fat (mono)

Barbecued Raspberry-Hoisin Chicken

INGREDIENTS
- 1 cup fresh or frozen raspberries
- 3/4 cup hoisin sauce, (see Ingredient Note)
- 5 tablespoons rice vinegar, divided
- 1 clove garlic
- 1 strip (2-by-1/2-inch) orange zest

- 1 tablespoon chopped fresh ginger
- 1/8 teaspoon freshly ground pepper
- Pinch of crushed red pepper
- 1 1/2 pounds boneless, skinless chicken thighs, trimmed, each cut into 3 crosswise strips
- 2 1/2 cups water
- 1 cup long- or medium-grain brown rice
- 1/3 cup thinly sliced scallion greens, divided

PREPARATION
1. Combine raspberries, hoisin sauce, 3 tablespoons rice vinegar, garlic, orange zest, ginger, pepper and crushed red pepper in a blender or food processor. Blend or process until smooth, about 1 minute. Set aside 1/4 cup for a dipping sauce.
2. Transfer the remaining marinade to a medium bowl and add chicken; stir to coat. Cover and refrigerate for at least 2 hours and up to 24 hours.
3. Combine water and rice in a medium saucepan and bring to a boil. Cover, reduce heat to a simmer and cook until most of the liquid has been absorbed, 40 to 50 minutes. Remove from the heat and let stand, covered, until ready to serve.
4. Preheat grill to medium-high or preheat the broiler to high.
5. Meanwhile, remove the chicken from the marinade, scrape off excess (discard marinade), and thread onto 4 skewers, distributing equally.
6. Grill the chicken until browned and cooked through, 3 to 4 minutes per side. If using the broiler, place the chicken on a broiler pan coated with cooking spray and broil 4 inches from the heat source until cooked through, about 5 minutes per side.
7. Just before serving, sprinkle the rice with the remaining 2 tablespoons vinegar and 1/4 cup scallions; fluff with a fork. Sprinkle the chicken and rice with the remaining scallions. Serve with the reserved dipping sauce.

TIPS & NOTES
- **Make Ahead Tip**: Marinate for up to 24 hours before grilling. | Equipment: 4 skewers
- **Ingredient Note:** Hoisin sauce is a thick, dark brown, spicy-sweet sauce made from soybeans and a complex mix of spices. Look for it in the Asian section of your supermarket.

NUTRITION
Per serving: 398 calories; 11 g fat (3 g sat, 4 g mono); 86 mg cholesterol; 44 g carbohydrates; 4 g added sugars; 28 g protein; 4 g fiber; 313 mg sodium; 376 mg potassium.

Nutrition Bonus: Selenium (54% daily value), Zinc (20% dv), Fiber (16% dv).
Carbohydrate Servings: 3
Exchanges: 2 starch, 1 other carbohydrate, 3 lean meat

Broccoli-Cheese Chowder

INGREDIENTS
- 1 tablespoon extra-virgin olive oil
- 1 large onion, chopped
- 1 large carrot, diced
- 2 stalks celery, diced
- 1 large potato, peeled and diced
- 2 cloves garlic, minced
- 1 tablespoon all-purpose flour
- 1/2 teaspoon dry mustard
- 1/8 teaspoon cayenne pepper
- 2 14-ounce cans vegetable broth, or reduced-sodium chicken broth
- 8 ounces broccoli crowns, (see Ingredient Note), cut into 1-inch pieces, stems and florets separated
- 1 cup shredded reduced-fat Cheddar cheese
- 1/2 cup reduced-fat sour cream
- 1/8 teaspoon salt

PREPARATION
1. Heat oil in a Dutch oven or large saucepan over medium-high heat. Add onion, carrot and celery; cook, stirring often, until the onion and celery soften, 5 to 6 minutes. Add potato and garlic; cook, stirring, for 2 minutes. Stir in flour, dry mustard and cayenne; cook, stirring often, for 2 minutes.
2. Add broth and broccoli stems; bring to a boil. Cover and reduce heat to medium. Simmer, stirring occasionally, for 10 minutes. Stir in florets; simmer, covered, until the broccoli is tender, about 10 minutes more. Transfer 2 cups of the chowder to a bowl and mash; return to the pan.
3. Stir in Cheddar and sour cream; cook over medium heat, stirring, until the cheese is melted and the chowder is heated through, about 2 minutes. Season with salt.

TIPS & NOTES
- **Make Ahead Tip**: Prepare through Step 2. Cover and refrigerate for up to 2 days or freeze for up to 2 months.
- **Ingredient note:** Most supermarkets sell broccoli crowns, which are the tops of the bunches, with the stalks cut off. Although crowns are more expensive than entire bunches, they are convenient and there is considerably less waste.

NUTRITION

Per serving: 205 calories; 9 g fat (4 g sat, 3 g mono); 21 mg cholesterol; 23 g carbohydrates; 9 g protein; 4 g fiber; 508 mg sodium; 436 mg potassium.
Nutrition Bonus: Vitamin C (61% daily value), Vitamin A (64% dv), Calcium (34% dv).
Carbohydrate Servings: 1 1/2
Exchanges: 1 starch, 1 vegetable, 1 high-fat meat

Rosemary & Garlic Crusted Pork Loin with Butternut Squash & Potatoes

INGREDIENTS
- 3 tablespoons chopped fresh rosemary, or 1 tablespoon dried
- 4 cloves garlic, minced
- 1 teaspoon kosher salt, divided
- 1/2 teaspoon freshly ground pepper, plus more to taste
- 1 2-pound boneless center-cut pork loin roast, trimmed
- 1 1/2 pounds small Yukon Gold potatoes, scrubbed and cut into 1-inch cubes
- 4 teaspoons extra-virgin olive oil, divided
- 1 pound butternut squash, peeled, seeded and cut into 1-inch cubes
- 1/2 cup port, or prune juice
- 1/2 cup reduced-sodium chicken broth

PREPARATION
1. Preheat oven to 400°F.
2. Combine rosemary, garlic, 1/2 teaspoon salt and 1/2 teaspoon pepper in a mortar and crush with the pestle to form a paste. (Alternatively, finely chop the ingredients together on a cutting board.)
3. Coat a large roasting pan with cooking spray. Place pork in the pan and rub the rosemary mixture all over it. Toss potatoes with 2 teaspoons oil and 1/4 teaspoon salt in a medium bowl; scatter along one side of the pork.
4. Roast the pork and potatoes for 30 minutes. Meanwhile, toss squash with the remaining 2 teaspoons oil, 1/4 teaspoon salt and pepper in a medium bowl.
5. Remove the roasting pan from the oven. Carefully turn the pork over. Scatter the squash along the other side of the pork.
6. Roast the pork until an instant-read thermometer inserted in the center registers 155°F, 30 to 40 minutes more. Transfer the pork to a carving board; tent with foil and let stand for 10 to 15 minutes. If the vegetables are tender, transfer them to a bowl, cover and keep them warm. If not, continue roasting until they are browned and tender, 10 to 15 minutes more.
7. After removing the vegetables, place the roasting pan over medium heat and add port (or prune juice); bring to a boil, stirring to scrape up any browned bits.

Simmer for 2 minutes. Add broth and bring to a simmer. Simmer for a few minutes to intensify the flavor. Add any juices that have accumulated on the carving board.
8. To serve, cut the strings from the pork and carve. Serve with the roasted vegetables and pan sauce.

TIPS & NOTES

- By placing the potatoes along one side of the roast and the squash along the other, you have the flexibility of removing one of the vegetables if it is done before the other.

NUTRITION
Per serving: 299 calories; 10 g fat (3 g sat, 5 g mono); 63 mg cholesterol; 23 g carbohydrates; 1 g added sugars; 25 g protein; 3 g fiber; 365 mg sodium; 451 mg potassium.
Nutrition Bonus: Vitamin A (110% daily value), Vitamin C (45% dv).
Carbohydrate Servings: 1 1/2
Exchanges: 11/2 starch, 3 lean meat

Fennel-Crusted Salmon on White Beans

INGREDIENTS
- 5 teaspoons extra-virgin olive oil, divided
- 1 bulb fennel, halved, cored and thinly sliced, plus 1 tablespoon chopped fennel fronds
- 2 15-ounce cans white beans, rinsed
- 2 medium tomatoes, diced
- 1/3 cup white wine
- 1 tablespoon Dijon mustard
- 1/2 teaspoon freshly ground pepper, divided
- 1 tablespoon fennel seeds
- 1 pound salmon fillet, skin removed (see Tip), cut into 2 portions

PREPARATION
1. Heat 2 teaspoons oil in a large nonstick skillet over medium heat. Add sliced fennel; cook, stirring occasionally, until lightly browned, about 6 minutes. Stir in beans, tomatoes and wine. Cook, stirring occasionally, until the tomatoes begin to break down, about 3 minutes. Transfer to a bowl; stir in chopped fennel fronds, mustard and 1/4 teaspoon pepper. Cover to keep warm.
2. Meanwhile, combine fennel seeds and the remaining 1/4 teaspoon pepper in a small bowl; sprinkle evenly on both sides of salmon.

3. Wipe out the pan. Add the remaining 3 teaspoons oil to the pan and heat over high heat until shimmering but not smoking. Add the salmon, skinned-side up, and cook until golden brown, 3 to 5 minutes. Turn the salmon over, cover and remove from the heat. Let stand until the salmon finishes cooking off the heat, 3 to 5 minutes more. Transfer the salmon to a cutting board and flake with a fork. Serve salmon on top of the warm bean mixture.

TIPS & NOTES
- **Tip:** To skin a salmon fillet: Place it on a clean cutting board, skin-side down. Starting at the tail end, slip the blade of a long knife between the fish flesh and the skin, holding the skin down firmly with your other hand. Gently push the blade along at a 30 degree angle, separating the fillet from the skin without cutting through either.

NUTRITION
Per serving: 306 calories; 13 g fat (2 g sat, 6 g mono); 45 mg cholesterol; 29 g carbohydrates; 0 g added sugars; 25 g protein; 9 g fiber; 467 mg sodium; 1019 mg potassium.
Nutrition Bonus: Folate (39% daily value), Fiber (36% dv), Potassium (29% dv), Vitamin C (25% dv), Iron (15% dv), Omega-3s.
Carbohydrate Servings: 1
Exchanges: 1.5 starch, 1 vegetable, 3 lean meat, 1 fat

Blueberries with Lemon Cream

INGREDIENTS
- 4 ounces reduced-fat cream cheese (Neufchâtel)
- 3/4 cup low-fat vanilla yogurt
- 1 teaspoon honey
- 2 teaspoons freshly grated lemon zest
- 2 cups fresh blueberries

PREPARATION
1. Using a fork, break up cream cheese in a medium bowl. Drain off any liquid from the yogurt; add yogurt to the bowl along with honey. Using an electric mixer, beat at high speed until light and creamy. Stir in lemon zest.
2. Layer the lemon cream and blueberries in dessert dishes or wineglasses. If not serving immediately, cover and refrigerate for up to 8 hours.

TIPS & NOTES
- **Make Ahead Tip**: Cover and refrigerate for up to 8 hours.

NUTRITION

Per serving: 156 calories; 7 g fat (4 g sat, 0 g mono); 22 mg cholesterol; 19 g carbohydrates; 6 g protein; 2 g fiber; 151 mg sodium; 189 mg potassium.
Nutrition Bonus: Vitamin C (15% daily value).
Carbohydrate Servings: 1
Exchanges: 1 fruit, 1 fat (saturated)

DAY 24
BREAKFAST

Healthy Pancakes
Strawberries (1 cup)
Low-fat vanilla yogurt (8 oz.)

LUNCH

Shrimp Salad-Stuffed Tomatoes
Roasted Pear-Butternut Soup with Crumbled Stilton or Wild Rice with Dried Apricots & Pistachios
Whole-wheat toast (1 slice)
Ginger-Orange Biscotti

SNACK

Banana (1 cup, sliced)
Skim milk (1 cup)

DINNER

Sausage, Mushroom & Spinach Lasagna or Chicken Divan
Sliced Tomato Salad
Steamed asparagus (1/2 cup)
Whole-wheat toast (1 slice)
Winter Fruit Salad

DAY 24 RECIPES

Healthy Pancakes

INGREDIENTS
- 2 1/2 cups whole-wheat flour
- 1 cup buttermilk powder, (see Note)
- 5 tablespoons dried egg whites, such as Just Whites (see Note)
- 1/4 cup sugar
- 1 1/2 tablespoons baking powder
- 2 teaspoons baking soda
- 1 teaspoon salt
- 1 cup flaxseed meal, (see Note)
- 1 cup nonfat dry milk

- 1/2 cup wheat bran, or oat bran
- 1 1/2 cups nonfat milk
- 1/4 cup canola oil and 1 teaspoon vanilla extract

PREPARATION
1. Whisk flour, buttermilk powder, dried egg whites, sugar, baking powder, baking soda and salt in a large bowl. Stir in flaxseed meal, dry milk and bran. (Makes 6 cups dry mix.)
2. Combine milk, oil and vanilla in a glass measuring cup.
3. Place 2 cups pancake mix in a large bowl. (Refrigerate the remaining pancake mix in an airtight container for up to 1 month or freeze for up to 3 months.) Make a well in the center of the pancake mix. Whisk in the milk mixture until just blended; do not overmix. (The batter will seem quite thin, but will thicken up as it stands.) Let stand for 5 minutes.
4. Coat a nonstick skillet or griddle with cooking spray and place over medium heat. Whisk the batter. Using 1/4 cup batter for each pancake, cook pancakes until the edges are dry and bubbles begin to form, about 2 minutes. Turn over and cook until golden brown, about 2 minutes longer. Adjust heat as necessary for even browning.

TIPS & NOTES
- **Notes:** Buttermilk powder, such as Saco Buttermilk Blend, is a useful substitute for fresh buttermilk. Look in the baking section or with the powdered milk in most markets.
- **Dried egg whites:** Dried egg whites are convenient in recipes calling for egg whites because there is no waste. Look for brands like Just Whites in the baking or natural-foods section of most supermarkets or online at bakerscatalogue.com.
- **Flaxseed meal:** You can find flaxseed meal in the natural-foods section of large supermarkets. You can also start with whole flaxseeds: Grind 2/3 cup whole flaxseeds to yield 1 cup.
- **Variations:** Chocolate-Chocolate Chip Pancakes: Fold 1/2 cup cocoa powder and 3 ounces chocolate chips into the batter. Blueberry: Fold 1 cup frozen blueberries into the batter. Banana-Nut: Fold 1 cup thinly sliced bananas and 4 tablespoons finely chopped toasted pecans into the batter.

NUTRITION

Per serving: 272 calories; 13 g fat (2 g sat, 6 g mono); 8 mg cholesterol; 27 g carbohydrates; 12 g protein; 5 g fiber; 471 mg sodium; 336 mg potassium.
Nutrition Bonus: Calcium (24% daily value), Fiber (20% dv)
Carbohydrate Servings: 1/2

Exchanges: 2 starch, 1 very lean meat, 2 fat (mono)

Shrimp Salad-Stuffed Tomatoes

INGREDIENTS
- 1 pound peeled cooked shrimp, (21-25 per pound; thawed if frozen), tails removed, chopped
- 1 stalk celery, finely diced
- 1/4 cup minced fresh basil
- 10 Kalamata olives, pitted and finely chopped
- 1 medium shallot, minced
- 2 tablespoons reduced-fat mayonnaise
- 1 tablespoon white-wine vinegar
- Pinch of freshly ground pepper
- 4 large ripe tomatoes, cored

PREPARATION
1. Combine shrimp, celery, basil, olives, shallot, mayonnaise, vinegar and pepper in a medium bowl. Stir to combine.
2. Carefully hollow out the inside of each tomato using a melon baller or small spoon; reserve the scooped tomato for another use (see Tip). To serve, fill each tomato with a generous 1/2 cup of the shrimp salad.

TIPS & NOTES
- **Make Ahead Tip**: Prepare the salad (Step 1). Cover and refrigerate for up to 1 day.
- Save the scooped-out tomato insides to use in fresh tomato soup or pasta sauce. Store in the refrigerator for up to 3 days or in the freezer for up to 6 months.

NUTRITION

Per serving: 192 calories; 6 g fat (1 g sat, 2 g mono); 230 mg cholesterol; 12 g carbohydrates; 0 g added sugars; 30 g protein; 2 g fiber; 585 mg sodium; 774 mg potassium.
Nutrition Bonus: Vitamin C (80% daily value), Iron (25% dv), Vitamin A (25% dv).
Carbohydrate Servings: 1
Exchanges: 1 vegetable, 3 1/2 very lean meat, 1 fat (mono)

Roasted Pear-Butternut Soup with Crumbled Stilton

INGREDIENTS
- 2 ripe pears, peeled, quartered and cored
- 2 pounds butternut squash, peeled, seeded and cut into 2-inch chunks

- 2 medium tomatoes, cored and quartered
- 1 large leek, pale green and white parts only, halved lengthwise, sliced and washed thoroughly
- 2 cloves garlic, crushed
- 2 tablespoons extra-virgin olive oil
- 1/2 teaspoon salt, divided
- Freshly ground pepper, to taste
- 4 cups vegetable broth, or reduced-sodium chicken broth, divided
- 2/3 cup crumbled Stilton, or other blue-veined cheese
- 1 tablespoon thinly sliced fresh chives, or scallion greens

PREPARATION
1. Preheat oven to 400°F.
2. Combine pears, squash, tomatoes, leek, garlic, oil, 1/4 teaspoon salt and pepper in a large bowl; toss to coat. Spread evenly on a large rimmed baking sheet. Roast, stirring occasionally, until the vegetables are tender, 40 to 55 minutes. Let cool slightly.
3. Place half the vegetables and 2 cups broth in a blender; puree until smooth. Transfer to a large saucepan. Puree the remaining vegetables and 2 cups broth. Add to the pan and stir in the remaining 1/4 teaspoon salt.
4. Cook the soup over medium-low heat, stirring, until hot, about 10 minutes. Divide among 6 bowls and garnish with cheese and chives (or scallion greens).

TIPS & NOTES
- **Make Ahead Tip**: Cover and refrigerate for up to 3 days or freeze for up to 1 month. Add more broth when reheating, if desired.

NUTRITION
Per serving: 235 calories; 10 g fat (5 g sat, 5 g mono); 11 mg cholesterol; 34 g carbohydrates; 6 g protein; 6 g fiber; 721 mg sodium; 700 mg potassium.
Nutrition Bonus: Vitamin A (350% daily value), Vitamin C (70% dv), Potassium (21% dv), Calcium (20% dv)
Carbohydrate Servings: 2
Exchanges: 1 starch, 1 vegetable, 1/2 fruit, 2 fat

Wild Rice with Dried Apricots & Pistachios

INGREDIENTS
- 7 cups water
- 1 cup wild rice, rinsed
- 2 teaspoons extra-virgin olive oil
- 1 small red onion, chopped

- 1 medium red bell pepper, seeded and diced
- 2 cloves garlic, minced
- 1 1/2 teaspoons ground cumin
- 1/2 cup dried apricots, diced
- 1/2 cup orange juice
- 1/4 teaspoon salt, or to taste
- Freshly ground pepper, to taste
- 2/3 cup thinly sliced scallion greens
- 1/3 cup shelled pistachios, coarsely chopped

PREPARATION

1. Bring water to a boil in a large saucepan. Add wild rice, cover, reduce heat to medium-low and cook at a lively simmer until the grains are tender and starting to split, 45 to 55 minutes. Drain in a fine sieve.
2. Shortly before the wild rice is ready, heat oil in a large nonstick skillet over medium-high heat. Add onion and cook, stirring often, until softened, 2 to 3 minutes. Add bell pepper, garlic and cumin; cook, stirring, for 1 minute. Add apricots, orange juice, salt and pepper; simmer until the apricots have plumped and the liquid has reduced slightly, 1 to 2 minutes. Stir in the wild rice. Remove from the heat and stir in scallion greens. Serve topped with chopped pistachios.

NUTRITION

Per serving: 224 calories; 5 g fat (1 g sat, 3 g mono); 0 mg cholesterol; 39 g carbohydrates; 0 g added sugars; 7 g protein; 5 g fiber; 104 mg sodium; 498 mg potassium.
Nutrition Bonus: Vitamin C (110% daily value), Vitamin A (35% dv), Fiber (20% dv).
Carbohydrate Servings: 2
Exchanges: 2 starch, 1 vegetable, 1 fat

Ginger-Orange Biscotti

INGREDIENTS
- 3/4 cup whole-wheat pastry flour
- 3/4 cup all-purpose flour
- 1 cup sugar, or 1/2 cup Splenda Sugar Blend for Baking
- 1/2 cup cornmeal
- 2 teaspoons ground ginger
- 1 teaspoon baking powder
- 1/2 teaspoon baking soda and 1/4 teaspoon salt
- 2 large eggs and 2 large egg whites
- 2 teaspoons freshly grated orange zest
- 1 tablespoon orange juice

PREPARATION

1. Preheat oven to 325°F. Line a baking sheet with parchment paper or a silicone baking mat.
2. Whisk whole-wheat flour, all-purpose flour, sugar (or Splenda), cornmeal, ginger, baking powder, baking soda and salt in a medium bowl. Whisk eggs, egg whites, orange zest and orange juice in a large bowl until blended. Stir in the dry ingredients with a wooden spoon until just combined.
3. Divide the dough in half. With dampened hands, form each piece into a 14-by-1 1/2-inch log. Place the logs side by side on the prepared baking sheet
4. Bake until firm, 20 to 25 minutes. Cool on the pan on a wire rack. Reduce oven temperature to 300°.
5. Slice the logs on the diagonal into cookies 1/2 inch thick. Arrange, cut-side down, on 2 ungreased baking sheets. Bake until golden brown and crisp, 15 to 20 minutes. (Rotate the baking sheets if necessary to ensure even browning.) Transfer the biscotti to a wire rack to cool.

TIPS & NOTES
- **Make Ahead Tip**: Store in an airtight container for up to 2 weeks.

NUTRITION
Per biscotti: 34 calories; 0 g fat (0 g sat, 0 g mono); 8 mg cholesterol; 8 g carbohydrates; 1 g protein; 0 gfiber; 34 mg sodium; 9 mg potassium.
Carbohydrate Servings: 1/2
Exchanges: 1/2 other carbohydrate
Nutrition Note: Per biscotti with Splenda: 0 Carbohydrate Servings; 28 calories; 5 g carbohydrate.

Sausage, Mushroom & Spinach Lasagna

INGREDIENTS
- 8 ounces whole-wheat lasagna noodles
- 1 pound lean spicy Italian turkey sausage, casings removed, or vegetarian sausage-style soy product
- 4 cups sliced mushrooms, (10 ounces)
- 1/4 cup water
- 1 pound frozen spinach, thawed
- 1 28-ounce can crushed tomatoes, preferably chunky
- 1/4 cup chopped fresh basil
- 1/4 teaspoon salt
- Freshly ground pepper, to taste
- 1 pound part-skim ricotta cheese, (2 cups)
- 8 ounces part-skim mozzarella cheese, shredded (about 2 cups), divided

PREPARATION

1. Preheat oven to 350°F. Coat a 9-by-13-inch baking dish with cooking spray.
2. Bring a large pot of water to a boil. Add noodles and cook until not quite tender, about 2 minutes less than the package directions. Drain; return the noodles to the pot, cover with cool water and set aside.
3. Coat a large nonstick skillet with cooking spray and heat over medium-high heat. Add sausage; cook, crumbling with a wooden spoon, until browned, about 4 minutes. Add mushrooms and water; cook, stirring occasionally and crumbling the sausage more, until it is cooked through, the water has evaporated and the mushrooms are tender, 8 to 10 minutes. Squeeze spinach to remove excess water, then stir into the pan; remove from heat.
4. Mix tomatoes with basil, salt and pepper in a medium bowl.
5. To assemble lasagna: Spread 1/2 cup of the tomatoes in the prepared baking dish. Arrange a layer of noodles on top, trimming to fit if necessary. Evenly dollop half the ricotta over the noodles. Top with half the sausage mixture, one-third of the remaining tomatoes and one-third of the mozzarella. Continue with another layer of noodles, the remaining ricotta, the remaining sausage, half the remaining tomatoes and half the remaining mozzarella. Top with a third layer of noodles and the remaining tomatoes.
6. Cover the lasagna with foil and bake until bubbling and heated through, 1 hour to 1 hour 10 minutes. Remove the foil; sprinkle the remaining mozzarella on top. Return to the oven and bake until the cheese is just melted but not browned, 8 to 10 minutes. Let rest for 10 minutes before serving. Vegetarian Variation: Use a sausage-style soy product, such as Gimme Lean, or simply omit the sausage altogether.

TIPS & NOTES

- **Make Ahead Tip**: Prepare through Step 5 up to 1 day ahead.
- **Ingredient Note:** Whole-wheat lasagna noodles are higher in fiber than white noodles. They can be found in health-food stores and some large supermarkets.
- **Vegetarian Variation:** Use a sausage-style soy product, such as Gimme Lean, or simply omit the sausage altogether.

NUTRITION

Per serving: 333 calories; 14 g fat (5 g sat, 3 g mono); 41 mg cholesterol; 28 g carbohydrates; 26 g protein; 7 g fiber; 655 mg sodium; 607 mg potassium.
Nutrition Bonus: Vitamin A (128% daily value), Calcium (23% dv), Iron (21% dv), Folate (19% dv), Potassium (17% dv).
Carbohydrate Servings: 1 1/2
Exchanges: 1 starch, 1 1/2 vegetable, 1 lean meat, 2 medium-fat meat

Chicken Divan

INGREDIENTS
- 1 1/2 pounds boneless, skinless chicken breast
- 1 tablespoon extra-virgin olive oil
- 2 cups diced leek, white and light green parts only (about 1 large; see Tip)
- 1/2 teaspoon salt
- 5 tablespoons all-purpose flour
- 1 14-ounce can reduced-sodium chicken broth
- 1 cup low-fat milk
- 2 tablespoons dry sherry (see Tip)
- 1/2 teaspoon dried thyme
- 1/2 teaspoon freshly ground pepper
- 2 10-ounce boxes frozen chopped broccoli, thawed, or 1 pound broccoli crowns (see Ingredient Note), chopped
- 1 cup grated Parmesan cheese, divided
- 1/4 cup low-fat mayonnaise
- 2 teaspoons Dijon mustard

PREPARATION
1. Preheat oven to 375°F. Coat a 7-by-11-inch (2-quart) glass baking dish with cooking spray.
2. Place chicken in a medium skillet or saucepan and add water to cover. Bring to a simmer over high heat. Cover, reduce heat to low and simmer gently until the chicken is cooked through and no longer pink in the center, 10 to 12 minutes. Drain and slice into bite-size pieces.
3. Heat oil in a large nonstick skillet over medium-high heat. Add leek and salt and cook, stirring often, until softened but not browned, 3 to 4 minutes. Add flour; stir to coat. Add broth, milk, sherry, thyme and pepper and bring to a simmer, stirring constantly. Add broccoli; return to a simmer. Remove from heat and stir in 1/2 cup Parmesan, mayonnaise and mustard.
4. Spread half the broccoli mixture in the prepared baking dish. Top with the chicken, then the remaining broccoli mixture. Sprinkle evenly with the remaining 1/2 cup Parmesan. Bake until bubbling, 20 to 25 minutes. Let cool for 10 minutes before serving.

TIPS & NOTES
- **Tips:** To clean leeks, trim and discard green tops and white roots. Split leeks lengthwise and place in plenty of water. Swish the leeks in the water to release any sand or soil. Drain. Repeat until no grit remains.
- Sherry is a type of fortified wine originally from southern Spain. Don't use the "cooking sherry" sold in many supermarkets—it can be surprisingly high in

sodium. Instead, purchase dry sherry that's sold with other fortified wines in your wine or liquor store.
- **Ingredient Note:** Most supermarkets sell broccoli crowns, which are the tops of the bunches, with the stalks cut off. Although crowns are more expensive than entire bunches, they are convenient and there is considerably less waste.

NUTRITION

Per serving: 308 calories; 10 g fat (4 g sat, 4 g mono); 76 mg cholesterol; 20 g carbohydrates; 35 g protein;4 g fiber; 712 mg sodium; 401 mg potassium.
Nutrition Bonus: Vitamin C (70% daily value), Vitamin A (35% dv), Calcium (30% dv), Folate (19% dv).
Carbohydrate Servings: 1
Exchanges: 1/2 starch, 3 vegetable, 3 lean meat

Sliced Tomato Salad

INGREDIENTS
- 4 tomatoes, sliced
- 1/4 cup thinly sliced red onion and 8 anchovies
- 1/2 teaspoon dried oregano
- Salt & freshly ground pepper, to taste
- 2 tablespoons extra-virgin olive oil
- 1 tablespoon white-wine vinegar

PREPARATION
1. Arrange tomato slices on a platter. Top with onion, anchovies, oregano, salt and pepper. Drizzle with oil and vinegar.

NUTRITION

Per serving: 44 calories; 1 g fat (0 g sat, 0 g mono); 3 mg cholesterol; 8 g carbohydrates; 0 g added sugars;3 g protein; 2 g fiber; 300 mg sodium; 403 mg potassium.
Nutrition Bonus: Vitamin C (35% daily value), Vitamin A (25% dv).
Carbohydrate Servings: 1/2
Exchanges: 1 vegetable, 1 1/2 fat

Winter Fruit Salad

INGREDIENTS
- 4 seedless oranges, peeled
- 3 pink grapefruits, peeled
- 1 pineapple, peeled, quartered, cored and sliced
- 2 star fruit, sliced and 1 pomegranate, cut in half and seeds removed

PREPARATION
1. Remove white pith from oranges and grapefruits; quarter the fruit lengthwise and cut into 1/4-inch slices. Place in a large bowl and toss with pineapple, star fruit and pomegranate seeds.

NUTRITION
Per serving: 110 calories; 0 g fat (0 g sat, 0 g mono); 0 mg cholesterol; 28 g carbohydrates; 0 g added sugars; 2 g protein; 4 g fiber; 2 mg sodium; 400 mg potassium.
Nutrition Bonus: Vitamin C (160% daily value), Vitamin A (20% dv), Fiber (16% dv).
Carbohydrate Servings: 1 1/2
Exchanges: 3 fruit

DAY 25
BREAKFAST
Spiced Apple Cider Muffins
Skim milk (1 cup)
Grapefruit (1/2)
LUNCH
Skim milk (1 cup)
Nouveau Niçoise or Seafood Salad with Citrus Vinaigrette
Wasa crispbread (1 cracker)
SNACK
Cottage Cheese Veggie Dip
Carrot sticks (1 cup)
DINNER
Turkey Cutlets with Peas & Spring Onions
Quick-cooking barley (1 cup)
Mixed Greens with Berries & Honey-Glazed Hazelnuts or Crunchy Pear & Celery Salad

DAY 25 RECIPES

Spiced Apple Cider Muffins
INGREDIENTS
STREUSEL
- 2 tablespoons packed light brown sugar
- 4 teaspoons whole-wheat flour
- 1/2 teaspoon ground cinnamon
- 1 tablespoon butter, cut into small pieces
- 2 tablespoons finely chopped walnuts, (optional)

MUFFINS
- 1 cup whole-wheat flour
- 1 cup all-purpose flour
- 1 1/2 teaspoons baking powder
- 1/2 teaspoon baking soda
- 1/4 teaspoon salt
- 1 tablespoon ground cinnamon
- 1/2 teaspoon ground nutmeg
- 1 large egg
- 1/3 cup packed light brown sugar
- 1/2 cup apple butter, such as Smucker's
- 1/3 cup maple syrup
- 1/3 cup apple cider
- 1/3 cup low-fat plain yogurt
- 1/4 cup canola oil

PREPARATION
1. Preheat oven to 400°F. Coat 12 muffin cups with cooking spray.
2. To prepare streusel: Mix brown sugar, whole-wheat flour and cinnamon in a small bowl. Cut in butter with a pastry blender or your fingers until the mixture resembles coarse crumbs. Stir in walnuts, if using.
3. To prepare muffins: Whisk whole-wheat flour, all-purpose flour, baking powder, baking soda, salt, cinnamon and nutmeg in a large bowl.
4. Whisk egg and brown sugar in a medium bowl until smooth. Whisk in apple butter, syrup, cider, yogurt and oil. Make a well in the dry ingredients; add the wet ingredients and stir with a rubber spatula until just combined. Scoop the batter into the prepared muffin cups (they'll be quite full). Sprinkle with the streusel.
5. Bake the muffins until the tops are golden brown and spring back when touched lightly, 15 to 25 minutes. Let cool in the pan for 5 minutes. Loosen edges and turn muffins out onto a wire rack to cool slightly before serving.

NUTRITION
Per muffin: 209 calories; 7 g fat (1 g sat, 3 g mono); 21 mg cholesterol; 34 g carbohydrates; 4 g protein; 2 gfiber; 162 mg sodium; 40 mg potassium.
Carbohydrate Servings: 2 1/2
Exchanges: 2 starch, 1 fat

Nouveau Niçoise

INGREDIENTS

- 8 cups water
- 8 ounces green beans, trimmed and halved
- 8 small red potatoes
- 2 eggs
- 1/4 cup minced shallots
- 1/4 cup red-wine vinegar
- 2 tablespoons Dijon mustard
- 1/4 teaspoon salt
- 1/4 teaspoon freshly ground pepper
- 3 tablespoons extra-virgin olive oil
- 6 cups mixed salad greens
- 2 6-ounce cans chunk light tuna, drained (see Note)
- 12 Nicoise or Kalamata olives

PREPARATION

1. Bring water to a boil in a 3- to 4-quart saucepan. Add green beans and cook until just tender and bright green, 1 to 2 minutes. Using a slotted spoon, transfer the beans to a colander, rinse under cold water and set aside in a large bowl. Carefully place potatoes and eggs into the boiling water. Cook the eggs until hard, 12 minutes. Using a slotted spoon, transfer the eggs to the colander, rinse under cold water until cool and set aside. Continue cooking the potatoes until fork-tender, 3 minutes more. Drain the potatoes; rinse under cold water until cool enough to handle.
2. Meanwhile, combine shallots, vinegar, mustard, salt and pepper in a small bowl. Slowly whisk in oil.
3. Cut the potatoes into quarters or eighths, depending on their size. Add to the bowl with the beans. Add greens, tuna and the dressing. Toss well. Peel the eggs and cut into wedges. Divide the salad among 4 plates. Top with egg wedges and olives. Serve immediately.

TIPS & NOTES

- **Make Ahead Tip**: Cook green beans, potatoes and eggs; dry, cover and refrigerate for up to 1 day.
- **Note:** Chunk light tuna, which comes from the smaller skipjack or yellowfin, has less mercury than canned white albacore tuna. The FDA/EPA advises that women who are or might become pregnant, nursing mothers and young children consume no more than 6 ounces of albacore a week; up to 12 ounces of canned light tuna is considered safe.

NUTRITION

Per serving: 436 calories; 16 g fat (3 g sat, 11 g mono); 159 mg cholesterol; 38 g carbohydrates; 0 g added sugars; 33 g protein; 6 g fiber; 547 mg sodium; 1140 mg potassium.
Nutrition Bonus: Vitamin C (90% daily value), Potassium (33% dv), Vitamin A (30% dv), Folate (26% dv), Iron (15% dv).
Carbohydrate Servings: 2
Exchanges: 2 starch, 2 vegetable, 3 very lean meat, 3 fat

Seafood Salad with Citrus Vinaigrette

INGREDIENTS
- 4 medium dry sea scallops, (see Ingredient note), quartered (about 3 ounces), tough muscle removed
- 1 small grapefruit, preferably ruby-red
- 1 small shallot, minced
- 3 tablespoons white-wine vinegar
- 1 teaspoon Dijon mustard
- Salt, to taste
- 1/4 teaspoon freshly ground pepper
- 2 tablespoons extra-virgin olive oil
- 6 ounces lump crabmeat
- 1 small head romaine lettuce, shredded (about 3 cups)
- 6 cherry tomatoes, halved (see Tip)
- 1 small avocado, peeled, pitted and diced

PREPARATION

1. Bring a small saucepan of water to a boil. Add scallops and cook until firm, opaque and just cooked through, about 1 minute. Drain and rinse under cold water until cool.
2. Slice 1/4 inch off the bottom and top of the grapefruit; stand it on a cutting board. Using a sharp paring knife, remove the peel and pith. Hold the fruit over a medium bowl and cut between the membranes to release individual grapefruit sections into the bowl, collecting any juice as well. Discard membranes, pith, peel and any seeds. Transfer just the grapefruit sections to a serving bowl.
3. Whisk shallot, vinegar, mustard, salt and pepper into the bowl with the grapefruit juice. Whisk in oil in a slow, steady stream. Add the scallops and crab to the dressing; toss well to coat.
4. Add lettuce, tomatoes and avocado to the bowl with the grapefruit; toss to combine. Add the seafood and dressing; toss gently.

TIPS & NOTES

- **Ingredient Note:** Be sure to request "dry" scallops (i.e., not treated with sodium tripolyphosphate, or STP) from your fish store. Sea scallops that have been subjected to a chemical bath are not only mushy and less flavorful, but will not brown properly.
- **Tip - Shopping for 2:** What if you want just six cherry tomatoes, not a whole container full? Shop the salad bar at your local supermarket. The produce may cost a little more, but you're guaranteed not to waste any of it since you'll buy just what you need.

NUTRITION

Per serving: 420 calories; 27 g fat (3 g sat, 11 g mono); 70 mg cholesterol; 23 g carbohydrates; 0 g added sugars; 28 g protein; 6 g fiber; 666 mg sodium; 900 mg potassium.
Nutrition Bonus: Vitamin A (130% daily value), Vitamin C (120% dv), Folate (35% dv), Potassium (30% dv).
Carbohydrate Servings: 1
Exchanges: 2 vegetable, 1 fruit, 4 lean meat, 2 fat (mono)

Cottage Cheese Veggie Dip

INGREDIENTS

- 1/2 cup low-fat cottage cheese
- 1/4 teaspoon lemon pepper
- 1/2 cup each baby carrots and snow (or snap) peas

PREPARATION

1. Combine cottage cheese and lemon pepper. Serve with carrots and peas.

NUTRITION

Per serving: 120 calories; 2 g fat (1 g sat, 0 g mono); 10 mg cholesterol; 14 g carbohydrates; 14 g protein; 2 g fiber; 561 mg sodium; 202 mg potassium.
Nutrition Bonus: Vitamin A (170% daily value), Vitamin C (30% dv), Calcium (25% dv).
Carbohydrate Servings: 1
Exchanges: 1 vegetable, 2 very lean meat

Turkey Cutlets with Peas & Spring Onions

INGREDIENTS

- 1/2 cup all-purpose flour
- 1/2 teaspoon salt, divided
- 1/4 teaspoon freshly ground pepper
- 1 pound 1/4-inch-thick turkey breast cutlets, or steaks

- 2 tablespoons extra-virgin olive oil, divided
- 4 ounces shiitake mushrooms, stemmed and sliced (about 1 1/2 cups)
- 1 bunch spring onions, or scallions, sliced, whites and greens separated
- 1 cup reduced-sodium chicken broth
- 1/2 cup dry white wine
- 1 cup peas, fresh or frozen, thawed
- 1 teaspoon freshly grated lemon zest

PREPARATION

1. Whisk flour, 1/4 teaspoon salt and pepper in a shallow dish. Dredge each turkey cutlet (or steak) in the flour mixture. Heat 1 tablespoon oil in a large nonstick skillet over medium-high heat. Add the turkey and cook until lightly golden, 2 to 3 minutes per side. Transfer to a plate; cover with foil to keep warm.
2. Add the remaining 1 tablespoon oil to the pan and heat over medium-high heat. Add mushrooms and onion (or scallion) whites and cook, stirring often, until the mushrooms are browned and the whites are slightly softened, 2 to 3 minutes. Add broth, wine and the remaining 1/4 teaspoon salt; cook, stirring occasionally, until the sauce is slightly reduced, 2 to 3 minutes. Stir in peas and onion (or scallion) greens and cook, stirring, until heated through, about 1 minute. Stir in lemon zest. Nestle the turkey into the vegetables along with any accumulated juices from the plate. Cook, turning the cutlets once, until heated through, 1 to 2 minutes.

NUTRITION

Per serving: 313 calories; 8 g fat (1 g sat, 5 g mono); 45 mg cholesterol; 23 g carbohydrates; 34 g protein; 3 g fiber; 571 mg sodium; 223 mg potassium.
Nutrition Bonus: Iron (15% daily value), Vitamin A & C (20% dv).
Carbohydrate Servings: 1
Exchanges: 1 starch, 1 vegetable, 4 lean meat, 1 fat

Mixed Greens with Berries & Honey-Glazed Hazelnuts

INGREDIENTS
NUTS
- 1 teaspoon extra-virgin olive oil
- 1 teaspoon honey
- 1/4 cup chopped hazelnuts, or walnuts

DRESSING
- 1/3 cup raspberries, blackberries and/or blueberries
- 2 tablespoons extra-virgin olive oil
- 1 tablespoon balsamic vinegar
- 1 tablespoon water

- 1 teaspoon Dijon mustard
- 1 small clove garlic, crushed and peeled
- 1/2 teaspoon honey
- 1/8 teaspoon salt, or to taste
- Freshly ground pepper, to taste
- 2 tablespoons finely chopped shallots

SALAD
- 10 cups mesclun salad greens, (about 8 ounces)
- 1 cup blackberries, raspberries and/or blueberries
- 1/2 cup crumbled feta, or goat cheese (4 ounces)

PREPARATION
1. To prepare nuts: Preheat oven to 350°F. Coat a small baking dish with cooking spray. Combine oil and honey in a small bowl. Add nuts and toss to coat. Transfer to the prepared baking dish and bake, stirring from time to time, until golden, 10 to 14 minutes. Let cool completely.
2. To prepare dressing: Combine berries, oil, vinegar, water, mustard, garlic, honey, salt and pepper in a blender or food processor. Blend until smooth. Transfer to a small bowl and stir in shallots.
3. To prepare salad: Just before serving, place greens in a large bowl. Drizzle the dressing over the greens and toss to coat. Divide the salad among 4 plates. Scatter berries, cheese and the glazed nuts over each salad; serve immediately.

TIPS & NOTES
- **Make Ahead Tip**: Cover and refrigerate the dressing (Step 2) for up to 2 days.

NUTRITION
Per serving: 232 calories; 17 g fat (4 g sat, 10 g mono); 17 mg cholesterol; 15 g carbohydrates; 7 g protein;6 g fiber; 349 mg sodium; 596 mg potassium.
Nutrition Bonus: Vitamin A (80% daily value), Vitamin C (60% dv), Calcium (20% dv).
Carbohydrate Servings: 1/2
Exchanges: 2 vegetable, 1 medium-fat meat, 2 fat

Crunchy Pear & Celery Salad

INGREDIENTS
- 4 stalks celery, trimmed and cut in half crosswise
- 2 tablespoons cider, pear, raspberry or other fruit vinegar
- 2 tablespoons honey
- 1/4 teaspoon salt

- 2 ripe pears, preferably red Bartlett or Anjou, diced
- 1 cup finely diced white Cheddar cheese
- 1/2 cup chopped pecans, toasted (see Tip)
- Freshly ground pepper, to taste
- 6 large leaves butterhead or other lettuce

PREPARATION

1. Soak celery in a bowl of ice water for 15 minutes. Drain and pat dry. Cut into 1/2-inch pieces.
2. Whisk vinegar, honey and salt in a large bowl until blended. Add pears; gently stir to coat. Add the celery, cheese and pecans; stir to combine. Season with pepper. Divide the lettuce leaves among 6 plates and top with a portion of salad. Serve at room temperature or chilled.

TIPS & NOTES

- **Make Ahead Tip**: Prepare salad without pecans up to 2 hours ahead. Stir in pecans just before serving.
- **Tip**: To toast chopped pecans, cook in a small dry skillet over medium-low heat, stirring constantly, until fragrant and lightly browned, 2 to 4 minutes.

NUTRITION
Per serving: 215 calories; 13 g fat (5 g sat, 4 g mono); 20 mg cholesterol; 20 g carbohydrates; 5 g protein; 4 g fiber; 240 mg sodium; 219 mg potassium.
Nutrition Bonus: Calcium (15% daily value)
Carbohydrate Servings: 1

DAY 26
BREAKFAST
Skim milk (1 cup)
Southwestern Omelet Wrap
Grapefruit (1/2)
LUNCH
Stir-Fry of Pork with Vietnamese Flavors or Provolone & Olive Stuffed Chicken Breasts
Quick Kimchi
Blueberries (1 cup)
Rolled Sugar Cookies
SNACK
Almonds (1 oz.)
Low-fat vanilla yogurt (8 oz.)

DINNER

Corn & Broccoli Calzones or Lentil & Chicken Stew
Arugula-Mushroom Salad
Sliced Tomato Salad
Mango Sorbet

DAY 26 RECIPES

Southwestern Omelet Wrap

INGREDIENTS
- 1 large egg
- 1 large egg white
- 1/2 teaspoon hot sauce, such as
- Freshly ground pepper, to taste
- 1 tablespoon chopped scallions
- 1 tablespoon chopped fresh cilantro, or parsley (optional)
- 2 tablespoons prepared black bean dip
- 1 9-inch whole-wheat wrap, (see Ingredient note)
- 1 teaspoon canola oil
- 2 tablespoons grated pepper Jack or Cheddar cheese
- 1 tablespoon prepared green or red salsa, (optional)

PREPARATION

1. Set oven rack 6 inches from the heat source; preheat broiler. Stir eggs, hot sauce and pepper briskly with a fork in a medium bowl. Stir in scallions and cilantro (or parsley), if using.
2. If black bean dip is cold, warm it in the microwave on High for 10 to 20 seconds. Place wrap between paper towels and warm in the microwave on High for about 10 seconds. Spread bean dip over the wrap, leaving a 1-inch border all around.
3. Brush oil over a 10-inch nonstick skillet; heat over medium heat. Add the egg mixture and cook, lifting the edges with a heat-resistant rubber spatula so uncooked egg will flow underneath, until the bottom is light golden, 20 to 30 seconds. Place the skillet under the broiler and broil just until the top is set, 20 to 30 seconds. Immediately slide the omelet onto the wrap. Sprinkle with cheese. Fold the edges over the omelet on two sides, then roll the wrap up and around the omelet. Serve immediately, with salsa, if desired.

TIPS & NOTES
- **Make Ahead Tip**: Wrap in plastic and refrigerate, overnight. To reheat, remove plastic wrap and rewrap in paper towel. Microwave at High for 1 to 2 minutes.

- **Ingredient Note:** You can find wraps designed for wrap sandwiches in the deli section of large supermarkets.

NUTRITION
Per serving: 318 calories; 17 g fat (5 g sat, 5 g mono); 201 mg cholesterol; 24 g carbohydrates; 18 gprotein; 2 g fiber; 678 mg sodium; 147 mg potassium.
Nutrition Bonus: Calcium (25% daily value), Vitamin A (15% dv).
Carbohydrate Servings: 1 1/2
Exchanges: 1 1/2 starch, 1 medium-fat meat, 1 high-fat meat, 1 fat (mono)

Stir-Fry of Pork with Vietnamese Flavors

INGREDIENTS
- 2 tablespoons finely chopped fresh ginger
- 2 serrano or jalapeño peppers, seeded and finely chopped
- 4 cloves garlic, finely chopped
- 3 tablespoons fish sauce, divided
- 2 tablespoons orange juice, divided
- 1 teaspoon cornstarch
- 1/2 teaspoon freshly ground pepper
- 1 pound pork tenderloin, trimmed and cut across the grain into 1/4-inch-thick slices
- 1 tablespoon sugar
- 3 teaspoons canola oil, divided
- 2 cups finely sliced onions, (2-4 onions)
- 1/4 cup sliced fresh cilantro leaves

PREPARATION
1. Combine ginger, peppers, garlic, 1 tablespoon of the fish sauce, 1 tablespoon of the orange juice, cornstarch and black pepper in a shallow dish. Add pork and toss to coat it with marinade. Set aside to marinate for 10 to 20 minutes.
2. Mix sugar, the remaining 2 tablespoons fish sauce and 1 tablespoon orange juice in a small bowl.
3. Heat a wok over high heat. Swirl in 1 teaspoon of the oil. Add onions and cook, stirring, until limp and caramelized, about 5 minutes. Transfer the onions to a plate. Wipe out the pan. Add the remaining 2 teaspoons oil to the pan and increase heat to high. Slowly drop in pork and stir-fry until browned and just cooked through, 2 to 3 minutes. Add the reserved fish sauce/orange juice mixture and the reserved onions; toss until the pork is coated with sauce. Sprinkle with cilantro and serve over rice.

NUTRITION
Per serving: 243 calories; 7 g fat (1 g sat, 4 g mono); 68 mg cholesterol; 19 g carbohydrates; 3 g added sugars; 25 g protein; 3 g fiber; 575 mg sodium; 615 mg potassium.
Nutrition Bonus: Selenium (44% daily value), Vitamin C (28% dv), Potassium (18% dv).
Carbohydrate Servings: 1
Exchanges: 1 1/2 vegetable, 3 lean meat

Provolone & Olive Stuffed Chicken Breasts

INGREDIENTS
- 1/4 cup shredded provolone cheese, preferably aged
- 3 tablespoons chopped California Ripe Olives
- Freshly ground pepper, to taste
- 4 boneless, skinless chicken breasts, (1-1 1/4 pounds total)
- 1 large egg white
- 1/2 cup plain dry breadcrumbs
- 1/2 teaspoon salt
- 2 teaspoons extra-virgin olive oil

PREPARATION
1. Preheat oven to 400°F. Lightly coat a baking sheet with sides with cooking spray.
2. Combine the provolone, olives and pepper in a small bowl.
3. Lightly beat the egg white with a fork in a medium bowl. Mix the breadcrumbs and salt in a shallow dish.
4. Cut a horizontal slit along the thin, long edge of a chicken breast half, nearly through to the opposite side. Open up each breast and place one-fourth of the cheese filling in the center. Close the breast over the filling, pressing the edges firmly together to seal. Repeat with remaining chicken breasts and filling. Hold each chicken breast half together and dip in egg white, then dredge in breadcrumbs. (Discard leftovers.)
5. Heat oil over in a large nonstick skillet medium-high heat. Add chicken and cook until browned on one side, about 2 minutes. Transfer chicken to the prepared baking sheet, browned-side up, and bake until it is no longer pink in the center or until an instant-read thermometer registers 170°F, about 20 minutes.

NUTRITION
Per serving: 242 calories; 9 g fat (2 g sat, 3 g mono); 68 mg cholesterol; 11 g carbohydrates; 0 g added sugars; 27 g protein; 1 g fiber; 572 mg sodium; 229 mg potassium.
Nutrition Bonus: Selenium (36% daily value)
Carbohydrate Servings: 1
Exchanges: 1/2 starch, 3 lean meat, 1 fat

Quick Kimchi

INGREDIENTS

- 1 small head napa (Chinese) cabbage, cored and cut into 1-inch squares (about 8 cups)
- 2 cloves garlic, minced
- 1/4 cup water
- 2 tablespoons distilled white vinegar
- 1 tablespoon toasted sesame oil
- 2 teaspoons fresh ginger, finely grated
- 3/4 teaspoon salt
- 1/2 teaspoon sugar
- 1/2 teaspoon crushed red pepper, red
- 3 scallions, sliced
- 1 carrot, peeled and grated

PREPARATION

1. Combine cabbage, garlic and water in a large saucepan and bring to a boil over high heat. Reduce heat to medium-low and cook, stirring once or twice, until tender, 4 to 5 minutes.
2. Meanwhile, whisk vinegar, oil, ginger, salt, sugar and crushed red pepper in a large bowl.
3. Add the cabbage, scallions and carrot to the bowl and toss to combine. Refrigerate for about 25 minutes before serving.

NUTRITION

Per serving: 37 calories; 2 g fat (0 g sat, 1 g mono); 0 mg cholesterol; 4 g carbohydrates; 0 g added sugars;1 g protein; 1 g fiber; 235 mg sodium; 47 mg potassium.
Nutrition Bonus: Vitamin A (50% daily value), Vitamin C (40% dv).
Exchanges: 1 vegetable

Rolled Sugar Cookies

INGREDIENTS

- 3/4 cup whole-wheat flour
- 3/4 cup unsifted cake flour
- 1 teaspoon baking powder
- 1/4 teaspoon salt
- 2 tablespoons butter
- 1/2 cup sugar, or 1/4 cup Splenda Sugar Blend for Baking
- 2 tablespoons canola oil and 1 large egg
- 1 1/2 teaspoons vanilla extract

PREPARATION
1. Set a rack in the upper third of the oven; preheat to 350°F. Coat 2 baking sheets with cooking spray.
2. Whisk whole-wheat flour, cake flour, baking powder and salt in a medium bowl.
3. Melt butter in a small saucepan over low heat. Cook, swirling the pan, until the butter turns a nutty brown, about 1 minute, and pour into a mixing bowl. Add sugar (or Splenda) and oil; beat with an electric mixer until smooth. Mix in egg and vanilla; beat until smooth. Add the flour mixture and mix on low speed until just combined. Divide the dough in half and press each piece into a disk.
4. Working with one disk at a time, roll dough on a lightly floured surface to a thickness of 1/8 inch. Cut out cookies with small (about 2- to 2 1/2-inch) cookie cutters. Place the cookies about 1/2 inch apart on the prepared baking sheets.
5. Bake the cookies in the upper third of the oven, 1 sheet at a time, until slightly golden on the edges, 5 to 7 minutes. Do not overbake. Transfer to wire racks to cool.

TIPS & NOTES
- **Make Ahead Tip**: Prepare the dough through Step 3; wrap well and refrigerate for up to 2 days or freeze for up to 1 month. (If frozen, return to room temperature before rolling out.) Store the cookies in an airtight container for up to 3 days or freeze for longer storage.

NUTRITION
Per cookie: 53 calories; 2 g fat (1 g sat, 1 g mono); 9 mg cholesterol; 8 g carbohydrates; 1 g protein; 0 gfiber; 35 mg sodium; 19 mg potassium.
Carbohydrate Servings: 1/2
Exchanges: 1/2 other carbohydrate
Nutrition Note: Per cookie with Splenda: 1/2 carbohydrate serving; 49 calories, 6 g carbohydrate.

Corn & Broccoli Calzones

INGREDIENTS
- 1 1/2 cups chopped broccoli florets
- 1 1/2 cups fresh corn kernels, (about 3 ears; see Tip)
- 1 cup shredded part-skim mozzarella cheese
- 2/3 cup part-skim ricotta cheese
- 4 scallions, thinly sliced
- 1/4 cup chopped fresh basil
- 1/2 teaspoon garlic powder
- 1/4 teaspoon salt
- 1/4 teaspoon freshly ground pepper

- All-purpose flour, for dusting
- 20 ounces prepared whole-wheat pizza dough, (see Tip), thawed if frozen and 2 teaspoons canola oil

PREPARATION

1. Position racks in upper and lower thirds of oven; preheat to 475°F. Coat 2 baking sheets with cooking spray.
2. Combine broccoli, corn, mozzarella, ricotta, scallions, basil, garlic powder, salt and pepper in a large bowl.
3. On a lightly floured surface, divide dough into 6 pieces. Roll each piece into an 8-inch circle. Place a generous 3/4 cup filling on one half of each circle, leaving a 1-inch border of dough. Brush the border with water and fold the top half over the filling. Fold the edges over and crimp with a fork to seal. Make several small slits in the top to vent steam; brush each calzone with oil. Transfer the calzones to the prepared baking sheets.
4. Bake the calzones, switching the pans halfway through, until browned on top, about 15 minutes. Let cool slightly before serving.

TIPS & NOTES

- **Tips:** To remove corn kernels from the cob: Stand an uncooked ear of corn on its stem end in a shallow bowl and slice the kernels off with a sharp, thin-bladed knife. This technique produces whole kernels that are good for adding to salads and salsas. If you want to use the corn kernels for soups, fritters or puddings, you can add another step to the process. After cutting the kernels off, reverse the knife and, using the dull side, press it down the length of the ear to push out the rest of the corn and its milk.
- Look for balls of whole-wheat pizza dough at your supermarket, fresh or frozen and without any hydrogenated oils.
- **Healthy Heart Variation:** To reduce saturated fat even further, use nonfat ricotta in place of the reduced-fat ricotta. 334 calories, 2 g saturated fat.

NUTRITION

Per calzone: 350 calories; 7 g fat (3 g sat, 3 g mono); 21 mg cholesterol; 50 g carbohydrates; 17 g protein;4 g fiber; 509 mg sodium; 250 mg potassium.
Nutrition Bonus: Vitamin C (35% daily value), Calcium (25% dv), Vitamin A (20% dv).
Carbohydrate Servings: 3
Exchanges: 3 starch, 1 medium-fat protein

Lentil & Chicken Stew

INGREDIENTS
- 3 teaspoons extra-virgin olive oil, divided
- 8 ounces boneless skinless chicken breast, diced
- 1 carrot, peeled and finely diced
- 4 cloves garlic, minced
- 1 teaspoon whole coriander seed, crushed (see Tip)
- 1/8 teaspoon salt
- 1/4 teaspoon freshly ground pepper
- 1 14-ounce can reduced-sodium chicken broth
- 1/2 cup French green or brown lentils, sorted and rinsed (see Note)
- 1 6-ounce bag baby spinach
- 1 tablespoon lemon juice
- 1 tablespoon chopped fresh dill

PREPARATION
1. Heat 1 teaspoon oil in a large saucepan over medium-high heat. Add chicken and cook, stirring once or twice until no longer pink in the middle, about 2 minutes. Transfer the chicken to a plate with a slotted spoon.
2. Add the remaining 2 teaspoons oil to the pan and heat over medium-low heat. Add carrot, garlic, coriander, salt and pepper and cook, stirring constantly, until fragrant, 30 seconds to 1 minute. Stir in broth and lentils, increase heat to medium-high and bring to a simmer. Reduce heat to maintain a simmer and cook, stirring occasionally, until the lentils are tender, 20 to 30 minutes (brown lentils take a little longer).
3. Add the cooked chicken, spinach and lemon juice and return to a simmer. Cook until heated through, 1 to 2 minutes. Stir in dill.

TIPS & NOTES
- **Make Ahead Tip**: Cover and refrigerate up to 3 days or freeze up to 3 months.
- **Tip:** Place whole spices in a plastic bag and crush with the bottom of a heavy skillet or pulse in a spice grinder.
- **Note:** French green lentils are firmer than brown lentils and cook more quickly. They can be found in natural-foods stores and some large supermarkets.

NUTRITION
Per serving: 369 calories; 11 g fat (2 g sat, 6 g mono); 50 mg cholesterol; 37 g carbohydrates; 0 g added sugars; 33 g protein; 10 g fiber; 520 mg sodium; 1140 mg potassium.
Nutrition Bonus: Vitamin A (260% daily value), Vitamin C (50% dv), Folate (43% dv), Potassium (33% dv).
Carbohydrate Servings: 2

Exchanges: 2 starch, 1 vegetable, 3 1/2 very lean meat, 1 1/2 fat

Arugula-Mushroom Salad

INGREDIENTS
- 1 clove garlic, peeled
- 1/4 teaspoon salt
- 1 tablespoon lemon juice
- 1 tablespoon reduced-fat mayonnaise
- 1 tablespoon extra-virgin olive oil
- 1 tablespoon chopped fresh parsley
- Freshly ground pepper, to taste
- 6 cups arugula leaves
- 2 cups sliced mushrooms

PREPARATION
1. Place garlic on a cutting board and crush. Sprinkle with salt and use the flat of a chefs knife blade to mash the garlic to a paste; transfer to a serving bowl. Whisk in lemon juice, mayonnaise, oil and parsley. Season with pepper. Add arugula and mushrooms; toss to coat with the dressing.

NUTRITION

Per serving: 62 calories; 4 g fat (1 g sat, 3 g mono); 1 mg cholesterol; 3 g carbohydrates; 0 g added sugars;2 g protein; 1 g fiber; 188 mg sodium; 235 mg potassium.
Nutrition Bonus: Vitamin C (15% daily value).
Exchanges: 1 vegetable, 1 fat (mono)

Sliced Tomato Salad

INGREDIENTS
- 4 tomatoes, sliced
- 1/4 cup thinly sliced red onion
- 8 anchovies
- 1/2 teaspoon dried oregano
- Salt & freshly ground pepper, to taste
- 2 tablespoons extra-virgin olive oil
- 1 tablespoon white-wine vinegar

PREPARATION
1. Arrange tomato slices on a platter. Top with onion, anchovies, oregano, salt and pepper. Drizzle with oil and vinegar.

NUTRITION

Per serving: 44 calories; 1 g fat (0 g sat, 0 g mono); 3 mg cholesterol; 8 g carbohydrates; 0 g added sugars;3 g protein; 2 g fiber; 300 mg sodium; 403 mg potassium.
Nutrition Bonus: Vitamin C (35% daily value), Vitamin A (25% dv).
Carbohydrate Servings: 1/2
Exchanges: 1 vegetable, 1 1/2 fat

Mango Sorbet

INGREDIENTS

- 3 ripe mangoes
- 1/2 cup sugar and 1/2 cup water
- 1/3 cup coarsely mashed banana, (1 small)
- 2 tablespoons lime juice

PREPARATION

1. Preheat oven to 350°F. Place whole mangoes in a shallow baking pan and roast until very soft, 70 to 90 minutes. Refrigerate until cool, about 1 hour.
2. Meanwhile, combine sugar and water in a small saucepan. Bring to a boil, stirring to dissolve sugar. Remove from heat and refrigerate until cold, about 1 hour.
3. When the mangoes are cool enough to handle, remove skin and coarsely chop pulp, discarding pit. Place the mango pulp and accumulated juices in a food processor. Add banana and lime juice; process until very smooth. Transfer to a large bowl and stir in the sugar syrup. Cover and refrigerate until cold, 40 minutes or overnight.
4. Freeze the mixture in an ice cream maker according to manufacturer's directions. (Alternatively, freeze the mixture in a shallow metal pan until solid, about 6 hours. Break into chunks and process in a food processor until smooth.) Serve immediately or transfer to a storage container and let harden in the freezer for 1 to 1 1/2 hours. Serve in chilled dishes.

TIPS & NOTES

- **Make Ahead Tip**: Store in an airtight container in the freezer for up to 1 week. Let soften in the refrigerator for 1/2 hour before serving. | Equipment: Ice cream maker or food processor

NUTRITION

Per serving: 108 calories; 0 g fat (0 g sat, 0 g mono); 0 mg cholesterol; 28 g carbohydrates; 1 g protein; 2 gfiber; 2 mg sodium; 159 mg potassium.
Nutrition Bonus: Vitamin C (40% daily value).

Carbohydrate Servings: 2
Exchanges: 2 fruit

DAY 27
BREAKFAST
Morning Smoothie
Whole-wheat toast (1 slice)
Plum spread
LUNCH
Skim milk (1 cup)
Tuna & Bean Salad in Pita Pockets or Chicken Parmesan Sub
Apple (1 cup, quartered)
SNACK
Ranch Dip & Crunchy Vegetables
Fat-free Chese slice
DINNER
Turkey Cutlets with Peas & Spring Onions or Asian "Salisbury" Steak
Brown rice (3/4 cup, cooked)
Arugula & Strawberry Salad
Mango Bread Pudding with Chai Spices

DAY 27 RECIPES

Morning Smoothie
INGREDIENTS
- 1 1/4 cups orange juice, preferably calcium-fortified
- 1 banana
- 1 1/4 cups frozen berries, such as raspberries, blackberries, blueberries and/or strawberries
- 1/2 cup low-fat silken tofu, or low-fat plain yogurt
- 1 tablespoon sugar, or Splenda Granular (optional)

PREPARATION
1. Combine orange juice, banana, berries, tofu (or yogurt) and sugar (or Splenda), if using, in a blender; cover and blend until creamy. Serve immediately.

NUTRITION
Per serving: 139 calories; 2 g fat (0 g sat, 0 g mono); 0 mg cholesterol; 33 g carbohydrates; 0 g added sugars; 4 g protein; 4 g fiber; 19 mg sodium; 421 mg potassium.

Nutrition Bonus: Vitamin C (110% daily value), Fiber (16% dv).
Carbohydrate Servings: 2
Exchanges: 2 fruit, 1/2 low-fat milk

Plum spread

INGREDIENTS
- 5 pounds plums, pitted and sliced (14-15 cups)
- 3 Granny Smith apples, washed and quartered (not cored)
- 1/4 cup white grape juice, or other fruit juice
- 2 tablespoons lemon juice
- 3/4 cup sugar, or Splenda Granular
- 1/4 teaspoon ground cinnamon, or ginger (optional)

PREPARATION
1. Place a plate in the freezer for testing consistency later.
2. Combine plums, apples, grape juice (or fruit juice) and lemon juice in a large, heavy-bottomed, nonreactive Dutch oven. Bring to a boil over medium-high heat, stirring. Cover and boil gently, stirring occasionally, until the fruit is softened and juicy, 15 to 20 minutes. Uncover and boil gently, stirring occasionally, until the fruit is completely soft, about 20 minutes. (Adjust heat as necessary to maintain a gentle boil.)
3. Pass the fruit through a food mill to remove the skins and apple seeds.
4. Return the strained fruit to the pot. Add sugar (or Splenda) and cinnamon (or ginger), if using. Cook over medium heat, stirring frequently, until a spoonful of jam dropped onto the chilled plate holds its shape, about 15 minutes longer. (See Tip.) Remove from heat and skim off any foam.

TIPS & NOTES
- **Make Ahead Tip**: Store in an airtight container in the refrigerator for up to 2 months. For longer storage, process in a boiling-water bath.

- **To test the consistency of the spread:** Drop a dollop of cooked spread onto a chilled plate. Carefully run your finger through the dollop. If the track remains unfilled, the jam is done.

NUTRITION
Per tablespoon with sugar: 14 calories; 0 g fat (0 g sat, 0 g mono); 0 mg cholesterol; 4 g carbohydrates; 0 g protein; 0 g fiber; 0 mg sodium; 30 mg potassium.
Exchanges: free food
Nutrition Note: Per tablespoon with Splenda: 0 Carbohydrate Servings; 12 calories; 3 g carbohydrate.

Tuna & Bean Salad in Pita Pockets

INGREDIENTS

- 1 clove garlic, crushed and peeled
- 1/4 teaspoon salt
- 1 tablespoon lemon juice
- 1 tablespoon extra-virgin olive oil
- 1/4 teaspoon crushed red pepper
- 1 15-ounce can great northern beans, rinsed
- 1 3-ounce can tuna packed in water, drained and flaked (see Note)
- 1 cup arugula leaves, coarsely chopped
- Freshly ground pepper, to taste
- 2 6-inch whole-wheat pita breads
- 2-4 large lettuce leaves
- 1/4 cup thinly sliced red onion

PREPARATION

1. With a chef's knife, mash garlic and salt into a paste. Transfer to a bowl. Whisk in lemon juice, oil and crushed red pepper. Add beans, tuna and arugula; toss to mix. Season with pepper.
2. Cut a quarter off each pita to open the pocket. (Save the trimmings to make pita crisps.) Line the centers with lettuce. Fill with tuna/bean salad and red onion slices

TIPS & NOTES

- **Note:** Chunk light tuna, which comes from the smaller skipjack or yellowfin, has less mercury than canned white albacore tuna. The FDA/EPA advises that women who are or might become pregnant, nursing mothers and young children consume no more than 6 ounces of albacore a week; up to 12 ounces of canned light tuna is considered safe.

NUTRITION

Per serving: 454 calories; 10 g fat (2 g sat, 6 g mono); 13 mg cholesterol; 66 g carbohydrates; 29 g protein;15 g fiber; 782 mg sodium; 842 mg potassium.
Nutrition Bonus: Fiber (59% dv), Folate (48% dv), Potassium (42% dv), Magnesium (33% dv), Iron (30% dv), Calcium (15% dv), Vitamin C (15% dv), Vitamin A. (15% dv).
Carbohydrate Servings: 3
Exchanges: 3 1/2 starch, 1 1/2 vegetable, 3 lean meat

Chicken Parmesan Sub

INGREDIENTS

- 1/2 cup all-purpose flour
- 1/2 teaspoon kosher salt
- 1/2 teaspoon freshly ground pepper
- 1 pound boneless, skinless chicken breasts (2 large breasts cut into 4 portions or 4 small breasts), (2 large breasts cut into 4 portions or 4 small breasts)
- 4 teaspoons extra-virgin olive oil, divided
- 2 6-ounce bags baby spinach
- 1 cup marinara sauce, preferably low-sodium (see Tip)
- 1/4 cup grated Parmesan cheese
- 1/2 cup shredded part-skim mozzarella
- 4 soft whole-wheat sandwich rolls, toasted

PREPARATION

1. Position oven rack in top position; preheat broiler.
2. Combine flour, salt and pepper in a shallow dish. Place chicken between 2 large pieces of plastic wrap. Pound with the smooth side of a meat mallet or a heavy saucepan until the chicken is an even 1/4-inch thickness. Dip the chicken in the flour mixture and turn to coat.
3. Heat 2 teaspoons oil in a large nonstick skillet over medium-high heat. Add spinach and cook, stirring often, until wilted, 2 to 3 minutes. Transfer to a small bowl.
4. Add 1 teaspoon oil to the pan. Add half the chicken and cook until golden, 1 to 2 minutes per side. Transfer to a large baking sheet. Repeat with the remaining 1 teaspoon oil and chicken; transfer to the baking sheet.
5. Top each piece of chicken with the wilted spinach, marinara sauce and Parmesan. Sprinkle with mozzarella. Broil until the cheese is melted and the chicken is cooked through, about 3 minutes. Serve on rolls.

TIPS & NOTES

- **Tip:** Refrigerate leftover marinara sauce for up to 1 week or freeze for up to 3 months.

NUTRITION

Per serving: 472 calories; 15 g fat (4 g sat, 6 g mono); 85 mg cholesterol; 48 g carbohydrates; 40 g protein;5 g fiber; 837 mg sodium; 923 mg potassium.
Nutrition Bonus: Vitamin A (160% daily value), Vitamin C (46% dv), Folate (43% dv), Magnesium (26% dv).
Carbohydrate Servings: 3
Exchanges: 3 starch, 1 vegetable, 4 1/2 very lean meat, 1 fat

Ranch Dip & Crunchy Vegetables

INGREDIENTS
- 1/2 cup nonfat buttermilk, (see Tip)
- 1/3 cup low-fat mayonnaise
- 2 tablespoons minced fresh dill, or 2 teaspoons dried
- 1 tablespoon lemon juice
- 1 teaspoon Dijon mustard
- 1 teaspoon honey
- 1/2 teaspoon garlic powder
- 1/8 teaspoon salt
- 6 cups vegetables, such as baby carrots, sliced red bell peppers, snap peas, broccoli and cauliflower florets, cucumber spears, grape tomatoes

PREPARATION
1. Whisk buttermilk, mayonnaise, dill, lemon juice, mustard, honey, garlic powder and salt in a medium bowl until combined. Serve the dip with vegetables of your choice.

TIPS & NOTES
- **Make Ahead Tip**: Cover and refrigerate the dip for up to 3 days.
- **Tip:** No buttermilk? You can use buttermilk powder prepared according to package directions. Or make "sour milk": mix 1 tablespoon lemon juice or vinegar to 1 cup milk.

NUTRITION

Per serving: 61 calories; 1 g fat (0 g sat, 0 g mono); 0 mg cholesterol; 11 g carbohydrates; 1 g added sugars; 3 g protein; 2 g fiber; 224 mg sodium; 196 mg potassium.
Nutrition Bonus: Vitamin C (100% daily value), Vitamin A (80% dv).
Carbohydrate Servings: 1
Exchanges: 1 1/2 vegetable, 1/2 fat

Turkey Cutlets with Peas & Spring Onions

INGREDIENTS
- 1/2 cup all-purpose flour
- 1/2 teaspoon salt, divided
- 1/4 teaspoon freshly ground pepper
- 1 pound 1/4-inch-thick turkey breast cutlets, or steaks
- 2 tablespoons extra-virgin olive oil, divided

- 4 ounces shiitake mushrooms, stemmed and sliced (about 1 1/2 cups)
- 1 bunch spring onions, or scallions, sliced, whites and greens separated
- 1 cup reduced-sodium chicken broth
- 1/2 cup dry white wine
- 1 cup peas, fresh or frozen, thawed
- 1 teaspoon freshly grated lemon zest

PREPARATION

1. Whisk flour, 1/4 teaspoon salt and pepper in a shallow dish. Dredge each turkey cutlet (or steak) in the flour mixture. Heat 1 tablespoon oil in a large nonstick skillet over medium-high heat. Add the turkey and cook until lightly golden, 2 to 3 minutes per side. Transfer to a plate; cover with foil to keep warm.
2. Add the remaining 1 tablespoon oil to the pan and heat over medium-high heat. Add mushrooms and onion (or scallion) whites and cook, stirring often, until the mushrooms are browned and the whites are slightly softened, 2 to 3 minutes. Add broth, wine and the remaining 1/4 teaspoon salt; cook, stirring occasionally, until the sauce is slightly reduced, 2 to 3 minutes. Stir in peas and onion (or scallion) greens and cook, stirring, until heated through, about 1 minute. Stir in lemon zest. Nestle the turkey into the vegetables along with any accumulated juices from the plate. Cook, turning the cutlets once, until heated through, 1 to 2 minutes.

NUTRITION
Per serving: 313 calories; 8 g fat (1 g sat, 5 g mono); 45 mg cholesterol; 23 g carbohydrates; 34 g protein; 3 g fiber; 571 mg sodium; 223 mg potassium.
Nutrition Bonus: Iron (15% daily value), Vitamin A & C (20% dv).
Carbohydrate Servings: 1
Exchanges: 1 starch, 1 vegetable, 4 lean meat, 1 fat

Asian "Salisbury" Steak

INGREDIENTS
- 12 ounces 90%-lean ground beef
- 3/4 cup finely diced red bell pepper
- 3/4 cup chopped scallions
- 1/4 cup plain dry breadcrumbs
- 4 tablespoons hoisin sauce, divided
- 2 tablespoons minced fresh ginger
- 3 teaspoons canola oil, divided
- 4 bunches or 2 4-ounce bags watercress, trimmed (16 cups)
- 1/2 cup Shao Hsing rice wine, (see Ingredient note) or dry sherry

PREPARATION

1. Place rack in upper third of oven; preheat the broiler. Coat a broiler pan and rack with cooking spray.
2. Gently mix beef, bell pepper, scallions, breadcrumbs, 3 tablespoons hoisin sauce and ginger in a medium bowl until just combined. Form the mixture into 4 oblong patties and place on the broiler-pan rack. Brush the tops of the patties with 1 teaspoon oil. Broil, flipping once, until cooked through, about 4 minutes per side.
3. Meanwhile, heat the remaining 2 teaspoons oil in a large skillet over high heat. Add watercress and cook, stirring often, until just wilted, 1 to 3 minutes. Divide the watercress among 4 plates. Return the skillet to medium-high heat, add rice wine (or sherry) and the remaining 1 tablespoon hoisin sauce and stir until smooth, bubbling and slightly reduced, about 1 minute. Top the watercress with the Salisbury steaks and drizzle with the pan sauce.

TIPS & NOTES
- **Ingredient Note:** Shao Hsing (or Shaoxing) is a seasoned rice wine available in most Asian specialty markets and some larger supermarkets' Asian sections.

NUTRITION
Per serving: 303 calories; 13 g fat (4 g sat, 6 g mono); 56 mg cholesterol; 18 g carbohydrates; 21 g protein; 2 g fiber; 392 mg sodium; 623 mg potassium.
Nutrition Bonus: Vitamin C (140% daily value), Vitamin A (70% dv), Potassium (18% dv), Iron (15% dv).
Carbohydrate Servings: 1
Exchanges: 1 other carb., 1 vegetable, 2.5 lean meat

Arugula & Strawberry Salad

INGREDIENTS
- 1/2 cup chopped walnuts
- 4 cups baby arugula, or torn arugula leaves
- 2 cups sliced strawberries, (about 10 ounces)
- 2 ounces Parmesan cheese, shaved and crumbled into small pieces (1/2 cup)
- 1/4 teaspoon freshly ground pepper
- 1/8 teaspoon salt
- 2 tablespoons aged balsamic vinegar, (see Ingredient note)
- 1 tablespoon extra-virgin olive oil

PREPARATION

1. Toast walnuts in a small dry skillet over medium-low heat, stirring frequently, until lightly browned and aromatic, 3 to 5 minutes. Transfer to a salad bowl; let cool for 5 minutes.
2. Add arugula, strawberries, Parmesan, pepper and salt. Sprinkle vinegar and oil over the salad; toss gently and serve at once.

TIPS & NOTES

- **Ingredient Note:** Aged balsamic vinegar (12 years or older) is a treat, but not an economical one. If you don't want to spring for a $40 bottle, use regular balsamic. Alternatively, bring 1/2 cup regular balsamic vinegar to a boil over high heat in a small skillet. Cook until the vinegar begins to thicken and become syrupy, 2 to 3 minutes.

NUTRITION

Per serving: 204 calories; 16 g fat (3 g sat, 5 g mono); 7 mg cholesterol; 10 g carbohydrates; 7 g protein; 3 g fiber; 251 mg sodium; 262 mg potassium.
Nutrition Bonus: Vitamin C (70% daily value), Calcium (20% dv).
Carbohydrate Servings: 1/2
Exchanges: 1/2 fruit, 1 vegetable, 1 lean meat, 2 1/2 fat

Mango Bread Pudding with Chai Spices

INGREDIENTS

- 4 cups stale (but not dry) white bread slices, cut into 1/2-inch cubes
- 2 large ripe mangoes, peeled (see Tip) and cut into 1/2-inch cubes (3 cups)
- 2 cups fat-free milk
- 2 eggs, lightly beaten
- 2 tablespoons light or dark rum, (optional)
- 1/2 cup packed dark brown sugar
- 1 teaspoon vanilla extract
- 1/2 teaspoon ground cinnamon
- 1/2 teaspoon ground cloves
- 1/2 teaspoon ground cardamom
- 1/2 teaspoon ground ginger
- 1/4 teaspoon ground black peppercorns
- 1/8 teaspoon salt

PREPARATION

1. Position rack in the center of the oven; preheat to 350ºF. Coat an 8-inch square baking dish with cooking spray.

2. Toss bread cubes and mangoes together in the baking dish.
3. Whisk milk, eggs, rum (if using), brown sugar, vanilla, cinnamon, cloves, cardamom, ginger, pepper and salt in a medium bowl. Pour over the bread and mangoes; allow the mixture to soak for about 5 minutes.
4. Bake the pudding until it is set and a knife inserted in the center comes out clean, about 1 1/4 hours. Serve warm for best flavor.

TIPS & NOTES
- **Tip:** How to cut a mango:
- 1. Slice both ends off the mango, revealing the long, slender seed inside. Set the fruit upright on a work surface and remove the skin with a sharp knife.
- 2. With the seed perpendicular to you, slice
- the fruit from both sides of the seed, yielding two large pieces.
- 3. Turn the seed parallel to you and slice the two smaller pieces of fruit from each side.
- 4. Cut the fruit into the desired shape.

NUTRITION
Per serving: 164 calories; 2 g fat (0 g sat, 1 g mono); 54 mg cholesterol; 34 g carbohydrates; 6 g protein; 2 g fiber; 180 mg sodium; 228 mg potassium.
Nutrition Bonus: Calcium (11% daily value).
Carbohydrate Servings: 2
Exchanges: 1/2 starch, 1/2 fruit, 1 other carbohydrate

DAY 28
BREAKFAST
Sunday Sausage Strata or Ham & Cheese Breakfast Casserole
Skim milk (1 cup)
Orange (1 large)
LUNCH
Chicken Salad Wraps
Skim milk (1 cup)
Blueberries (1 cup)
SNACK
Fat-free cheese (1 slice)
Toasted Pita Crisps
DINNER
Pizza-Style Meatloaf or Barbecue Pulled Chicken
Steamed aparagus (1/2 cup)
Baked potato (1 medium)

Creamy Herb Dip
Red & White Salad
Buttermilk Biscuits
Chewy Chocolate Brownies

DAY 28 RECIPES

Sunday Sausage Strata

INGREDIENTS
- 1/2 pound turkey breakfast sausage, (four 2-ounce links), casing removed
- 2 medium onions, chopped (2 cups)
- 1 medium red bell pepper, seeded and diced (1 1/2 cups)
- 12 large eggs
- 4 cups 1% milk
- 1 teaspoon salt, or to taste
- Freshly ground pepper, to taste

- 6 cups cubed, whole-wheat country bread, (about 7 slices, crusts removed)
- 1 tablespoon Dijon mustard
- 1 1/2 cups grated Swiss cheese, (4 ounces)

PREPARATION
1. Coat a 9-by-13-inch baking dish (or similar shallow 3-quart baking dish) with cooking spray.
2. Cook sausage in a large nonstick skillet over medium heat, crumbling with a wooden spoon, until lightly browned, 3 to 4 minutes. Transfer to a plate lined with paper towels to drain. Add onions and bell pepper to the pan and cook, stirring often, until softened, 3 to 4 minutes.
3. Whisk eggs, milk, salt and pepper in a large bowl until blended.
4. Spread bread in the prepared baking dish. Scatter the sausage and the onion mixture evenly over the bread. Brush with mustard. Sprinkle with cheese. Pour in the egg mixture. Cover with plastic wrap and refrigerate for at least 2 hours or overnight.
5. Preheat oven to 350 degrees F. Bake the strata, uncovered, until puffed, lightly browned and set in the center, 55 to 65 minutes. Let cool for about 5 minutes before serving hot.

TIPS & NOTES
- **Make Ahead Tip**: Prepare through Step 4 the night before serving.

NUTRITION

Per serving: 255 calories; 13 g fat (45 g sat, 4 g mono); 229 mg cholesterol; 19 g carbohydrates; 17 gprotein; 2 g fiber; 513 mg sodium; 380 mg potassium.
Nutrition Bonus: Vitamin C (72% daily value), Calcium (23% dv).
Carbohydrate Servings: 1
Exchanges: 2/3 starch, 1/3 milk, 1/2 vegetable, 1 very lean protein, 1 1/3 medium-fat protein

Ham & Cheese Breakfast Casserole

INGREDIENTS
- 4 large eggs
- 4 large egg whites
- 1 cup nonfat milk
- 2 tablespoons Dijon mustard
- 1 teaspoon minced fresh rosemary
- 1/4 teaspoon freshly ground pepper
- 5 cups chopped spinach, wilted (see Tip)
- 4 cups whole-grain bread, crusts removed if desired, cut into 1-inch cubes (about 1/2 pound, 4-6 slices)
- 1 cup diced ham steak, (5 ounces)
- 1/2 cup chopped jarred roasted red peppers
- 3/4 cup shredded Gruyère, or Swiss cheese

PREPARATION
1. Preheat oven to 375°F. Coat a 7-by-11-inch glass baking dish or a 2-quart casserole with cooking spray.
2. Whisk eggs, egg whites and milk in a medium bowl. Add mustard, rosemary and pepper; whisk to combine. Toss spinach, bread, ham and roasted red peppers in a large bowl. Add the egg mixture and toss well to coat. Transfer to the prepared baking dish and push down to compact. Cover with foil.
3. Bake until the custard has set, 40 to 45 minutes. Uncover, sprinkle with cheese and continue baking until the pudding is puffed and golden on top, 15 to 20 minutes more. Transfer to a wire rack and cool for 15 to 20 minutes before serving.

TIPS & NOTES
- **Make Ahead Tip**: Prepare casserole through Step 2; refrigerate overnight. Let stand at room temperature while the oven preheats. Bake as directed in Step 3.
- **Tip:** To wilt spinach, rinse thoroughly with cool water. Transfer to a large microwave-safe bowl. Cover with plastic wrap and punch several holes in it. Microwave on High until wilted, 2 to 3 minutes. Squeeze out excess moisture before adding the spinach to the recipe.

NUTRITION

Per serving: 286 calories; 10 g fat (4 g sat, 3 g mono); 167 mg cholesterol; 23 g carbohydrates; 23 gprotein; 4 g fiber; 813 mg sodium; 509 mg potassium.
Nutrition Bonus: Vitamin A (70% daily value), Folate (37% dv), Calcium (30% dv), Vitamin C (20% dv).
Carbohydrate Servings: 1 1/2
Exchanges: 1 starch, 1 vegetable, 2 medium-fat meat

Chicken Salad Wraps

INGREDIENTS
- 1/2 cup lemon juice
- 1/3 cup fish sauce, (see Ingredient note)
- 1/4 cup sugar
- 2 cloves garlic, minced
- 1/4 teaspoon crushed red pepper
- 8 6-inch flour tortillas
- 4 cups shredded romaine lettuce
- 3 cups shredded cooked chicken, (12 ounces)
- 1 large ripe tomato, cut into thin wedges
- 1 cup grated carrots, (2 medium)
- 2/3 cup chopped scallions, (1 bunch)
- 2/3 cup slivered fresh mint

PREPARATION
1. Whisk lemon juice, fish sauce, sugar, garlic and crushed red pepper in a small bowl until sugar is dissolved.
2. Preheat oven to 325° F. Wrap tortillas in foil and heat in the oven for 10 to 15 minutes, until softened and heated through. Keep warm.
3. Combine lettuce, chicken, tomato, carrots, scallions and mint in a large bowl. Add 1/3 cup of the dressing; toss to coat.
4. Set out the chicken mixture, tortillas and the remaining dressing for diners to assemble wraps at the table. Serve immediately.

TIPS & NOTES
- **Ingredient note:** A pungent, soy sauce-like condiment used throughout Southeast Asia, fish sauce is made from fermented, salted fish. Available in large supermarkets and in Asian markets.
- To warm tortillas in a microwave, stack between two damp paper towels; microwave on high for 30 to 60 seconds, or until heated through.

NUTRITION

Per serving: 439 calories; 9 g fat (2 g sat, 4 g mono); 89 mg cholesterol; 49 g carbohydrates; 40 g protein; 5 g fiber; 1018 mg sodium; 783 mg potassium.
Nutrition Bonus: 140% dv vitamin a, 31 mg vitamin c (50% dv), 179 mcg folate (45% dv), 4 mg iron (25% dv).
Carbohydrate Servings: 3
Exchanges: 3 stach, 1 vegetable, 3 lean meat

Toasted Pita Crisps

INGREDIENTS
- 4 whole-wheat pita breads
- Olive oil cooking spray, or extra-virgin olive oil

PREPARATION
1. Preheat oven to 425°F.
2. Cut pitas into 4 triangles each. Separate each triangle into 2 halves at the fold. Arrange, rough side up, on a baking sheet. Spritz lightly with cooking spray or brush lightly with oil. Bake until crisp, 8 to 10 minutes.

TIPS & NOTES
- **Make Ahead Tip:** Store in an airtight container at room temperature for up to 1 week or in the freezer for up to 2 months.

NUTRITION

Per crisp: 23 calories; 0 g fat (0 g sat, 0 g mono); 0 mg cholesterol; 4 g carbohydrates; 0 g added sugars; 1 g protein; 1 g fiber; 43 mg sodium; 14 mg potassium.
Exchanges: 1/3 starch

Pizza-Style Meatloaf

INGREDIENTS
- 1 teaspoon extra-virgin olive oil
- 1 medium onion, sliced
- 1 red or yellow bell pepper, sliced
- 4 ounces mushrooms, sliced
- 1/4 cup chopped fresh basil
- 1 pound lean ground beef
- 1 clove garlic, minced
- 1/3 cup seasoned (Italian-style) breadcrumbs
- 1/3 cup low-fat milk and 1/2 teaspoon salt
- 1/2 cup prepared marinara sauce
- 1/4 cup shredded sharp Cheddar cheese

PREPARATION
1. Preheat oven to 400°F. Coat a 12-inch pizza pan with cooking spray and place it on a large baking sheet with sides.
2. Heat oil in a large skillet over medium heat. Add onion, bell pepper, mushrooms and basil; cook, stirring, until softened, about 10 minutes.
3. Meanwhile, combine beef, garlic, breadcrumbs, milk and salt in a large bowl. Mix well.
4. Transfer the meat mixture to the prepared pan. With dampened hands, pat into a 10-inch circle. Top with marinara sauce. Spoon the vegetable mixture over the sauce and sprinkle with cheese.
5. Bake until the meat is browned and the cheese has melted, about 30 minutes. Drain off any fat. Cut into wedges and serve.

TIPS & NOTES
- **Make Ahead Tip**: Equipment: Use a perforated pizza pan so excess fat drips away.

NUTRITION

Per serving: 195 calories; 8 g fat (3 g sat, 2 g mono); 53 mg cholesterol; 11 g carbohydrates; 20 g protein; 2 g fiber; 471 mg sodium; 414 mg potassium.
Nutrition Bonus: Vitamin C (48% daily value), Zinc (27% dv), Selenium (21% dv), Vitamin A (18% dv).
Carbohydrate Servings: 1
Exchanges: 1 other carbohydrate, 21/2 lean meat

Barbecue Pulled Chicken

INGREDIENTS
- 1 8-ounce can reduced-sodium tomato sauce
- 1 4-ounce can chopped green chiles, drained
- 3 tablespoons cider vinegar
- 2 tablespoons honey
- 1 tablespoon sweet or smoked paprika
- 1 tablespoon tomato paste
- 1 tablespoon Worcestershire sauce
- 2 teaspoons dry mustard
- 1 teaspoon ground chipotle chile
- 1/2 teaspoon salt
- 2 1/2 pounds boneless, skinless chicken thighs, trimmed of fat
- 1 small onion, finely chopped
- 1 clove garlic, minced

PREPARATION

1. Stir tomato sauce, chiles, vinegar, honey, paprika, tomato paste, Worcestershire sauce, mustard, ground chipotle and salt in a 6-quart slow cooker until smooth. Add chicken, onion and garlic; stir to combine.
2. Put the lid on and cook on low until the chicken can be pulled apart, about 5 hours.
3. Transfer the chicken to a cutting board and shred with a fork. Return the chicken to the sauce, stir well and serve.

TIPS & NOTES

- **Make Ahead Tip**: Cover and refrigerate for up to 3 days or freeze for up to 1 month.
- For easy cleanup, try a slow-cooker liner. These heat-resistant, disposable liners fit neatly inside the insert and help prevent food from sticking to the bottom and sides of your slow cooker.

NUTRITION

Per serving: 364 calories; 13 g fat (3 g sat, 5 g mono); 93 mg cholesterol; 32 g carbohydrates; 4 g added sugars; 30 g protein; 4 g fiber; 477 mg sodium; 547 mg potassium.
Nutrition Bonus: Zinc (18% daily value), Vitamin A (16% dv)
Carbohydrate Servings: 1/2
Exchanges: 1/2 other carb., 4 lean meat

Creamy Herb Dip

INGREDIENTS

- 1/4 cup reduced-fat cream cheese, (Neufchâtel), softened (2 ounces)
- 2 tablespoons buttermilk, or low-fat milk
- 2 tablespoons chopped fresh chives, or scallions
- 1 tablespoon chopped fresh dill, or parsley
- 1 teaspoon prepared horseradish, or more to taste
- Pinch of sugar
- 1/8 teaspoon salt
- Freshly ground pepper, to taste

PREPARATION

1. Place cream cheese in a small bowl and stir in buttermilk (or milk) until smooth. Mix in chives (or scallions), dill (or parsley), horseradish, sugar, salt and pepper.

TIPS & NOTES

- **Make Ahead Tip**: Cover and refrigerate for up to 4 days.

NUTRITION

Per tablespoon: 20 calories; 2 g fat (1 g sat, 0 g mono); 5 mg cholesterol; 1 g carbohydrates; 0 g added sugars; 1 g protein; 0 g fiber; 72 mg sodium; 18 mg potassium.
Exchanges: free food

Red & White Salad

INGREDIENTS
CHAMPAGNE VINAIGRETTE
- 1 shallot, peeled and quartered
- 1/4 cup champagne vinegar or white-wine vinegar
- 1/4 cup extra-virgin olive oil
- 1 tablespoon Dijon mustard
- 3/4 teaspoon salt
- Freshly ground pepper to taste

RED & WHITE SALAD
- 4 cups thinly sliced hearts of romaine
- 2 heads Belgian endive, cored and thinly sliced
- 1 bulb fennel, trimmed, cored, quartered and thinly sliced
- 1 15-ounce can hearts of palm, drained, halved lengthwise and thinly sliced
- 1/2 head radicchio, cored, quartered and thinly sliced
- 1 red apple, cored and cut into matchsticks
- 1 cup thinly sliced radishes
- Freshly ground pepper to taste

PREPARATION
1. To prepare the vinaigrette: Combine shallot, vinegar, oil, mustard, salt and pepper in a blender. Puree until smooth. (Whirring this dressing in the blender gives it a creamy consistency. If you don't have a blender just mince the shallots, then whisk the ingredients in a medium bowl.)
2. To prepare the salad: Toss romaine, endive, fennel, hearts of palm, radicchio, apple and radishes together in a large salad bowl. Add vinaigrette and toss to coat. Season with pepper.

TIPS & NOTES
- **Make Ahead Tip**: Cover and refrigerate vinaigrette (Step 1) for up to 1 week; prepare salad without dressing, cover and refrigerate for up to 4 hours. Toss with vinaigrette just before serving.

NUTRITION

Per serving: 92 calories; 6 g fat (1 g sat, 5 g mono); 0 mg cholesterol; 10 g carbohydrates; 0 g added sugars; 3 g total sugars; 2 g protein; 3 g fiber; 364 mg sodium; 326 mg potassium.
Nutrition Bonus: Vitamin C (28% daily value)
Carbohydrate Servings: 1/2
Exchanges: 1 1/2 vegetable, 1 1/2 fat

Buttermilk Biscuits

INGREDIENTS
- 3/4 cup buttermilk
- 1 tablespoon canola oil
- 1 cup whole-wheat pastry flour
- 1 cup all-purpose flour
- 1 tablespoon sugar
- 1 1/2 teaspoons baking powder
- 1/2 teaspoon baking soda
- 1/2 teaspoon salt
- 1 1/2 tablespoons cold butter, cut into small pieces
- 1 tablespoon milk, for brushing

PREPARATION
1. Preheat oven to 425 degrees F. Coat a baking sheet with cooking spray.
2. Combine buttermilk and oil. Whisk whole-wheat flour, all-purpose flour, sugar, baking powder, baking soda and salt in a large bowl. Using your fingertips or 2 knives, cut butter into the dry ingredients until crumbly. Make a well in the center and gradually pour in the buttermilk mixture, stirring with a fork until just combined.
3. Transfer the dough to a floured surface and sprinkle with a little flour. Lightly knead the dough 8 times, then pat or roll out to an even 3/4-inch thickness. Cut into 2-inch rounds and transfer to the prepared baking sheet. Gather any scraps of dough and cut more rounds. Brush the tops with milk.
4. Bake the biscuits for 12 to 16 minutes, or until golden brown. Transfer to a wire rack and let cool slightly before serving.

NUTRITION

Per biscuit: 104 calories; 3 g fat (1 g sat, 1 g mono); 4 mg cholesterol; 18 g carbohydrates; 3 g protein; 1 gfiber; 216 mg sodium; 35 mg potassium.
Carbohydrate Servings: 1
Exchanges: 1 starch, 1/2 fat

Chewy Chocolate Brownies

INGREDIENTS
- 16 whole chocolate graham crackers, (8 ounces) (see Ingredient notes)
- 2 tablespoons unsweetened cocoa powder
- 1/4 teaspoon salt
- 2 large eggs
- 1 large egg white
- 1/3 cup packed light brown sugar, or 3 tablespoons
- 1/3 cup granulated sugar, or 3 tablespoons
- 2 teaspoons instant coffee granules
- 2 teaspoons vanilla extract
- 2/3 cup chopped pitted dates
- 1/4 cup semisweet chocolate chips

PREPARATION
1. Preheat oven to 300°F. Coat an 8-by-11 1/2-inch baking dish with cooking spray.
2. Pulse graham crackers into crumbs in a food processor or place in a large plastic bag and crush with a rolling pin. You should have about 2 cups crumbs. Transfer to a small bowl; add cocoa and salt and mix well.
3. Combine eggs, egg white, brown sugar (or Splenda) and granulated sugar (or Splenda) in a large bowl. Beat with an electric mixer at high speed until thickened, about 2 minutes. Blend in coffee granules and vanilla. Gently fold in dates, chocolate chips and the reserved crumb mixture. Scrape the batter into the prepared baking dish, spreading evenly.
4. Bake the brownies until the top springs back when lightly touched, 25 to 30 minutes. Let cool completely in the pan on a wire rack before cutting.

TIPS & NOTES

- **Make Ahead Tip**: Store in an airtight container for up to 3 days or freeze for longer storage.
- **Ingredient Notes:** To avoid trans-fatty acids, look for brands of graham crackers that do not contain partially hydrogenated canola oil, such as Mi-Del chocolate snaps or Barbara's Chocolate Go-Go Grahams.
- **Substituting with Splenda:** In the Test Kitchen, sucralose is the only alternative sweetener we test with when we feel the option is appropriate. For nonbaking recipes, we use Splenda Granular (boxed, not in a packet). For baking, we use Splenda Sugar Blend for Baking, a mix of sugar and sucralose. It can be substituted in recipes (1/2 cup of the blend for each 1 cup of sugar) to reduce sugar calories by half while maintaining some of the baking properties of sugar. If you make a similar blend with half sugar and half Splenda Granular, substitute this homemade mixture cup for cup.

- When choosing any low- or no-calorie sweetener, be sure to check the label to make sure it is suitable for your intended use.
- Easy cleanup: Dessert pans can be a headache to clean. Skip the soaking and scrubbing by lining your pan with parchment paper before you bake.

NUTRITION
Per brownie: 93 calories; 2 g fat (0 g sat, 0 g mono); 18 mg cholesterol; 15 g carbohydrates; 2 g protein; 1 gfiber; 72 mg sodium; 60 mg potassium.
Carbohydrate Servings: 1
Exchanges: 1 other carbohydrate

7 DAY 1500 CALORIE MEAL PLAN 1 (WITH RECIPES)

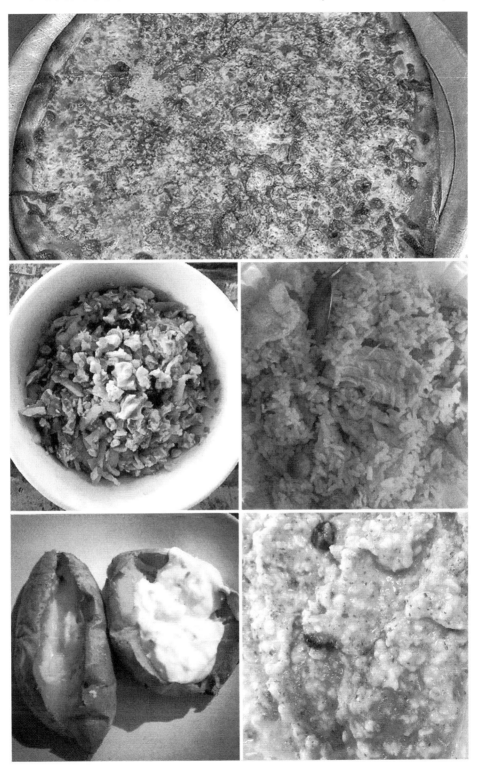

DAY 1

Breakfast

1 Poached egg, a handful of baby spinach, finely chopped onion and 1 teaspoon olive oil spread on wholewheat toast.

Snack

2 Naartjies and 10 pistachio nuts.

Lunch

Tuna Salad Lettuce Wraps: A tin of tuna mixed with low-fat mayonnaise, lemon juice and fresh dill. Serve in lettuce leaves and a side of 6 corn thins, baby carrots and tomatoes.

Snack

1 Fruit kebab with half a cup of low-fat yoghurt.

Dinner

Baked Sweet Potato: One 180g Sweet Potato (microwave for 10 minutes), split open and topped with 1 teaspoon olive oil margarine, finely chopped spring onion, shredded lettuce and 6 tablespoons cooked ostrich mince.

DAY 2

Breakfast

1 Cup cooked oats with half a cup low-fat milk, topped with a grated apple, cinnamon and 4 chopped raw almonds.

Snack

- 3 Provitas
- 2 Teaspoons peanut butter

Lunch

A seeded roll (spread witha teaspoon of olive oil margarine) filled with 3 slices of mozzarella cheese (30g) and 2 slices of ham, along with a side salad.

Snack

An apple and 3-4 strips lean biltong.

Dinner

Tuna & Tomato Pasta (1 cup cooked pasta). Serve with a side salad.

DAY 3

Breakfast

2 Slices of rye toast spread with a teaspoon of olive oil margarine and topped with a quarter cup of fat-free cottage cheese and tomato slices. Half a grapefruit.

Snack

1 Crumble bar.

Lunch

A whole wheat pita bread filled with 2 scrambled eggs, lettuce, tomato, cucumber, mustard and a quarter avocado.

Snack

3 Slices of pineapple and 4 slices of ham.

Dinner

Spicy Chicken Fillets with brown or basmati rice and assorted roasted vegetables.

DAY 4

Breakfast

Bircher Muesli.

Snack

A 1/3 cup of pretzels and 10 peanuts.

Lunch

4 Tablespoons hummus with 2 thin slices rye bread and assorted finger salads (e.g. cherry tomatoes, baby carrots, snap peas, cucumber sticks, etc.)

Snack

Fruit smoothie.

Dinner

Mince and Butternut Pilaf with green beans on the side.

DAY 5

Breakfast

1 Slice of whole wheat toast spread with olive oil spread and anchovette.

2 Cups fresh fruit salad with half a cup low-fat yoghurt.

Snack

A banana and 4 almonds.

Lunch

A tin of tuna combined with half a cup couscous, half a cup sweetcorn, assorted salad ingredients and 2 tablespoons salad dressing.

Snack

1 Papino with half a cup low-fat yoghurt.

Dinner

Homemade Pizza: 1 Soft tortilla wrap topped with 2 tablespoons salsa, 60g mozzarella and slices of tomato. Add rocket after baking for 7 minutes at 200 C.

DAY 6

Breakfast

A cup of All-Bran flakes with half a cup low-fat milk, topped with a banana and 2 teaspoons pumpkin seeds.

Snack

A 30-Day Muffin with 2 lowfat cheese wedges.

Lunch

Chicken Rice Bowl: 1 Cup of brown rice, layered with chopped lettuce, cherry tomatoes and spring onion. Top with half a grilled chicken breast and 30g grated cheddar. Add fresh lemon juice and olive oil as dressing.

Snack

A peach.

Dinner

Extra lean burger patty (120g) or chicken breast (120g) marinated in periperi sauce and grilled. Place on a seeded roll topped with caramalised onion, gherkins, tomato and cucumber. Serve with a side salad.

DAY 7

Breakfast

2 Slices of whole wheat bread with baked beans, tomato, mushrooms. One piece of fruit.

Snack

A closed handful of trail mix (dried fruit and mixed seeds).

Lunch

Open Sandwich: Top 2 slices of rye bread with 60g mozzarella cheese, sundried tomatoes, red pepper, chilli and coriander. Grill until the cheese has melted.

Snack

2 Kiwis and half a cup lowfat yoghurt.

Dinner

3 Salmon cakes and mashed potato (half a cup) with steamed broccoli and cauliflower.

RECIPES FOR 7 DAY 1500 CALORIE MEAL PLAN

30-Day Muffins
makes 24 muffins

Ingredients:
- 2 eggs
- 80 ml oil
- 500 ml fat-free milk
- 200 ml seedless raisins
- 625 ml cake flour
- 375 ml soft brown sugar
- 500 ml All-Bran flakes
- 5 ml salt
- 12,5 ml bicarbonate of soda
- 5 ml vanilla extract

Method:
1. Beat eggs and sugar well.
2. Add oil and mix well.
3. Add the raisins, flour, All-Bran, salt and vanilla extract. Mix well.
4. Mix bicarb with the milk.
5. Leave in the fridge overnight (or for up to 30 days).
6. When ready to bake, stir the mixture well.
7. Prepare muffin tray - either use cupcake cases or spray with non-stick cooking spray.
8. Spoon the mixture into muffin tray.
9. Bake at 180 C for 10-12 minutes.

Bircher Muesli
serves 1

Ingredients:
- 1 cup rolled oats
- half a cup low-fat milk
- 2 teaspoons coconut curls
- 2 teaspoons sunflower seeds
- 45 ml Greek yoghurt
- honey, to taste (optional)
- handful of fresh berries

Method:
1. Put oats in a bowl and cover with milk.
2. Cover the bowl and refrigerate overnight.
3. Place the coconut curls in a dry non-stick pan over medium-high heat and toast until golden. To serve, spoon oats into a bowl, top with yoghurt, sprinkle with sunflower seeds and coconut.
4. Add berries and drizzle with honey (optional).

Tips:
You can store the soaked oats in an airtight container in the fridge for up to a week. Toast larger quantities of coconut curls and refrigerate them in a Zip-lock bag for those hurried weekday mornings. You can use frozen berries or grated apple instead of fresh berries.

Crumble Bars
makes 40 bars

Ingredients:
- 150 g softened butter
- 160 g soft brown sugar
- 1 egg
- 1 teaspoon vanilla extract
- 2 cups cake flour
- 1 teaspoon baking powder
- 1 cup oats
- half a teaspoon salt
- 1 teaspoon cinnamon
- 130 g smooth jam e.g apricot, strawberry, raspberry, etc.

Method:
1. Cream the butter and sugar together.
2. Add the egg and vanilla extract and mix well.
3. Sift the flour and baking powder and combine with the mixture. Mix well.
4. Add the oats, salt and cinnamon and mix (it's easier with your hands) until it forms a soft, crumbly dough.
5. Press three quarters of the dough on a greased 26 cm x 38 cm baking tray.
6. Brush the jam evenly over the dough with a pastry brush. Make a small ball with the rest of the dough and grate it evenly over the jam layer.
7. Bake at 180 C for 20-25 minutes.
8. Let it cool for a few minutes and cut it into 40 rectangular or square (as desired) bars.

Fruit Smoothie
makes 1 smoothie

Ingredients:
- 100 g frozen berries e.g. blueberries, raspberries, strawberries, etc.
- half a banana
- half a cup low-fat fruit yoghurt
- ice, as desired

Method:
1. Cut and blend all ingredients together in a blender.

Note:
You can really tailor your smoothie to your taste, i.e. use your favourite fruits, make it as thick or thin as desired, etc.
- Add ice cubes for texture.
- To thicken and boost the soluble fibre content (great for lowering cholesterol) add oats to your smoothies.
- Peel fruit only when absolutely necessary. For example, citrus fruit, bananas or pineapples should be peeled, but you can keep the peel on apples, peaches, grapes etc.
- Store fruit chunks in the freezer and add them to smoothies without thawing. Berries, peeled bananas, peeled mango, peaches and pears freeze well.

Spicy Chicken Fillets
serves 4

Ingredients:
- 4 garlic cloves, crushed
- 150 ml fat-free plain yoghurt
- 1 tablespoon grated onion
- 1 chilli, de-seeded & finely diced
- 1 teaspoon each of ground coriander, cumin, fenugreek, paprika and ginger
- a pinch of dry mustard powder
- 4 chicken breast fillets, cut in large strips
- lime wedges

Method:
1. Mix together the garlic, yoghurt, onion, chilli, spices and mustard. Add the chicken and marinade overnight.
2. Grill the chicken for 3-4 minutes on each side
3. Serve with the lime wedges, brown or basmati rice and vegetables or salad.

Tuna and Tomato Pasta
serves 4

Ingredients:
- 5 ml olive oil
- 1 onion, chopped
- 1 garlic clove, crushed
- 1 chilli, chopped (optional)
- 1 x 170 g tin tuna chunks in brine, drained
- 2 x 400 g tins tomatoes
- 250 g wholewheat pasta - spaghetti
- freshly ground black pepper
- handful of fresh basil leaves

Method:
1. Heat a large frying pan over medium heat and grease with non-stick cooking spray.
2. Fry the onion until soft, add the garlic and chilli, and fry for a further minute.
3. Add the tuna and fry until heated through.
4. Add the tomatoes and simmer for 20 minutes.
5. Cook the pasta according to the package instructions. Drain and mix through the tuna sauce. Season with black pepper.
6. Top with fresh basil and serve.

Salmon Cakes
makes 9 salmon cakes - serves 3

Ingredients:
- 3 slices of whole wheat bread, crusts removed
- 1 egg
- 15 ml sweet chilli sauce + extra 15 ml Dijon mustard
- small handful of chives, chopped
- zest and juice of half a lemon
- a handful of fresh coriander leaves, chopped + extra for serving
- 2 x 213 g tins of salmon, bones and skins removed
- freshly ground black pepper
- cake flour for dusting

Method:
1. Crumb the bread and mix the egg, sweet chilli sauce, mustard, chives, lemon zest and juice, and coriander through.
2. Flake the salmon, mix through and season with black pepper.
3. Cover your hands well in flour and shape the mix into 9 salmon cakes.
4. Heat a large pan over a medium-high heat, lightly grease with non-stick cooking spray and fry the salmon cakes for 3 minutes on each side until golden brown.
5. Serve with extra sweet chilli sauce and coriander leaves.

7 DAY 1400 CALORIE MEAL PLAN

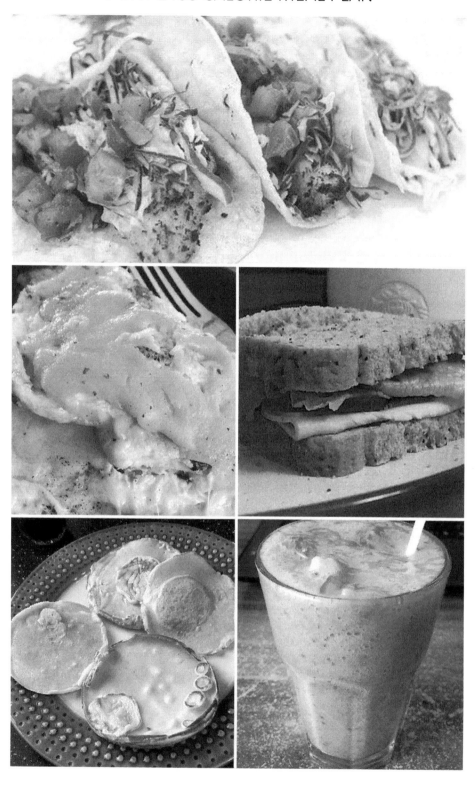

DAY 1

Breakfast: Veggie omelet: Cook 1 egg white in a pan with 2 tsp canola, peanut, or olive oil; 1/2 c spinach leaves; 1/2 c mushrooms; and onion, garlic, and herbs as desired. Top with 1/4 c reduced-fat cheese. Serve with 1 slice whole grain toast spread with 1 tsp canola-oil margarine and 1/2 c fat-free milk.

Lunch: Mixed-up salad: Toss 2 c vegetable greens, 3/4 c low-fat cottage cheese, and 1/2 c mandarin orange slices with 2 Tbsp light Italian dressing. Top with 2 Tbsp chopped almonds or walnuts. Serve with 5 whole grain crackers (such as Triscuits).

Snack: Yogurt: 6 oz light, fat-free, or low-fat flavored yogurt.

Dinner: Grilled fish tacos: Place 2 oz grilled fish and 1 c shredded cabbage, seasoned with rice vinegar, between 2 corn tortillas. Top with 2 Tbsp light sour cream. Serve with 2 c veggies (such as eggplant, mushrooms, green beans, and onions) marinated in 2 Tbsp light Italian dressing and 1 tsp olive oil, then grilled.

Snack: Hummus and crackers: 2 Tbsp hummus on 2 whole grain rye crispbreads.

DAY 2

Breakfast: Pancakes: Top 3 buckwheat or whole wheat pancakes (6" diameter) with 1 tsp canola oil margarine and 1 Tbsp 100% fruit spread (or 2 Tbsp sugar-free syrup). Serve with 1 c fat-free milk or calcium-enriched soy or rice beverage.

Lunch: Tuna sandwich: Mix 2 oz water-packed tuna with 2 tsp regular mayonnaise and 4 chopped large black olives. Spread on 2 slices reduced-calorie whole grain bread. Top with lettuce leaf and 1 sm sliced tomato (1/2 c).

Snack: Yogurt parfait: 1 c fat-free plain yogurt topped with 3/4 c fresh blueberries or blackberries.

Dinner: Chicken with veggies: Grill 3 oz chicken breast sprinkled with herb seasoning (such as Mrs. Dash Garlic & Herb Seasoning Blend) and 1 c vegetables (such as mushrooms, zucchini, yellow squash, and bell peppers) tossed in 2 tsp olive oil. Serve with 2/3 c cooked wild rice.

Snack: Apple and peanut butter: 1 sm apple, sliced and spread with 2 tsp all-natural peanut butter.

DAY 3

Breakfast: Oatmeal: Top 1 c cooked oatmeal with 2 Tbsp walnut halves. Add ground cinnamon and/or sugar substitute to taste. Serve with 1/2 c fat-free milk or calcium-enriched soy beverage.
Lunch: Grilled chicken salad: Toss 2 c mixed greens with 1/2 c diced tomato, 1/2 c sliced cucumbers, and 1/4 c diced carrots, and top with 2 oz grilled chicken breast. Drizzle with avocado-yogurt dressing (combine 1/4 c mashed avocado, 1/2 c fat-free plain yogurt, and vinegar and herbs to taste). Serve with 2 slices whole grain crispbread crackers.
Snack: Cheese and fruit: 1 oz string cheese and 1 sm pear or other fruit.
Dinner: Meat and potatoes: Roast 3 oz beef or pork tenderloin in oven with 1/2 c potato and 1 1/2 c nonstarchy vegetables (such as cauliflower, carrots, broccoli, eggplant, zucchini, and yellow squash) with onion and garlic tossed in 1 Tbsp olive oil.
Snack: Fruit and nuts: 1 med orange and 2 Tbsp cashews.

DAY 4

Breakfast: Super white egg: Break 1 whole egg in small skillet coated with 2 tsp canola oil. Add 1 egg white (or 1/4 c egg substitute) around outside of whole egg and cook over low heat. Top with 2 Tbsp chopped tomato or salsa. Serve with 1 slice reduced-calorie, high-fiber whole grain toast spread with 1 tsp canola margarine and 1 c fat-free milk or calcium-enriched soy beverage.
Snack: Yogurt and dried fruit: 6 oz fat-free yogurt and 4 dried apricot halves.
Lunch: Pile 'er high turkey-and-ham sandwich: Spread 2 slices reduced-calorie, high-fiber whole wheat bread with 1 Tbsp light mayonnaise (or 1 tsp regular mayo and 1 Tbsp mustard), if desired. Layer on 1 oz each of turkey, ham, and low-fat cheese. Top with 1/2 c shredded romaine lettuce and 1/2 sliced tomato. Serve with 16 baby carrots dipped in 1 Tbsp low-fat ranch dressing.
Dinner: Chicken and broccoli stir-fry: Sauté 4 oz chicken (or lean beef) and 2 c broccoli, carrots, and onions in 1 Tbsp olive oil and 2 Tbsp light teriyaki stir-fry sauce. Serve over 1/3 c cooked brown rice.
Snack: Popcorn: 3 c light microwave popcorn.

DAY 5

Breakfast: Cereal: Combine 1 c whole grain flaxseed-enriched cereal, 1 c fat-free milk, and 2 Tbsp almonds.

Lunch: Cheese quesadilla: Sprinkle 2 oz reduced-fat shredded cheese onto 1 whole wheat tortilla, fold in half, and microwave on medium power for 30 to 45 seconds. Top with 1 c chopped lettuce and tomato, 1/4 c salsa, 2 Tbsp avocado, and 1 Tbsp light sour cream.

Snack: Peanut butter and banana: 1 med banana, sliced in half and spread with 1 Tbsp all-natural peanut butter.

Dinner: Soup-and-salad combo: Heat 1 c canned beef-barley soup ("healthy" type) and serve with spinach salad: Toss 2 c fresh spinach with 2 Tbsp shredded reduced-fat mozzarella cheese and 1 Tbsp olive oil-and-balsamic-vinegar dressing.

Snack: Cookies and milk: 2 fig cookies and 1 c fat-free milk or calcium-enriched soy or rice beverage.

DAY 6

Breakfast: Fruit smoothie: In a blender, add 1 c fat-free milk or calcium-enriched soy or rice beverage, 6 oz fat-free plain yogurt, 1/2 c strawberries or other fresh fruit, 2 Tbsp chopped walnuts, and 2 Tbsp flax meal. Add ground cinnamon and/or sugar substitute to taste. Blend for 15 seconds.

Lunch: No-taco salad: Mix 2 oz grilled fish, chicken, or lean beef; 1/3 c brown rice; and 1/2 c cooked red, black, or pinto beans. Sprinkle with 1 oz reduced-fat shredded cheese and microwave on medium power for 45 seconds. Top with 1/2 c salsa and 1 Tbsp light sour cream. Serve over 2 c mixed lettuce greens.

Snack: Fruit and yogurt: 1 c watermelon (or other melon in season) and 3/4 c fat-free light yogurt.

Dinner: Grilled fish: Grill 3 oz salmon and top with 1/2 c chopped melon and mango. Serve with 2 c fresh spinach tossed with 2 Tbsp chopped pecans, sliced red onions, and 1 Tbsp oil-and-vinegar dressing. Serve with 1 c fat-free milk.

Snack: Fruit and cheese: 1 med pear, sliced, with 1 oz spreadable light cheese.

DAY 7

Breakfast: Peanut butter-banana toast: Spread 1 slice reduced-calorie whole grain toast with 2 Tbsp all-natural peanut butter and top with 1/2 med sliced banana. Serve with 1/2 c fat-free milk or calcium-enriched soy beverage.

Lunch: Chicken Caesar salad: Toss 3 c romaine lettuce with 2 oz skinless chicken, sliced, and 1/2 c mandarin oranges (juice- or water-packed, drained). Drizzle with 2 Tbsp reduced-fat Caesar dressing and top with 1 Tbsp Parmesan cheese. Serve with 1 oz whole grain crackers.

Snack: Fruit and nuts: 1 c apple slices and 1/4 c walnut halves.

Dinner: Steak and potatoes: Broil 4 oz top sirloin and serve with 1/2 oven-baked potato (slice potato lengthwise, drizzle with 1 tsp olive oil, and bake cut side down) and garlic-roasted asparagus (toss 10 med asparagus spears in 1 tsp olive oil and chopped garlic, then bake at 400?F for 20 minutes).

Snack: Crackers and milk: 3 graham cracker squares and 1 c fat-free milk.

ANOTHER 7 DAY MEAL PLAN

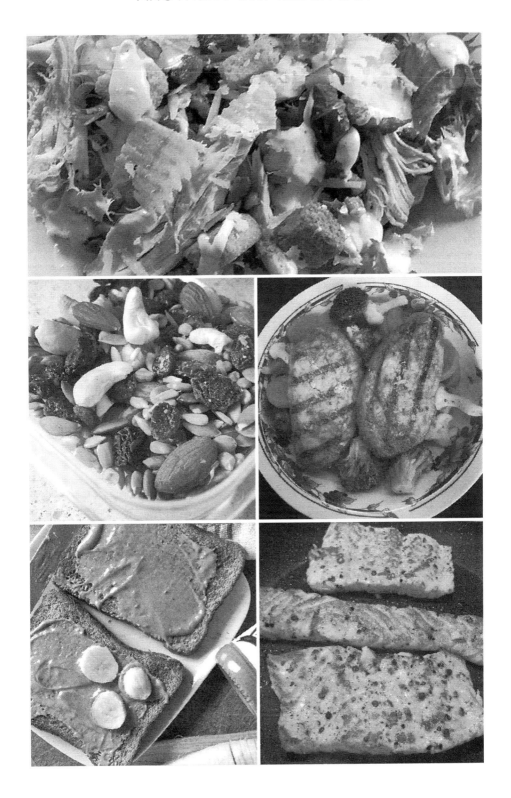

DAY 1

Breakfast: Superwhite egg Break 1 whole egg into a small frypan coated with 2 tsp canola oil. Add 1 egg white around outside of whole egg and cook over low heat. Top with 2 tbs chopped tomato or salsa. Serve with 1 slice wholegrain toast spread with 1 tsp reduced-fat canola margarine and 1 cup skim milk.
Snack: Yoghurt and dried fruit 200 g fat-free yoghurt and 4 dried apricots.
Lunch: Grilled-vegie sandwich (above) Puree 100 g chargrilled red capsicum (skin removed) with 1 tbs water, 1 tsp dried chilli flakes and 1/4 tsp paprika. Chargrill 100 g tofu; slices of nonstarchy vegies, such as zucchini, eggplant and capsicum; and 1 wholegrain roll. Spread roll with 1 tsp mayonnaise and top with vegies, tofu and capsicum 'sauce' to serve.
Dinner: Pan-grilled Mediterranean salmon Pan-fry 1/2 diced Spanish onion, 1 chopped garlic clove, 1/2 tsp crumbled dried sage and 1 tsp canola oil until onion softens. Add 120 g cannellini beans, 1/4 cup reduced-salt chicken stock and 1 cup spinach. Cook until spinach wilts. Serve with 90 g pan-grilled salmon and top with chilli flakes, if desired.
Snack: Popcorn 3 cups light microwave popcorn.

DAY 2

Breakfast: Pancakes Top 3 wholemeal-flour pancakes (15-cm diameter) with 1 tsp reduced-fat canola spread and 1 tbs 100%-fruit spread. Serve with 1 cup skim milk.
Lunch: Tuna sandwich Mix 95 g tinned tuna (in water) with 2 tsp reduced-fat mayonnaise and 4 large chopped black olives. Spread on 2 slices wholegrain bread. Top with leafy greens and 1 small sliced tomato (1/2 cup).
Snack: Yoghurt parfait 1 cup fat-free plain yoghurt topped with 3/4 cup fresh blueberries or blackberries.
Dinner: Chicken with vegies Grill 90 g chicken breast sprinkled with herb seasoning and 2 cups nonstarchy vegetables, such as mushrooms, zucchini, yellow squash and capsicum, tossed in 2 tsp olive oil. Serve with 2/3 cup cooked wild rice.
Snack: Apple and peanut butter 1 small apple, sliced and spread with 2 tsp natural peanut butter.

DAY 3

Breakfast: Porridge Top 1 cup cooked porridge with 2 tbs walnut halves. Add ground cinnamon, sugar substitute or both, to taste. Serve with 1/2 cup skim milk.

Lunch: Grilled-chicken salad Toss 2 cups mixed leafy greens with 1/2 cup diced tomato, 1/2 cup sliced cucumber and 1/4 cup diced carrots. Top with 60 g grilled-chicken breast and serve with avocado-yoghurt dressing (1/4 cup mashed avocado, 1/2 cup fat-free plain yoghurt, and balsamic vinegar and herbs to taste). Serve with 2 wholegrain rye crispbreads, such as Ryvitas.

Snack: Cheese and fruit 30 g cheese stick and 1 small pear or other fruit.

Dinner: Pasta primavera Cook 60 g wholemeal pasta until al dente, reserving pasta water. Pan-fry 1 chopped garlic clove, 1/2 chopped onion and 1 finely chopped carrot until soft, adding pasta water, 1 spoonful at a time, if vegies stick to pan. Stir through 1/4 cup frozen peas and 1/4 cup artichoke hearts in brine (rinsed). Warm through. Serve vegies tossed with pasta, fresh basil and 1 tsp grated parmesan cheese.

Snack: Fruit and nuts 1 orange and 2 tbs cashews.

DAY 4

Breakfast: Open egg sandwich Top 1/2 multigrain English muffin with 110 g blanched spinach, 1/2 cup sliced tomato, 1 sliced hard-boiled egg and 1 tbs reduced-fat mayonnaise. Season with herbs as desired and grill until mayo is lightly browned.

Lunch: Mixed salad Toss 2 cups leafy greens, 3/4 cup low-fat cottage cheese and pieces of 1 medium mandarin with 2 tbs light Italian dressing. Top with 2 tbs chopped almonds or walnuts. Serve with 5 wholegrain crackers.

Snack: Yoghurt 200 g low-fat flavoured yoghurt.

Dinner: Grilled fish tacos Place 60 g grilled fish and 1 cup shredded cabbage, seasoned with a little rice-wine vinegar, in 2 corn tacos. Top with 2 tbs light sour cream. Serve with 2 cups vegies, such as eggplant, mushrooms, green beans and onions, marinated in 2 tbs light Italian dressing and 1 tsp olive oil, then grilled.

Snack: Hummus and crackers 2 tbs hummus on 2 wholegrain rye crispbreads, such as Ryvitas.

DAY 5

Breakfast: Cereal 1 cup high-fibre wholegrain breakfast cereal, 1 cup skim milk and 2 tbs nuts.

Lunch: Cheese quesadilla Sprinkle 60 g reduced-fat shredded cheese onto 1 wholemeal tortilla, fold in half and microwave on medium for 30 to 45 seconds. Top with 2 cups chopped leafy greens and tomato, 1/4 cup salsa, 2 tbs avocado and 1 tbs light sour cream.

Snack: Peanut-butter banana Slice 1 medium banana in half and spread with 1 tbs natural peanut butter.

Dinner: Soup-and-salad combo Heat 300 g lamb-and-vegetable soup (such as Pitango Organic lamb soup). Serve with spinach salad: toss 2 cups fresh spinach with 2 tbs shredded reduced-fat mozzarella cheese and 1 tbs olive-oil-and-balsamic-vinegar dressing.

Snack: Orange frappé with strawberries Combine 1/4 cup reduced-fat ricotta cheese with 1 1/2 tsp honey and 1/2 tsp orange zest until smooth. Serve with 1/4 cup sliced strawberries and top with a touch of grated dark chocolate, if desired.

DAY 6

Breakfast: Fruit smoothie In a blender, add 1 cup skim milk, 200 g fat-free plain yoghurt, 1/2 cup strawberries or other fresh fruit, 2 tbs chopped walnuts and 2 tbs LSA (linseed, sunflower seed, almond) mix. Add ground cinnamon or sugar substitute to taste. Blend for 15 seconds.

Lunch: Mexican salad Toss 60 g grilled fish, chicken or lean beef with 1/3 cup brown rice and 1/2 cup kidney beans. Sprinkle with 1 tbs reduced-fat shredded cheese; microwave for 45 seconds. Top with 1/2 cup salsa and 1 tbs light sour cream. Serve over 2 cups leafy greens.

Snack: Fruit and yoghurt 1 cup watermelon and 250 g fat-free yoghurt.

Dinner: Grilled fish Grill 90 g salmon and top with 1/2 cup chopped melon and mango. Serve with 2 cups fresh baby spinach tossed with 2 tbs chopped nuts, sliced Spanish onion and dressing (1 tsp oil combined with 2 tbs vinegar). Serve with 1 cup skim milk.

Snack: Fruit and cheese 1 medium pear, sliced, with 1 tbs spreadable light cheese.

DAY 7

Breakfast: Peanut-butter-and-banana toast. Spread 1 slice wholegrain toast with 2 tbs all-natural peanut butter; top with 1/2 medium sliced banana. Serve with 1/2 cup skim milk.

Lunch: Chicken caesar salad Toss 3 cups leafy greens with 60 g sliced skinless chicken and pieces of 1 medium mandarin. Drizzle with 2 tbs reduced-fat caesar dressing and top with 1 tbs parmesan cheese. Serve with a slice of multigrain bread.

Snack: Cookies and milk 3 plain sweet biscuits and 1 cup skim milk.

Dinner: Chicken roll-ups (pictured) Sauté 110 g chicken, 1 tbs minced ginger, 1/4 cup sliced tinned water chestnuts and 2 cups of chopped spring onions and carrots in 1 tbs olive oil and 2 tbs hoisin sauce. Serve in 3 iceberg-lettuce leaves.

Snack: Fruit and nuts 1 cup apple slices with 1/4 cup walnut halves.

ABOUT THE AUTHOR

I am an engineering student and I write kindle books in my spare time. I enjoy writing informative books that provide useful information that is to the point. I like to provide people with value and I hope that this book provides you with new information about diabetes. Your support is much appreciated and I hope that you take the time to give me your feedback.

Made in the USA
Middletown, DE
15 June 2017